Daniel A. Lichtenstein

Lung Ultrasound in the Critically Ill

The BLUE Protocol

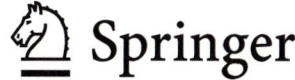

Daniel A. Lichtenstein
Hôpital Ambroise Paré
Service de Réanimation Médicale
Boulogne (Paris-West University)
France

ISBN 978-3-319-15370-4   ISBN 978-3-319-15371-1   (eBook)
DOI 10.1007/978-3-319-15371-1

Library of Congress Control Number: 2015941278

Springer Cham Heidelberg New York Dordrecht London
© Springer International Publishing Switzerland 2016
This work is subject to copyright. All rights are reserved by the Publisher, whether the whole or part of the material is concerned, specifically the rights of translation, reprinting, reuse of illustrations, recitation, broadcasting, reproduction on microfilms or in any other physical way, and transmission or information storage and retrieval, electronic adaptation, computer software, or by similar or dissimilar methodology now known or hereafter developed.
The use of general descriptive names, registered names, trademarks, service marks, etc. in this publication does not imply, even in the absence of a specific statement, that such names are exempt from the relevant protective laws and regulations and therefore free for general use.
The publisher, the authors and the editors are safe to assume that the advice and information in this book are believed to be true and accurate at the date of publication. Neither the publisher nor the authors or the editors give a warranty, express or implied, with respect to the material contained herein or for any errors or omissions that may have been made.

Printed on acid-free paper

Springer International Publishing AG Switzerland is part of Springer Science+Business Media (www.springer.com)

"The lung: a major hindrance for the use of ultrasound at the thoracic level."

TR Harrison
Principles of Internal Medicine, 1992, p. 1043

"Ultrasound imaging: not useful for evaluation of the pulmonary parenchyma."

TR Harrison
Principles of Internal Medicine, 2011, p. 2098

"Most of the essential ideas in sciences are fundamentally simple and can, in general, be explained in a language which can be understood by everybody."

Albert Einstein
The evolution of physics, 1937

"Le poumon…, vous dis-je !" (The lung… I tell you!)

Molière, 1637

(continued)

These extracts were introducing the Chapter on lung ultrasound of our 2005 Edition.

The present textbook is fully devoted to this application.

A ma famille, mes enfants, le temps que je leur ai consacré était en concurrence avec ces livres qui ont aussi été ma vie. Trouver l'équilibre entre une vie de famille idéale et la productivité scientifique a été un défi permanent. Les défauts qu'on pourra trouver dans le présent ouvrage ne seront dûs qu'à une faiblesse dans la délicate gestion de cet équilibre. Mon père n'aurait pas cru, en 1992, époque de la première édition, qu'il verrait celle-ci; cet ouvrage lui est dédié. Ma mère sera heureuse de voir d'en haut cet achèvement d'une vie.

A Joëlle

Our life is a gift from God; what we do with that life is our gift to God.

Contents

Part I The Tools of the BLUE-Protocol

1 Basic Knobology Useful for the BLUE-Protocol (Lung and Venous Assessment) and Derived Protocols 3
Preliminary Note on Knobology. Which Setting for the BLUE-Protocol? Which Setting for the Other Protocols (FALLS, SESAME, etc.) and Whole Body Critical Ultrasound? 3
Step 1: The Image Acquisition. 4
Step 2: Understanding the Composition of the Image. 6
Step 3: Image Interpretation. 8
References 9

2 Which Equipment for the BLUE-Protocol? (And for Whole-Body Critical Ultrasound). 1 – The Unit 11
The Seven Requirements We Ask of an Ultrasound Machine Devoted to Critical Care – A Short Version for the Hurried Reader 12
A Longer Version: The Seven Requirements We Ask of an Ultrasound Machine Devoted to Critical Care 12
The Coupling System: A Detail? 17
Data Recording 18
How to Practically Afford a Machine in One's ICU 18
What Solutions Are There for Institutions Already Equipped with Laptop Technologies? 19
Which Machines for Those Who Work Outside the Hospital and in Confined Space? 19
The Solution for the Future 20
Some Basic Points and Reminders 21
Appendix 1: The PUMA, Our Answer to the Traditional Laptops 21
References 22

3 Which Equipment for the BLUE-Protocol 2. The Probe 23
The Critical Point to Understand for Defining the "Universal Probe" in Critical Care: The Concept of the Providential (Optimal) Compromise 23

vii

	How to Scientifically Assess This Notion of "Domain of Interpretability"? Our High-Level Compromise Probe.......	25
	Why Is Our Microconvex Probe Universal	28
	The Strong Points of Having One Unique Probe..............	29
	The Usual Probes of the Laptop Machines	31
	Some Doctors Prefer to Swap the Probes for Each Application, and Not Use the Universal Probe. Why?	33
	Pericardial Tamponade: Time for a Nice Paradox, Just One Illustration of What is "Holistic Ultrasound"	33
	What to Say to Those Who Still Have Only the Three Usual Probes?	34
	An Unexpected (Temporary) Solution?.....................	34
	Important Notes Used as Conclusion......................	35
	Reference	35
4	**How We Conduct a BLUE-Protocol (And Any Critical Ultrasound): Practical Aspects**..........	37
	Disinfection of the Unit: Not a Futile Step	38
	When Is It Time to Perform an Ultrasound Examination	42
	Since When Do We Perform These Whole-Body Ultrasound Examinations: Some Historical Perspectives.................	42
	References	42
5	**The Seven Principles of Lung Ultrasound**.................	45
	Development of the First Principle: A Simple Method	45
	Development of the Second Principle: Understanding the Air-Fluid Ratio and Respecting the Sky-Earth Axis	46
	The Third Principle: Locating the Lung and Defining Areas of Investigation	47
	The Fourth Principle: Defining the Pleural Line	47
	The Fifth Principle: Dealing with the Artifact Which Defines the Normal Lung, the A-Line............................	47
	The Sixth Principle: Defining the Dynamic Characteristic of the Normal Lung, Lung Sliding........................	47
	Development of the Seventh Principle: Acute Disorders Have Superficial, and Extensive, Location	47
	Reference	49
6	**The BLUE-Points: Three Points Allowing Standardization of a BLUE-Protocol**.....................................	51
	The Concept of the BLUE-Hands	51
	Lung Zones, Their Relevance in the BLUE-Protocol, Their Combination with the Sky-Earth Axis for Defining Stages of Investigation...	52
	Some Technical Points for Making Lung Ultrasound an Easier Discipline......................................	53
	Standardization of a Lung Examination: The BLUE-Points..	53
	Standardization of a Lung Examination: The Upper BLUE-Point...................................	54

Standardization of a Lung Examination:
The Lower BLUE-Point.................................. 54
The PLAPS-Point... 54
Location of the Lung in Challenging Patients 56
Other Points? The Case of the Patient in the Prone Position..... 56
BLUE-Points and Clinical Information 56
Aside Note More Devoted to Pulmonologists 57
Philosophy of the BLUE-Points: Can the Users Do Without?.... 57
Reference 58

7 An Introduction to the Signatures of Lung Ultrasound 59
   1. The pleural line...................................... 59
   2. The A-line.. 59
   3. Lung sliding 59
   4–7. The quad sign, sinusoid sign, shred sign,
        and tissue-like sign 59
   8. Lung rockets 59
   9. Abolished lung sliding 59
   10. The lung point..................................... 59
Other Signs... 60
Note 60

8 The Pleural Line... 61
The Pleural Line: The Basis............................... 61
Standardizing Lung Ultrasound: Merlin's Space.............. 63
Standardizing Lung Ultrasound: Keye's Space 63
Standardizing Lung Ultrasound: The M-Mode-Merlin's Space .. 64
Reference 64

9 The A-Profile (Normal Lung Surface): 1) The A-Line....... 65
The Artifact Which Defines the Normal Lung Surface:
The A-line 65
Note 66
Other Artifacts 66
Some History 66
Reference 66

10 The A-Profile (Normal Lung Surface): 2) Lung Sliding 67
Lung Sliding: A New Sign, a New Entity
in the Respiratory Semiology............................. 67
Normal Lung Sliding in the Healthy Subject,
a Relative Dynamic: The Seashore Sign 68
Lung Sliding, Also a Subtle Sign Which Can Be
Destroyed by Inappropriate Filters or So-Called
Facilities. The Importance of Mastering Dynamics
and Bypassing These Facilities 69
The Various Degrees of Lung Sliding,
Considering Caricaturally Opposed States 69
Lung Sliding in the Dyspneic Patient. The Maximal Type.
Critical Notions Regarding the Mastery of the B/M-Mode...... 70

	Dyspnea and the Keyes' Sign.	70
	Lung Sliding in the Ventilated Patient. The Minimal Type.	
	Critical Notions Regarding the Mastery of the Filters.	72
	Lung Sliding: Three Degrees, but a Dichotomous	
	Sign Anyway	76
	Can One Quantify Lung Sliding?	76
	How About Our Healthy Volunteer?	76
	References	78
11	**Interstitial Syndrome and the BLUE-Protocol: The B-Line** . .	79
	A Preliminary Definition: What Should Be Understood by	
	"Interstitial Syndrome"?	79
	The Usual Tools for Diagnosing Interstitial Syndrome	80
	Elementary Sign of Interstitial Syndrome, the B-Line	80
	The Seven Detailed Criteria of the B-Lines.	81
	Physiopathologic Meaning of the B-Lines	81
	How Do We Explain the Generation of the B-Line?	
	Is It Really "Vertical," Not a Bit Horizontal?.	82
	Accuracy of the B-Line?	84
	Comet-Tail Artifacts That May Mimic the B-Lines.	84
	Additional Features of the B-Lines	85
	References	86
12	**Lung Rockets: The Ultrasound Sign**	
	of Interstitial Syndrome.	87
	Lung Rockets, Preliminary Definitions	87
	The Data of Our Princeps Study and the Real Life	87
	Pathophysiological Explanation of Lung Rockets,	
	Clinical Outcome.	88
	Characterization of the Lung Rockets in Function	
	of Their Density: Morphological Patterns	88
	The Clinical Relevance of the Lung Rockets	
	in the Critically Ill, Some Illustrations.	89
	Normal Locations of B-Lines and Lung Rockets	92
	Pathological Focalized Lung Rockets	92
	A Small Story of Lung Rockets to Conclude: Notes About Our	
	Princeps Papers	92
	References	94
13	**Interstitial Syndrome in the Critically Ill: The B-Profile**	
	and the B'-Profile.	95
	The Ultrasound Transudative Interstitial Syndrome (B-Profile) . .	95
	The Ultrasound Exudative Interstitial Syndrome (B'-Profile). . . .	95
	The Language of the BLUE-Protocol, Its Main Principle	96
	Reference.	96
14	**Pneumothorax and the A'-Profile**.	97
	Warning for the Reader	97
	Pneumothorax, How Many Signs?.	97
	Determination of the A'-Profile	98

	The Lung Point, a Sign Specific to Pneumothorax	102
	Additional Signs of Pneumothorax	103
	Evaluation and Evolution of the Size of Pneumothorax	104
	Pitfalls and Limitations	104
	For the Users of Modern Laptop Machines	106
	The Essential in a Few Words	106
	An Endnote	106
	References	108
15	**LUCI and the Concept of the "PLAPS"**	**109**
	The "PLAPS Code"	110
	One Major Interest of PLAPS	110
16	**PLAPS and Pleural Effusion**	**111**
	The Technique of the BLUE-Protocol	111
	The Signs of Pleural Effusion	111
	Value of Ultrasound: The Data	114
	Diagnosing Mixt Conditions (Fluid and Consolidation) and Diagnosing the Nature or the Volume of a Pleural Effusion: Interventional Ultrasound (Thoracentesis)	114
	Pseudo-pitfalls	115
	Additional Notes on Pleural Effusions	115
	References	116
17	**PLAPS and Lung Consolidation (Usually Alveolar Syndrome) and the C-profile**	**117**
	Some Terminologic Concepts	117
	Why Care at Diagnosing a Lung Consolidation, Whereas the Concept of "PLAPS" Allows Energy Saving?	118
	One Ultrasound Peculiarity of Lung Consolidations: Their Locations	118
	Ultrasound Diagnosis of a Lung Consolidation	118
	Other Signs Not Required for the Diagnosis of Lung Consolidation in the BLUE-Protocol but Useful for Its Characterization	120
	Accuracy of the Fractal and Tissue-Like Signs	121
	The C-Profile and the PLAPS	121
	Pseudo-Pitfalls	121
	References	122
18	**The BLUE-Protocol, Venous Part: Deep Venous Thrombosis in the Critically Ill. Technique and Results for the Diagnosis of Acute Pulmonary Embolism**	**123**
	Why Is This Chapter Long and Apparently Complicated?	123
	For the Very Hurried Readers: What Is Seen from the Outside at the Venous Step of the BLUE-Protocol?	123
	When to Make Use of Venous Ultrasound in the BLUE-Protocol	123

	To Who Can This Chapter Provide New Information?	124
	The Developed BLUE-protocol	139
	Limitations of Venous Ultrasound (Reminder)	140
	Some Main Points for Concluding	140
	References	141
19	**Simple Emergency Cardiac Sonography: A New Application Integrating Lung Ultrasound**	**143**
	So Still No Doppler in The Present Edition?	144
	At the Onset, Two Basic Questions	144
	The Signs of Simple Emergency Cardiac Sonography Used in the BLUE-Protocol: What Is Required?	145
	The Signs of Simple Emergency Cardiac Sonography Used in the FALLS-Protocol: What Is Required?	145
	The Signs of Simple Emergency Cardiac Sonography Used in Cardiac Arrest (the SESAME-Protocol)	148
	Signs of Simple Emergency Cardiac Sonography Not Used in the BLUE-Protocol, FALLS-Protocol, Nor SESAME-Protocol	148
	A Preview of More Complex Cardiac Applications Which Are Not Used in Our Protocols and Rarely in Our Daily Clinical Practice	149
	Before Concluding: How to Practice Emergency Echocardiography When There Is No Cardiac Window	151
	Repeated as Previously Announced, Our Take-Home Message	152
	Appendix	152
	References	153

Part II   The BLUE-Protocol in Clinical Use

20	**The Ultrasound Approach of an Acute Respiratory Failure: The BLUE-Protocol**	**157**
	The Spirit of the BLUE-Protocol	157
	The Design of the BLUE-Protocol	158
	The BLUE-Profiles: How Many in the BLUE-Protocol?	158
	Some Terminology Rules	160
	The Results	161
	Pathophysiological Basis of the BLUE-Protocol	162
	The Decision Tree of the BLUE-Protocol	162
	The Missed Patients of the BLUE-Protocol. What Should One Think? An Introduction to the Extended BLUE-Protocol	162
	When Is the BLUE-Protocol Performed	163
	The Timing: How Is the BLUE-Protocol Practically Used	164
	The BLUE-Protocol and Rare Causes of Acute Respiratory Failure	164
	Frequently Asked Questions Regarding the BLUE-Protocol	164

	A Whole 300-Page Textbook Based on 300 Patients............	165
	How Will the BLUE-Protocol Impact Traditional Managements?...............................	165
	A Small Story of the BLUE-Protocol	165
	References	166
21	**The Excluded Patients of the BLUE-Protocol: Who Are They? Did Their Exclusion Limit Its Value?**	167
	The Exclusion of Rare Causes: An Issue?...................	167
	Patients Excluded for More Than One Diagnosis: An Issue?	168
	Patients Excluded for Absence of Final Diagnosis: An Opportunity for the BLUE-Protocol	168
	References	169
22	**Frequently Asked Questions Regarding the BLUE-Protocol**......................................	171
	Why Isn't the Heart Featuring in the BLUE-Protocol?.........	171
	Are Three Minutes Really Possible?	172
	Why Is the Lateral Chest Wall Not Considered?..............	172
	Didn't the Exclusion of Patients Create a Bias Limiting the Value of the BLUE-Protocol?	173
	Is the BLUE-Protocol Only Accessible to an Elite?	173
	Can the BLUE-Protocol Allow a Distinction Between Hemodynamic (HPE) and Permeability-Induced (PIPE) Pulmonary Edema?	173
	How About Patients with Severe Pulmonary Embolism and No Visible Venous Thrombosis?......................	173
	Why Look for Artifacts Alone When the Original Is Visible?....	173
	What About Pulmonary Edema Complicating a Chronic Interstitial Lung Disease (CILD)?.................	173
	What About the Mildly Dyspneic Patients (Simply Managed in the Emergency Room)?	174
	Challenging (Plethoric) Patients?	174
	What Happens When the BLUE-Protocol Is Performed on *Non-Blue* Patients?	174
	Will the BLUE-Protocol Work Everywhere?.................	174
	Will Multicentric Studies Be Launched for Validating the BLUE-Protocol?...................................	174
	What Is the Interest of the PLAPS Concept?................	175
	By the Way, Why "BLUE"-Protocol?	175
	References	175
23	**The BLUE-Protocol and the Diagnosis of Pneumonia**	177
	Pathophysiological Reminder of the Disease................	177
	The Usual Ways of Diagnosis	177
	When Is the BLUE-Protocol Performed? Which Signs? Which Accuracy?.....................................	177
	Value of the BLUE-Protocol for Ruling Out Other Diseases	178

	Ultrasound Pathophysiology of Pneumonia................	178
	Why Not 100 % Accuracy? The Limitations of the BLUE-Protocol. How Can They Be Reduced?.........	179
	Miscellaneous	179
	References	179
24	**BLUE-Protocol and Acute Hemodynamic Pulmonary Edema**.....................................	181
	Pathophysiological Reminder of the Disease................	181
	The Usual Ways of Diagnosis	181
	So Why Ultrasound?...................................	181
	When Is the BLUE-Protocol Applied? Which Signs? Which Accuracy?......................................	182
	Value of the BLUE-Protocol for Ruling Out Other Diseases	182
	Ultrasound Pathophysiology of Acute Hemodynamic Pulmonary Edema (AHPE).............................	182
	Why Not 100 % Accuracy? The Limitations of the BLUE-Protocol	184
	A Small Story of the BLUE-Diagnosis of Hemodynamic Pulmonary Edema in the BLUE-Protocol.....	185
	References	185
25	**BLUE-Protocol and Bronchial Diseases: Acute Exacerbation of COPD (AECOPD) and Severe Asthma**...............	187
	Pathophysiological Reminder of the Disease................	187
	The Usual Ways of Diagnosis	187
	How Does the BLUE-Protocol Proceed? Which Signs? Which Accuracy?......................................	187
	Value of the BLUE-Protocol for Ruling Out Other Diseases	187
	Ultrasound Pathophysiology of AECOPD or Asthma..........	188
	Why Not 100 % Accuracy? The Limitations of the BLUE-Protocol	188
	Miscellaneous	188
	Reference..	188
26	**BLUE-Protocol and Pulmonary Embolism**................	189
	Pathophysiological Reminder of the Disease................	189
	The Usual Ways of Diagnosis	189
	When to Proceed to the BLUE-Protocol? Which Signs? Which Accuracy?......................................	190
	Value of the BLUE-Protocol for Ruling Out Other Diseases	191
	Ultrasound Pathophysiology of Pulmonary Embolism	191
	Why Not 100 % Accuracy? The Limitations of the BLUE-Protocol	191
	Miscellaneous	193
	References	193

27	**BLUE-Protocol and Pneumothorax**.............................	**195**
	Why and How the Ultrasound Diagnosis of Pneumothorax, Just This, Can Change Habits in Acute Medicine.............	195
	Pathophysiological Reminder of the Disease.................	196
	The Usual Ways of Diagnosis	196
	When Does the BLUE-Protocol Proceed? Which Signs? Which Accuracy?.......................................	196
	Value of the BLUE-Protocol for Ruling Out Other Diseases	196
	Ultrasound Pathophysiology of Pneumothorax	196
	Why Not 100 % Accuracy? The Limitations of the BLUE-Protocol. How to Circumvent Them	197
	Some Among Frequently Asked Questions	197
	Pneumothorax Integrated in the LUCI-FLR Project	198
	References	198

Part III   The Main Products Derived from the BLUE-Protocol

28	**Lung Ultrasound in ARDS: The Pink-Protocol. The Place of Some Other Applications in the Intensive Care Unit (CLOT-Protocol, Fever-protocol)**	**203**
	Peculiarities of the Ventilated Patient in the ICU..............	203
	The BLUE-Protocol for *Positive Diagnosis* of ARDS..........	204
	Lung Ultrasound for *Quantitative Assessment* of ARDS........	204
	Long-Staying Patients in the ICU: What to Do with These So Frequent PLAPS?.........................	208
	Diagnosis of Pulmonary Embolism in ARDS: The CLOT-Protocol	209
	Fever in the ICU: The Fever-Protocol	213
	References	215
29	**The LUCI-FLR Project: Lung Ultrasound in the Critically Ill – A Bedside Alternative to Irradiating Techniques, Radiographs and CT**	**217**
	Lung Ultrasound and the Traditional Imaging Standards in the Critically Ill: The LUCI-FLR Project	217
	Overt and Occult Drawbacks of Thoracic Tomodensitometry....	218
	Some Legitimate Indications for Traditional Imaging..........	222
	The HICTTUS, a Small Exercise, an Interesting Outcome......	222
	The LUCI-FLR Project in Action: Example of the Pneumothorax	223
	The LUCI-FLR Project in Action: Example of the Pulmonary Embolism	223
	The LUCI-FLR Project in Action: Example of the Pregnancy with Acute Ailments......................	224
	LUCI-FLR Project Can Reduce Irradiation? Fine. But if There Is No Available Irradiation?....................	224
	References	224

30	**Lung Ultrasound for the Diagnosis and Management of an Acute Circulatory Failure: The FALLS-Protocol (Fluid Administration Limited by Lung Sonography) – One Main Extension of the BLUE-Protocol**	227
	A Few Warnings	227
	Evolution of Concepts Considering Hemodynamic Assessment in the Critically Ill. Which Is the Best One? And for How Long?	228
	Can We Simplify Such a Complex Field? The Starting Point of the FALLS-Protocol	232
	Three Critical Pathophysiological Notes for Introducing the FALLS-Protocol	232
	Three Critical Tools Just Before Using the FALLS-Protocol	234
	Practical Progress of a FALLS-Protocol	235
	Aside Note of Nice Importance	238
	The Case of the B-Profile on Admission. Which Management? Are We Still in the FALLS-Protocol? The Place of the Caval Veins	238
	FALLS-Protocol: Again a Fast Protocol. Its Positioning with Respect to the Early Goal-Directed Therapy and Its Recent Troubles	242
	Weak Points of the FALLS-Protocol: The Limitations and Pseudo-limitations	244
	FAQ on the FALLS-Protocol	244
	A Schematical Synthesis of the FALLS-Protocol	251
	An Attempt of (Very) Humble Conclusion	252
	Some Small Story of the FALLS-Protocol	252
	Glossary	254
	Appendix A	255
	References	255
31	**Lung Ultrasound as the First Step of Management of a Cardiac Arrest: The SESAME-Protocol**	261
	The Concept of Ultrasound in Cardiac Arrest or Imminent Cardiac Arrest, Preliminary Notes	261
	SESAME-Protocol: Another Fast Protocol	262
	Practical Progress of a SESAME-Protocol	264
	Interventional Ultrasound in the SESAME-Protocol	269
	Limitations of the SESAME-Protocol	269
	Frequently Asked Questions on the SESAME-Protocol	270
	The SESAME-Protocol: Psychological Considerations	271
	Critical Notes for Concluding	271
	Appendix 1: Our Adapted Technique for Pericardiocentesis	274
	References	274

Part IV Extension of Lung Ultrasound to Specific Disciplines, Wider Settings, Various Considerations

32 Lung Ultrasound in the Critically Ill Neonate 277
  Lung Ultrasound in the Newborn: A Major Opportunity 277
  The Design of Our Study............................... 278
  Basic Technique...................................... 278
  The Signs of Lung Ultrasound (Seen and Assessed in Adults)
  and Rough Results.................................... 278
  Demonstration of the Potential of Ultrasound
  to Replace the Bedside Radiography as a Gold Standard 280
  Some Comments 281
  Limitations and Pseudo-limitations of Lung Ultrasound
  in the Newborn...................................... 282
  Various Diseases Seen in the Neonate and the Baby........... 282
  Safety of Lung Ultrasound in the Newborn.................. 283
  One FAQ: How About the Intermediate Steps Between
  Neonates and Adults?................................. 283
  Lung Ultrasound in the Neonate, Conclusions 283
  References 284

33 Lung Ultrasound Outside the Intensive Care Unit.......... 287
  Specialties Dealing with Critical Care..................... 287
  Other Medical Specialties 291
  "Last But Not Least": LUCIA – Lung Ultrasound
  for the Critically Ill Animals, Lung Ultrasound for Vets 294
  References 294

34 Whole Body Ultrasound in the Critically Ill (Lung, Heart, and Venous Thrombosis Excluded) 295
  Basics of Critical Abdomen.............................. 295
  Basics in Any Urgent Procedure in the Critically Ill 297
  Basics of Subclavian Venous Line Insertion 298
  Basics of Optic Nerve (and Elevated Intracranial Pressure) 302
  Basics of Soft Tissues 302
  Basics of Airway Management (and a Bit of ABCDE).......... 303
  Basics on Sepsis at Admission........................... 303
  Basics on Fever in the Long-Staying Ventilated Patient 304
  Basics of Basics on Trauma............................. 304
  Basics on Acute Deglobulization......................... 304
  Basics on Non-pulmonary Critical Ultrasound in Neonates
  and Children.. 305
  Basics on Futuristic Trends 305
  Basic Conclusion..................................... 306
  References 307

35	**The Extended-BLUE-Protocol**	309
	What Is the Extended BLUE-Protocol, Three Basic Examples	310
	The Extended BLUE-Protocol: An Opportunity to Use the Best of the Clinical Examination	312
	Pulmonary Embolism: How the Extended BLUE-Protocol Integrates Lung Consolidations? When Should Anterior Consolidations Be Connected to This Diagnosis?	312
	Distinction Between Acute Hemodynamic Pulmonary Edema and ARDS	312
	Distinction Between Pulmonary Edema and the Few Cases of Pulmonary Embolism with Lung Rockets	314
	Distinction Between Bronchial Diseases and Pulmonary Embolism with No DVT	314
	Distinction Between Hemodynamic Pulmonary Edema and Exacerbation of Chronic Lung Interstitial Disease	315
	The "Excluded Patients" of the BLUE-Protocol Revisited by the Extended BLUE-Protocol	315
	Pneumonia, More Advanced Features for Distinction with Other Causes of Lung Consolidation	316
	Obstructive Atelectasis, a Diagnosis Fully Considered in the Extended-BLUE-Protocol	318
	Noninvasive Recognition of the Nature of a Fluid Pleural Effusion	320
	One Tool Used in the Extended BLUE-Protocol: Bedside Early Diagnostic Thoracentesis at the Climax of Admission	321
	Lung Puncture	322
	Doppler in the Extended BLUE-Protocol?	323
	The Extended BLUE-Protocol, an Attempt of Conclusion	324
	References	325
36	**Noncritical Ultrasound, Within the ICU and Other Hot Settings**	327
	Noncritical Ultrasound Inside the ICU	327
	Outside the ICU	328
	References	332
37	**Free Considerations**	333
	Critical Ultrasound, Not a Simple Copy-Paste from the Radiologic Culture	333
	Lung Ultrasound in the Critically Ill: 25 Years from Take-Off, Now, the Sleepy Giant Is Well Awake (Better Late Than Never!)	333
	Seven Common Places and Misconceptions About Ultrasound	335
	The Laptop Concept: An Unnecessary Tool for a Scientific Revolution, Why?	338

Critical Ultrasound, a Tool Enhancing
the Clinical Examination 342
The SLAM 344
And How About US? 347
References 347

38 A Way to Learn the BLUE-Protocol 349
A Suggestion for the Training 350
The Approach in Our Workshops: How to Make Our
Healthy Models a Mine of Acute Diseases and How
to Avoid Bothering Our Poor Lab Animals 351
References 353

**39 Lung Ultrasound: A Tool Which Contributes in Making
Critical Ultrasound a Holistic Discipline and Maybe
a Philosophy** 355
Endnote 1 356

40 Suggestion for Classifying Air Artifacts 359

41 Glossary 365

Index 371

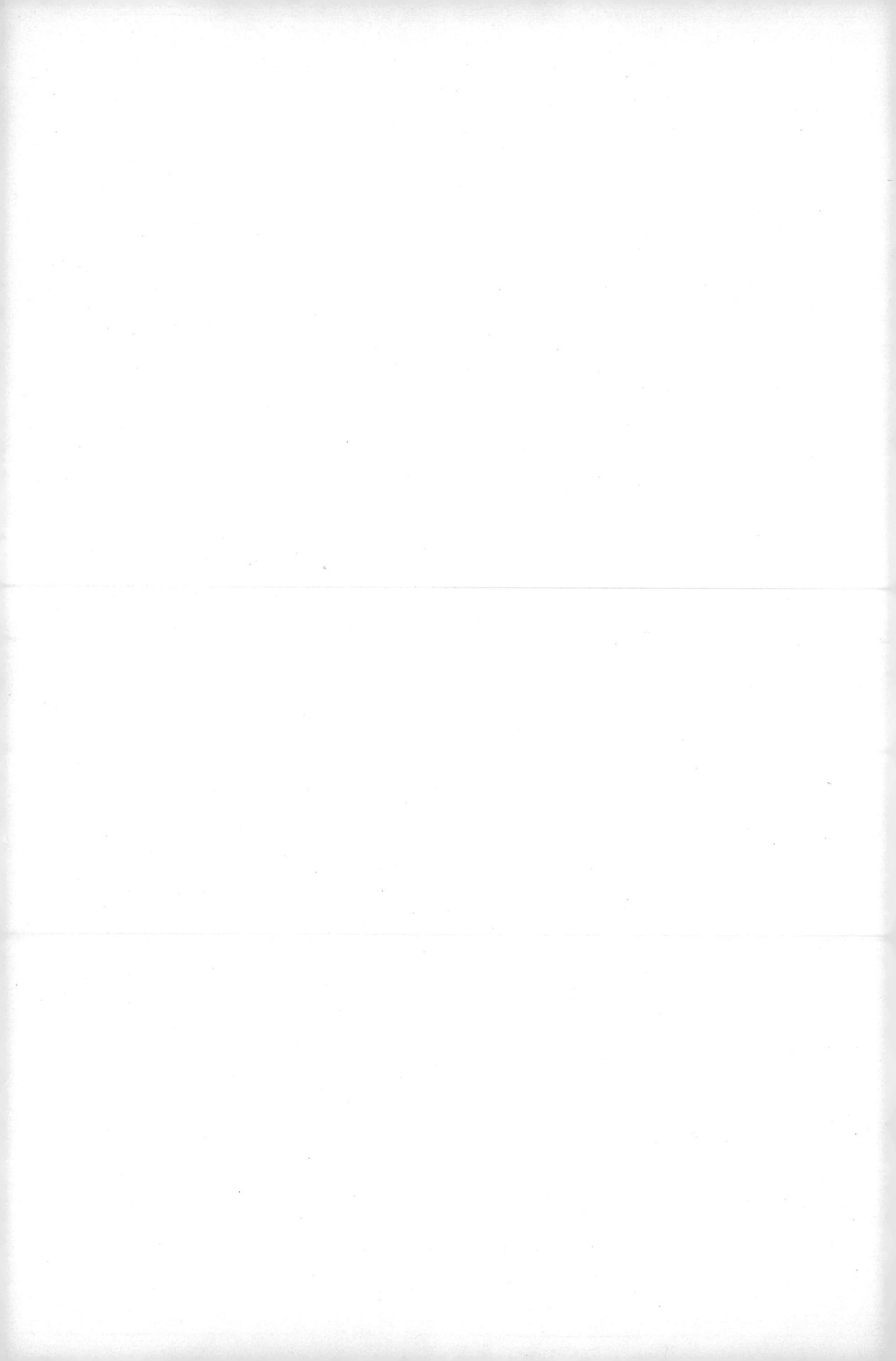

List of Videos

Video 10.1   The A-profile. A standard lung sliding. See the ribs, the bat sign, and the pleural line, and note the sparkling at the pleural line, spreading below. Note also the A-line. Example of A-profile, indicating a normal lung surface. It is seen in healthy subjects and a group of diseases (pulmonary embolism, severe asthma, exacerbation of COPD, etc.). Above the pleural line, the parietal layers are quiet: no dyspnea

Video 10.2   Some examples of dyspnea in asthmatic or COPD patients, where no B-line is here for helping. The Keye's sign is displayed at various degrees on M-mode. Focusing only on the real-time, the lung dynamic can be difficult to distinguish from the overall dynamic. Sometimes even on M-mode, the distinction is challenging and subtle signs are of major help (see Fig. 10.3)

Video 10.3   The effect of a summation filter. Standard lung sliding. Yet see how suddenly it gets markedly decreased, at the 6th second. The whole of the image is possibly "worked," nice to see, but the lung sliding has quite vanished. The setting "SCC," second line, has been activated ("1" if fully activated, "4" if not). Now, imagine a patient with a minimal lung sliding, plus such a filter: the condition for a difficult discipline is created

Video 10.4   The lung pulse. Patient with abolished lung sliding for any reason but not because of a pneumothorax. First, a B-line is visible. Second and mostly, even in its absence, a cardiac activity can be detected, 98 bpm. Example of lung pulse recorded at the right lower BLUE-point

Video 10.5   A stratosphere sign without pneumothorax. Young patient under mechanical ventilation for toxic coma. If looking carefully to the M-mode, lung sliding appears abolished, with a typical stratosphere sign. CEURF advises to always begin with the real time: a very discrete lung sliding can be visualized. No B-line is present, for helping. Sometimes (for not yet elucidated reasons), in spite of a M-mode shooting line at the center of the real-time image, a discrete lung sliding does not generate the expected seashore sign on the M-mode. We are between the pseudo-A'-profile and the A'-profile (as often in medicine).

Note several points. Note that the filter "SCC" has been optimized, i.e., suppressed (position 4). Imagine that, if not, the real time should have never shown this minimal lung sliding. Note, at the bottom of the M-mode image, some sand is displayed (not exactly the Peyrouset phenomenon); this sand is far from the pleural line (unknown meaning, minor event). A comprehensive analysis would show the same pattern through the whole chest wall and above all no lung point. This additional detail prevents to wrongly evoke a pneumothorax. To summarize here: no pneumothorax

Video 11.1 Typical Z-lines. Note how these comet-tail artifacts arising from the pleural line are standstill, ill-defined, not white like the pleural line but rather grey, short, with an A-line discreetly visible. Several are visible simultaneously. They will in no way be confused with B-lines and lung rockets (see videos 13.1 and 13.2 for comparison). Here, dyspneic COPD patient

Video 13.1 The B-profile. Lung rockets are associated with frank lung sliding. Patient with hemodynamic pulmonary edema

Video 13.2 The B'-profile. These lung rockets are here associated with a quite complete abolition of lung sliding. This is a typical B'-profile, seen in a patient with ARDS

Video 14.1 Basic A'-profile. Historical image, a pneumothorax diagnosed with the ADR-4000 (a 1982 technology). Note from top to bottom the absence of dyspnea, the pleural line (clearly defined using the bat sign), perfectly standstill – no lung sliding, and the Merlin's space occupied by four exclusive A-lines

Video 14.2 Pneumothorax and stratosphere sign. Left, a pneumothorax using a Hitachi-405 (1992 technology). Right, both Keye's space and M-Merlin's space display stratified lines, generating the stratosphere sign. Note this basic feature: both images move together, a feature not possible in very modern machines

Video 14.3 Dyspnea, the Keye's sign and the Avicenne sign. In this dyspneic patient, the abolition of lung sliding, on real time, is not that obvious, because of the muscular contractions, superficial to the pleural line. The Merlin's space displays subtle A-lines. On M-mode, the Keyes' space shows a parasite dynamic from muscular contractions. These accidents are displayed in the M-M space without any change when crossing the pleural line: the Avicenne sign, demonstrating the abolished lung sliding with no confusion

Video 14.4 Pneumothorax and the lung point. Dyspneic patient. The probe, searching for a lung point because of an A'-profile, finds suddenly, near the PLAPS-point in this patient, a sudden change, from a lateral A'-profile (no lung sliding, only A-lines) to a transient lateral B-profile (fleeting lung sliding, fleeting lung rockets), in rhythm with respiration during the acquisition. This is the pathognomonic sign of pneumothorax. Example here of lateral lung point

Video 14.5	No pneumothorax despite severe subcutaneous emphysema. The image (ill-defined, unsuitable acquisition parameters) first shows the Cornu's sign; then the operator tries to withdraw the gas collections. At 15", a hyperechoic line is identified, first oblique (the probe was not fully perpendicular). The probe stabilizes it on the screen, making it horizontal at 21". A lung sliding is visible. At 25", the M-mode shows a seashore sign, i.e., definite absence of pneumothorax
Video 16.1	Minute pleural effusion and the "butterfly syndrome." This video clip shows a pleural effusion, minute but indisputable: the quad sign and sinusoid sign are clearly displayed. Those who were reading the note in Chap. 11 regarding the sub-B-lines will not be confused. When the question is "Where is the pleural line?" many novices show the lung line, as if they were attracted, *hypnotized* by this brilliant and dynamic line. On the contrary, the real pleural line is this discreet line located at its standardized location, half a centimeter in this adult below the rib line, and, mostly, standstill. Reminder, the pleural line is the parietal pleura, always
Video 18.1	The lower femoral vein. Detection, compression (V-point), and escape sign. Transversal scan at the right lower femoral vein. The femur is easily detected. Inside, tubular structures are isolated. One has marked coarse calcifications and should be the artery. The other is larger, ovoid more than round, and should be the femoral vein. Carmen maneuver (seconds 3–8) has correctly showed these were tubes – definitely the vascular pair, what else? The simple observation shows that the supposed vein has a marked echogenicity and is irregular and motionless: the thrombosis is quite certain. On compression (see at the bottom of the image the print of the Doppler hand through the posterior skin (seconds 25–34)), all soft tissues shrink. From skin to vein, they shrink from 4 to 2.5 cm. During this compression, the vein "escapes" a travel of 5 mm, while its cross-section remains 7–8 mm. Positive escape sign. This is, definitely, an occlusive deep venous lower femoral thrombosis
Video 18.2	Calf analysis. How it is done practically, what the operator can see on the screen, how the vessels appear without, then under compression. 0": the product is applied, then the probe, with a Carmen maneuvre, and the probe is stabilized on the best site. 7": vision of the landmarks, two bones, one interosseous membrane, the tibial posterior muscle vessels. 11", the Doppler hand comes, and both thumbs join, locating (blindly) the Doppler hand at the correct height. During this maneuvre, the eye of the operator does not leave the screen (15"). The Doppler hand leaves the probe hand, and proceeds with smooth compressions (25" and 30"). 37"-41", first compression with full venous collapse. 46"-52", second compression. For experts, the anterior

	tibial group is visible, much smaller, just anterior to the membrane. See that functional arteries are spontaneously standstill here, but become systolic under compression (roughly 110 bpm).
Video 28.1	Jugular internal floating thrombosis. In this jugular internal vein, this 1982 technology, associated with a low-quality digitalization, shows however a floating thrombosis with systolodiastolic halting movements: the mass is obviously attracted by the right auricular diastole. One guesses the severity of these findings. The small footprint probe of this ADR-4000 was inserted on the supraclavicular fossa, allowing to see the Pirogoff confluence
Video 30.1	Standard search for a tension pneumothorax. The probe is quietly applied at anterior BLUE-points, or nearby (it does not matter a lot, since the pneumothorax is supposed to be substantial). Note the Carmen maneuver, searching for B-lines, therefore increasing the sensitivity of the A-line sign
Video 30.2	Inferior caval vein. In this patient who had the providence of a good window, the IVC can be seen behind the gallbladder (head of patient on left of image). No respiratory variation, suggesting a reasonable fluid therapy. See the ebb and flow of microparticles within the lumen, with inspiratory changes of direction (backward), using this 1982 technology
Video 31.1	Pericardial tamponade. This video clip shows for the youngest a basic pericardial tamponade from a subcostal window. The heart is recognized, beating, and surrounded by an external line: pericardial effusion is diagnosed. This effusion is substantial (20 mm at the inferior aspect). The right cardiac cavities are collapsed, indicating here a tamponade
Video 31.2	Asystole. Nothing much to be written here. A few seconds were necessary for recording this loop. This is a fresh cardiac arrest, maybe the visible floating sludge is a sign of recent arrest (good neurological recovery after ROSC in this hypoxic arrest)
Video 34.1	Pneumoperitoneum. Real-time (*left*) shows an absolute abolition of gut sliding. M-mode (*right*) shows an equivalent of the stratosphere sign (some accidents can be seen, but not arising from the very peritoneal line
Video 34.2	Mesenteric infarction. These completely motionless GI loops can be seen in mesenteric ischemia or infarction
Video 34.3	GI tract hemorrhage. Massive amounts of fluid within the GI tract indicate here a GI-tract hemorrhage. Note some free fluid in this postoperative case. The patient had a cardiac arrest, of hemorrhagic cause, detected at Step 3 of the SESAME-protocol, i.e., after 15 s
Video 35.1	A fully standstill cupola (in a necrotizing pneumonia). This video illustrates Fig. 29.3, in the LUCIFLR project (showing ultrasound superior when compared to CT), and Fig. 17.6, which shows the real dimensions of a consolidation. Here, the diaphragmatic cupola, perfectly exposed, is fully motionless –

	in a ventilated patient. It can therefore not be any phrenic palsy, as argued by some for explaining the frequent abolition of lung sliding in pneumonia. Look for the abolished lung sliding, fully redundant with the standstill cupola – or conversely too. Necrotizing pneumonia in a ventilated 76-year old man
Video 35.2	The dynamic air bronchogram. In this huge lung consolidation, which quite fully impairs lung sliding, several among the multiple air bronchograms have an inspiratory centrifuge excursion – a sign correlated with a nonretractile consolidation. Here, pneumonia due to pneumococcus in a 42-year-old man (1982 technology)
Video 36.1	One can see clearly the cupola, thanks to the pleural effusion above. Note that the deep part seems absent; this is just a tangency artifact (nothing to do with a rupture)
Video 36.2	This clip shows three interesting points. It is done in a healthy subject who breathes slowly for didactic reasons. (1) We do not see any diaphragm. We see only lung (left) and liver (right). (2) However, we know exactly where is the diaphragm: in between. (3) And we have the most important information: this diaphragm works perfectly, no palsy. See its elevated amplitude. This example shows that we should learn priority targets before the diaphragm by itself

Lung Ultrasound in the Critically Ill (LUCI) and Critical Ultrasound: How Did All This Happen? A (Not So) Short Introduction

It was a sunny afternoon after a pleasant night shift, May 1996, Café Danton, Boulevard Saint-Germain (Paris 6th). Sitting at a cozy table, we opened our vintage computer and created a file, the first of a series of patients investigated for acute respiratory failure. A canvas was initiated. Case after case, it was modified: complexified here, simplified there. The BLUE-protocol was coming to life. Time passed and a number of cases were gathered, the manuscript was submitted, the manuscript was rejected, and then rejected again and again before finally being accepted 12 years later. And that sunny day in 1996 was preceded by 11 other years.

We now write a book fully devoted to the most vital organ, unlike our 1992, 2002, 2005, 2010, and 2011 editions. From general ultrasound to whole-body ultrasound, we come now to lung ultrasound in the critically ill, or LUCI. So how did this happen? And how could one imagine, long before it became a standard of care, the story of lung ultrasound in the critically ill?

Lung ultrasound?

Imagine human beings with transparent lungs.

Imagine a lung accessible to ultrasound. Could we see fluid (alveolar, interstitial) inside this fluid-free organ? Could we monitor fluid therapy at the bedside, in harmony with cardiac data?

We don't need to imagine any longer. Since its advent in the 1950s, ultrasound has been able to make the lung transparent. With the development of the real-time ultrasound scanner in 1974, we have been able to do it even better.

The integration of the lung changes almost every step of traditional ultrasound: from the choice of equipment, probe, applications, disciplines, and training priorities to its very philosophy. This is the paradox of LUCI.

A Brief History of Critical and Lung Ultrasound: The Birth of a New Discipline

One hundred and eighteen years after Lazzaro Spallanzani's study on bats, the wreckage of the *Titanic* initiated the birth of ultrasound. Paul Langevin created a type of sonar in 1915 for detecting icebergs. It was used in the 1920s by fishermen (to detect whales), by the military (to detect submarines), and by industry in the 1930s in the manufacture of metals and tires. Eventually, in the 1940s, physicians considered a possible extension. The father of medical ultrasound (if we choose to omit Karl Dussik, who studied human skulls in Austria in 1942, dark times for medical research, and described as brain structures what appeared to be simple reverberation artifacts) seems to be André Dénier, a modest man who published in *la Presse Médicale* in 1946. From the 1950s on, ultrasound use made great strides in obstetrics (Ian Donald) and cardiology (Inge Edler), and the field was established. The heart was the domain of cardiologists; the uterus, obstetricians; and the rest was for the radiologists. Technological advances lead to improvements, such as real-time scanning in 1974 (Walter Henry and James Griffith). Critically ill patients, however, remained forgotten, in a no-man's land.

So when was *critical ultrasound* created? It is surprising to see that, even today, a number of doctors are persuaded that it came along the advent of the laptop machines (this textbook quietly invalidates this myth). It is true that a commercial revolution made ultrasound suddenly appear in emergency and intensive care rooms. This "new" technology was adopted rapidly, as if physicians were ashamed not to have had this simple idea before. Ironically, a piece, and not just any piece, was missing. In this frenzy of self-appropriating the technique, the most important organ was skipped: the lung. This is the paradox of LUCI.

We do not know who discovered critical ultrasound. In our 1993 article, submitted in 1991, we described a whole-body use, including the lung (a critical organ like any other), by the intensivist in charge of the patient, for critical or routine needs, followed by immediate therapeutic or diagnostic changes; a "24/7/365" use in a field where each minute matters, where there is not always time to call a specialist. Likewise, we don't know who brought first this concept into a clinical practice. Our own small story began in 1983.

1983. Hospital Laënnec, Paris, a sunny Saturday morning. We were kindly asked to bring a woman to the radiology department for an ultrasound test. A student, we had no choice but to agree. The radiologist quietly proceeded, and, so simply, we saw the *inside* of the belly. This was a thunderbolt, a *coup de foudre*. We realized, this is a visual tool for doctors. We also believed that ultrasound should go to the patient, not the other way around.

1984. We learned ultrasound's very basis in a standard radiology department, while initiating an intensivist career.

1985. We worked our first night shifts as an intensivist at François Fraisse ICU, Hospital Delafontaine, Saint-Denis. The responsibility was huge and heavy. This was our challenge: to decrease the risk of erroneously managing these very sick patients. The radiology department was not far from our ICU. Was completely desert after 11 PM. We were tempted to approach one of the machines, discreetly unplug it, and take it to the ICU (these heavy units had wheels!). The transgression was committed, and, little by little, the "monster" was clandestinely domesticated.

1986. We had become familiar with the habit of "borrowing" the machine. It was a night in March, and one of our patients was not well and was not benefitting from our care. It was midnight, and, thinking fast, we crept to the radiology department. All was quiet, not a noise (just the rain outside), nobody was there. We unplugged the machine and brought it to the ICU, Bed 1.

There was supposedly no fluid in the thorax, but there actually was! Action was necessary, there was simply no choice (there was no local computed tomography in 1986, and, even so, our patient was too unstable). In spite of the rules, a needle was inserted in the thorax. Amounts of purulent pleural effusion were withdrawn. The obstacle to the venous return decreases, the signs of circulatory failure seem to improve. The ultimate rendez-vous is not for this night. We bring the machine back to the radiology dept, clean the finger prints, replug it back in. Perhaps, on this dark night in 1986, a new standard of care was born. If similar acts were performed in the same setting (full night, bedside use, etc.) by some other doctor, we would love to shake his or her hand.

1989. We saw that ultrasound could impact critical medicine, but we could not continue "stealing" a unit from the radiology department. Where could we find a suitable ICU with *on-site* ultrasound? There was no need to move across the Atlantic; it was within biking distance at Boulogne (Paris-West). The road to discovery was made by successive encounters. Jean-François Lagoueyte helped us to discover medicine. William Loewenstein gave us the "fatal" taste of critical care. At François Fraisse ICU, we met Bruno Verdière, who introduced us to Alain Bernard, through whom we met Gil Roudy. He helped us by opening the doors of Ambroise-Paré's ICU, where François Jardin developed this pioneering vision: on-site ultrasound for cardiac assessment. There, in our day-and-night research, feeling free to apply the probe everywhere, we discovered, one after another, the countless applications that changed the approach to the critically ill.

1992. The field and limits of critical ultrasound were described in our first textbook (since we did not find any, we simply wrote our own). Today, you find these applications in all courses. Some were classical but did not really benefit the time-dependent patient (e.g., finding free abdominal blood). Some were specific to the critically ill (subclavian vein cannulation). Some were modern (optic nerve). Some were "fantasy" (lung). Some were futuristic (mingling lung with heart). There was no secret to writing our book. The inspiration came by simply always asking, "How can this tool be of help to the patients?" Instead of going to bed on these hot nights, there was endless work in building our research. Thanks to the ideas of Paul Langevin, André Dénier, and François Jardin, the father of echocardiography in the ICU, a discipline was born, the basis humbly gathered in 160 pages, one application or more per page ("1,001 Reasons of Practicing Critical Ultrasound" was the malicious label of Young-Rock Ha in his Korean translation).

Scared was the right word: managing a patient based on what these strange images told, or seemed to tell, was not insignificant. Mainly, we were scared to realize how much this visual tool could impact so many areas of medicine. Yet we did not care about the numerous obstacles. To begin with, there were human factors: the concept sounded so *weird* to our colleagues (mostly academicians). Time was lost. They were intrigued (or another word, maybe) to see an intensivist borrowing the tool of "specialist." And when they saw this person applying the probe at the *lung*, making it a priority target, they were … a little more intrigued (to not use a much worse word). Every time we proudly showed them our "baby," no one had time, or they used the indisputable argument: "If this were possible, it should long have been known." That being said, they found the solution and returned, reassured, to their daily routine. Critical time was lost. Ultrasound was reserved for radiologists (to count gallstones) or cardiologists (to assess complex valvular diseases), making two opposing worlds, both very far from ours. Only a few pragmatic (not academic) colleagues, such as Gilbert Mezière, Agnès Gepner, Eryk Eisenberg, and Philippe Biderman, immediately saw the potential and used it. Remember that, at the time, CT was a rarity and D-dimers did not exist. This was the time for an absolute revolution, and we (our small group) were the "kings of the night," but outlaws at daylight. Just the price to pay when you innovate.

Because ultrasound generates *images*, it was "logically" placed (with the exception of the heart and fetus) in the hands of radiologists: they were experts, but not accustomed to *touching* patients (especially in the night or on weekends), nor were they trained to make diagnoses based on artifacts, that is, undesirable parasites. Consequently, this elegant tool was used for almost all organs, *lung excluded*. An issue? Not at all! In the 1980s, CT appeared, and they found a serious tool, keeping ultrasound as a minor discipline, used to see gallstones during office hours. These experts had decreed lung ultrasound's unfeasibility in the most prestigious textbooks, burying it alive! And the following generations quietly followed. This mistake will possibly seem funny (using temperate words) in the history of medicine. We don't blame them; they had so many things to do. But they also succeeded in slowing down publications able to remedy this mistake (once the tool was in the right hands), and this caused more harm.

Before dealing with this harm. How did ultrasound of the lung happen? Initially, it is true, we saw only "snow" or "fog," like on an old TV at night. Yet we had the leisure to spend days and nights on it. This was just (insatiable) curiosity, wondering why these futile parasites were sometimes horizontal, sometimes vertical, until the day when, scanning a young patient with an acute interstitial pneumonia, we had a revelation. Maybe these "parasites" were a language. A language that we just did not understand. In our quest to define critical ultrasound, it appeared that the lung would be the major part. These ultrasound beams were so smart and also able to "cross" the lung. With observations, assessments, time for hope and disillusions, then simplifications, nomenclatures, standardization, we arrived at the point where a simple approach using a simple machine, a simple probe, and simple signs was legitimate. This initiated a work of endless submissions. We aimed at rapidly publishing the lung first, the absolute priority. This was a mistake.

This mistake (*defining* critical ultrasound before widespreading it) prevented us from popularizing nonpolemic fields since 1985 (like peritoneal blood detection – without acronym). Discovering was rather easy, but publishing was almost impossible. We did not publish the majority of our discoveries in the peer review literature. Our reviewers were cautious. We have always respected their work, even if it resulted in breaking our research. Countless teams throughout the world can thank them: while we were stuck with this impossible to publish work on the lung, these authors were able to quietly publish and publish some more. Leaderships emerged here and there in emergency ultrasound. We are glad for them: our "cake" was too big for one mouth. What remains today from this cake is a minute part – just the lung! This is good as it is. Too many papers in too few hands is probably not good. We are glad to have made so many doctors happy and famous (far more than the number of patients we have saved!). We have now brothers and sisters all over the world who all "think ultrasound." This is great, let us not be too demanding! We know how pleasant it is to publish. In addition, we see the endless work (invitations, etc.) generated by the few articles we were able to publish. For this, also, we thank those who published our discoveries.

The dark consequences of our countless rejections were that mainly laptop machines were invading our hospitals. These machines were chosen by experts, while researchers in the shadows (those who created the field) were judged unworthy of this responsibility. Emergency doctors discovered the worst aspects of the tool: the appearance of being small, a complicated knobology, poor resolution, endless start-up time, cost, "facilities" such as harmonics, and time lag – the worst for lung ultrasound! This revolution was a poor copy and paste of radiologic and cardiologic cultures. Since 1992 and even 1982, we had in hand a tool that could make this revolution really *disruptive*, using a holistic philosophy. Our simple, beloved Japanese unit was more suitable than these laptops. To begin with, it was just slimmer! This is another incredible paradox of critical and lung ultrasound. In parallel, many misconceptions became common (e.g., today, for many emergency physicians, the definition of interstitial syndrome is based on the detection of more than three B-lines). Such distorsions may be spread widely and quickly via the Internet, but are here... *wrong*. This situation created the conditions for writing our textbook, devoted to giving to experts support to be even better. This means for us, instead of a good nap, an endless work in the times to come.

This textbook comes at a convenient time. The words "lung ultrasound" are no longer scary. The previous dogma resulted in disastrous effects on choices of equipment. How can one explain the weird delay in the recognition of critical and lung ultrasound? The human factor possibly explains everything: a doctor who thinks he is good does not need to invest in a new field, especially if it comes from the mist. We give a piece of advice to researchers: begin young! Our story illustrates the words of Max Planck, who said, "an idea wins, not because its detractors are convinced, but because they eventually... die" and Stuart Mill, who stated that "all innovators had to pass through three steps: ridicule; observation; application".

How Does LUCI Make Critical Ultrasound a Holistic Discipline

We did not create lung ultrasound but a holistic ultrasound, with the lung at the center. We may provocatively assert that there is no lung ultrasound, there is just critical ultrasound, integrating the lungs. Lung ultrasound comes in harmony within critical ultrasound. LUCI encompasses more than just the lung. Integrated with simple cardiac data, it provides answers in the hemodynamic field (FALLS-protocol). Some even think that those who come to CEURF (Le Cercle des Echographistes d'Urgence et de Réanimation Francophones) sessions should forget their previous culture (from Rafik Bekka). This is a bit strong, but we do ask them to temporarily put aside all their knowledge (Doppler, cardiac output, etc.) to catch the spirit of the FALLS-protocol, integrate it, and then return to their previous habits with a bit or more of the CEURF vision.

The challenge in creating a truly holistic innovation was to transform a scary machine into a simple clinical tool, used 24/7/365 by simple clinicians. We used not only science but tools such as a piece of cardboard with holes to hide the useless buttons and highlight the *three* useful ones (i.e., creating, 25 years earlier, the innovation recently developed by a popular Dutch brand: a magic button with two levels: expert and basic). Button or cardboard, never mind, the expert knobology of ultrasound could be skipped. Far from daring any comparison with René Laënnec, simply inspired by his great work, we built our instrument. Laënnec was the father of the stethoscope, of course, but mostly of a new science based on observation. It was the step before the modern era initiated by Claude Bernard. Laënnec had a difficult life, and he began from nothing, which is an impossible task for those who change something in medicine (such a serious profession). With lung ultrasound, the work had to begin from less than nothing. There "was no lung ultrasound." It developed against a dogma; this was another challenge.

Some precious colleagues from various centers, including Raul Laguarda in Boston, Beth Powell and Jeff Handler in Toronto, Mike Welsh in Indianapolis, and German Moreno-Aguilar in Colombia, have efficiently transmitted the holistic spirit of lung ultrasound in the manner of CEURF.

LUCI: A Tool for Whom?

We have never designed who had to hold the probe. It was more important to show what was possible to see; for example, the lung. The historical experts (the radiologists) had a major opportunity, which they did not take advantage of in time. This is a pity because, knowing the basis, they could transmit the method immediately. These times are passed, and now the tool is in the hands of clinicians. We hope that LUCI will be used by all physicians dealing with the lung. This means, as an utmost priority, intensivists, pediatricians (neonatologists, PICUs, etc.), and pre-hospital doctors. Next is anesthesiology, emergency medicine, pulmonology, cardiology, and many others (see Chap. 33). This change will impact a number of unexpected disciplines.

Still a Single-Author Textbook?

Luciano Gattinoni told us of his preference for these books. It means more work for the author, but provides a homogeneous content, avoiding repetitions (or worse, contradictions). The coordination is optimized, as well as the thickness: a maximal quantity of information in a minimal volume. The writing by a single author was the key for reaching this target.

Of interest, our specific equipment allows an approach based on absolute simplicity. One of our challenges was to change ultrasound into a clinical tool, making each step easier for non-"experts." This textbook shows a winning combination (machine, probe, signs, etc.). Simple machines, available as early as 1982, and a different distribution of priorities (lung first) allowed more than just a transfer of "competencies." Self-taught in critical ultrasound (because nothing existed), free of any influence, we had a major privilege: creating signs as we saw them, for example, not defining pleural effusions as "anechoic collections." When all teams have our equipment and protocols, then many expert multi-author books, similar to this one, will be available.

This book contains unpublished material, that is, "ideas" for other teams. Why? There are roughly three ideas per page, which is not far from 1,000 in a single textbook. We have succeeded in publishing roughly one paper per year (a mini-disaster), making for two dozen papers, or roughly 2.5 % of our goal. Make a calculation: send out 1,000 manuscripts (with five anticipated rejections for each, i.e., 5,000 mailings) or just one textbook. What would *you* do? We chose to write, all in one, the ideas that we will never publish. The readers have a choice: read our non-peer-reviewed experience, tested by 30 years of full-time intensive experience, with permanent confrontations with reality, acceptance of failures, and pertinent criticisms; or wait for each article to be published. The lucid author offers these applications to keep in mind the most important: we deal with patients. This is our small gift to the community. Interested teams will just have to randomly open the book and begin a clinical study; we are ready to help them.

All authors have always, without exception, only one unique target: being useful to the patients. This is true for all. Most are great, most publish good articles, some publish amazing quantities, even if we could see in some a subtle art of visibility, or some curious cases of self-proclamation, sometimes again the art of pushing open doors. We were unable to comprehensively quote all authors, and we deeply apologize for this. In our first underground period, we had plenty of time but nothing to read. Now, publications are countless, to the point that we have only time to read their titles. Just note:

1. An explosive number of papers were the result of the recent (and unnecessary) intrusion of the laptop machines in emergency rooms. These publications usually show that emergency physicians can do as radiologists, after a defined number of examinations. Such articles are laudable, but this has nothing to do with the present textbook. Some are quoted.
2. Works that confirm published points are reassuring but will not modify the content of this textbook. Similarly, articles showing that a sign that worked in 100 patients works in 1,000 or 10,000 won't add anything new. They just confirm that it works. Some are quoted anyway.
3. Many articles extensively develop points that were found in modest textbooks in one simple sentence (e.g., the diagnosis of hemoperitoneum, not far from a religion for many emergency physicians, was dealt with in 12 lines in our 1992 textbook). Some are quoted.

To conclude this section, the author apologizes for possible errors or omissions, and will as always pay close attention to any remark.

LUCI: A Permanently Evolving Field. Additional Notes to This Edition

We mentioned LUCI after our clinical debut (1985), a time for gathering expertise. Once the 12 signatures were described (1989–1990), assessed (1990–1993), and published (from 1993 to 2006), successive evolutions were made. The main clinical relevance of LUCI was published: the BLUE-protocol in 2008. The hemodynamic potential of LUCI was published (FALLS-protocol) in 2009 and 2012. These protocols aimed at simplifying echocardiography. Our work on the neonate (our main priority) was finally published in 2009 and heralded by the LUCI-FLR (Lung Ultrasound in the Critically Ill Favoring Limitation of Radiographies) project for reducing medical irradiation. The holistic power of lung ultrasound was best illustrated in 2014 with the SESAME-protocol (cardiac arrest). Holistic ultrasound, a technical (not mystical) concept, indicates that, without the lung, critical ultrasound cannot be a complete discipline.

Rarely a month passes without new findings. During the production of this book, our research did not suddenly stop. Following are points that came too late to be included.

Additions to This Edition
Chapter 2, on the unit. Some colleagues (Lindsay Bridgford, Sydney) informed us that the batteries of these laptops are not devoid of severe issues.
Chapter 3, on the probe. In the search for a compromise for those who do not have our universal probe, we tend to favor the abdominal probes. Yet the effort of holding a heavy probe prevents keeping it perfectly still, generating minute parasites at the Keye's space, which can destroy the subtle semiology of the seashore sign. Finding a good compromise is really difficult.
Chapter 12. Some B-lines seem to have one top and two ends (in the absence of a filter such as harmonics). See, in Fig. 12.1, the second B-line from the left. This pattern (the bifid B-line) should be considered as one B-line.
Chapter 17. Please note that atelectasis is a lung consolidation but not really an alveolar syndrome (alveoli are collapsed).
Chapter 17. Comet-tail artifacts arising from the fractal line of a non-translobar lung consolidation are not B-lines. We could temporarily call them "fractal comet-tails." Consequently, a fractal comet-tail is a sign of lung consolidation.
Chapter 18, page 138. Calf veins are sometimes not visible simply because the leg is lying on the bed. The use of the Doppler hand at the first step, creating a "negative compression," should make more calf vein volume appear.

Chapter 30. How much fluid therapy is to be used in septic shock? Read the chapter well: not one drop!

Chapter 31, on cardiac arrest. Machines unable to record a sequence if the patient ID was not previously inserted are not in the spirit of critical ultrasound.

Chapter 31. One application among hundreds for lung sliding. The pneumothorax is sought for before cardiac compressions (because they can break ribs) and just after return of spontaneous circulation management for the same reason. According to recent recommendations, patients with cardiac arrest should no longer be ventilated. We ask, why not? However, those who follow these recommendations must be prepared to perform CPR for hours without making the diagnosis of pneumothorax, which can be provided by the SESAME-protocol in a few seconds.

Chapter 33. One more discipline has shown interest: palliative medicine, where the tools are scarce (nice reminder of Gabriel Carvajal Valdy).

What Is New in This Edition

The more space the lung took, the more the book adapted. The CEURF protocols (BLUE, FALLS, SESAME, Pink, CLOT, and Fever) are fully detailed. Compared with previous editions, each chapter has been completely rewritten, divided, and redesigned. A detailed venous protocol, the best of the simple heart, was again refined. "Traditional" areas (critical belly, blood in the abdomen, procedures, etc.) were made much shorter. Gyneco-obstetrics, appendicitis, and other topics with little to do with a book on lung ultrasound were deleted. Again, the rare situations were sacrificed to the profit of daily life. Propaganda talks (i.e., why to do ultrasound) are gone: the community has understood.

What is unchanged is the spirit of simplicity, a basis of holistic ultrasound, pushed to its limits without compromising the patient' safety. There are still no Doppler images. Regarding our wish to decrease radiation, expressed in 1992 (before these dangers were officially pinpointed), an entire chapter is now devoted to a standardized way of achieving this aim (the LUCI-FLR project) through our dear target: the lung.

Lung Ultrasound: An Accessible Discipline, or Not?

By considering the thickness of this book (which we made as thin as possible), one may think that LUCI is an expert discipline. Yet only one-fifth describes the "alphabet": the rest is for applications. Once an alphabet is mastered, one can create words, sentences, then books, newspapers, poetry, and so on at will.

Our aim is to make LUCI not more complicated than it actually is. If one takes a unit, a probe, and settings that make things complicated, then, yes, one builds a complex discipline. Acrobatic airplanes are not built like commercial ones. Many laptops allegedly devoted to critical care have been designed like commercial airplanes.

Lung ultrasound is simple mainly because the lung is a superficial organ, and the diseases are superficial, that is, accessible. The signs have been standardized to be as simple as possible (quad sign, fractal sign, etc.). Lung ultrasound is accessible if one learns step-by-step. This minimal investment pays off: those who focus on a single item, for instance, lung sliding to simply rule out pneumothorax, will use LUCI 10 times a day in 10 disciplines. The adjunct of one other simple sign (e.g., lung rockets) multiplies the potential, and so on up to full mastery.

Those who do us the honor of reading this textbook will tell us and their peers whether it succeeded in answering the challenge and in improving, even just a little, this area of medicine.

Part I
The Tools of the BLUE-Protocol

Basic Knobology Useful for the BLUE-Protocol (Lung and Venous Assessment) and Derived Protocols

Notions of the physical properties of ultrasound are not indispensable for the user (as we wrote in our 1992, 2002, 2005, 2010, and 2011 editions). Interested readers will find them in any ultrasound textbook.

We will discuss here the notions useful for understanding critical ultrasound. Every maneuver which favors simplicity will be exploited. Space will be used for explaining why only one setting is used; why, at the lung or venous area, only one probe orientation is favored; and how to easily improve the image quality.

Preliminary Note on Knobology. Which Setting for the BLUE-Protocol? Which Setting for the Other Protocols (FALLS, SESAME, etc.) and Whole Body Critical Ultrasound?

An ultrasound machine includes a various number of buttons, cursors, functions, etc. In our routine, we use only *three* functions:
1. The gain
2. The depth
3. The B/M-mode

The sole use of these three buttons converts any complex unit into a simple stethoscope (since 1982).

The setting is a basic point. Our setting is not "Lung", but "Critical Ultrasound." This concept, which initiates the SESAME-protocol, allows us to see the heart, veins, and belly (and lung) with a single approach, a single probe [1]. Our setting is, briefly, always the same. No filter, no facility. The next chapter will develop this point.

Some revolutionary machines use this concept with electronic control (basic/expert level), which is fine, but we did the same for a lesser cost, with a simple piece of cardboard (or thick plastic) and a cutter for making holes and hiding those scary, useless buttons, respectively. Since 1982, these machines were suddenly transformed into user-friendly units. A genuine stethoscope, making novice users at ease.

We quite never touch the countless pre- and post-processing possibilities nor all modern facilities, mainly harmonics (see Chap. 2). Annotations are useless when the examination is *not* made by a radiologist (or technician) for a doctor: the spirit of critical ultrasound.

The B/M mode seems insignificant. Technical misconceptions can contribute in losing lives, especially for diagnosing pneumothorax in difficult conditions (i.e., the most critical ones precisely). We will see in Chaps. 8, 10, and 14 that the modern manufacturers are usually unable to provide a left image in real time, and a right image in M-mode: side by side and without freezing the real-time image. This configuration, easily found in the 1980's technology, is a critical basis in lung ultrasound.

Read if you have time the interesting Anecdotal Note 1 of Chap. 28, proving that lung ultrasound could have been perfectly developed since the 1960s.

Opinions about sophisticated modes, harmonics, etc., are debated in Chap. 37. For the freeze button, read Anecdotal Note 1.

Step 1: The Image Acquisition

Whatever the unit (even with pocket machines), the mastery of the spatial dimension is probably the major difficult point of ultrasound. When the probe is moved, significant changes appear on the screen – very unsettling at the beginning. How to understand what happens on the screen should be mastered in priority. We travel through the third dimension. These changes will be integrated and become automatic with practice. The other step (interpreting the image) is much easier. The spatial control also makes the superiority of ultrasound, i.e., the possibility, by a slight change, of answering the clinical question. Even if we assume that in the current times physicians have all access to basic programs which explain this delicate step, the aim of CEURF is to simplify this step too.

For achieving this simplification, we will suppress movements we never do. Tilting the probe for instance. For anterolateral lung venous (belly, optic nerve, etc.) ultrasound, our probe is always perpendicular to the skin (Fig. 1.1). The two exceptions are (1) the heart, subcostal and apical views, (2) the posterior aspect of the lung in ventilated patients, where the probe tries to be as perpendicular as possible (see description of the PLAPS-point in Chap. 6). Being quite always perpendicular suppresses other movements, i.e., simplifies ultrasound (and is what we daily do).

Our microconvex probe has a sectorial scanning, displaying a trapezoidal image, the probe head being on top.

We assume that what is at the left, the right, the superficy, and the depth of the image is integrated. Note that for lung ultrasound, we adopted the radiological convention, head to the left, feet to the right, unlike the echocardiographists (roughly the only element that we took from the radiologic culture). Critical ultrasound should be

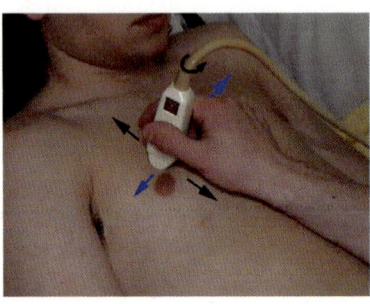

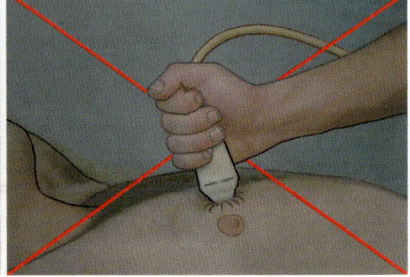

Fig. 1.1 How we hold the probe, how we don't. *Left*: Like with a fountain pen, the operator can stay hours without any fatigue, and the image is stable on the screen. The probe is applied at zero pressure, which is comfortable for the patient and mandatory for any venous analysis as well as the optic nerve. The probe is (reversibly) stable on the skin, not slippery using Ecolight, which decreases the energy needed for keeping it stable. The probe is perpendicular to the skin. It is applied longitudinally. Three main movements are *arrowed*. These *blue arrows* indicate the Carmen maneuver (this movement is done from left to right in this scan moving the skin on the underskin). If the probe was transversally applied, the Carmen maneuver would be from head to feet. The turning arrow indicates rotation of the probe (like screwdriving). The black arrows indicate a scanning looking like changing gears of an automobile (of major importance to the trainee for reaching the good position). *Right*: The pressure is not controlled (a very bad habit in venous ultrasound), and this position will generate fatigue. More severe, the hand is not stable; this will disturb the practice of a discipline based on the analysis of dynamics

homogenized: lung with head left, heart with head right makes no sense.

The operator must apply the probe on the skin, then search for the best image. For that, a good acoustic window must be found. This is really easy, never a problem for the lung, ironically. First, any perpendicular scan at any point of the chest wall provides the same basic image: the lung is "everywhere," just below the skin. Second, the gas is not a hindrance here. This completely changes the traditional rules of ultrasound. At the heart, the abdomen, etc., we admit that this step is challenging (although countless tricks are available).

Once a structure is detected more or less, subtle movements of the probe will optimize the image.

How We Hold the Probe Basically

Critical ultrasound analyzes vital structures, i.e., permanent movements. The operator's hand must be standstill (Fig. 1.1): the dynamic should be generated by the patient alone (never the operator's hand). Figure 1.1 shows how we do not hold the probe. Uncontrolled movements of the probe create dynamics which bring nothing. Ecolight®, our contact product, allows to save energy usually lost for stabilizing a slippery probe (Chap. 2). We find critical to hold the (microconvex) probe like a fountain pen between the thumb and index fingers (+/− medium etc.), with the operator's hand quietly applied on the patient's skin. For many parts, we work at "Zero pressure": the probe is applied to the skin until an image appears on the screen. This minimal pressure warrants absence of pain (or cardiac trouble when working onto the eyelid), absence of fatigue (in prolonged examinations), and absence of errors (too much initial energy will result in squashing veins).

Some beginners hold the probe too tight. This probe must be withdrawn without effort from the operator's hand by another person. One secret is the suppleness of the hand. Often, the young user is discouraged since he got a suboptimal image, whereas the experienced user comes nonchalantly after and obtains a much nicer image. Yet the difference is often due to minimal changes. Whereas the probe keeps its mark on the young user's hand (like, almost always, the joystick of a first flight – a sign of intense crispation), the experienced user holds it slightly and is not afraid to move it liberally. The Carmen maneuver (see just below) is to our knowledge the best way to dramatically improve an image.

The Elementary Movements

One secret for a steep learning curve is to study them one by one. Associating rotating and scanning movements would be challenging at the debuts. We use three elementary movements (Fig. 1.1). Instead of complex words (pivoting, translating), we use familiar comparisons.
1. *Changing a gear* (from 1st to 2nd speed). Sliding a longitudinal probe in a craniocaudal axis, from a rib to the lower intercostal space, positions the pleural line between the two ribs.
2. *Screwdriving*. Rotation on its main axis: the study of a vessel on its short axis (for DVT detection) then on its long axis (for cannulation).
3. *Painting a wall*. All probes (apart from cardiac) can be assimilated to brushes, with 2 axes. The *Carmen maneuver* is a simple movement that we permanently make. It is like using a large brush, but with the probe nearly standstill, just using the gliding of the skin over the underskin (making a centimetric amplitude to each side). Our contact product helps in "sticking," reversibly, the probe to the skin. This subtle maneuver allows us to have immediate control of the image: it helps in optimizing the image quality when scanning an intercostal space or any other area. It shows immediately a vascular couple that was not obvious on a static view, making Doppler far less useful, at least for helping locating the vessels.

The Second Hand in Critical Ultrasound

At CEURF, critical ultrasound is performed with both hands. The second hand is permanently used for countless uses. It helps for slightly turning the patient's back for prompting a posterior lung analysis (Fig. 6.4). It makes the venous compression possible in reputed noncompressible areas (Fig. 18.16). It helps the probe's hand to push the gas in an abdominal scan (Fig. 28.7). It takes the compress soaked with our contact product, making the operator ready to extend the field of investigation with no loss of time.

This is why we do not share the general enthusiasm generated by the pocket machines, where the spots always show smiling faces holding the machine in one hand, the probe in another (read Anecdotal Note 5 of Chap. 18).

Longitudinal or Transversal Scans?

Ultrasound can be made easy or difficult. Choosing longitudinal or transversal scans is part of this policy. Note that, strictly speaking, longitudinal and transversal are terms which refer to the craniocaudal and left-right locations of the human being. Axial and cross-sectional scans refer to structures with one long axis and one short axis (vessels, heart, kidneys, intestines, gallbladder, etc.).

The BLUE-protocol advises to scan the lung *always* longitudinally, the veins *always* in their short axis. By considering only one axis per structure, the difficulty is divided by two.

Figure 18.1 shows that most veins are roughly parallel to the longitudinal and transversal axes. For studying a vein, the choice of an axial approach is a bit similar to the violin practice, the cross-sectional approach to the guitar (Fig. 1.2). Violin is more demanding than guitar, where the pitch is self-adjusted. Studying a vessel through its cross-sectional scan is easy: once the probe is applied, the vascular couple is immediately recognized. If not, the Carmen maneuver makes it. Even if the hand of the operator moves, using this maneuver, the vessel

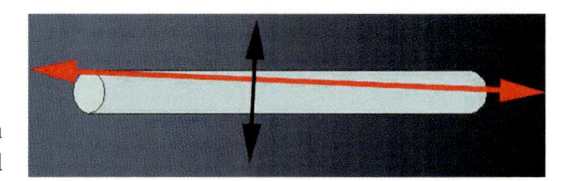

Fig. 1.2 Long vs. short axis. Cross-sectional vs. axial scan. This figure shows these two incidences for approaching a tubular structure – with a slight drift. Whereas the cross-sectional scan (*black*, 3°) is roughly insensitive to this drift, the axial scan (*red*, just 2°) is much more affected. Slight movements can make the vein disappear out of plane, at worst simulating a positive compression maneuver, and all in all make ultrasound a more difficult discipline. Cross-sectional scans are easy like guitar (long axis difficult like violin): the vein is always promptly visible on the screen (one is free to prefer violin anyway)

remains stable in the gunsight. Making an axial approach requires millimetric precision. Some operators even halt breathing. At the lung area, the practice of transversal/oblique scans (in the rib axis) would make ultrasound a difficult exercise.

Step 2: Understanding the Composition of the Image

We assume the readers have enough experience for knowing what are the white, gray, and black components of the images. We assume they master the words echoic, hypoechoic, hyperechoic, and acoustic window. An acoustic window can be physiological (bladder for the analysis of the uterus) or pathological (pleural effusion used to study the thoracic aorta).

Gain

Optimal control of gain is obtained with experience. At the lung, this step can be standardized. Radiologists have long defined the best gain as giving a gray (healthy) liver and a black (healthy) gallbladder content. We can do the same with lung ultrasound: the best gain gives black shadows of ribs, grey parietal tissues, and white pleural line (Fig. 1.3). In the units we use, the

Step 2: Understanding the Composition of the Image

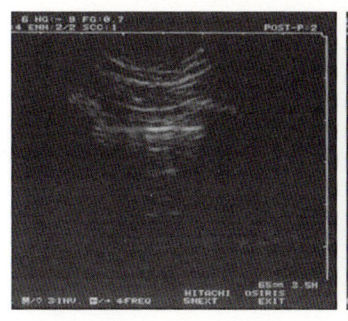

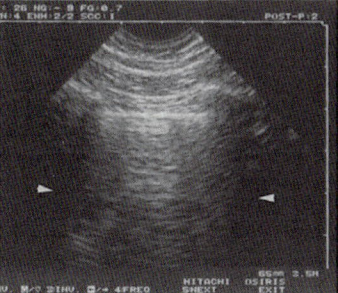

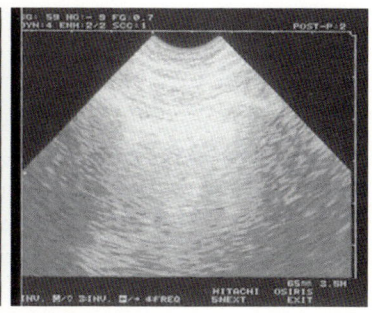

Fig. 1.3 Standardized gain for lung ultrasound. Longitudinal scan of the lung. *Left*: The gain is too low. Details are lost. *Middle*: The gain is optimal, clearly showing the pleural line. *Right*: The gain is too high: superficial areas are saturated

proximal, distal, and global gains can be adjusted. That said, we modify only the global gain, from time to time, and quite never the proximal and distal gains.

We very quickly remind the components of the echogenicity:
- Parenchyma, venous thrombosis, lung consolidation, hematoma, and gallbladder sludge are echoic.
- Abscess and necrosis are less echoic.
- Pure fluid collection or circulating blood is anechoic. Some artifacts are anechoic (acoustic shadow of bones).
- Some artifacts are hyperechoic (repetitions of air mainly).
- Interface, surface of ribs, gas, and cardiac valve appear white.

Deep fat is hyperechoic such as mesenteric fat (allowing us to perfectly locate the mesenteric artery). We did not invest a lot in this field, but, for those interested, commercial oil is anechoic, and commercial butter has a tissular, liver-like pattern.

Artifacts: One Basis of Lung Ultrasound

The analysis of artifacts (traditionally a hindrance in the ultrasound's world, a foe to eradicate with no mercy) is the basis of critical ultrasound.

Artifacts are created by the principle of propagation of the ultrasound beam. The beam is stopped by air and bones. How to recognize an artifact is the easiest part: these are images with regular, straight, and geometric shape, usually vertical or horizontal, more precisely converging to the head of the probe (the top of the screen) like parallels or meridians. This is the common point to nearly all artifacts. Real images have totally different shape: anatomic, never fully regular, and suitable for measurements (e.g., lung consolidation).

Some words should be familiar.

Reverberation or repetition artifacts. They are the basis of lung ultrasound, generating the A-lines and B-lines, mainly. The profiles of the BLUE-protocol with artifacts (A, A', B, B' profiles) create a complete acoustic barrier below the pleural line: they obliterate any information located deeper.

Acoustic shadows. They are anechoic barriers, arising behind bone structures, also hiding deeper information (see Fig. 8.1). The rib shadows are basic landmarks of lung ultrasound.

In thoracic ultrasound, a longitudinal view makes an alternance of artifacts: acoustic shadows behind the ribs, reverberation artifacts behind the pleural line, either horizontal (A-lines) or vertical (B-lines), again shadow of the rib, etc. This is (probably) a main factor which originated the dogma of the unfeasibility of lung ultrasound [2].

The acoustic enhancement is a popular artifact which we quite never use. Never in LUCI, exceptionally for venous scanning, just before compressing apparently empty veins. Therefore, no figure is provided (see if needed Fig. 1.7 of our 2010 Edition). It indicates the fluid nature of a mass in traditional ultrasound (the liver parenchyma is more echoic behind the gallbladder than lateral to it).

Dynamics: The Other Basis of Lung Ultrasound

Critical ultrasound scans vital organs: lungs, heart, vessels, and bowel mainly. A common feature to any vital structure is a permanent dynamic, from birth to death. The brain? Read Anecdotal Note 2. A vital structure that does not move is *dead* or dying. The M-mode button allows demonstration of any dynamic on a frozen picture. Almost all diagnoses at the lung area consider the dynamic dimension: pulmonary edema, pneumothorax, pneumonia, pleural effusion, complete atelectasis, among others. This textbook shows examples of pathological dynamics in pneumoperitoneum, mesenteric infarction (Chap. 34), and floating thrombosis.

Dimensions

Dimensions can be accurately measured by freezing the image and adjusting electronic calipers. Yet in critical ultrasound, there is not so much time, nor *need*, for measurements (see through this book).

Step 3: Image Interpretation

Only the operator's familiarity with the field, enriched by reading the literature and personal experience, will indicate which conclusions can be drawn. For instance, a lung consolidation at the anterior chest wall will have a specific meaning. Previously, this operator has carefully learned to choose an appropriate machine, an appropriate probe, switch on the ultrasound unit, check for the proper gain, by-pass useless modes, hold the probe correctly, locate the lung surface, and recognize this consolidation through its specific sign (the fractal sign).

Impediments to Ultrasound Examination

First have in mind that the most sophisticated machines, as well as the most flashy pocket machines, are unable to cross the bones, dressings, and air.

At the Lung Area

Air at the lung level was traditionally considered an absolute obstacle; now all doctors know that this dogma was wrong. What is true is that the air immediately visible at the lung surface prevents us to see deeper. This is one of the paradoxes of LUCI: not a big issue (principle N° 7, see Chap. 5).

The real obstacles are really few. Huge dressings that cannot be withdrawn easily are the main one. Subcutaneous emphysema is a hindrance for beginners (and for experts in advanced stages); see how to deal with it in Chap. 14 on pneumothorax. Images are more easy to define when the BLUE-points are followed (*see* Chap. 6), and the scapula is not put by mistake on strategic areas (see note, p. 53). Only in exceptional cases, an image remains difficult to interpret.

Lung Apart

In the rest of the body, mainly the abdomen, there are so many organs that, we agree, ultrasound may appear an esoteric fog for the beginner's eyes.

Gas and ribs interrupt the image. This drawback of ultrasound, one of the rare, is not found with radiography, CT or MRI.

Bowel gas is, per se, an inescapable obstacle. However, a gas can move, like a cloud previously hiding the sun. Before concluding that the examination is impossible, the approaches must be diversified: one must sometimes wait and try again. Both operator's hands may be able to shift the gas (see Fig. 28.7). For getting rid of the gas, our maneuver is slight expiratory pressure, maintaining the pressure during next inspiration, then exert a slightly superior pressure, and so on – with patience and method – this is the most pacific and efficient way.

Thick bones are absolute obstacles. Fine bones (maxillary bones, scapula) are transparent to the ultrasound beam. Using these windows, ultrasound extends its territory throughout the entire body.

Subcostal organs (liver and spleen) can be entirely hidden by the ribs and cannot be analyzed using the abdominal approach. Our universal probe scans through the intercostal spaces, creating an incomplete vision – but fully adapted to the information required in the critically ill.

Obese (currently, the elegant term is "challenging") patients are traditionally not candidates for ultrasound (nor CT nor any imaging modality). The devoted Chap. 33 will show that the problem is surprisingly limited.

Extensive dressings, devices, G-suits, cervical collars, etc., are real hindrances.

In daily practice, a really non contributive examination is rare. All in all, ultrasound answers a clinical question with a clear analysis in 80–90 % of cases [3]. At superficial areas (lung, veins, optic nerve, etc.), the answer is quite always possible.

Anecdotal Notes

1. *The freeze function*
   The freeze button is apparently insignificant. If one operator (sonographer) provides a static image, and another operator (radiologist) interprets this image (i.e., US used at the US sauce), the potential of critical ultrasound is not exploited. Our philosophy stems from deactivating the freeze function. Critical ultrasound is a real-time discipline.

2. *The brain, a vital organ?*
   Some would argue that the brain does not move. We answer that the brain, our most precious organ, is not a vital organ (life is possible without). Critical ultrasound just tries to always use the right word. Here, this is just a detail which does not change any action, but words should have a major relevance when a new discipline is defined.

References

1. Lichtenstein D (2014) How can the use of lung ultrasound in cardiac arrest make ultrasound a holistic discipline. The example of the SESAME-protocol. Med Ultrason 16(3):252–255
2. Friedman PJ (1992) Diagnostic procedures in respiratory diseases. In: Harrison's principles of internal medicine, 12th edn. McGraw-Hill, New York, p 1043
3. Lichtenstein D (2002) Particularités d'un examen échographique chez le patient de réanimation. In: L'échographie générale en réanimation. Springer, Paris/Berlin/Heidelberg, pp 11–16

Which Equipment for the BLUE-Protocol? (And for Whole-Body Critical Ultrasound). 1 – The Unit

> If we give the paternity of the ultrasound revolution to the laptop machines, the merit of the physicians who developed critical ultrasound at the bedside before the advent of these technologies (using smaller equipment, superior in many respects) would not be considered.

> With its use of complicated machines (even laptops) with complicated techniques and nonsuitable probes, ultrasound *remains* a complicated discipline. The use of pocket machines will not make critical ultrasound simpler. Their small size does not eliminate the main steps (or difficulty): probe handling, image acquisition, and image interpretation. Most hypermodern machines, which destroy real time (instant response) and artifacts, can harm lung ultrasound.

> The essential thing with laptop technology is to note the width and not the height of the unit. This is because obstacles are lateral, not above. Remember that the unit always remains on its cart (an excellent accessory, by the way). We need narrow units, not laptops.

This chapter should be read carefully by users who want to understand what holistic ultrasound is (and, for example, practice the SESAME-protocol, the use of ultrasound in cardiac arrest). Each word of this chapter (and the next one covering the probe) is important. The reader may not understand the importance until he or she faces a cardiac arrest (dealt with in Chap. 31).

As in the 2010 edition, this chapter will be neutral, only describing facts (and repeating them, if necessary); more personal opinions are given in Chap. 37. Some readers may be surprised to see described here a 1992 technology unit. Perhaps "1992" sounds slightly antique, but if we add that the last update (just cosmetic) was done in 2008, they will read the text with more attention. This machine, fully adapted for critical care, has not yet been replaced, and we will describe why we still use it.

Critical ultrasound heralds a new discipline (that we can call *visual medicine*). The simpler we make it, the more widespread its use will be. When we wrote our 1992 textbook, interested physicians had in mind traditional, cumbersome, complex machines. When we wrote the 2005 edition, all physicians had in mind laptop machines, which had roughly the same width (including the cart, usually 60 cm) and a smaller height (which is of no interest within hospitals). As we write the present edition, all physicians have in mind the pocket machines, which are easier to steal and more cumbersome than apparent, for their image quality is not always optimal.

We understand that users are attached to their machines. If they are persuaded that the modern, up-to-date machines (which do not integrate the lung) are better than older ones, let them appreciate their machines. Some are even persuaded that laptop technology was what made the birth of critical ultrasound possible. The most courageous will see for themselves and make their own opinions, if they realize that the craze for these machines results from a slight confusion: a machine with small height (i.e., a laptop) is of no interest to those who work inside hospitals. *Smaller* machines existed long before – and worked better.

The Seven Requirements We Ask of an Ultrasound Machine Devoted to Critical Care – A Short Version for the Hurried Reader

We continue using a machine manufactured in 1992 (last update 2008) because of seven critical criteria. Are they present in the today's laptop machines? Sharp reading of this chapter (and the section on laptops in Chap. 37) answers this question.

1. *The size.* Our unit is small: a width of 29 cm, a critical point in a setting where each centimeter counts. Its intelligent cart fits the machine exactly, making an efficient width of 32 cm. The cart is an important piece. It is mounted on wheels, and these wheels allow transportation of even heavy material (our machine weighs 12 kg) with two fingers, from the intensive care unit (ICU) to the emergency room (ER), between a patient and the ventilator, and so on. The wheels are the key factor in the revolution.
2. *The image quality.* The image comes from a cathode ray tube providing analog resolution (as demonstrated by all figures in this book).
3. *Its switch-on time.* Seven seconds, which is just enough time to take the probe, the contact product, and begin scanning, in time-dependent settings as well as multiple daily managements.
4. *Flat design.* The keyboard is flat and its design is compact, allowing efficient cleaning, a critical requirement between patients.
5. *Simple technology.* The three main buttons are easy to find in extreme emergencies. The absence of a destructive filter and of Doppler explain its cost-effectiveness.
6. *The probe.* Its large-range, 5-MHz microconvex probe is suitable for whole-body analysis and qualifies as universal. This small probe can be applied anywhere without need for change.
7. *The cost.* We appreciate the low cost of this system, a basic point, because it has allowed easy purchase by hospitals, thus saving lives, since 1992.

A nonscientific point, apart from these seven: its aesthetics. Combined with the technical advantages, it gives the feeling of a *harmonious* tool. Those readers familiar with the Millennium Falcon of *Star Wars* will recognize our unit: rustic perhaps, but the fastest in the galaxy.

A Longer Version: The Seven Requirements We Ask of an Ultrasound Machine Devoted to Critical Care

We now go into more detail. These seven criteria contribute to making critical ultrasound an easy daily tool.

First Basic Requirement: A *Really* Short Size

It is important to find a location for the machine between the patient and the ventilator. Each centimeter is important. The critical dimension (for those who have high ceilings, i.e., those who work in hospitals) is the width (Fig. 2.1). We invite colleagues to measure the width of their machine (using the instrument in Fig. 28.2). We use our 1992 (updated 2008) machine every day because of its small width, 29 cm by itself, 32 cm with the smart cart, no matter its height,

A Longer Version: The Seven Requirements We Ask of an Ultrasound Machine Devoted to Critical Care

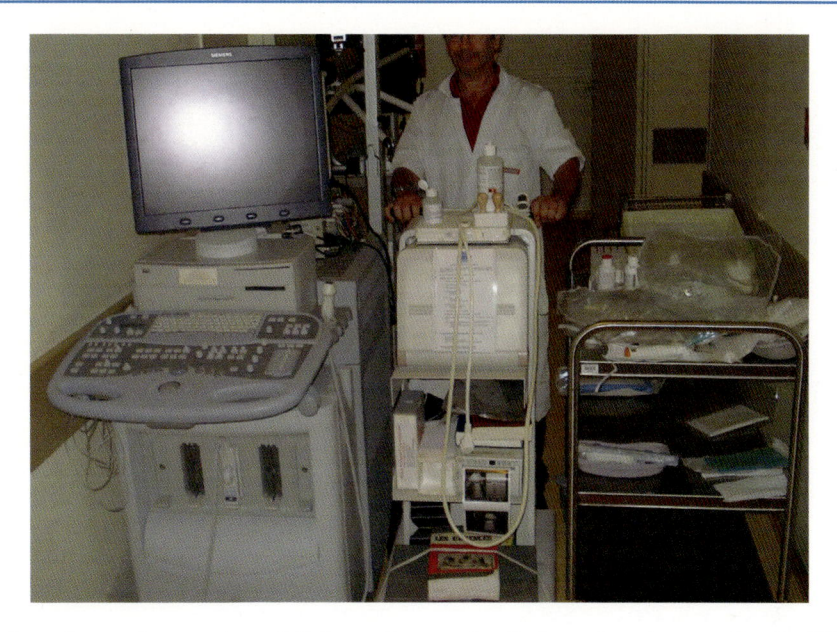

Fig. 2.1 A figure that speaks more than a full chapter. In all the hospitals in the world, the ceilings are high enough. The obstacles come from devices that strangle us *laterally*, preventing the machine from being brought rapidly on site. Each saved centimeter makes the difference. This unit is much thinner than laptops (the big machine at one side is not so large compared with a standard laptop machine; just measure for yourself)

and it fits between beds without problem. This is one of the paradoxes of critical ultrasound.

The PUMA concept highlights our vision. It is fully detailed in the Appendix 1. For doctors working outside the hospital (in airplanes, etc.), please see below.

Second Basic Requirement: Intelligent Image Quality

The figures in this book show why we respect our 1992 image quality, generated by analog technology (cathode ray tube). The weight of the cathode ray tube is not a problem because it is carried by the wheels of the cart. Figure 2.2 shows our definition of a suitable resolution.

What is holistic ultrasound? Having a cathode ray tube provides the best image quality *and* provides a top (there is no top with laptop machines). This top can support objects, allowing one to decrease the lateral volume, arrive faster on-site, and save more lives.

Third Basic Requirement: Short Start-Up Time

In cardiac arrest, or in multiple routine daily uses, the start-up time plays a basic role. With our 1992 technology, it is 7 s. Each additional second is an issue. There is no complicated program to start-up. It is pure visual medicine.

Fourth Basic Requirement: Access to an Intelligent Microconvex Probe

The probe is perhaps the most important part of critical ultrasound – the bow of the violin. The traditional culture requires cardiac phased-array (2.5 MHz) probes for the heart, abdominal (3.5 MHz) probes for the abdomen, vascular (7.5 MHz) probes for the vessels, and endovaginal probes for the vagina. We use none of these probes. We considered a distinct chapter was worthwhile, and the next one is fully devoted to this critical point.

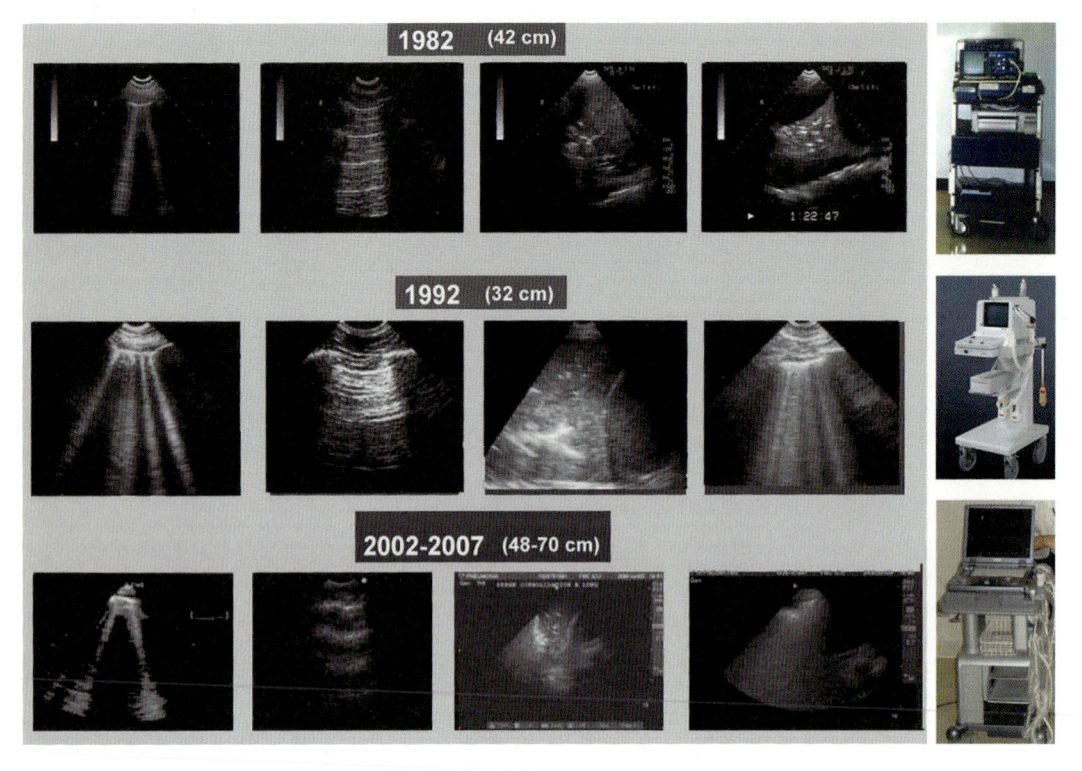

Fig. 2.2 A backward step of 25 years. A nice revolution (the laptops), but a questionable resolution. This figure summarizes a small drama in the history of (lung) ultrasound. From top to bottom (top, our ADR-4000) (middle, our Hitachi 405); note in the bottom line how the image quality has worsened. The bottom line (modern laptop) shows the way many physicians discovered lung ultrasound. Please just compare: a backward jump of 25 years for no gain of space

Fifth Basic Requirement: Compact Design – for Efficient Cleaning

We respect our current patient and also our future ones. Accordingly, the cleaning of the machine is a critical point in the ER, and even more so in the ICU, not to mention the pediatric ICU. Our 1992 machine has a *flat* keyboard, which can be efficiently washed in a few seconds. Its compact and smooth body with the unique probe is also rapidly cleaned if necessary (see Chap. 4).

Sixth Basic Requirement: Intelligent, Simple Technology

This section is long but is worth knowing. How can a higher technology be of lower quality than previous ones? This point, at the center of critical ultrasound, is also one of its main paradoxes. Sophisticated programs have been conceived that slightly improve tissular imaging (a minor benefit for us) and greatly worsen lung imaging, which is most critical.

As an example, imagine two simple radio sets. Select the same channel, one on FM to your left, one on LW to your right. You will immediately hear that the FM sound is clearer, but the sound of LW comes sooner. If your main interest is to get the information as soon as possible, and if you are able to hear the info anyway, the antique LW technology will be superior. Critical ultrasound is a different discipline with specific requirements.

The Point About Doppler – The DIAFORA Concept

We do not use Doppler. This will be commented upon throughout this textbook, for each classical application. Additional comments are found in Chap. 37, in the section on Doppler, where we explain how Doppler possibly killed, indirectly.

The main problem with Doppler is the cost (it triples the cost of the machine), making ultrasound out of reach for most hospital budgets for decades. This factor delayed a revolution that could have occurred in 1982 (ADR-4000®).

Our daily use is centered around life-saving or current applications. Observations have shown that Doppler is sometimes required, but only in rare occasions for extreme emergency use. We therefore developed the concept of the *Doppler Intermittently Asked from Outside in Rare Applications* – DIAFORA– to indicate that we are not opposed to it. We just ask, from time to time, for an outside operator with a complex machine to come to the bedside (Anecdotal Note 1). More than half the time, this does not contribute to the patient's care (study in process).

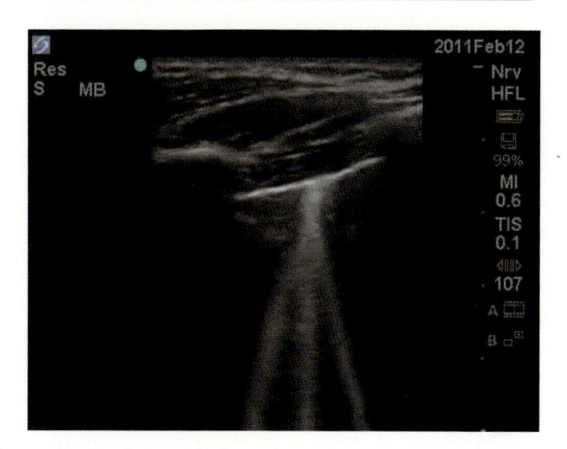

Fig. 2.3 Lung rockets? Typical example of how modern technologies can confuse. For an experienced user, it is obvious that only one B-line is visible here, multiplied by the multibeam concept (harmonics, etc.). A younger user will possibly see three comet-tail artifacts, conclude there is an interstitial syndrome, and manage the patient accordingly (healthy model here)

Filters, Harmonics, Etc., All Facilities Imagined by Modern Machines

These "facilities" were worked out by engineers, who are smart, but they are not physicians, especially intensivists, involved in holistic, lung ultrasound. Let us look at them one by one.

Filters

Filters are good for radiologists because they provide images that are nice to look at. For critical ultrasound, especially lung ultrasound, they create a hindrance. They prevent real-time dynamic analysis of vital organs, lungs, heart, and vessels. Filters create a time lag that is not compatible with dynamic analysis. The multibeam mode is perhaps the most destructive filter for lung ultrasound. The more manufacturers suppress artifacts, the more they bury lung ultrasound *alive*. The recent profusion of modes is possibly a necessary adaptation to the poor resolution of the laptop flat-screen technology, an attempt to reach the quality of the previous *analog* equipment. We inactivate all filters. We bypass persistence filters, dynamic noise filters, and average filters. We don't see the benefit of harmonics and shut off this function, too. This kind of filter can fool young users, who have heard that "multiple comet-tail artifacts are a sign of pulmonary edema" (Fig. 2.3). As a rule, we bypass *all* filters. Critical ultrasound is performed using natural images.

What about facilities for challenging patients? If some modern modes advocate making them well echoic, we are not opposed to their use. We fear that they improve tissular echogenicity (not a major target, as parenchymal studies do not come first in critical ultrasound) to the detriment of lung ultrasound. This is one reason to invoke the DIAFORA.

Harmonics can possibly provide nice images to look at, especially of nonmobile organs. We use again the concept of the perfect compromise (see the next chapter, on the probe, especially Figs. 3.1 and 3.2). It is true that, in some areas, the image will be slightly less easy to interpret because of background noise, parasites. However, our sole question is, does it remain within the domain of possible interpretation? If so, we accept to have sometimes a lower quality, and most of the time the optimal quality. For the large majority of targets aimed at in critical ultrasound, this is the winning choice. Lung first. The concept of the perfect compromise, of vital relevance in cardiac arrest mainly, is illustrated in the self-explanatory Figs. 3.1 and 3.2.

The Function Focus

We have never understood what changes in the image.

Contrast-Enhanced Ultrasound

This mode is possibly interesting, although it requires sophisticated, costly software. We promise to involve ourselves in this mode once all the potentials of simple critical ultrasound are covered.

Computer Technology

This condemns the user to a long switch-on time (minutes, far from our 7-s time) and the permanent risk of bugging. It is devoted to sophisticated cardiological programs, which we do not use.

M-Mode

This is a critical function, allowing ideal use of lung ultrasound. It will be detailed in Chaps. 10 and 14. Simply put, lung ultrasound requires two images exactly side by side. All other settings are either suboptimal or confusing, with deleterious risks.

The Setting "Lung"?

Which setting do we advise for the BLUE-protocol? In the past, we were accustomed to see the sempiternal settings "vascular," "abdominal," "gyneco-obstetrical," "urology," "cardiac," and so on. Now, we have begun to see the word "LUNG" on some modern machines. This vision gives us mixed feelings. Looking at the entire donut, this seems like a victory: at last, now that the community widely believes in lung ultrasound, manufacturers have begun to follow. Focusing on the hole of the donut, we wonder what is the setting "LUNG"? What is behind it? How far did they go? We did not assess this setting personally and are unable at the time being to recommend one or another of these machines.

The setting we use, the same for the whole body, is not a "lung" setting. It is the "null" setting. We need to see altogether the lungs, veins, heart, belly, and so on, without any adaptation. And this is what we actually do. No filter, no harmonic, no time lag, none of these "facilities" that are a hindrance for lung and venous ultrasound. Our setting, ready for the worst (cardiac arrest, SESAME-protocol), is used daily for routine tasks (e.g., venous line insertion, checking for bladder distension, etc.). Read Chap. 31 on cardiac arrest.

Robustness?

Manufacturers' advertisements claim that their machines can fall down without (immediate) damage. This can be of interest during wartime but not in our setting. We are not accustomed to letting our beloved unit fall down. This is one of the countless reasons why the cart is a major part of the unit.

Cable Length

This detail could be inserted above under point 4 (the probe), or 5 (compact design). The length of the cables is anything but a minor detail, especially when they are numerous. Smart cables do not trail. Cables lying on the ground make a nice nest for all the microbes that proliferate there and jump on the cables to discover new horizons. Most importantly, in an emergency, when the machine is moved in haste, there is the risk of a wheel being suddenly blocked by the cable, provoking, of course, the destruction of the cable and an immediate tip-over of the machine (at best on the doctor's foot, resulting in lessening the damage to the machine). This creates three victims: the machine, the physician, and the patient. An appalling vision, which has already happened.

Imagination should be at work here, too. The cable length is an important detail that should be easily fixed.

The Cart and Its Wheels: A Piece of Major Relevance

For those who work in hospitals (i.e., more than 95 % of us), the cart is critical. It brings together the ultrasound unit, the probe, the contact product, the procedural equipment, the disinfectant, and more. The cart is equipped with a major, even old, technology: the *wheel*. The wheel was available 5500 years ago in Mesopotamian cultures. Thanks to the wheel, our 12-kg machine is easily transported from bed to bed, from ICU to ER. The laptop machines, proudly purchased from hand to hand, always stay on their cart, which is, by the way, a necessary thing. Therefore, the cart cancels the advantage of miniaturization, *which is not a problem if the unit plus the cart are narrow.*

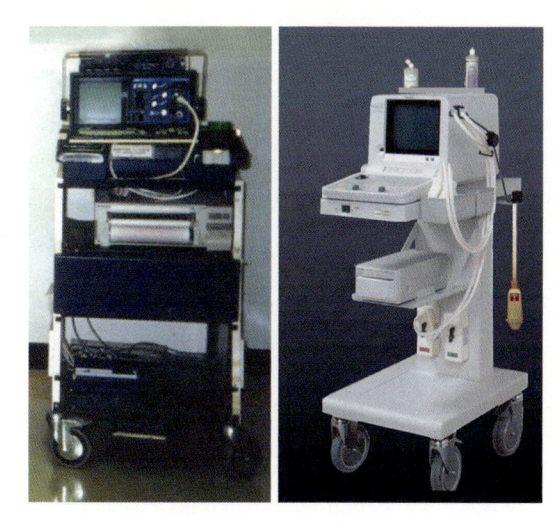

Fig. 2.4 The ADR-4000® and the Hitachi 405. Our references: two respectable collector machines, yet perfectly mobile to the bedside and able to achieve the ultrasound revolution since 1982 (*left*) and 1992 (*right*). Both are small in width (*left*, 42 cm, *right*, 32 cm), and both have wheels, the key to the revolution. Please also see Fig. 2.2, showing how fine were these machines for developing lung ultrasound

Since 1982, the ADR-4000® has had these wheels and a 42-cm width (Fig. 2.4). These features have allowed the authors to define critical ultrasound at the point of care [1]. The resolution was suitable for all critical diagnoses (only limited by the optic nerve), and we can state that the year 1982 was the point for the ultrasound revolution in the critically ill.

Our intelligent cart fits the unit exactly and does not take up useless space laterally. The important Fig. 4.3 shows how the space is exploited for setting the main elements (probe, contact product, disinfectant) on top of our cathode ray tube, instead of having these cumbersome lateral devices. The cart protects the machine. The overall weight makes it difficult to steal.

Seventh Basic Requirement: A Cost-Effective Purchase

This is the consequence of the points 2 (analog technology), 4 (unique probe), and 6 (simple technology without Doppler, harmonics, etc.). The cost-effectiveness is critical, since every saved dollar (euro, rupee, etc.) saves additional lives. Our unit and its probe were the cost of an unsophisticated automobile.

One Word to Summarize Again Our Seven Requirements

Smart readers have seen that each part of this machine interacts with the others. The cart fits the machine. The cathode ray tube gives optimal resolution. The cathode ray tube is made light thanks to the wheels. The wheels allow the machine to go to the bedside. The cathode ray tube allows exploiting the top, i.e., benefiting from a small width, one probe finding a natural place on this top. This universal probe allows fast whole-body ultrasound with easy cleaning, and so on. One word for characterizing this type of completion: *harmony*.

The Coupling System: A Detail?

Since the dawn of ultrasound, doctors have used a gooey coupling medium between probe and skin, which is not the most glamorous part of ultrasound. Ecolight®, a system we created several years ago, eliminates the problems of the traditional gel. The image quality is exactly the same (all figures in this textbook were acquired using it) and it has the following advantages:

1. Stability: Critical ultrasound is a dynamic discipline, where only the patient's structures are under analysis. The gel creates a slippery field. It is more difficult to stay stable once a good window has been found (echocardiographic users permanently make this effort). Ecolight® makes a nonslippery contact, and the probe is well applied to the skin just by using gentle pressure. Therefore, the effort of holding the probe is minimal. If the user wants to scan, the pressure should simply be relieved.
2. Speed: Ecolight® is poured on an adapted compress always kept near the field, and one travels from lung to legs, for example, with less than two seconds per change: a critical time savings.

3. A major advantage in cardiac arrest is that no slippery gel needs to be wiped off for efficient thoracic compression. After one or two minutes, more than sufficient in critical ultrasound to make a diagnosis (B-profile, etc.), Ecolight® vanishes, leaving no trace on skin, nothing to clean, and no culture medium, as can be the case with traditional gels.
4. A less important advantage is the eradication of the gurgling noises (reminiscent of undesirable digestive noise) generated by stressed hands, never appropriate in these dramatic settings.
5. Another minor advantage is the comfort of making a clean examination, far from the traditional mess (see Fig. 37.1). This is our daily vision of ultrasound: a clean field. Morning visions of the dried gel from the night before that was not wiped off and, on occasion, things (hair) stuck to the probe, are part of the past.

Ecolight® is harmless and odorless. Based on equimolecular combination, its adiabatic properties allow quick warming (if passed under hot water), which is appreciated by the conscious patient. Recently patented, soon distributed, our "gelless gel" is one example among others of holistic ultrasound.

Data Recording

In an emergency, we find it suitable (for the novice users) to record the examination. It saves time, as there is no need to take pictures. The movie can be read subsequently, and data are easier to read than on static images. All the videos that we exhibited in hundreds of congresses come from VHS cassettes, a technology around since 1976. The VHS recorder is part of our PUMA. With VHS, time for recording is unlimited, not restricted to 6 s as with standard laptops. For the purposes of teaching, we have converted our sequences to digital technology since 2000. Previously, we lectured using plastic slides and VHS. Many colleagues have witnessed lung sliding this way since 1989. This quietly proves that analog or digital recording is not at all the problem. Modern technologies (smartphones, Twitter, USB outputs, etc.) are interesting but are *not* the key to the ultrasound revolution. The revolution had to happen in the brains. Remote ultrasound? Read Anecdotal Note 2.

How to Practically Afford a Machine in One's ICU

We currently see three approaches:
1. Buying a new machine. Please note that if one thinks in terms of width and not height, the choice is extremely large (buying laptops is not mandatory, especially in areas where space is an issue: ICUs, ERs, operating rooms ORs).
2. Buying a second-hand machine. Occasionally a radiology department gets rid of obsolete units and leaves them to whoever wants them. These "old" machines can save lives, and some of them can be excellent. Remember that cathode ray tubes give better resolution than digital screens and that the weight is not an issue, thanks to the wheels.
3. Stealing one. The possibility of stealing a machine is an option that must be considered, now that ultrasmall machines have invaded our hospitals. These lines have been written with serious intentions, and we want to make colleagues aware of this scenario, which occurs regularly in respectable institutions. Fixing a portable unit solidly on a cart is the solution, which immediately invalidates the (pseudo) advantage of the ultraminiature technology. Consequently, the user will benefit from all disadvantages of laptop machines, with no advantage (see Chap. 37). *Please, consider this basic point.*

Should We Share a Unit Between Several Departments?

One will face technical and human issues. Machines designated to be "universal," i.e., shared by several disciplines in the same hospital, are based upon a misconception. They are universal only in light of traditional ultrasound (cardiologic, urologic, etc.). Therefore, they have integrated all possible technologies. Because these machines are (for unknown reasons) laptops, thus remaining small in height (the useless dimension), they use high-cost technologies, which are useless once the necessity of a cart has been understood.

A critical care institution must have, permanently, its own machine. The intensivist must have priority access. Shared machines usually belong to one department, and the others must ask to use it, creating hierarchical relations, not a good point for the philosophy of simple ultrasound.

What Solutions Are There for Institutions Already Equipped with Laptop Technologies?

Do not worry! Laptop machines can be used, and they are good. Their owners must be happy with them. They are lucky to have ultrasound rather than nothing. Any kind of machine can give pieces of information. Specialized ICUs (cardiac and neurosurgical ICUs) probably need Doppler, so let us welcome it for simplifying. But in daily life, simple units can be used with advantage. In "normal" ICUs (ERs, ORs) equipped with up-to-date machines, each component can create difficulty, which can range from slight to extreme. Difficulties that add on to each other (e.g., a 3-min start-up time plus 60-cm width plus a dirty keyboard plus nonergonomic probes plus filters that are impossible to bypass) are a frequent occurrence in the landscape of today's ultrasound. Lung ultrasound will not be made easier there.

Accustomed to working with a perfectly profiled tool since 1992, we gave it the value "0." We will delight ourselves by comparing it with modern technologies and subtracting points (CEURF units) for each difficulty.

- Each centimeter in width >32 cm (cart included): subtract one point.
- Each decrease in resolution preventing accurate use. From the ideal 100 %, one point per percent.
- Each button to be cleaned is a hindrance: one point per button.
- Each second >7 for start-up reduces the chances for the patient. One point per second, 60 points per minute (no discount).
- Each millimeter of probe footprint > 10 × 20 mm: the access to difficult parts, hard to reach, is decreased. Ten points per square centimeter.
- Each millimeter of length of the probe > 8.8 cm makes posterior analysis more difficult: 10 points per centimeter.
- Each probe not suitable for holistic ultrasound (i.e., one probe for the whole body) is a factor of cost and lost time, especially if the perfect one for the lungs is missing: 20 points.
- Each filter that is impossible to bypass: 15 points.
- Each additional dollar > $14,000 makes the purchase more difficult: One point for every $100.
- Mess of cables lying on the ground near the wheels: 100 points per cable.

Some laptop machines have *simultaneously* a width > 32 cm, a resolution image < 100, a number of buttons > 3, a start-up time > 7 s, a probe length > 8.8 cm, not the suitable probe shape and property, and a cost > $14,000. We calculated in one of the current giants −830 CEURF units. This number is not an opinion, it is a fact.

Calculate your own score and see whether the community has gained or lost an opportunity to discover a simple discipline. If your score is extremely negative, the solution is already on the way (read below).

Which Machines for Those Who Work Outside the Hospital and in Confined Space?

The few doctors who work in airplanes (and helicopters, ambulances, or spaceships) will be interested in hand-held machines, an absolute revolution, in these particular settings where each centimeter counts in the *three dimensions* (Fig. 2.5). No cart is needed here for transporting laptop machines weighing sometimes 6 kg.

In our part-time work as a flying doctor, we used successive units. From 1995 to 1997, we used the rudimentary 3.5-kg battery-powered Dymax TM-18, built in Pittsburgh, and this unit was used in passing for conducting the first world

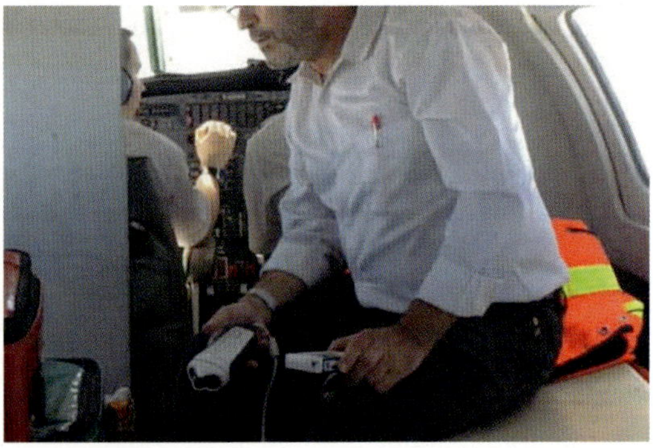

Fig. 2.5 The place of hand-held machines. When space is really a hindrance (airborne missions in small jets), light ultrasound machines are a blessing. Thanks to Anne Nikolsky for the picture

experience of extra-hospital critical ultrasound [2] from our medical helicopter (see Fig. 33.1).

From 1999 to 2013, we used the Tringa S-50 from Pie Medical (Maastricht, Netherlands), a compact 1.9-kg machine made in accordance with our wishes, using a flat screen and one quite universal probe (creating a substantial gain in size and weight). It was 15×12.5×13 cm in dimension (see Fig. 33.2). The image quality was not great, it is true (75 % from our ideal), but suitable for lung and venous imaging. It held, with the probe, the contact product, emergency procedures material, even the charger, in a 26×17×19 cm market bag that opened at the top, i.e., a perfect bag providentially found on the Boulevard Saint-Michel (Paris 6th, left river side, free ad).

We currently use an Australian 0.4-kg pocket machine for these airborne missions. Its technology is optimized for critical ultrasound, with a kind of microconvex probe, no Doppler, two buttons allowing one to perform BLUE, FALLS, and SESAME-protocols, and an image quality, especially for lungs and veins, reminiscent of the quality we have worked with since 1992. Not all "pocket machines" have this image quality. These technologies are a providence in such settings,

and we accept minor and inherent drawbacks (small size of screen and need for holding the central unit with one hand - fixing this small machine to a cart makes no sense). One extreme solution is to lay the central unit on the ground of the aircraft. Remember that *critical ultrasound is done with both hands*. In cardiac arrest or any other emergency or routine, both hands constantly interact (e.g., venous compression in strategic areas such as the lower femoral veins). Using Ecolight for each change of area, the user works with clean, gel-free hands. We would have more difficulties accepting these drawbacks hundreds of times a day in a hospital use. And do not forget our warning, some lines above, regarding the risk of theft.

The Solution for the Future

Many physicians acquired their first experience with machines that appeared of lesser quality than the one we have advocated for decades, even if they have other facilities (which we don't use). Using these technical interfaces, the full power of holistic ultrasound did not completely appear to them. We simply bet that, with time, the need will increase to the point that one machine per ICU (and others), even "top level," will appear insufficient. We calculate that the small machine devoted for cardiac arrest, BLUE-protocol, and the whole-body approach for 100 applications (venous line insertion, etc.) should be used and answer the questions in more than 85 % of cases. For the remaining causes, the sophisticated machines can be switched on.

When physicians can afford an additional unit, they have a choice. If they buy the same as they already have, they will just have two of the same laptop machines. If they buy one of the kind we describe, they will rediscover critical ultrasound. We suggest that key opinion leaders try our system, at least once, to facilitate this future. They will become even greater experts.

Do you think our 1992/2008 upgraded unit appears antique? Try it. As a marketing strategy, in light of the field covered by this textbook, we could write: "Tomorrow's medicine using yesterday's tools."

Some Basic Points and Reminders

- The important dimension (for optimal mobility) is the lateral width, not the height.
- The cathode ray tube technology (which is not heavy, thanks to the wheels of the cart) provides the best image quality and has allowed bedside use since 1982.
- A flat keyboard is easy to quickly disinfect.
- An immediate start-up time (7 s.).
- An intelligent cart does not annihilate the advantages of miniaturization.
- One probe can accomplish whole body use (e.g., our 0.6–17 cm range microconvex probe).
- Doppler and other sophisticated modes (harmonics, etc.) are not used in our setting. Filters can yield major issues.

Anecdotal Notes

1. *Duplex Doppler*
    We have also imagined a simple, low-cost alternative: a continuous Doppler probe, which we arranged to couple with our real-time probe, to locate the vessel, then the Doppler signal. We never found time to build a serious device for coupling the two probes (indicating that we did not feel urgent need for using this potential).
2. *Remote ultrasound*
    We had a talk with a giant (there are several) in emergency ultrasound, trying for the Nth time to show him the advantages of our simple system. He argued that there are not remote capabilities with this antique machine. Simply filming the screen with any mobile phone would eliminate this (non)problem.

Appendix 1: The PUMA, Our Answer to the Traditional Laptops

An ultrasound unit has three dimensions: depth, width, and height. The width is critical for rapidly reaching the bedside, which is why we do not favor large laptops (50–70 cm). The height must be considered using the *cart*, allowing one to work comfortably at human level. A laptop machine is a few centimeters in height but the space below (up to 100,000 cc) is empty space. The PUMA exploits every cubic centimeter available. Since 1982 (ADR-4000) and 1992 (Hitachi-405), we have fully exploited this space for inserting all useful equipment, to the point that our cart can be considered a Polyvalent Ultrasound and Management Apparatus (PUMA). We just developed the 4th dimension: imagination.

The PUMA is our answer to the current laptop market. The PUMA is *not* an ultrasound unit. It *includes* an ultrasound unit.

The PUMA exploits each floor (Fig. 2.6). Basic life-support equipment at the lobby (25-cm high), extreme emergency procedural equipment at the first floor (for treating tension pneumothorax, pericardial tamponade, immediate central venous cannulation, etc.) (10 cm), some refresher textbooks on the second floor, of help to the youngest users (5 cm), etc., at the imagination of the user. On the fourth floor, you find an ultrasound machine, 27-cm high, with the keyboard at the perfect ergonomic height for clinical use. On the top of the PUMA, you have a *top*. This top bothers nobody and is highly useful, since this is the area where are fixed the (unique) probe, the contact product, and the disinfectant. They are fixed using adapted holes within polystyrene that we built ourselves, allowing these items not to fall when the cart is moved (Fig. 2.6, and see details in Fig. 4.3). This avoids the loss of

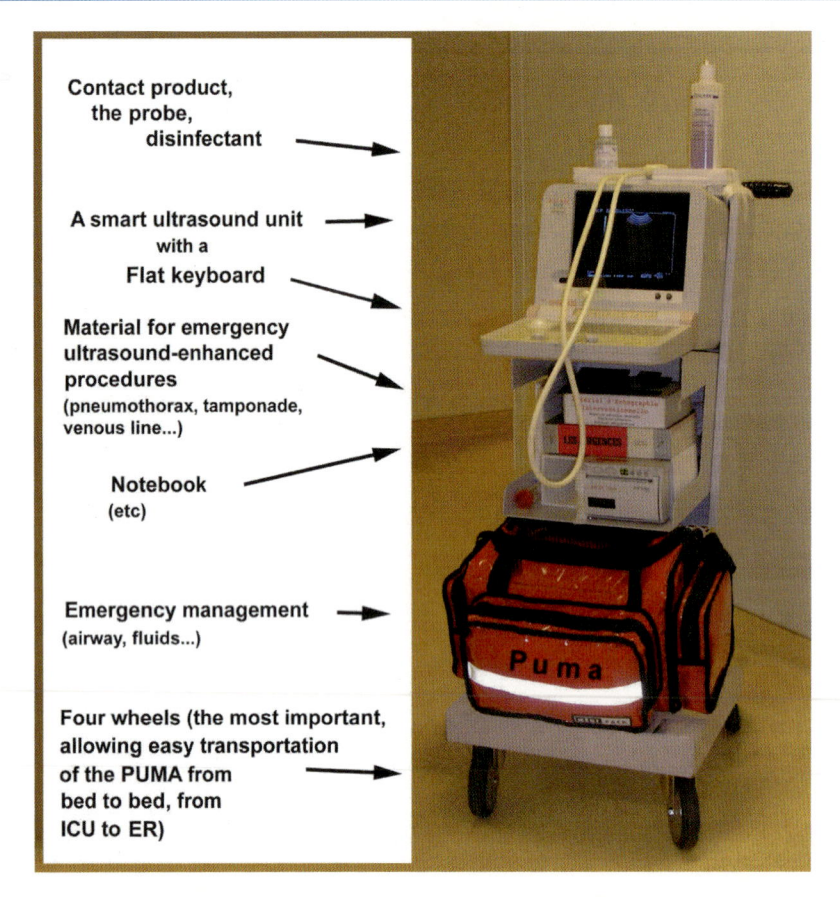

Fig. 2.6 The PUMA concept. This figure shows that ultrasound is only a part of patient management. The concept of the PUMA (Polyvalent Ultrasound and Management Apparatus) allows major procedures in the critically ill. It does not yet make coffee (which may be considered, to relax the team once the patient is promptly stabilized), but inserting a coffee machine at the highest level would be technically possible. This wink just indicates that the height is not a limiting factor. In other words, laptop machines are not a major key for developing critical ultrasound in our hospitals. Note, at the upper floor, how the three tools are solidly fixed, preventing any fall (see diving view in Fig. 3 of Chap. 4)

time: time for picking objects up from the dirty ground, time for disinfecting them, or, if not, time for managing patients with the nosocomial infections that may occur as a result. This is not high tech, this is just a bit of imagination. The PUMA: another face of holistic ultrasound.

References

1. Lichtenstein D, Axler O (1993) Intensive use of general ultrasound in the intensive care unit, a prospective study of 150 consecutive patients. Intensive Care Med 19:353–355
2. Lichtenstein D, Courret JP (1998) Feasibility of ultrasound in the helicopter. Intensive Care Med 24:1119

Which Equipment for the BLUE-Protocol 2. The Probe

> The microconvex probe: a universal probe for the BLUE-protocol, the FALLS-protocol, the SESAME-protocol, and many others. A providence in cardiac arrest and routine daily tasks. Probably the probe of the future for critical ultrasound. Definitely one of the main paradoxes generated by critical ultrasound.

We could make this chapter very short and simple: just try our 1992 probe, or just see Fig. 3.1, a nice summary, and make an opinion. In daily practice, we start up our unit, take our probe, and scan the whole body, quietly or fast, in function of the emergency. We were a bit surprised by the length and complexity of writing of this chapter, which obliged us at making a deep analysis of the current situation. There is a lot to say for explaining that the usual three probes are, again, a use of the radiological or cardiological cultures without adaptation.

Intensivists who have not been educated in the spirit of holistic ultrasound are often cardio-centered (and use vascular probes for vascular access). Here, the reader should forget any preconception and carefully read this chapter. When he or she will have rendezvous with the SESAME-protocol (i.e., cardiac arrest, where each second matters), this reading will show particularly useful [1]. We use a probe which appears universal and should be that of the critical care physician. Since some institutions still have ultrasound machines with the traditional three probes, but not the universal one, we will demonstrate how one probe can be, paradoxically, superior to three others.

This chapter is sensitive, we know it may upset some key-opinion leaders, we know this may slow down the widespread of the message of a vision which will be soon or late a standard.

The Critical Point to Understand for Defining the "Universal Probe" in Critical Care: The Concept of the Providential (Optimal) Compromise

What is required from a probe? A correct vision of what is en face, this is all. Unfortunately, the price to pay for this is a shape non-suitable if too large, or a too small range, obliging to have several probes. In critical care, changing a probe costs time and money, and *asepsis faults are quite unavoidable*. Here, the smaller size in all dimensions is critically important: small footprint for avoiding any hindrance (dressings, nonlinear areas), small length for assessing the posterior part of the lung. None of the three usual probes of laptop machines answers to this requirement.

The users must realize two points, not really misconceptions, the term is too tough, but we did not find any other. Critical ultrasound analyzes first superficial fields; however, the first millimeters are not critically important. A very deep penetration (36 cm) is not critically important.

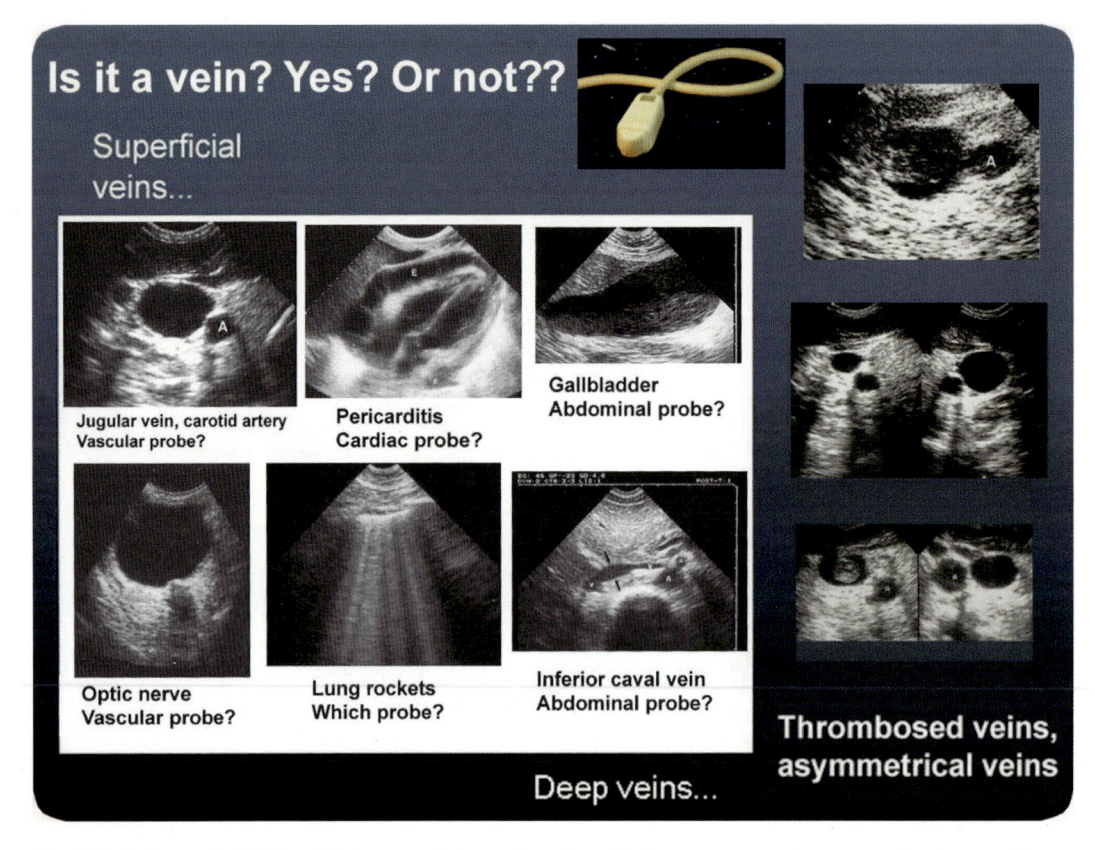

Fig. 3.1 Is it a vein? This slide, extracted from the CEURF courses, shows how one single probe can inform on superficial as well as deep veins, and besides the lung, heart, belly, even retroperitoneum and optic nerve. In two words, the whole body. Look at the image quality and the clinical information, and make your opinion

In critical ultrasound, superficial areas are first on focus. But not the first millimeters (the real raison d'être of the linear probes)

As a striking feature of critical ultrasound, the most critical data are extracted from the analysis of superficial areas usually (aorta and IVC being some exceptions). The lung (the most important part) first. But also most of the venous network (internal jugular, subclavian, femoral, etc.), peritoneum, and optic nerves are areas both superficial and relevant to analyze. The SESAME-protocol has distinguished the pericardium, a superficial structure, from the heart for this reason (and some others). As regards the heart, the ventricles are more superficial than the auricles, which are of lesser importance. In plethoric patients, deep abdominal analysis (pancreas, etc.) is often disappointing even with traditional ultrasound, and these patients are eventually referred to CT: our concept has taken this important detail into consideration.

This point is important: we need superficial, but *not too* superficial. The raison d'être of these vascular probes is the good quality of the first mms. Yet these 5 first mms, in the critically ill, are usually of no interest. We have paid attention in our daily practice in adults, to the critical zones. They are deeper than 1 cm (pleural line, most veins, etc.), rarely between 6 and 9 mm (some veins), and never below 5 mm. There is no critical target in this zone, apart from very rare and quite always not urgent cases (tracheal analysis in skinny patients, radial artery cannulation). In other words, those who are persuaded that these 5 first mm are important make a misconception (sorry for this word) which will be paid; see also below (for the same reason).

Regarding the far penetration, in most cases of investigations in critical holistic ultrasound, the lung is included and answers to questions usually pertaining to cardiac cultures. Here, attention is paid on basic items: the pericardium, LV, and RV. The fine analysis of the auricles can be done later usually, at opened hours.

How to Scientifically Assess This Notion of "Domain of Interpretability"? Our High-Level Compromise Probe

How can one probe be suitable for all areas? We just see since decades that it works (we tried to contact the Japanese engineer who made it in 1992). Figure 3.1 is a indisputable answer by the image.

When we write that some areas are "less well" seen than others, here comes the critical notion of the optimal compromise. Let us make an experience: take again the two radio sets used in Chap. 2, proving how modernity does not always provide improvements. Make again the manipulation (one in FM, one in LW). Do you hear well on the LW channel? Do you recognize the song? The words? If the answer is yes, clearly, you have demonstrated that LW has the required quality (while providing faster information). The difference is futile if you just want to hear radio, but critical if you want a fast information. Willing to have a better (and here, useless) quality yields dramatic regressions, i.e., the traditional three probes and their heavy issues: cost, ergonomy, dirt, imperfect quality for the lung, and huge waste of time in extreme emergencies or daily routine. Therefore, the only question the physician should ask is: "Does the quality of this given image remain within the domain of interpretation?" If the answer is yes, the user will have most of the time, for critical targets (the lung/veins first, then simply the heart and belly, i.e., the large majority of targets), the optimal quality: the winning choice. Our probe is more than a compromise; it is a providence: it is providential since quite all (93 %) of these critical targets will be seen with the "FM quality" (speed in addition), and a few (6 %) with the "LW quality." See below how these numbers came.

Similarly, look at Fig. 3.2. It shows an animal. A dog or a cat? A cat definitely. The first image is heavy. If the question is to have a beautiful image

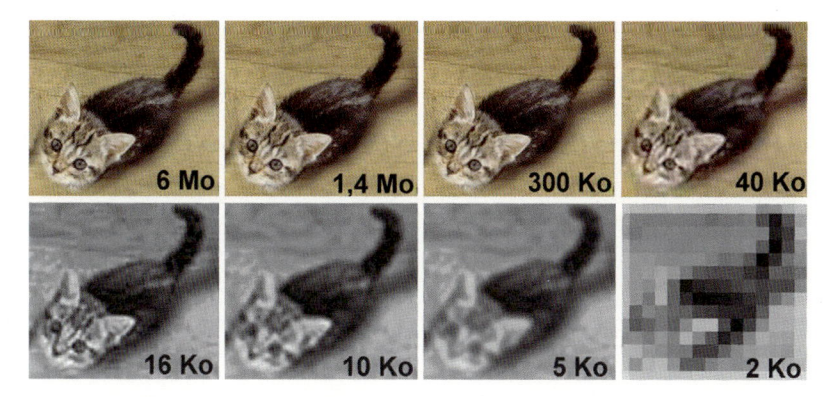

Fig. 3.2 Cat or dog? A simple manipulation. The 6 Mo image is heavy, for no advantage. We can decrease and decrease the weight without damage to the diagnosis: we still recognize the little cat, up to 10 Ko, i.e., 600 times lighter. At 5 Ko in gray scale, 1,200 times lighter, the risk of confusion just begins. Colored or gray scale, this is still a kitten. At 2 Ko, it is true, the resolution is not acceptable, one may confuse (with a scorpion, a stocky whale or any other image coming to your imagination). The weight of the 6 Mo image is the equivalent of the price to pay in terms of multiple probe equipment. Since we can do with light images without loss of safety for the patient, just imagine the impact for critical ultrasound

which can be enlarged on a wall, it fits, thanks to its heavy weight. If the question was to distinguish this animal from a dog, the answer can be done, immediately, with a 600x lighter weight with no damage to the target recognition. Below a certain value (×1200), the recognition begins to be chancy. Far before this step, we achieved considerable decrease of weight. The same is applied to our universal probe. Our concept of the optimal compromise is critical as well for the management of cardiac arrest, where there is no option at all, as our daily routine work.

The figures dispatched in this textbook are not always perfect, but they always answer to the clinical questions. Maybe this probe will not show perfect images everywhere (retroperitoneum in fat people, the first mm of soft tissues).

This is what has initiated our concept of the optimal compromise. We will explain one of the main paradoxes in critical ultrasound, by considering the areas of interest (the lung, heart, etc.) in the function of their strategic importance (the lung comes first) and the frequency of assessment (the lung comes first), drawing a diagram (Fig. 3.3). To give an example, aortic dissection would have a high height (dangerous disease) and a narrow basis (rare event), i.e., a small surface in our graph. A pneumonia is highly lethal, and rather frequent: large surface. This diagram is indicative for the daily life of an intensivist.

This diagram shows that one probe (ours) is perfect for making 93 % of the daily work (with the "FM quality," speed in addition) and also able to see, with inferior but anyway *sufficient quality* (the "LW quality"), the majority (say, 6 %) of the 7 % other points. This is the absolute future of the critical care. The user will accept to work, from time to time, with a quality inferior but perfectly suitable for answering the question. The concept of the optimal compromise, of vital relevance in cardiac arrest mainly, is illustrated in a self-speaking image (Fig. 3.2).

There is a paradox (one more): we could maybe say "Our target is not to have beautiful images, but diagnostic images," but even though, it appears that our probe has a perfect image resolution for the most important targets (the lung, veins, belly, heart *almost well*); see by yourselves through this textbook and see again Fig. 3.1. The "almost" (for the heart) is perfectly suitable for us, even if cardiologists will probably disdain such a probe, instinctively. Let them think so.

Those who would like to see perfectly these few 7 % would be condemned to buy the three usual probes – in addition to the microconvex, irreplaceable for cardiac arrest (Chap. 31). For the roughly 1 % remaining field which we cannot explore, and is never urgent, don't forget this precious DIAFORA option, defined in the previous Chapter (shortly: once a month, call radiologists with sophisticated, large machines full of probes for these very restricted applications). And it is good to work together in addition.

One anecdote from a nice friend, intensivist in India, summarizes a lot. He told us: "I see better those tracheas with a vascular probe." Absolutely, he was right, the image was not bad. But please pay attention:

1. He was right for a not frequent application (one can ask a machine from outside).
2. We saw from our eyes the price he (many of us) had to pay everyday: the large machine,

Fig. 3.3 The concept of the optimal compromise. These four images, and the fifth, integrating the areas, indicate how we assess the universality of a probe. The severity of the diseases is multiplied by their frequency, for providing a clinical relevance. The heart appears as important (height) but not as frequent (width) as the lung, because pure cardiologic diseases are not the most frequent. Note the white, not full areas of images C, A, L, and M. Just some examples. In Image C, the white 2nd box, all cases with absent cardiac window decrease the power of this probe (we made here an optimistic white box). In Image A, the white 4th box corresponds to these postsurgical abdomens covered with stomies, dressings, etc.: large probes are a disadvantage. In Image L, 3rd box: all veins not assessable using the traditional vascular probe. In the bottom image summarizing the C, A, L, M images, see how restricted is the domain of the "vascular" probe, how universal is the one of our microconvex probe

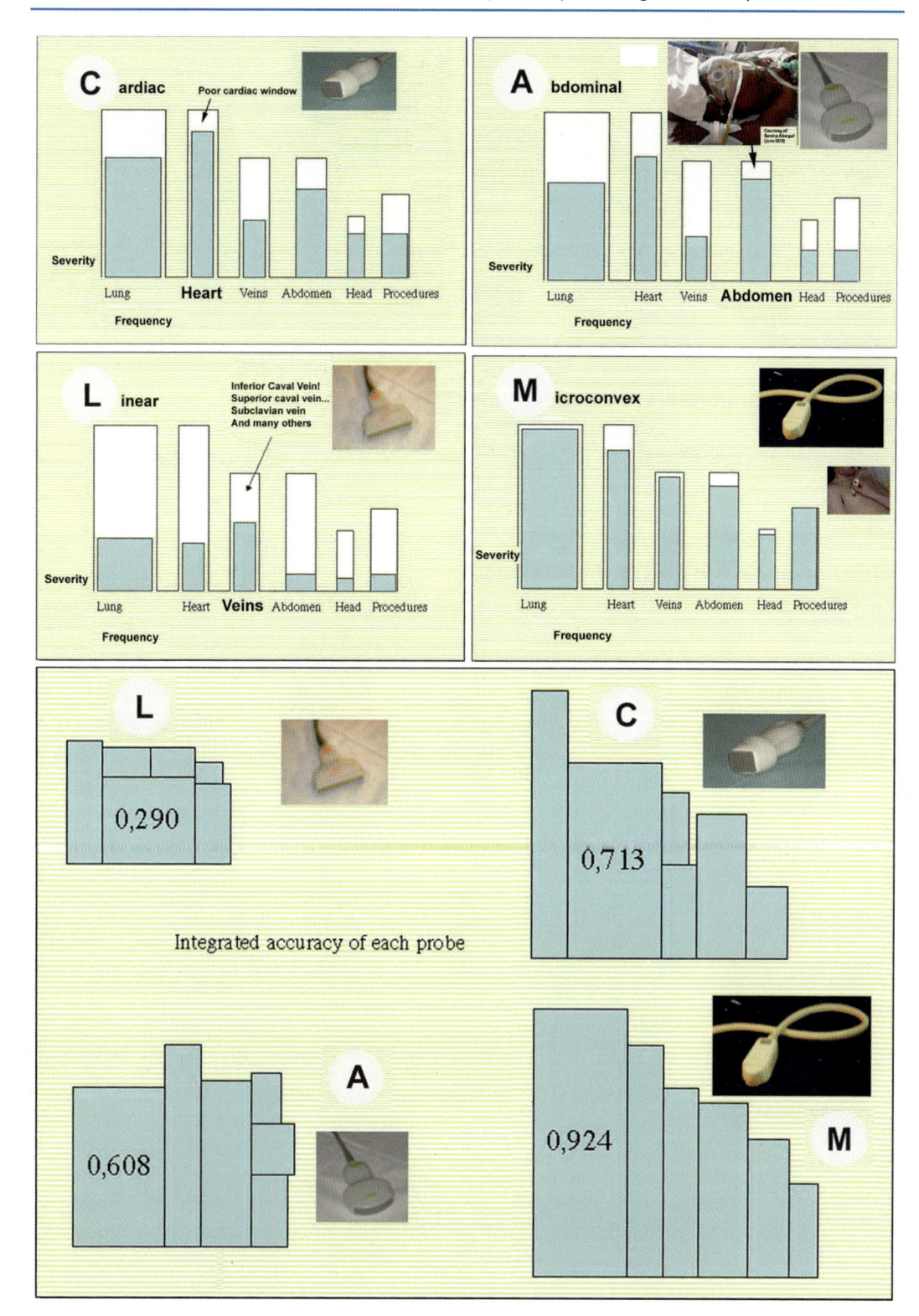

How to Scientifically Assess This Notion of "Domain of Interpretability"? Our High-Level Compromise Probe

Integrated accuracy of each probe

- L: 0,290
- C: 0,713
- A: 0,608
- M: 0,924

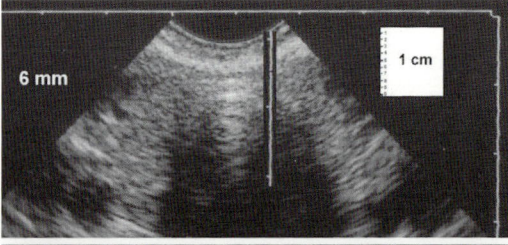

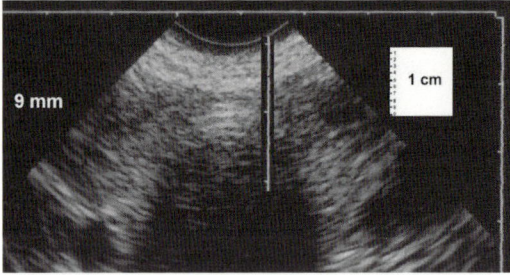

Fig. 3.4 A trachea seen using a microconvex probe. The trachea in this transversal scan is a bit near to the skin (6 mm). The use of some tofu, or any equivalent, makes it now 9 mm. Images taken using our 1992 microconvex probe

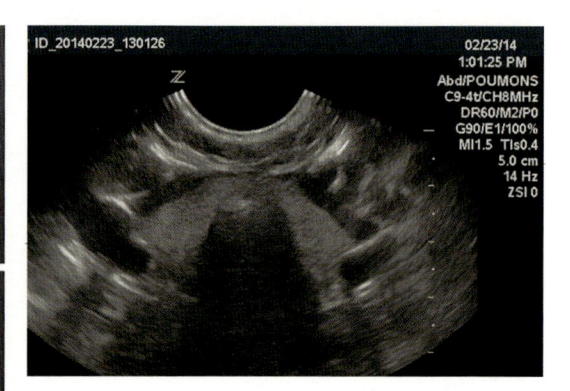

Fig. 3.5 Trachea seen using another microconvex probe. Those who really need to have a sharp vision of the trachea and don't want to make any compromise (such as using our jellyfish system) can however use the microconvex philosophy: look at this image acquired using an up-to-date microconvex probe and make your opinion

plenty of probes, an endless start-up time, cables making an inextricable mass (full of microbs usually), lying on the dirty ground (and the risk of the cable damage from the wheels, and the risk of sudden machine tipover), probes impossible to use rapidly and logically in the case of a cardiac arrest, and lateral stands which increase the width of these machines not to deal with the overall cost. All this for looking to a trachea.

3. He did not compare his vascular probe with our simple microconvex probe (Fig. 3.4). For sure, cardiac probes and abdominal probes will never be suitable. Even in very skinny patients, if our probe happens to miss the first mm, we share a very simple solution: making the area a bit far from the probe by using an acoustic device. It works like standard glasses for near vision. Let us call it temporarily "jellyfish," from the French name (old radiologists should remember this device, impossible to find currently, but easy to replace by alternatives that are easy to purchase). We will see them later for not breaking the rhythm. In this Indian ICU or elsewhere, this will show the tracheal rings with a quality similar to the sound quality of the LW radio: sufficient. For these few "low-resolution" but sufficient image quality, we have a unique whole-body approach, optimal (FM) for critical targets and sufficient (LW) for the others, with a clean, compact unit. This also is a holistic ultrasound. We prefer to make our compromise at the (very) (relative) detriment of the trachea, used from time to time and quite always in nonemergency ambiance.

4. If he really wanted a perfect image quality, the solution is fully available: some modern units have reached a nice score when compared to our reference: minus 101 CEURF units, including – 70 just for the cost and – 26 for the 33 s of start-up time (our equipment has zero "C.U."). But they have the quite perfect microconvex probe, with an impressive resolution, better than ours, in the first millimeters (Fig. 3.5).

Why Is Our Microconvex Probe Universal

We benefit since 1992 from a universal probe that is able to answer to all problems (Fig. 3.6). It is slightly better than the great 1982's sectorial probe we used on the ADR-4000 (Fig. 3.7).

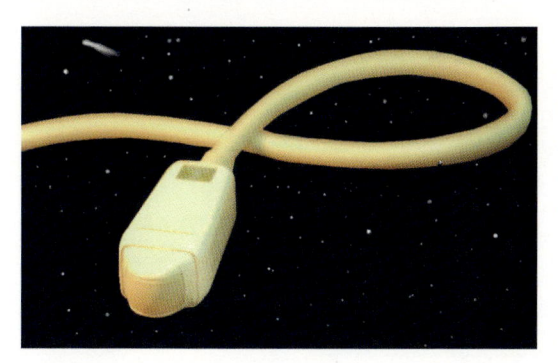

Fig. 3.6 Our universal microconvex probe. This probe is 80 g light, 88-mm long and has a 12×20 mm footprint. The frequency is 5 MHz, but this probe just shows, from 6 to 170 mm of penetration, what is in the explored field, regardless if the surface is linear or not. A simple probe, which changes the landscape of critical ultrasound

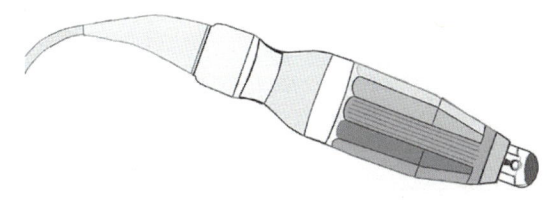

Fig. 3.7 The sectorial probe of the ADR-4000. This 1982 probe (drawn by our care, since we don't have any longer a photograph of it) looks antique, but allowed us anyway to define the *whole* of critical ultrasound and LUCI. It was a bit long, it is true. Using modern probes, there is not *one* more application we invented, optic nerve included, venous cannulation included; the work is now just easier and faster

The Range

It is 0.6–17 cm. This exceptional range allows us to see a huge majority of disorders of high interest. Figure 3.1 is a demonstration by the image, and Fig. 3.8 by a scientific approach (Fig. 3.8).

The Footprint

Its microconvex head has a really small footprint. There is a 10-mm-large linear part and a 20-mm-large curved part. It can therefore be applied on all these small, difficult areas: the intercostal spaces for the lung, supraclavicular fossa (lung, superior caval vein), suprasternal area (aorta, right pulmonary artery), jugular vein with short neck and tracheostomy, the subclavian vein, the popliteal area, the calf, and not to forget the heart. As to large areas (abdomen), they are analyzed as well without hindrance – especially in postoperative patients covered with dressings, devices, and stomies, and where a free access really lacks sometimes.

See the images of venous ultrasound in Chaps. 18 and 30: all deep veins can be seen. Superficial veins? Take our jellyfish (see above).

The Length

Our smart microconvex probe is 88 mm short. This length favors the investigation of the posterior lung wall in the supine, ventilated patient (PLAPS-point, a detail which allows to postpone thoracic CT, see Chap. 6), or the popliteal fossa, with less effort than with longer probes. Each centimeter and millimeter contributes in making the ultrasound easier. Using 12–15-cm-long probes is definitely boring for daily routine lung analysis.

The body of the probe is convenient, ergonomic, and held like a pen.

The Strong Points of Having One Unique Probe

Using a unique, universal probe has heavy advantages. We want to remain positive, so just imagine the contrary of these advantages, if you have in mind to purchase the usual three probes:

1. The unique probe allows fast protocols. Once the machine is switched on, the user wastes no time for selecting a probe or adjusting the settings. This is critical for acute respiratory failure, cardiac arrest, and also multiple daily uses.
2. It reduces the cost of the equipment and makes its purchase easy, i.e., saving lives more easily. Each saved $ (euro, roupie, etc.) saves more lives exactly the opposite way of the one of Doppler, which has killed patients (read relative notes in Chap. 37).

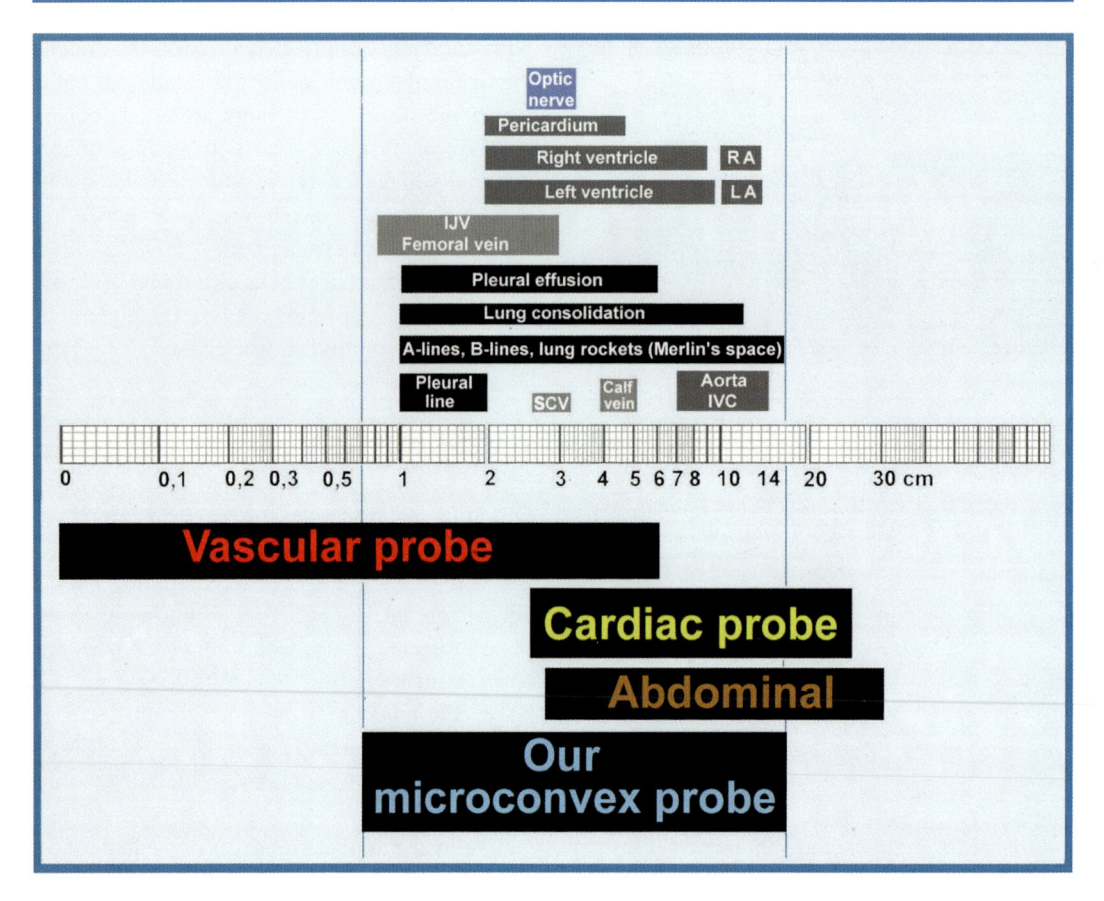

Fig. 3.8 The universal range of our microconvex probe. This figure quietly proves that our microconvex probe has a universal field in critical care. Using a logarithmic scale for convenience, we have inserted quite all our targets and then compared the range of various probes. One can see that critical ultrasound is rather the science of the superficial, but, as clearly demonstrated here, not too superficial

3. This is mandatory for performing clean ultrasound. One unique probe, with one cable, can be efficiently cleaned, then stored (clean), on a (clean) stand. One probe allows us to avoid this image of battlefield (this jungle of cables, which have to be changed in haste). Cleaning each probe during an examination obliges to clean the probes and the stands and the cables, *during* each probe change (meaning, interrupting the examination, washing one's hands for each probe cleaning, etc.). This is impossible to ask to a user. The alternative is to close the eyes, generating one of the main issues of ultrasound: crossed infections. Chapter 4 shows the way we make clean critical ultrasound.
4. Ironically, none of the usual three probes is perfect for a fast lung examination.
5. This favors simplicity – a golden rule of critical ultrasound.

By the Way, Our Probe: Which Frequency?

On our probe, it is written "5 MHz." But this number makes little sense. What we see is its unique, wide range (6–170 mm). Many "5 MHz microconvex probes" do not display this range. This means satisfactory analysis of a jugular or subclavian vein as well as the inferior caval vein, and 100 other examples (see all images of this textbook) (Fig. 3.8).

The Usual Probes of the Laptop Machines

The cardiologists use cardiac probes and are happy with them. The radiologists use the abdominal probe and are happy with it. The vascular doctors use linear probes and are happy with them. The gyneco-obstetricians use the transvaginal probe and are very happy with it. We, intensivists (and all specialties dealing with the critically ill), are not the least specialty, are we? Why should we adapt to specialists' habits? We are specialists as a whole, where the lung is the main target. For a fast and accurate whole-body approach, we don't have time to swap probes, first.

The lung precisely regards many disciplines (pediatricians, pulmonologists, cardiologists, nephrologists, internists, family doctors, etc.). Each of the traditional probes provides fractional data (abdominal probe for pleural-alveolar characterization, cardiac probe for posterior analysis in challenging patients, vascular probe if others cannot show lung sliding, abdominal again for assessment of artifacts length).

The Cardiac Probe

This probe has a good ergonomy. Small length, small footprint. Yet the resolution is really cardio-centered. It is usually suboptimal for key targets such as the lungs and veins, and subtle others. Some are providentially better than others; please check if you can see a bit of lung sliding in any type of patients (skinny, etc.) in any condition (acute dyspnea, mechanical bradypnea).

Supposedly perfect for the heart, it is without the slightest interest each time the patient has no cardiac window. The success of these probes rises from a misconception if one does not know the power of lung ultrasound (BLUE-protocol, FALLS-protocol, SESAME-protocol, and others).

Pericardial tamponade? A nice paradox, dealt with in Chap. 31 on cardiac arrest, is intentionally developed below; this is really too important.

The Abdominal Probe

It has not too bad resolution but really a poor ergonomy and a poor superficial penetration.

Too deep for most veins and for the lung surface; too cumbersome for the lung; heavy, large (8 cm), and requiring a crispated hand for holding it, and confined to large areas (abdomen by definition), this is really not our choice. It is maybe good for measuring the size of a liver – this is typically a culture for radiologists, not for the intensivist. However, if the choice is given for driving a whole-body analysis, we would use it better than the two others, probably.

The Linear Probe

We write "linear" instead of vascular. These probes are to our opinion the worst. They come from a misconception based on radiological traditions, including the assumption that the first mm is important to analyze.

We wrote "linear" because linear, they are, definite. But vascular? They can assess just some veins (the most superficial only, on linear areas only, in permitted orientations only): a rather restricted field. They can be used for the lung surface, but just for lung sliding (provided the patient is not too plethoric). They are unable to analyze correctly most Merlin's spaces. Look out, this image quality is not always spectacular: in many hospitals, a policy has favored the purchase of low-quality, "low-cost" laptop machines (but 4 times more costly than the ones we advocate); therefore, Doppler may be required for distinguishing, for instance, vein from artery: the deadly coil is initiated.

These users will have to change this probe in extreme emergency and stress, when they assess other veins (e.g., inferior caval vein) and of course the rest of the body. Scientific data are shared in Chap. 18 on DVT, free talks in Chap. 37. These probes are relics of the industrial (premedical) era of ultrasound, in the 1930s–1950s. We are not linear. Even if we were *snakes,* the most linear creatures, such probes would be suitable for longitudinal assessment, but not so well for

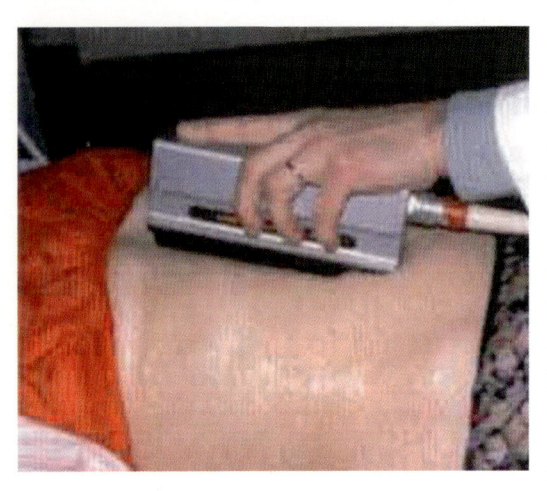

Fig. 3.9 The vascular probe philosophy. This probe, fortunately quite impossible to find nowadays (apart from dealing in improbable antiques), indicates however well the spirit of ultrasound inherited from generation to generation of radiologists, and suddenly given without adaptation to other physicians, those who precisely deal with critical care. We have a major tool for visual medicine; we must make it adapted to our use – not the opposite

transversal scans. Once the large 65-mm-footprint probe is applied, the physician is prisoner of the anatomy, restricted to some areas more linear than others, and must adapt the probe to the area (Fig. 3.9). The neck and upper chest wall areas are highly strategic areas. In the critically ill patient once in the ICU, they are of really restricted access, full of concavities and obstacles. If we add a short neck plus an IJV cannulation dressing plus a tracheostomy, with the cord, *here*, applying a vascular probe at the IJV is a challenge. Small angulations are made difficult or impossible. How can 65 mm of linear footprint be inserted on such areas remains a mystery for us. In addition, compressing a vein using a large linear probe makes a rough compression (not focused like our small footprint probe). Definitely, for studying human beings, the idea of linear probes is a weird concept.

Some advocate vascular probes for vascular access. They should try ours, easy to handle, with suitable footprint; see all details in Chap. 34.

Using our microconvex probes, doctors will rediscover ultrasound.

The following *vessels* are hardly or not accessible to "vascular" probes: the subclavian vein, the innominate vein; the superior caval vein; the inferior caval vein; the iliac vein; the low femoral vein; the popliteal vein in supine patients; the calf veins in their short axis, especially by anterior approach in supine, critically ill patients; and the whole aorta, abdominal *and* thoracic. In other words, more than half of the vascular network. Vascular probes? Now make your opinion: are they well labelled? The CEURF clearly states that vascular probes are not suitable for vascular assessment, especially in the critically ill. One proof: with such probes in hand, 65 statements were necessary in a recent I.C.C. on vascular access. The reader will see in Chap. 34, in the corresponding section, how basically simple it is with our microconvex probe.

For having by any means the control of very superficial areas (0–5 mm), we would face a serious, lethal issue. The result of this belief would be to complicate a discipline which can be done much simpler and more efficient. For no advantage, users will have a non-ergonomic probe, limited in depth, devoted to be changed in the haste. Would these 5 first mm need to be assessed, for these rare applications, our very solution, the modern "jellyfish," can be used for a lesser cost. See Fig. 3.4 and read the caption about the *tofu*, our jellyfish for a lesser cost, one Euro instead of buying a 10.000 $, cumbersome probe. One Euro per day (far less in fact) makes the equivalent of one (suboptimal) probe per 30 years. See a nice other example for those who want to see the radial artery in Chap. 31, Fig. 31.4.

Some users working in the ER may contest: "But we need to see the foreign bodies." We can answer a lot. First, this is not critical ultrasound. Then, if the foreign body is that superficial (<5 mm), use your eyes. Then, they can still use our modern jellyfish, but if they do this all day long in their ERs, let them do as they feel. Last option, an intelligent, up-to-date microconvex probe with even more superficial resolution (Figs. 3.5 and 3.10).

Note for the anesthesiologists who are now all using ultrasound, a real craze, for looking at the nerves. All use these vascular probes, with all problems seen above, and they have also now to deal with the complex issues of anisotropy. They want to see nerves? Figure 3.10 shows a

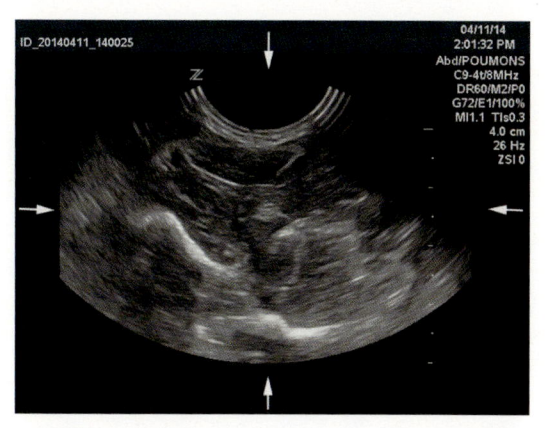

Fig. 3.10 The median nerve. Those who really need to have a sharp vision of the nerves and don't want to make any compromise can however use the microconvex philosophy. Look at this image acquired using an updated (*and suitable*) microconvex probe and make your opinion. How do you like the vision of this median nerve? Arrows inserted at a distance, for not disturbing this image. And possibly, with the microconvex probe, no issue with anisotropy

median nerve, using a basic microconvex probe. Scanning nerves from time to time, we don't know what is this strange phenomenon of "anisotropy." We guess it is one more issue generated by some refraction phenomena from these linear probes, like at the optic nerve, which in most publications was confused with a vulgar acoustic shadow.

Let them now make an opinion.

> **Note**
> Each probe makes the cost of a fine, standard automobile.

Some Doctors Prefer to Swap the Probes for Each Application, and Not Use the Universal Probe. Why?

It is true, not all machines devoted to critical ultrasound are equipped with the universal probe. Why? How are doctors positioned with this issue? We made deep investigations.

1. Some just don't know it. Nothing to say, but inform them.
2. Some had no choice: they have bought the usual three probes, not this one. Here, there is nothing to do but wait to collect the sum of money (or selling the probes to whoever is interested).
3. Some users complained that this probe is slippery (when plenty of gel), more than the large abdominal ones. They don't know Ecolight®, our product described in Chap. 2. Using it, nothing is slippery, the user has all advantages of this small probe: holistic ultrasound.
4. Some key-opinion leaders argue that they just don't like it. They had a microconvex probe in hands and they don't appreciate it. We took time for understanding what happened there. One day (it was in a slovenian course) we understood: those manufacturers of the recent and explosive laptop market made, in a haste, probes that were microconvex is true, but having none of our two main qualities, they had a poor resolution or they had a poor penetration, usually 8 cm, exceptionally 10. Given these critical details, we understand the positions of these few KOL. We are not at ease with these probes too. They cannot be considered "universal." They are just gadgets. To make it clear, we must write "our" instead of "the" microconvex probe, an insignificant label, for being clear.

Pericardial Tamponade: Time for a Nice Paradox, Just One Illustration of What is "Holistic Ultrasound"

A discipline is holistic when it is necessary to understand each of its components for being able to understand its whole. The definition of holistic ultrasound includes the choice of a probe able both to diagnose a pericardial tamponade and to efficiently guide the pericardiocentesis. You are now dealing with a pericardial tamponade, with imminence of cardiac arrest. The cardiac probe made the diagnosis it is true. But you are condemned to perform the pericardiocentesis using a probe unsuitable for needle detection. Even if you had time, which probe would you use instead? The abdominal? The ergonomy of the subcostal angle is not optimal. The linear? Here, the user pays both the ergonomy (too large) and the penetration (too short). Consequently they developed complex protocols for seeing the needle (contrast with microbubbles in the syringe, costly needles, etc.), while your patient initiates a bradycardia. This is an issue we never faced.

What to Say to Those Who Still Have Only the Three Usual Probes?

During several years, they will have to make the ultrasound revolution with this.

Can one use linear probes for the lungs?

Lives can certainly be saved using them. The users must just accept to have restricted access to the nonlinear areas and the deep structures; therefore, they need to swap probes, i.e., buy them, disinfect them, store them, take care of not letting the cable trail, etc. The user must be expert in swapping probes very rapidly if suddenly facing a cardiac arrest. The user must accept to have limited access to the longitudinal approach (the one which makes lung ultrasound easy), limited criteria for distinguishing B-lines from Z-lines, and limited access in obese patients. The user must accept, when cannulating a deep vein, to practice a complicated profession (65 statements). Some advocate that lung sliding is easier to detect. Our Japanese microconvex probe makes perfectly the work (see in particular Figs. 1, 3, 7–9 of Chap. 10). We talked with respected giants of emergency ultrasound who argued that Italian articles on lung ultrasound used linear probes, we just answered we saw exactly the same patterns (e.g., thickened pleural line) with ours.

The cardiac probes?

Same kind of remark, see the paragraph on pericardiocentesis. Some probes can make a bit of lung ultrasound, the owner can still try.

The abdominal probe?

This is probably the one we would use in first intention if we had no choice, but we would not be at ease. Clearly we would have to swap the probes regularly for other targets (veins, heart, "difficult" lung).

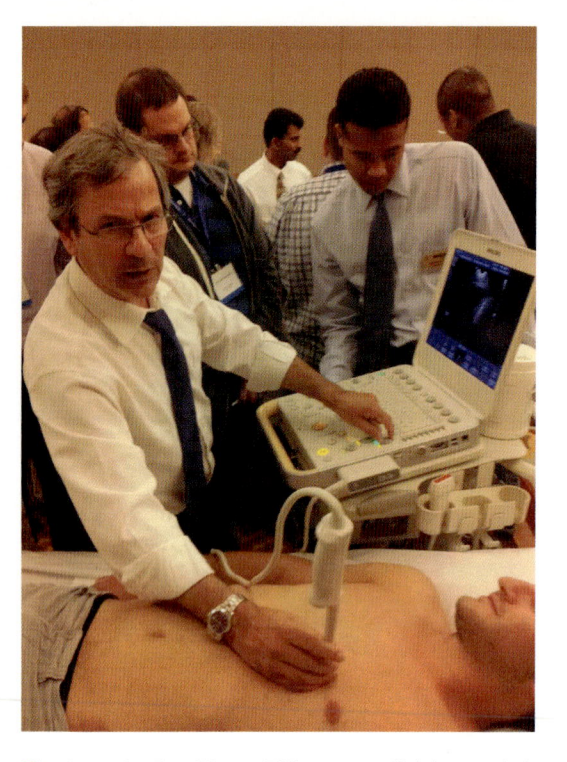

Fig. 3.11 At Las Vegas. This nervy, slightly puzzled sonographer had no other choice, for a demonstration of LUCI somewhere in Nevada, but taking this rather cumbersome probe, with it is true a suitable head, reminder of a microconvex probe. Most importantly, the image became clearly interpretable, and this unfortunate patient was saved, so to speak

All in all, when we have to animate workshops with the sempiternal three probes, we spend our time swapping probes, not finding the ideal one, not finding a real compromise. Some desperate solutions can sometimes rise in the heat of troubles, when nothing works (Fig. 3.11).

An Unexpected (Temporary) Solution?

Our best advise for helping the locomotive to go on the right rails would be to sell the vascular plus the abdominal probes, allowing to buy instead one microconvex probe, even not with the universal range – provided the resolution is suitable. An 8–10-cm range probe would be easy to find.

The physicians would use this microconvex probe for all those superficial tasks which make a majoritary part of critical ultrasound, they would use the cardiac probe for the heart, and also for all these rough abdominal assessments. They would still have, of course, to swap the probes during a SESAME-protocol. Just, outside this extreme setting, just making this slight and reasonable change for no added cost, they would already rediscover ultrasound.

Important Notes Used as Conclusion

The words "cardiac arrest" appear 12 times in the text. This does not mean that we are obsessed by a condition which comes from time to time, not all the time, and is far from summarizing holistic ultrasound. Our message is of critical simplicity: the use of ultrasound in cardiac arrest (13 now) is exactly the same, *with no adaptation*, as in hundreds daily, more quiet applications, with the same probe, the same settings: venous line insertion, dyspnea or shock assessment, abdominal routine scanning, etc. Ready for the worst, this probe makes the routine work with the same ease. This is holistic ultrasound, typically.

Reference

1. Lichtenstein D (2014) How can the use of lung ultrasound in cardiac arrest make ultrasound a holistic discipline. The example of the SESAME-protocol. Med Ultrason 16(3):252–255

How We Conduct a BLUE-Protocol (And Any Critical Ultrasound): Practical Aspects

What happens when a BLUE-protocol is performed or when any ultrasound test is done on a critically ill patient?

First, we see an "unusual" patient. Unusual is a term from the traditional perspective of the radiologist or the cardiologist. Our patient is in high distress (dyspneic, agitated, etc.) or already sedated. As opposed to ambulatory patients, who can be positioned laterally with inspiratory apnea for studying the liver, or sitting for pleural effusions, or again with legs down for venous analysis, etc., no cooperation is awaited. Apnea cannot be obtained: the patient is either mechanically ventilated, or dyspneic, or encephalopathic.

Then, we have to access the patient. When surrounded by multiple life-support devices (ventilator, hemodialysis, pleural drainage, etc.), the machine must be as narrow as possible. This is why we keep on using our 32-cm-width (with cart) 1992 machine. This is why laptops, which may be 5 cm high but 50, 60, or worse wide (we measured up to 76 cm), are not our preference (especially in extreme emergencies). Each saved lateral cm makes our work easier. In hospitals, ceilings are high enough – the height is *not a problem*.

Usually, lung ultrasound in a dyspneic patient is perfectly feasible using our unsophisticated, instant response system.

The barrier is lowered. We don't need to tear away the electrodes because our nurses have been taught to apply them at nonstrategic areas, i.e., the shoulders and sternum. The ECG is not disturbed. This slight detail makes one less useless loss of time (and costs).

Now, just before scanning our patient, we can note a remarkable and providential feature of ultrasound in the critically ill: most can be done in the supine position. The supine patient offers wide access to the most critical areas: the optic nerve, maxillary sinus, anterior and lateral areas of the lungs, most deep veins, heart, abdomen, etc. Turning a patient 90° is never easy nor fully harmless nor fast (and the BLUE-protocol is a fast protocol). The "hidden side" of the ventilated patient, i.e., the posterior disorders (effusion, consolidation), is a usual limitation, which we deeply reduce by optimizing the tools for making this setting like any other. The choice of our unique 88-mm-long probe is the main key for reducing the hidden face of the lung. For assessing the PLAPS-point (detection of most pleural effusions and posterior consolidations), the elbows are gently spread from the chest in order to facilitate a slight rotation.

Then, the scanning begins. With our compress soaked with Ecolight on the patient's skin (the bed would "drink" it and oblige to more soakings, i.e., loss of time) and our probe in hand, we scan what is required: the lungs and the veins for the BLUE-protocol and the heart first for the FALLS-protocol. We follow standardized points for expediting the protocol and make more comprehensive scanning once the clinical question is answered (time permitting). Each change of area (e.g., from deep lungs to femoral veins) takes two seconds: no time for swapping the probe and no time for taking the bottle of gel; we just take our soaked compress and treat the next area to scan. We always use both hands, permanently.

In good conditions, the whole body can be analyzed in less than 10 min using our probe (the BLUE-protocol takes 3 min or less; sometimes it is concluded after 5 s). The examination can be recorded in real time without losing time taking figures. When the question is focused (e.g. left pneumothorax or not), a few seconds are required. Table 4.1 shows a suggestion of ultrasound report made with this spirit.

The critically ill patient is – in a way – privileged with respect to ultrasound. The sedation facilitates all interventional procedures. Traditional obstacles (the gas barrier) turn into advantages since lung ultrasound is the main topic of this textbook. Our study showed a 92 % feasibility for all usual targets [1].

Disinfection of the Unit: Not a Futile Step

Prevention of cross-infections is a major care in the ICU, and this regards ultrasound. When we see these laptops plenty of buttons, we wonder how they can be kept clean. Our protocol is logical and easy to follow, aiming at a 95 % efficiency (96 % would need much more work; 97 % would be followed by nobody, resulting in dirty machines). We just ask to the user to create some good sense reflexes.

For instance, one may either say "do not touch useless things with contaminated hands" or make the list of the mistakes: pushing the machine by the hand for centimetric moves (we use our feet at low areas), leaving the contact product on the bed (it should never leave the cart), touching for no reason the on-site bottle of disinfectant, etc. Then, the reflexes become automatisms.

Our compact equipment really helps. Its keyboard is flat, no protrusion of buttons. Its unique probe is easily cleaned (several intricate probes, no). Such equipments exist since 1982 (ADR-4000).

We define as "dirty areas" the few parts which will be touched during an examination, probe, keyboard, and contact product, if used several times (Fig. 4.1). We define as "clean areas" all other parts of the ultrasound machine and avoid to touch them without strong reason during the examination.

Once the work is finished, the patient is covered again and the barrier up again; we leave the probe on the bed when the patient is quiet (if not, we leave the probe in a special place). We come back with clean hands. Our on-site disinfectant product (in a dedicated place, never handled during the examination) is poured onto a simple not woven compress which allows an efficient work. The stock of compresses is located in a "clean area" of the machine. Traditional moist wipes are not as efficient as our system of well-soaked compress. Then, the work of disinfection is simple: only the "dirty parts" are cleaned:

1. The flat keyboard is cleaned in a few seconds (Fig. 4.2).
2. The (unique) probe is cleaned from the cable to the probe. The cleaned probe is then inserted onto the stand. The stand is clean by definition because the user always cleans the probe before laying it on the stand. An efficient cleaning of a stand is difficult.
3. The contact product, if used twice, is cleaned (sophisticated note: the body of the bottle, easy to clean, is a "dirty area." The top, everything but flat, is difficult to clean and is defined as a "clean area," never to be touched during an examination. Once hands are clean, it is easy to take the bottle from the clean top and wipe the dirty body, making no asepsis fault).

It is not forbidden to touch "clean areas" of the unit without necessity. Putting soiled hands on clean areas, leaving the contact product bottle lying on the bed, or again handling the disinfectant by soiled hands is allowed, provided the user carefully cleans everything after examination. This is just a loss of energy. When the steps are done in a logical order, the cleaning time is estimated at 30 s and the unit remains clean.

Which disinfectants do we pour on our compress? We do not like to see products devoted for the grounds; they may be too detergent for our subtle equipment, especially the delicate silicone part. Manufacturers have always given us obscure

Table 4.1 Usual report of whole-body critical ultrasound

Hôpital
Ambroise-Paré

Service de
Réanimation Médicale

ULTRASOUND REPORT

| NAME   Day **DATE 2008**   xxx A.M/P.M |

D. Lichtenstein   Unit: Hitachi EUB-405 - probe 5 MHz microconvex   Birth date   Setting   Day XX
Clinical question :
Conditions, patient's echogenicity :   correct   **OR ELSE** (1)
Ventilatory status and position :   mechanical/spontaneous ventilation   Tidal volume   PEEP   02   Eupnea/dyspnea
Patient sedated or not   Curarization or not   supine position   semi recumbent   armchair   other
Various items for research design (auscultation data, description of radiography)

Thorax
    Right lung
        - Anterior analysis:
            - Upper BLUE-point :
                - peak lung sliding: present   abolished
                - artifacts :   exclusive or predominant A lines **OR ELSE**
            - Lower BLUE-point :
                - same items
        - Lateral analysis :
            - lateral: B lines **OR ELSE**
            - pleural effusion:
            - alveolar consolidation:
            - phrenic point : Cupola: eutopic   **OR ELSE**.   Amplitude xxx mm
        - Semiposterior analysis :
            - PLAPS-point : PLAPS (+ details) or not -   **OR ELSE**
        - Stage 4 analysis :
            - apex analysis:
            - comprehensive posterior scanning:
    Left lung
        - same items
Mediastinum
    Thoracic aorta (initial, arch, descending aorta) :   normal **OR ELSE**
    Right pulmonary artery :   visible   **OR ELSE**
    Vena cava superior :   visible   **OR ELSE**
    Heart (two-dimensional approach).   Easy examination **OR ELSE**
        Pericardium : sub- normal (2) **OR ELSE**
        Left ventricle :   text
            - diastolic caliper   - systolic caliper
            - i.e. : global contractility :   low   normal   exagerated
            - dilatation :   absent   moderate   substantial
        Right ventricle: text
            - volume: normal enlarged
            - free wall: thin   thick   **OR ELSE**
            - contractility
        Other elements :   text

Deep veins
Two-dimension, without Doppler, controlled compression method
    Internal jugular (dominant: right **or** left) :   free   **OR ELSE**   On-site catheter Yes No
    Subclavian: free   **OR ELSE**   On-site catheter Yes No
    IVC: correct exploration, empty vessel   **OR ELSE**
    Iliac: correct exploration, empty vessel   **OR ELSE**
    Femoral: free   **OR ELSE**

(continued)

Table 4.1 (continued)

  Popliteal: free   **OR ELSE**
  Calf: at least partially (%) compressible   **OR ELSE**

Head
Right (left) optic nerve: Caliper   xxx   (hM)   Micro-bulging : yes / no   Sinuosity checked: yes / no
Maxillary sinus (supine / erect patient) (nasogastric probe yes / no)   **Right (left)** :   Sinusogram absent **OR** present   If present: complete **OR** incomplete

Abdomen
  Examination : optimal / suboptimal   (reasons: body habitus, gas, dressings, others)
  Fluid peritoneal effusion: absent   **OR ELSE**
  Pneumoperitoneum :   absent   (gut sliding present and/or splanchnogram) **OR ELSE**
  Stomac :   full   empty   gastric probe visible in situ   **OR ELSE**
  Small bowel :   peristalsis present or abolished or not accessible   Wall: thin   **OR ELSE**
  Caliper: normal   **OR ELSE**   Contents: anechoic or echoic   Unaccessible bowel
  Colon   Same items   Search for air-fluid levels
  Aorta :   regular   **OR ELSE**
  Inferior vena cava :   Expiratory size at the left renal vein = xxx mm   Patency :
  Adrenal :   analyzed   **OR ELSE**
  Kidneys :   nondilated pelvis   **OR ELSE**
  Bladder :   full   empty   correctly drained   **Uterus** :
  Gallbladder :   No elective pain   Not enlarged (nn x nn mm)   Wall not thickened (mm)
  Wall regular homogeneous   Contents anechoic, or sludge (%)   No satellite peritoneal effusion
  OR ABSENCE OF THESE ITEMS
  Liver : no visible acute anomaly - no portal gas - on comprehensive or limited examination   **OR ELSE**
  Biliary tract :   fine   **OR ELSE**
  Spleen :   normal size   **OR ELSE**   Homogeneous pattern **OR ELSE**
  Portal system :   no anomaly   **OR ELSE**
  Pancreas :   normal in size and echostructure   **OR ELSE**
  Retroperitoneum :   analyzed   **OR ELSE**
  Other remarkable elements seen:

Miscellaneous
Musculo-fat ratio. Thickness of the crural muscle (right tigh):

SYNTHESIS

  A practical synthesis is written (time permitting) in a style allowing any physician, even without ultrasound culture, to understand the main points of the clinical situation. It focuses on immediate management changes.
  Notes for the textbook :
  (1) an item which has not been filled (in the heat of the night management e.g.) does not create ambiguity thanks to the words "or else"
  (2) If minimal pericardial effusion, keep "sub"

The style of this report has been designed for expediting its writing. It contains data pertinent to the initial examination of an unstable patient as well as routine examinations in stable, ventilated patients: a kind of photographic reference, useful for later examinations. Positive as well as negative items are specified. Serendipitous findings with immediate or delayed (aneurism) consequences are recalled here

Disinfection of the Unit: Not a Futile Step

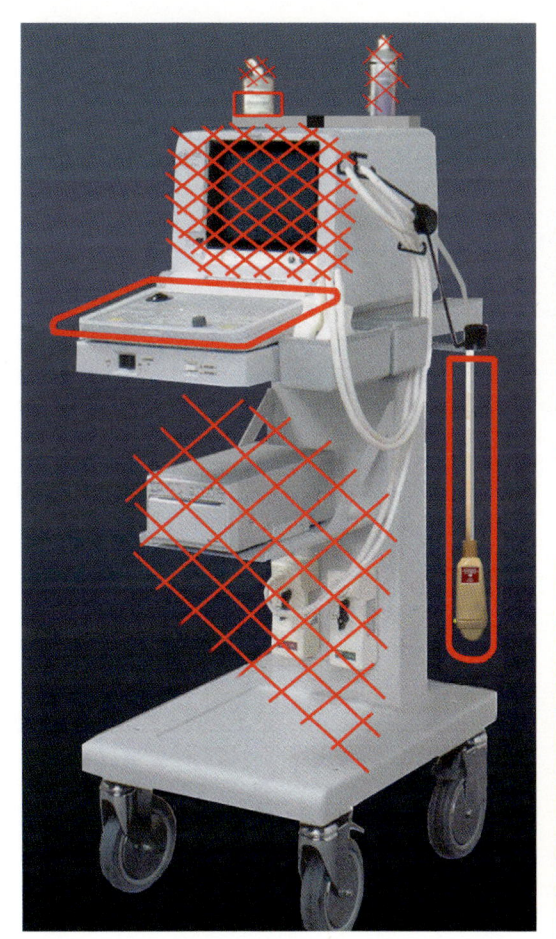

Fig. 4.1 Bacteriological partition of our unit. Only the *circled parts* need to be touched and should therefore be disinfected after use. See this flat keyboard, immediately cleaned. One single probe can efficiently be cleaned before insertion on its stand. There is no need to touch any of the other parts (*with crosses*) during the examination (or if so, they should just be cleaned after)

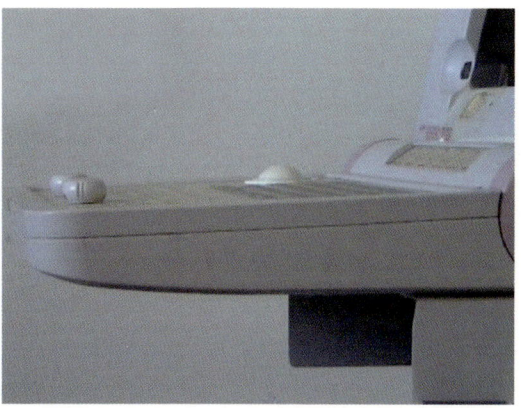

Fig. 4.2 A flat screen. This kind of screen, available in our 1982 ADR-4000 and 1992 Hitachi-405, is cleaned in a few seconds

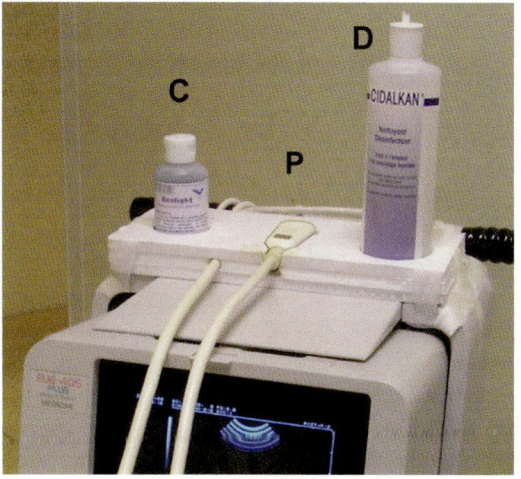

Fig. 4.3 How the top of our unit is optimized. This simple figure shows several points. First, our analogic unit, not a laptop, has a top, and we can see how this top is exploited, optimal space management in the usual dimension, the width: three tools, including one single probe (*P*), allowing to avoid these lateral stands which expand the width of the laptop (and other) machines, one (gelless) contact product (*C*), and one disinfectant (*D*) well tolerated since years and years by the probe. Second, it shows how the three tools we permanently use are solidly fixed on allotted holes, preventing any fall during transportation. Third, the unique probe concept allows precisely this configuration, avoiding these lateral stands which take lateral space (see through the textbook). Fourth, here is featuring the 2008 update of our 1992 technology (they just added some cosmetic changes: this purple color on the body).

answers. We were obliged to take some risk and build up experience with years. We have been using a 60 % alcohol-based alkylamine bactericidal spray with neutral tensioactive amphoteric pH on the microconvex probe of our Hitachi EUB-405 unit since 1995, and our probe has still not shown any damage (Fig. 4.3). Some authors have proposed 70 % alcohol as a simple and efficient procedure [2], but a majority of authors find it risky for the probes and not effective enough. An aldehyde-based and alcohol-based spray has been advocated [3], but this is a questionable approach if this blend fixes the proteins. The gel is a culture medium for bacteria. Many constraining procedures have been designed for carefully withdrawing all marks of gel. Some advocate an absorbent towel between two patients [4]. In the ICU, this solution seems clearly questionable. Since we do not use gel, these complicated procedures can be forgotten.

When Is It Time to Perform an Ultrasound Examination

The simple admission to an ICU is a sign of gravity. Ultrasound is fully part of the physical examination and is practiced during (sometimes after) (sometimes before, in cardiac arrest) this basic step. Only beneficial information can emerge from it (read Anecdotal Note 1). The utility of ultrasound has been proven in the critically ill. We expect each patient to benefit from several examinations during any long stay – not to say everyday or more.

For being schematical, the first contact provides the initial diagnosis. It includes any procedure, either diagnostic (puncture of suspect site) or venous line insertion. The following step is the follow-up, done ad lib, for early detection of the usual complications (pneumonia, sinusitis, thromboses, etc.). Routine, repeated ultrasound tests in the ICU are like taking a "photograph" of the patient. A test limited to one point (e.g., full bladder) takes a few seconds. The CLOT-protocol is a typical application of this concept (developed in Chap. 28).

Since When Do We Perform These Whole-Body Ultrasound Examinations: Some Historical Perspectives

Our hospital is probably the first where an ultrasound unit, belonging to the ICU for cardiac investigations (the efficient work of François Jardin), was used on the whole body by the intensivist, for immediate management. Our princeps study, sent in 1991, found a 22 % utility rate with immediate therapeutic changes in consecutive patients [5]. This percentage is confirmed in clinical settings [6] as well as, interestingly, the 31 % rate in a study considering unexpected autopsy findings from ICU patients [7]. Our 22 % rate was a minimal, since it did not include unpublished applications, i.e., mainly lung ultrasound and other fields (optic nerve, sinusitis, etc.), *nor* the benefit of repeated examinations for monitoring critically ill patients (venous thromboses, e.g.), *nor* cardiac results, *nor* interventional procedures, *nor* negative findings with immediate change in management (e.g., postponing CT when the question was answered), *nor* the decrease in radiations (X-rays), *nor* postponing of painful tests (arterial blood gas), etc. Performed today, this study would clearly quadruple this initial value of 22 %.

> **Anecdotal Note**
> 1. In ancient times, but far after the era of clinical ultrasound, it was not rare to see in prestigious institutions the admission of a patient by a team who knew the work and did not need bedside ultrasound. The patient, definitely critically ill, worsened day after day in spite of the therapy (done from a wrong diagnosis), eventually the team decided to practice an ultrasound test (at worst, sending the patient to the radiology department and to an inexperienced radiologist) (at best in the ICU by a skilled ICU member), and the diagnosis was done, just a bit late, once the inflammatory cascade was ongoing. We use the past, because we hope such a scenario would be difficult to find, nowadays.

References

1. Lichtenstein D, Biderman P, Chironi G, Elbaz N, Fellahi JL, Gepner A, Mezière G, Page B, Texereau J, Valtier B (1996) Faisabilité de l'échographie générale d'urgence en réanimation. Réan Urg 5:788
2. O'Doherty AJ, Murphy PG, Curran RA (1989) Risk of Staphylococcus aureus transmission during ultrasound investigation. J Ultrasound Med 8:619–621
3. Pouillard F, Vilgrain V, Sinègre M, Zins M, Bruneau B, Menu Y (1995) Peut-on simplifier le nettoyage et la désinfection des sondes d'échographie? J Radiol 76(4):217–218
4. Muradali D, Gold WL, Phillips A, Wilson S (1995) Can ultrasound probes and coupling gel be a source of

References

nosocomial infection in patients undergoing sonography? Am J Rœntgenol 164:1521–1524
5. Lichtenstein D, Axler O (1993) Intensive use of general ultrasound in the intensive care unit, a prospective study of 150 consecutive patients. Intensive Care Med 19:353–355
6. Manno E, Navarra M, Faccio L, Motevallian M, Bertolaccini L, MfochivÃ A, Pesce M, Evangelista A (2012) Deep impact of ultrasound in the intensive care unit: the ICU-sound protocol. Anesthesiology 117(4):801–809
7. Combes A, Mokhtari M, Couvelard A, Trouillet JL, Baudot J, Henin D, Gibert C, Chastre J (2004) Clinical and autopsy diagnoses in the ICU: a prospective study. Arch Intern Med 164(4):389–392

The Seven Principles of Lung Ultrasound

Lung ultrasound is a standardized domain. Each of its components is based upon pathophysiological realities. As for any novelty, a new terminology had to be considered. The one used in the BLUE-protocol favors fast communication, in the spirit of aviation language: maximal information in minimal time.

In this quest, a maximal effort has been done for helping memory. Logic and culture were mixed together. As an example, the term "B-line" should spontaneously suggest interstitial syndrome to any physician. Confusions were avoided for the best. The terms A-lines, B-lines, and up to Z-lines have been chosen on purpose with each time a precise idea helping memorization. We checked that the bat sign, seashore sign, lung sliding, quad sign, sinusoid sign, tissue-like sign, shred sign, lung rockets, stratosphere sign, lung point, BLUE-protocol, etc., did not yield confusion in the medical terminology. The standardization of the method is favored by following seven principles:

1. A simple method is suitable for lung ultrasound. A two-dimensional unit without filters or facilities is the most appropriate.
2. The thorax is an area where air and water are intimately mingled.
3. The lung is the largest organ in the human body.
4. All signs arise from the pleural line.
5. Lung signs are mainly based on the analysis of the artifacts.
6. The lung is a vital organ. Most signs are dynamic.
7. Nearly all acute disorders of the thorax come in contact with the surface. This explains the potential of lung ultrasound, which is paradoxical only at first view.

Development of the First Principle: A Simple Method

Two peculiar points highlight lung ultrasound.

First, sophisticated units – usually devoted for cardiac explorations – are not ideal. The large size of these cardiac units, the image resolution, the start-up time, the probe shape, the complexity of the technology, and the high cost can be hindrances for bedside use devoted to critically ill patients The machine that we use, manufactured in 1992, last (cosmetic) update 2008, is perfect for lung – and whole body – analysis. We provide some figures allowing the reader to compare our 1992 resolution with laptop models from the twenty-first century (see Fig. 2.2). One figure in particular may explain one of the main reasons of the delay of use of lung ultrasound in many ICUs (Fig. 5.1).

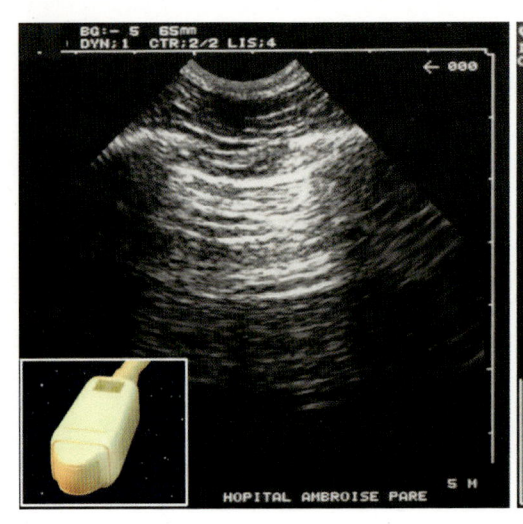

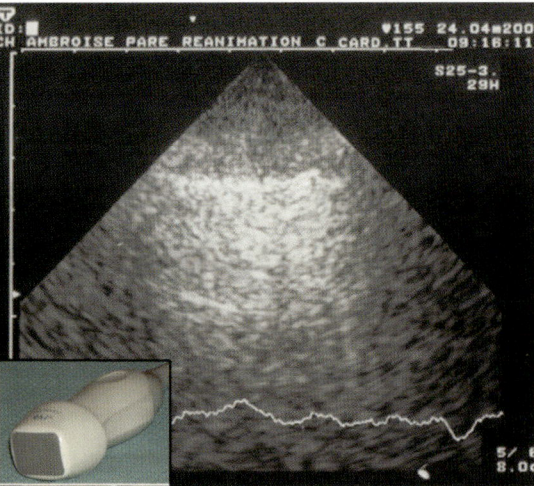

Fig. 5.1 Cardiac probes. This figure shows (*right image*) how lung ultrasound appeared to many intensivists who had standard echocardiography units. One can understand that they were not fully encouraged to go beyond. Compare with our 1992 machine (*left*)

Second, the pleural line and the normal signs arising from it (A-lines and lung sliding) are the same at any part of the thorax. The lung is a simple organ, unlike the heart, the abdomen (which contains more than 21 organs), or a fetus.

Development of the Second Principle: Understanding the Air-Fluid Ratio and Respecting the Sky-Earth Axis

Air and fluids coexist in the lung. Air rises, fluids sink. Lung ultrasound requires precisions on the patient's position with respect to the sky-earth axis and the area where the probe is applied. Pneumothorax is nondependent, interstitial syndrome usually nondependent, alveolar consolidation usually dependent, and fluid pleural effusion fully dependent.

The critically ill patient can be examined in supine, semirecumbent, or sometimes lateral position, rarely in an armchair, and on occasion in the prone position. Dependent disorders can become nondependent in the prone position.

The mingling between air and fluids generates the artifacts because of the high acoustic impedance gradient. Air completely stops the ultrasound beam (acoustic barrier); fluid is an excellent medium that facilitates its transmission. The air-fluid ratio differs completely from one disease to another. We used to describe the disorders from pure fluid to pure air, i.e., pleural effusion (pure fluid), lung consolidation, from atelectasis (mostly fluid) to pneumonia (some air), interstitial syndrome (mostly air), the normal lung (slightly hydrated), and pneumothorax (pure air) (Fig. 5.2).

In pleural effusion, the air-fluid ratio is 0.

In lung consolidation, the air-fluid ratio is very low, roughly 0.1 (due to some air bronchograms).

In interstitial syndrome, the air-fluid ratio is very high, roughly 0.95 (air is mingled with minute interstitial edema).

In decompensated COPD or asthma, air is the major component, and the ratio is higher, roughly 0.98.

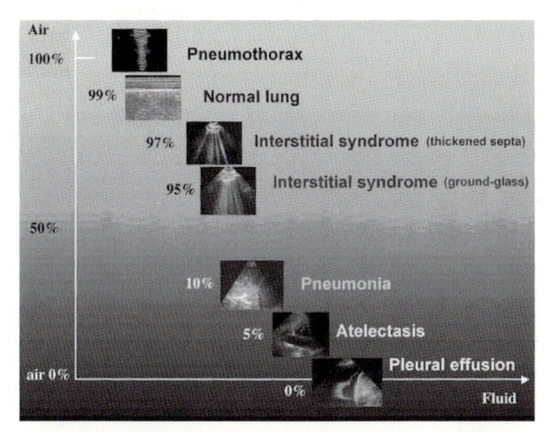

Fig. 5.2 The air-fluid ratio curve. The main disorders – and the normal lung – feature between pure air and pure fluid. Note, between pneumothorax and interstitial syndrome, the position of the normal lung. In order not to complicate this graph, we did not feature anaerobic empyema, which contains minute amounts of gas (and has echoic content)

The normal lung should logically be located here, the air-fluid ratio being roughly the same, 0.98.

In pneumothorax, the air-fluid ratio is 1.

The Third Principle: Locating the Lung and Defining Areas of Investigation

This deserves a whole chapter to make subheadings more visual. The principle is to make a lung ultrasound examination as standardized as an ECG. This principle is linked to the 7th, which defines where the diseases are. Like the ECG, we will define 6 basic points of analysis, three per lung: the *BLUE-points* (Chap. 6).

The Fourth Principle: Defining the Pleural Line

This is the time to take the probe. The pleural line is the basis of lung ultrasound, developed in Chap. 8.

The Fifth Principle: Dealing with the Artifact Which Defines the Normal Lung, the A-Line

This is the time to analyze the resulting image; this is developed in Chap. 9.

The Sixth Principle: Defining the Dynamic Characteristic of the Normal Lung, Lung Sliding

The lung is a vital organ and therefore moves permanently, from birth to death. This is developed in Chap. 10.

Development of the Seventh Principle: Acute Disorders Have Superficial, and Extensive, Location

Two providential features make lung ultrasound an accessible discipline:

(a) The lung is a *superficial* organ. The critical disorders are just near the probe.

The superficial extension of most disorders to the pleural line explains the 98–100 % feasibility of lung ultrasound in the critically ill. Pleural effusions and pneumothorax always reach the pleural line (no necessary study for proving it – read any CT). Acute lung consolidations touch the chest wall in nearly all cases (see Chap. 17). Acute interstitial syndrome extends superficially. The interstitial syndrome detected at the lung surface is a representative sample of deeper interstitial syndrome. Figure 5.3 explains how these disorders are sharply detected. As opposed to bedside radiography, which creates a summation of pleural, alveolar, and interstitial changes, ultrasound distinguishes each of them. The next chapters will show that each acute disorder gives a particular signal: lung consolidation from pneumonia to atelectasis, interstitial disorders, abscess, even pulmonary embolism, etc.

Pneumothorax	Normal lung surface	Interstitial syndrome	Lung consolidation	Pleural effusion
air	air / air / air	air / air / air		
100%	98%	95%	10%	0%
AIR/no fluid	AIR/fluid	AIR/fluid	air/FLUID	no air/FLUID

Air-fluid ratio

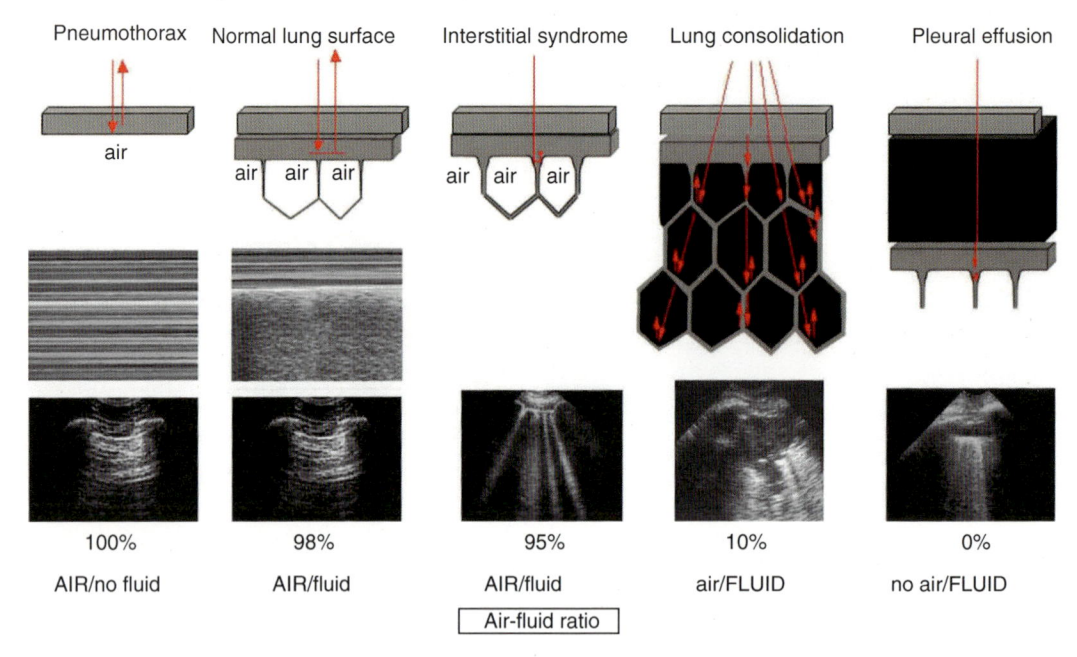

Fig. 5.3 How the main disorders generate specific signs. This figure demonstrates the basis of lung ultrasound according to the air-fluid ratio. Pneumothorax (pure air): the pleural line is drawn only on the parietal pleura. Pure air abuts the pleural line. This yields A-lines. The absence of visceral pleura yields abolition of lung sliding (stratosphere sign). Normal lung surface (99 % air): the dynamics of the visceral pleura generates lung sliding. The normal interlobular septa are too fine for generating B-lines. The visceral pleura contains a layer of cells, with minimal hydric content (sufficient for creating lung sliding). Interstitial edema (95 % air): these subpleural interlobular septa are thickened and surrounded by alveolar gas. The beam penetrates this small mixed system, is trapped after less than one millimeter, and tries to come back at the probe head, but is trapped again, this resulting in persistent to and fro movements, generating one small line at each movement, resulting in a long, vertical looking hyperechoic line, the B-line (an hydro-aeric artifact). Although enlarged, the septum is still too small to be directly visualized. Lung consolidation (3 % air): numerous alveoli are filled with fluid (transudate, exudate, etc.). They are separated by (deep) interlobular septa which, thin or thick, generate multiple reflecting interfaces, resulting in a tissue-like pattern. The whole is traversed by the ultrasound beam, resulting in a lump image of lung consolidation. The correct term should therefore be alveolar-interstitial syndrome. There is no place here for the generation of any comet-tail artifact. Note the irregular end of this (nontranslobar) consolidation, the shred (or fractal) line, which generates the shred or fractal sign. Pleural effusion (pure fluid): the two layers of the pleura are separated by fluid – resulting in a homogeneous pattern (traditionally anechoic, but not for the critical causes: empyema, hemothorax). This image is enclosed by four regular borders, especially the lower one, the lung line, which generates the quad sign

(b) The acute lung disorders are usually *extensive*. Therefore, a few standardized points are sufficient (dealt with in Chap. 6). This property makes LUCI easy, allowing to expedite our fast protocols: time-consuming, chancy scannings are unnecessary as opposed to the heart or abdominal organs. Pleural effusions and pneumothoraces develop in a free cavity and, like sheets of paper, have several dimensions. Even if they are "minute," they are also extensively applied at the wall. Acute interstitial syndrome is in our experience quite always extensive. Lung consolidations make a slight exception, although most cases are located at standardized areas (PLAPS-point). Some can be located anywhere else and be small.

Figure 5.4 shows that only ten signs are required for diagnosing normal lung surface, pleural effusion, lung consolidation, interstitial syndrome, and pneumothorax.

These are the seven principles of lung ultrasound. Although long described, they received constant improvements aiming at gaining efficiency and simplicity [1].

Fig. 5.4 The ten basic signs for the lung part of the BLUE-protocol. The first sign, from the left and the top, is the basis (the bat sign). The second and third are signs of normality (A-lines and lung sliding). The rest are pleural effusion (quad sign, sinusoid sign), lung consolidation (shred sign, tissue-like sign), interstitial syndrome (lung rockets), and pneumothorax (stratosphere sign and lung point – the A-line sign is already featuring). The only color is the one of the background, for esthetic purpose. No space for Doppler in LUCI. Nice figure indeed (which inspired some manufacturers)

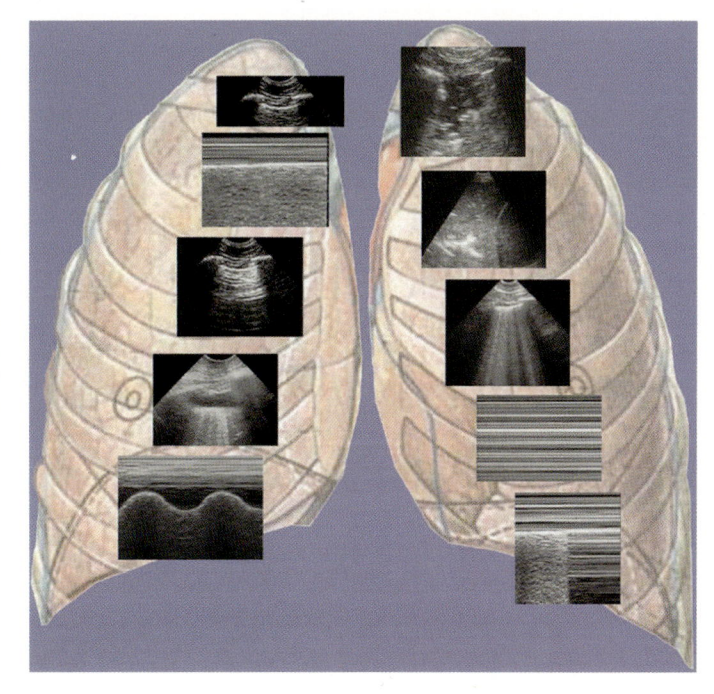

Reference

1. Lichtenstein D (1997) Lung ultrasound: a method of the future in intensive care? (Editorial). Rev Pneumol Clin 53:63–68

The BLUE-Points: Three Points Allowing Standardization of a BLUE-Protocol

> For exploring the most voluminous organ, three points allow standardized protocols, expedite the investigation of critically ill patients, and warrant the accuracy published in the BLUE-protocol native article.

The lung is our most voluminous organ (skin apart): about 1,500 cm^2 surface and 17 % of the body skin area. Where to apply the probe may appear as a quandary. We could answer simply but not efficiently "at the same places as the stethoscope." Some experts simplify the problem but complicate the technique by advocating comprehensive scans. In critical settings, time is too precious. The 7th principle of LUCI states that the life-threatening disorders have usually an extensive projection. Apart from some small and aberrant lung consolidations (read Anecdotal Note 1), the daily profiles are extensive: pulmonary edema (even moderate), pneumothorax (even small), pleural effusion, etc. This remarkable property allows to use standardized points for expediting a BLUE-protocol. A basic empiricism associated with a long research has allowed us to define the BLUE-points [1]. We defined six BLUE-points, exactly like the 6 thoracic electrodes of standard ECG. There are three points per lung, two anterior and one semiposterior (Anecdotal Note 2).

The Concept of the BLUE-Hands

This concept allows to immediately locate the lung on any patient, from skinny to bariatric ones, from firm youngsters to old, tired ladies, and from babies to giants. The physician first compares both hand sizes (the term BLUE-hands refers to the patient). Between 1.65 and 1.85 m, the difference is insignificant. Then, the physician applies the "upper" hand, just below the clavicle, with tip of fingers at the midline (Fig. 6.1). Therefore, the upper hand is *oblique*. The physician then applies the "lower" hand, just below the upper one, thumbs excluded. The geometry of the hands makes the lower finger of the lower hand naturally transverse on the thorax.

Once this is done, the anterior lung is located, in almost all cases, exactly facing both hands. The lower finger of the lower hand indicates the lower anterior border of the lung (i.e., what we may call the phrenic line). The BLUE-points replace our previous concepts (read Anecdotal Note 3).

The BLUE-protocol was designed for exploring supine or semirecumbent patients without bothering them too much. The anterior and lateral chest walls are rather accessible. The posterior wall, of high relevance, requires more technical subtleties.

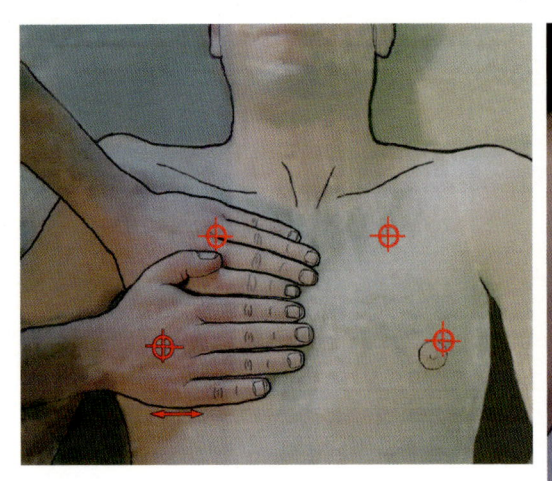

Fig. 6.1 The anterior BLUE-points. The *upper hand* is applied with the little finger against the lower border of the clavicle (in its long axis). The finger tips touch the midline. The *lower hand* is applied below the first one. The thumbs do not count. The upper BLUE-point is at the root of the middle and ring fingers of the upper hand (*upper cross*). The lower BLUE-point is in the middle of the palm of the lower hand (*lower cross*). In this subject, the lower BLUE-point is near the nipple. This definition makes a symmetric analysis usually avoiding the heart. The lower edge of the lower hand roughly indicates the phrenic line (*arrow*), i.e., the end of the lung. Note that the shape of the hands has been studied in order to correct the obliquity of the clavicle, yielding a roughly transversal phrenic line. Figure 1.1 shows an examination at the lower BLUE-point, in a supine patient at Earth level, defining a Stage 1 examination (1' in actual fact, since the subject is in semirecumbent)

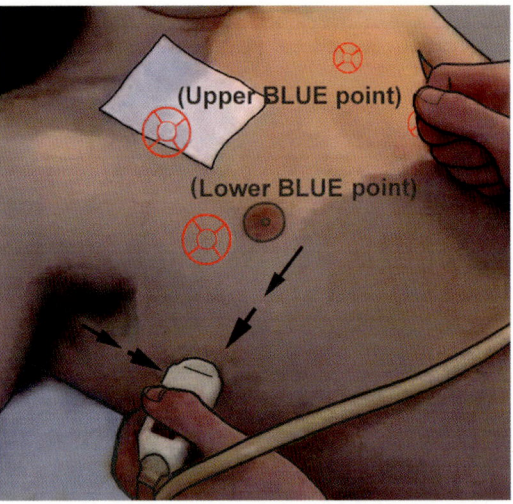

Fig. 6.2 Phrenic point. This figure shows a Stage 2 examination, i.e., a lateral continuation of the Stage 1. The probe here is at the intersection between the middle axillary line (*vertical arrow*) and the phrenic line (*horizontal arrow*): the phrenic point

Lung Zones, Their Relevance in the BLUE-Protocol, Their Combination with the Sky-Earth Axis for Defining Stages of Investigation

The anterior zone, defined using the BLUE-hands, is of utmost relevance, defining in a few seconds half of the profiles of the BLUE-protocol.

The lateral zone, defined from the anterior to the posterior axillary line, is not used in the BLUE-protocol, for reasons of redundancy. It may be however useful on occasion (if PLAPS-point is hard to reach) (Fig. 6.2).

The posterior zone, i.e., all that is behind the posterior axillary line, may appear of limited access in supine patients, a kind of twilight zone, a hidden face of the moon, etc., because the patient's weight squashes the bed. The aim of the PLAPS-point is to make this zone accessible, precise, and easy (without searching for a help, turning difficult patients, losing time for unleashing the hands, etc.).

We define stages by considering these areas and the fact that the patient is seen in the supine position and (for most of us) at Earth level. The notion of stages specifies that the finding is done at Earth level, a kinda tribute to Scott Dulchavsky and Andrew Kirkpatrick, who investigate astronauts.

Stage 1 investigates the anterior wall in supine patients.

Stage 2 adds the lateral wall.

Stage 3 adds the external part of the posterior wall (zone "3").

In *Stage 4*, the patient must be positioned laterally, or seated, in order to comprehensively study the posterior chest wall. Stage 4 also includes the apex. Only a microconvex probe can efficiently do this. With Stage 4, ultrasound is nearly as competitive as CT.

Some Technical Points for Making Lung Ultrasound an Easier Discipline

One major interest of the BLUE-points is to define points far enough from the abdomen. The advantages are as follows:
- Energy for explaining what the diaphragm looks like (although not a big issue) is avoided, at least initially.
- Energy for explaining how to recognize a diaphragm in challenging patients (a bigger issue) is avoided.
- Energy for explaining how to distinguish a pleural from a peritoneal effusion is avoided.
- Energy for explaining signs we don't use (e.g., spinal sign) is avoided.
- Energy for explaining how to distinguish a basithoracic lung consolidation from some common abdominal fat (or organ) is avoided. Without any notion of probe location, it can be a challenge (Fig. 6.3).

We guess that many users would be frustrated not to see the diaphragm. Its anterior insertion is located at the lowest finger of the BLUE-hands, defining the phrenic line. One main point must be understood. Using our perpendicular approach, we do not need to see the diaphragm: its location and dynamics are much more important. The diaphragm insertion is the location where the image displays on inspiration a thoracic structure at the left of the screen (i.e., air barrier or pleural or alveolar disorders) and on expiration an image of the liver (or spleen) at the right of the screen. We then know exactly where the diaphragm is (and how it works) without any direct visualization, sparing energy.

Following the BLUE-points prevents some mistakes, such as applying the probe too low. If applying it on the zones 2 and 4 of (color) Fig. 1 of the international consensus conference on lung ultrasound (2012), for instance, the users would regularly see the liver/kidney interface (which may look at very first sight as a diaphragm), would be happy to recognize the "diaphragm," would diagnose a huge lung consolidation (the… liver) above, and would prescribe antibiotics to a patient who has nothing to do with a diagnosis of pneumonia (and will remain untreated).

We should avoid to position patients with their hand behind their head, as often done for inserting chest tubes. In this position, the scapula comes in the field, generating an image really difficult to understand.

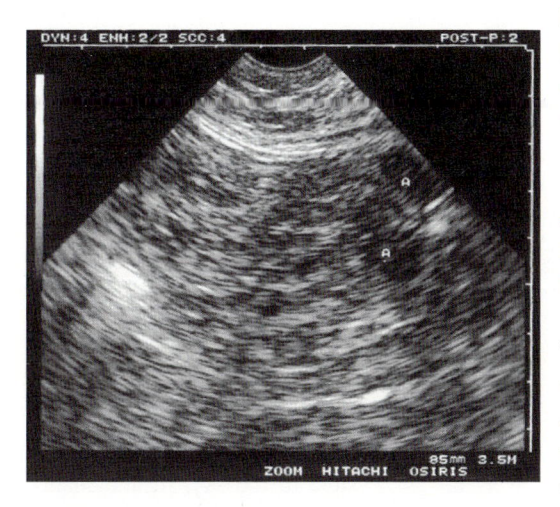

Fig. 6.3 Abdominal fat. Such an image given to a reader without the notion on where it was taken (here, far more podal than the lower BLUE-point or PLAPS-point) could mislead this reader for a lung consolidation. This abdominal fat may be distinguished, but this would require complicated knowledge: a waste of energy

Standardization of a Lung Examination: The BLUE-Points

There are 6 BLUE-points, three per lung. Like the 6 standard derivations of the ECG, the concept of the BLUE-points should help the users when they apply their probe on the largest organ of the body (read caption of Figs. 6.1 and 6.2). The label upper and lower BLUE-points assumes a Stage 1 (supine) or 1' (semirecumbent) analysis (if not, position has to be specified). They aim at following the trapezoidal shape of the lung.

Standardization of a Lung Examination: The Upper BLUE-Point

It is defined between the 3rd and 4th finger of the upper BLUE-hand, at their palmar insertion.

Standardization of a Lung Examination: The Lower BLUE-Point

It is defined at the middle of the palm of the lower BLUE-hand. This allows to avoid the heart in most cases, while having a symmetric definition. The lower BLUE-point is near to the nipple in the adult and far below in the neonate, but works at any age. When the heart occupies the lower BLUE-point, the probe should be placed more laterally.

The little finger of the lower BLUE-hand indicates the phrenic line (Fig. 6.2). The continuation of this line and its intersection with the middle axillary line define the phrenic point, locating the usual lateral place of the cupola (which can vary if there is atelectasis or lung overdistension).

The PLAPS-Point

This paragraph is long. Several details make this point more complicated than the anterior ones. One of the multiple benefits is the possibility to postpone a transfer to CT.

PLAPS is a practical abbreviation (a bit of an onomatopoeia, since PLAPS often looks like "splashes") for posterolateral alveolar and/or pleural syndrome. See Chap. 15. The PLAPS-point is posterior (Fig. 6.4). PLAPS is sought for in a Stage 3 examination, i.e., in *supine* (or semirecumbent) patients. The PLAPS-point is designed for detecting most alveolar or pleural disorders. Its basic description is simple: "the intersection between the posterior axillary line and the transversal line continuing posteriorly the lower BLUE-point." The reality is more complex:
1. Critically ill patients are usually supine, ventilated, sedated, and curarized. The bed makes a physical hindrance to the progression of the probe at the back and above all to a 100 % perpendicular approach of the probe on the posterior chest wall (a general rule in LUCI). A long probe would be a major issue to this maneuver. We aim at showing the maximal of this posterior wall. The probe head must point as far as possible to the sky, in accordance with the principle N°2. We wish at shooting at the lung (probe being considered like a gun) and not the parietal layers (Fig. 6.5).

Several solutions are now showed for optimizing this step:
- Using the shortest probe. Each cm of saved length is providential for analyzing more

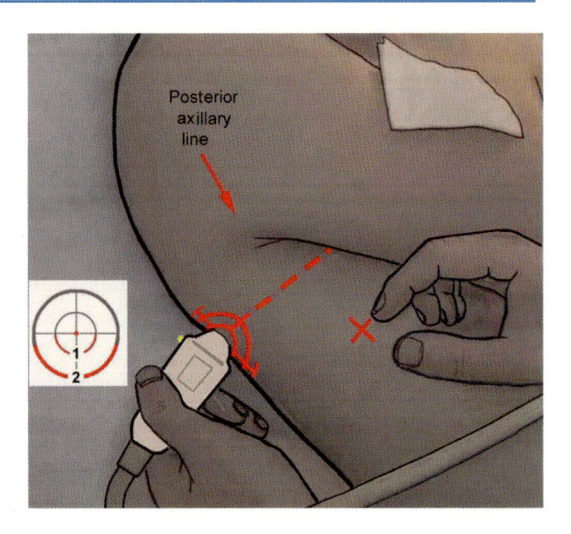

Fig. 6.4 PLAPS-point. This figure shows a probe applied at the PLAPS-point: this is a Stage 3, which adds this external part of the posterior area, using a short probe. This is the intersection between the transversal line continuing the lower BLUE-point (*dotted line*) and the longitudinal posterior axillary line (*arrow*) or, as seen here, as far as possible behind. This figure shows how the back of the patient is made slightly accessible by taking the elbow and rotating the thorax to the left, here. We gain precious centimeters of posterior exploration, with the probe head as perpendicular as possible and mostly pointing (as far as possible) to the sky, i.e., suitable for detecting small effusions in supine patients. Rigid beds require more of this maneuver, since the operator's hand cannot make a "hole" in the bed. The PLAPS-point immediately detects small and large pleural effusions (and 90 % of cases of lung consolidations in the critically ill). On the target to the left, the numbers 1 and 2 indicate the down extensions of the PLAPS-point. Using the PLAPS-point, the probe is just above the diaphragm, i.e., in full lung area. *PLAPS*: posterolateral alveolar and/or pleural syndrome. The right index of the operator points on the phrenic point (cross)

The PLAPS-Point

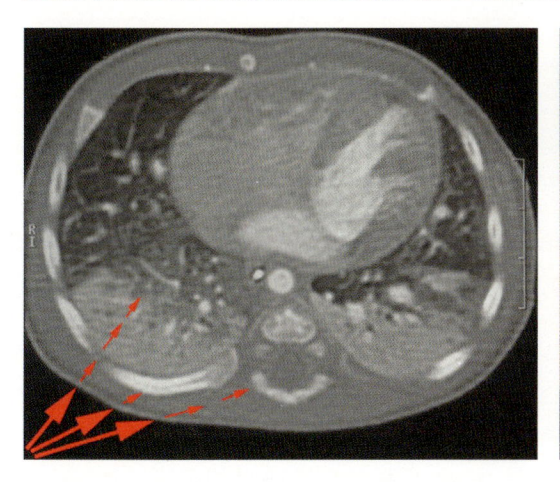

Fig. 6.5 PLAPS-point and perpendicularity of the probe. The *left red arrow* is a little perpendicular to the chest wall and will display the lung consolidation quite well. The *right red arrow* goes through soft tissues and will never show lung ultrasound patterns. Intermediate images will give ill-defined images. The operator should care at applying the probe as far as possible perpendicular to the wall

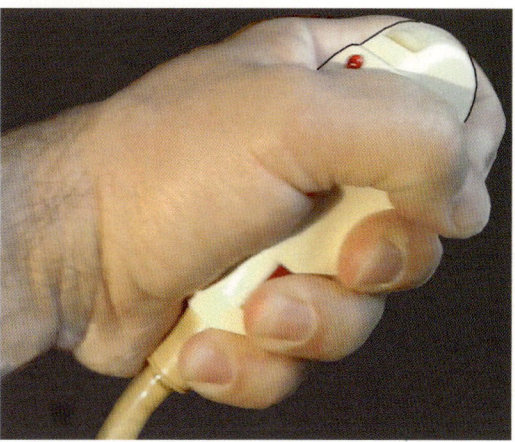

Fig. 6.6 PLAPS-hand. For PLAPS-point explorations, the probe must be held this way, like a tennis racket. See in the text why

   the posterior lung (i.e., developing LUCI). Our microconvex probe is 88 mm long.
   - Making a kind of "hole" in the bed. The hand depresses the bed to gain important cm. Rigid beds make this gesture more difficult.
   - Slightly turning the patient by putting the ipsilateral arm above the thorax and pushing slightly the elbow toward the midline. This opens a few (sometimes providential) degrees (Fig. 6.4). Turning the patient too much would maybe locate a small effusion at the mediastinal pleura, preventing to locate it posteriorly.
   - Our last solution for being 100 % perpendicular to the pleural line: just inserting a TEE probe posteriorly, a maneuver pompously labeled the BAPLUTEEP maneuver (bedside assessment of posterior lung using transesophageal echography probes).
2. How to hold the probe is diametrically opposed to the anterior way, where there is no constraint. Here, we have no visual control on the probe. We will hold it like a tennis racket, firmly, using the whole hand (Fig. 6.6). Like orbital walls that protect an eye, the thumb and index will protect the probe head. This allows to softly feel the skin and avoid a harmful pressure (for the patient *and* for the probe). The cable of the probe should also be protected from excessive curvature, and the hand, holding a short probe, will be able to protect both head and cable.
3. The probe should be as perpendicular as possible: this allows to have well-defined, standardized images of lung ultrasound signatures (lung line, fractal line, etc.); it ensures the best correlations with measurements (a tangential probe would overestimate dimensions).
4. The image acquisition. It can be useful to slightly rotate the probe for correcting the obliquity of the ribs. A clear bat sign must be displayed for locating the pleural line with confidence.
5. For optimizing this approach, the variable geometry of the PLAPS-points must be studied.
   - As regards the horizontal component, the short probe is inserted as far as possible medially (toward the rachis), after the posterior axillary line, depending on the body habitus, the possibility to slightly turning the patient's back. The shorter the probe, the easier the PLAPS-point.
   - As regards the vertical component, a negative examination makes already ultrasound as accurate as radiography. But the user wants more.

- The "extended PLAPS-point": one intercostal downward defines a first extension of the PLAPS-point (Fig. 6.4). Finding a PLAPS there makes ultrasound superior to radiograph. Logically, if no PLAPS has been found at the native PLAPS-point, a PLAPS found at this first extension must have a *small volume*.
- The second extension (one more intercostal space down), done if the first extension is negative, makes ultrasound as accurate as CT. If a PLAPS is present, its volume will be logically very small, just above the cupola. If a large image appears on the screen, it cannot be a PLAPS: this is the liver. This detail (useful in challenging patients) makes ultrasound easy.

The aim of the PLAPS-point is to have the probe located at the thorax. Too cranial would miss small juxta-phrenic lesions and too podal would make sometimes an insertion of the probe at the abdomen, showing structural images which can mimic consolidations, such as the liver, spleen, or fat. It is much simpler to avoid these structures than trying to explain why they are not a lung consolidation (Fig. 6.3). Using the notion of extended PLAPS-point, the operator will descend and detect the diaphragm easily. The principle of this flexible approach allows to define PLAPS with maximal accuracy and minimal explanations.

The user is free to use a lateral analysis first, more easy than the PLAPS-point in some ventilated patients. If large effusions or consolidations are detected this way, the BLUE-protocol is concluded as well.

Location of the Lung in Challenging Patients

The lung volume is the same in batriatric and thinner patients, yet all this fat may make it difficult to locate it. The BLUE-hands allow to confidently locate the anterior lung and acquire an information rather easily. Although the PLAPS-point will be strictly defined, the image acquisition is more difficult. We use some principles inspired from air navigation. If there is a doubt about the diaphragm, the user will scan podally and identify a large mass podally that will maybe look also ill defined. This tissular mass is supposedly the spleen, but may be a lung consolidation. If the user scans downward, and detects an organ, also ill-defined, but looking, even from far, to a kidney, the probability of a kidney surrounded by a spleen is major. And the phrenic location is confidently done.

Other Points? The Case of the Patient in the Prone Position

The simplest way we found was to consider the scapula. The point just inside its internal border at half way would be an equivalent of the upper BLUE-point (upper prone point?). The point at its lower end would fit for the lower BLUE-point (lower prone point?). A horizontal line drawn from one or two fingers above the point where the lower rib reaches the rachis usually indicates the diaphragm, at least in young adults (Fig. 6.7).

Regarding the whole thorax, we could have added many other points, but, from Sybile Merceron's words, "too many points kill the points." We agree.

BLUE-Points and Clinical Information

The upper and lower BLUE-points immediately indicate anterior interstitial syndrome.

The upper BLUE-point immediately indicates pneumothorax in semirecumbent, dyspneic patients.

The lower BLUE-point immediately indicates pneumothorax in supine, ventilated patients.

The PLAPS-point immediately indicates the huge majority of pleural effusions, whatever their size, and 90 % of locations of acute lung consolidations. Obviously, substantial effusions or consolidations are detected at the phrenic point.

Philosophy of the BLUE-Points: Can the Users Do Without?

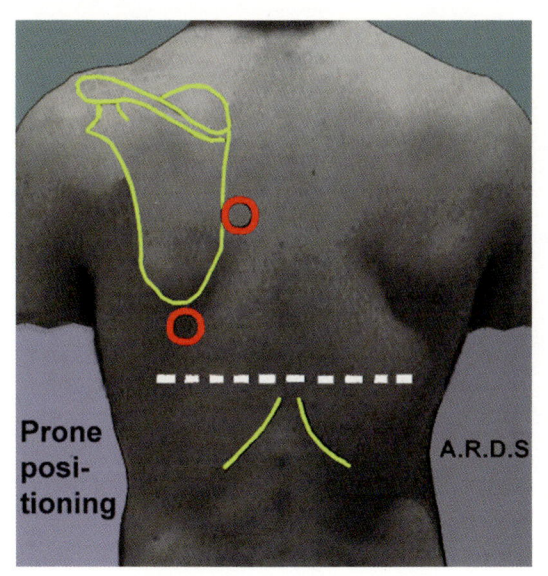

Fig. 6.7 The prone points, suggestion. Patient in the prone position. The upper prone point is located just inside the middle of the scapula. The lower prone point is just below the scapula. We determine the junction between the lung and abdomen, in young adults, at one or two cm above the point where the last ribs reach the rachis

Aside Note More Devoted to Pulmonologists

Of minor interest to the intensivist, the upper BLUE-point is roughly located at the upper lobe or culmen, the lower BLUE-point at the middle lobe (lingula), and the PLAPS-point at the lower lobe. In the prone position, one can correlate the upper third to the upper lobe, the middle to the Fowler segment of the lower lobe, and the lower third to the basal pyramid of the lower lobe.

Philosophy of the BLUE-Points: Can the Users Do Without?

Yes, the operator is always free to insert the probe at will of course.

Specifically designed for the BLUE-protocol, the BLUE-points make lung ultrasound simple. They are standardized and reproducible, associating clinical efficiency and easiness of use. They were carefully designed for optimizing the search for pleural or alveolar disorders, even small. One main idea is (reminder) to be far enough from the abdomen. The BLUE-points follow the principle N°7 of LUCI: most disorders have substantial extension. A disorder not seen behind a rib will for sure be seen also above or below. Interstitial syndrome, pneumothorax, and pleural effusion especially will be detected as well at a given BLUE-point than just beside and even at any other area (the only exception would be a minute isolated consolidation). Therefore, the BLUE-points are indicative, but also very flexible. If a BLUE-point is not accessible (dressing, subcutaneous device, electrode applied by not trained paramedical team, etc.), applying the probe just beside is faster than tearing the electrode or training the nursing team to put them at the shoulders (which should be ideal). As indicated on page 7, the ribs hide maybe *half* of the lung surface (at a given phase), but one can do perfectly with the other half.

Anecdotal Notes

1. Are small consolidations relevant?

    If the patient management critically depends on the detection of small consolidations, here, we agree that the lung ultrasound test should be comprehensive. This is *not* the case in the BLUE-protocol (this is more achieved in the extended BLUE-protocol).

2. ECG

    We find such definitions frequently in medicine, such as the 9 areas which score the abdomen, the four breast quadrants, etc. Regarding the ECG, when we just see how the electrodes are placed by some students, we just hope that the users will do better and read the user's guide with conscience (to begin with, the one of Einthoven, published in 1903, awarded 21 years later).

3. Previous points

    We defined the lower lung border in the adult between zero and two/three fingers below the nipple line. This landmark was valuable only in adult males, had too wide range, and was difficult to imagine in the case of saggy breasts, while young men have a phrenic line 3 fingers below the nipple line. In the neonate, the nipple is located higher (five fingers). The BLUE-hands are valuable at any age. Previously, we divided the anterior wall in four quadrants, like a breast.

Reference

1. Lichtenstein D, Mezière G (2011) The BLUE-points: three standardized points used in the BLUE-protocol for ultrasound assessment of the lung in acute respiratory failure. Crit Ultrasound J 3:109–110

An Introduction to the Signatures of Lung Ultrasound

7

For performing lung ultrasound in the critically ill, we have counted 12 main signs. Only the first ten are used in the BLUE-protocol (the two others are the dynamic air bronchogram and the lung pulse).

1. The pleural line
2. A-lines
3. Lung sliding
4. The quad sign
5. The sinusoid sign
6. The shred sign
7. The tissue-like sign
8. Lung rockets
9. Abolished lung sliding
10. The lung point

1. The pleural line

This is the basis of any lung examination.

2. The A-line

This fundamental horizontal artifact demonstrates air in the thorax (living or dead air, the next sign will tell).

3. Lung sliding

This sign demonstrates the physiological dynamic of the lung toward the chest wall. It gives in M-mode the seashore sign.

4–7. The quad sign, sinusoid sign, shred sign, and tissue-like sign

There are signs of pleural effusion and lung consolidation. The concept of PLAPS makes one sign of four, resulting in expediting the BLUE-protocol and its learning curve.

8. Lung rockets

Defined by three B-lines (or more) between two ribs, these fundamental artifacts indicate interstitial syndrome. Diffuse lung rockets indicate diffuse interstitial syndrome, of prime relevance in the critically ill.

9. Abolished lung sliding

It suggests pneumothorax (as well as a multitude of other conditions). This is demonstrated using the vision, in real time. If needed, the M-mode confirms the trouble, displaying the stratosphere sign.

10. The lung point

This sign, showing sudden lung signs at a given area, is pathognomonic to pneumothorax.

Other Signs

The dynamic air bronchogram and the lung pulse, detailed in Chap. 35, are not used in the BLUE-protocol. They are of high relevance in more advanced levels of LUCI, since they allow to distinguish infections from atelectatic lungs, schematically and among other uses.

Countless other signs can be described on structural patterns, i.e., among others, septations within effusions and necrosis within consolidations.

Note

"Lung sliding" is not really the opposite of "abolished lung sliding." Lung sliding is a basic sign seen in some diseases (mainly pulmonary embolism); abolished lung sliding is seen in other diseases (mainly pneumothorax). In a shocked patient, lung sliding indicates particular diseases more than others. This makes ten signs all in all.

The Pleural Line

8

The previous chapters detailed the first three of the seven main principles of lung ultrasound, just evoking the four last. Now it is time to take the probe. Chapter 1 showed how we hold it and how we don't. The probe is perpendicular to the anterior chest wall and tries to stay perpendicular at the PLAPS-point.

Principle N°4 tells that in LUCI, all signs come from the pleural line. This is an apparently easy statement, but the pleural line must be carefully defined, in all circumstances, especially in agitated, dyspneic, bariatric patients, subcutaneous emphysema, and shaky environments. In bariatric patients who are agitated because of a severe pneumothorax associated with subcutaneous emphysema, all this in an airborne mission, the rules of LUCI should minimize the difficulties.

Any BLUE-protocol must begin by a correct recognition of the pleural line. We do not use transversal scans. This would make lung ultrasound more difficult, since slight movements (of physician or patient) would deeply change the image acquisition (see Fig. 1.2).

Our 5 MHz microconvex probe is perfect for this part of lung investigation.

The Pleural Line: The Basis

General Remarks

The thorax is built by the ribs and lungs. A longitudinal scan in adults makes an alternance of the rib surface on roughly 2 cm, the lung surface on roughly 2 cm, the rib on 2 cm, etc.

The rib is recognized easily: arciform hyperechoic structure and then acoustic shadow.

Between the top of 2 ribs, one can draw a "rib line."

The lung surface, i.e., the visceral pleural, is normally against the parietal pleural, and both make the pleural line in normal subjects. This is the line visible less than a cm below the rib line in standard adults. This distance is roughly 1/2 cm anteriorly, a little more posteriorly. At any age including neonates, the pleural line is located at roughly 1/4–1/3 of the distance between the two rib borders.

The pleural line appears as a hyperechoic, roughly horizontal line (when the probe is correctly applied, tangential), in actual fact slightly bended because of intrinsic distorsion of the image (visible as well with sectorial as linear probes). The pleural line should be visible in any circumstance, apart from huge surgical emphysema (Fig. 8.1).

The pleural line indicates the interface between the soft tissues (fluid-rich) of the wall and the lung tissue (gas-rich), i.e., the lung-wall interface. It shows the parietal pleura in all cases and the visceral pleura, i.e., the lung surface, only when there is no pneumothorax (nor pulmonectomy). The pleural cavity is normally virtual. The pleural line makes the parietal and visceral pleuras one line. With our 5 MHz probe, we do not distinguish the two layers, which is not a problem.

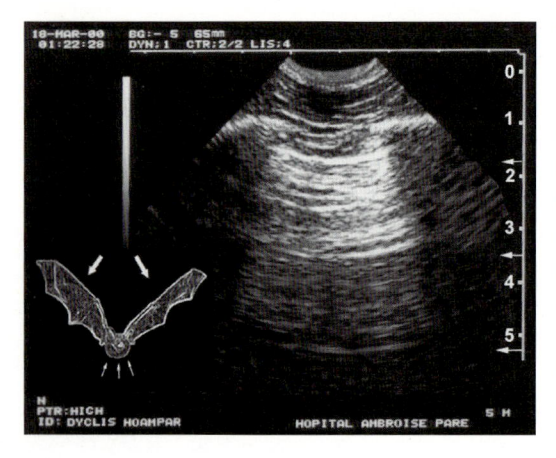

Fig. 8.1 The bat sign. The right vertical scale is centimetric. The ribs (cm 1) are recognized by their arciform shape with frank posterior acoustic shadow. A horizontal line below the rib line (1/2 cm in the adult) is highlighted (1.75 cm). This is the pleural line, which basically indicates the parietal pleura (and usually the visceral pleura). The upper rib, pleural line, and lower rib shape a kind of bat flying facing us, hence the bat sign, a basic landmark in lung ultrasonography. We made this figure without *arrow*, for keeping it preserved (see Figs. 9.1 and 10.1, for more details)

Pleural Line and the Bat Sign

The pattern created by the upper rib (left wing), pleural line (belly), and lower rib (right wing) has been labeled the bat sign, the basic first step in any lung ultrasound. It allows to precisely locate the lung surface using a stable landmark. Using longitudinal scans, the pleural line is always under control, even in hard conditions.

The concept of the bat sign avoids confusions with all other horizontal hyperechoic lines, i.e., superficial aponeuroses or deep repetition lines (A-lines, sub-A-lines, see below).

The visible length of the pleural line in adults, between two rib shadows (the belly of the bat), is roughly 2.5 cm (since the concept of a sectorial scan makes a triangular image).

In the neonate, the bat sign has exactly the same proportions (see Fig. 32.2).

The term "bat sign" appears in our publications in 2001 [1].

Variant of the Bat Sign

The "young bat sign." If the probe is applied near the sternum (inside the BLUE-points), the cartilage generates an ovoid structure that is traversed by the beam. We associated this pattern to the image of the young bat (with the idea that the bones are not yet calcified). In some cases where this may disturb (challenging examination), a shift of the probe to the outside will find the familiar landmark of the ribs.

Subcutaneous Emphysema: The Mocelin Variant

Amounts of gas invade the soft tissues in this case, and this prevents to detect the pleural line: subcutaneous emphysema is a main hindrance to LUCI. There is a possible reply. Bones are present, making a rigid deeper plan. Provided it does not harm the patient, we apply the probe with a pressure toward the rib cage in order to hide the gas. This can result in suddenly detecting an ill-defined bat sign. This sign, called the "bat in the fog," can be as precious as is the sudden detection of the runway through the fog for a stressed pilot lost in the fog (Fig. 8.2 and video 14.5).

Like in aviation rules again, the emergency can change the academic rules. In very difficult cases, to see a dynamic at the pleural line is precious, because it allows to locate precisely this pleural line (even if the ribs are not clearly visible). In other words, one uses lung sliding as a sign indicating the pleural line. This nonacademic way, called the Mocelin variant (from a Brazilian CEURFer), should be carefully used and must not be a habit, just a tool used in extreme difficulties. If we detect the pleural line *because* there is a lung sliding, this will prevent us to get accustomed to immediately detect a pneumothorax, which is, in the extreme emergency, one of the basis of LUCI. The pleural line should be recognized without any dynamic reference, only using the bat sign, as far as possible.

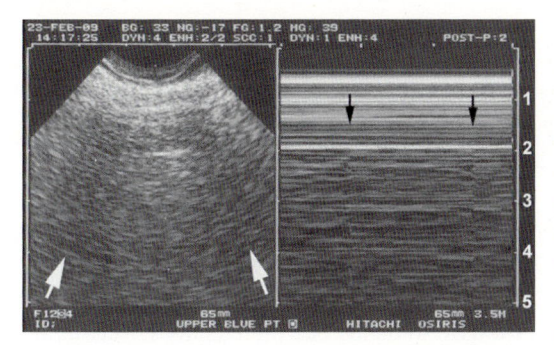

Fig. 8.2 The bat in the fog and T-lines. Many items are seen in this apparently challenging figure. This patient had a rather severe subcutaneous emphysema – after a trauma. The left image (real time) was quite impossible to interpret. After pressing the probe toward the rib cage, one has the feeling to detect ill-defined images which may correspond to acoustic shadows of the ribs (rising *white arrows*). Below what is possibly the rib line, a hyperechoic, horizontal line, ill-defined too, is visible, possibly the pleural line (2.0 cm of the right vertical scale). On the right, M-mode image, very slight accidents are visible, coming exactly from this line (*black arrows*) or, seen from *bottom to top*, stopping exactly at this line (2.0 cm of right scale). They shape the letter "T." They are definitely T-lines, i.e., an extreme equivalent of discreet lung pulse (see these terms in corresponding Chap. 10). In this really challenging file, from a traumatized patient with subcutaneous emphysema, and in spite of this extreme hindrance, one could define the rib shadows and the pleural line (the "bat in the fog") and a lung pulse. The rules of critical ultrasound make no space for confusion: there is no pneumothorax

Standardizing Lung Ultrasound: Merlin's Space

Once a probe is applied on an intercostal space and once the pleural line is identified, it is easy to build a space which has critical relevance in LUCI. This is the space located between the pleural line, the shadow of the ribs, and the lower border of the screen. It was called Merlin's space (from a question of Elisabeth Merlin, CEURFer from Oceania).

Merlin's space is normally occupied by air artifacts. Although always considered indesirable, they are under extreme attention in LUCI (principle N° 5). For the sake of rapid communication, air artifacts were given short names using alphabetic classification (we describe 12 of them at the pleural line: A-, B-, C-, F-, I-, J-, N-, O-, P-, T-, X-, and Z-lines). This is simpler than appearing at first view. Other artifacts are described above the pleural line (E-, S-, W-line), in other parts of the body (sub-B-, G-, R-, U-, V-lines), or outside the body (H-, K-lines). Most are either horizontally or vertically oriented.

All signs of LUCI arise at the very level of the pleural line (see Fig. 5.3). When the pleural layers are separated, the visceral pleura is either hidden by the air (in the case of a pneumothorax) or perfectly visible (in the case of a pleural effusion).

Standardizing Lung Ultrasound: Keye's Space

For making basic phenomena more easy to standardize, we have defined a virtual space, generated by the M-mode. The pleural line separates an upper rectangle and a lower one. This upper rectangle, limited downward by the pleural line (upward and laterally by the borders of the image), has been coined *Keye's space* (from Linda Keyes, CEURFer from Colorado) (Fig. 8.3). What happens in Keye's space is superficial to the lung.

In quiet breathing, Keye's space can be described as a stratified pattern. During dyspnea, accidents are visible within.

Just note a critical detail: the pleural line is perfectly defined without any confusion on the real-time image, using the bat sign. Using our 1992 machine (last update 2008), the pleural line is at exactly the same level, with no space for confusion, on the right M-mode image, with no lag as seen in quite all laptop machines. This means that, for searching the pleural line on the right image, one has just to continue the point where it appears (in the M-mode shooting line, supposedly at the middle) to the right image. Not configurating the modern machines this way would violate principle N°1 of LUCI: simplicity.

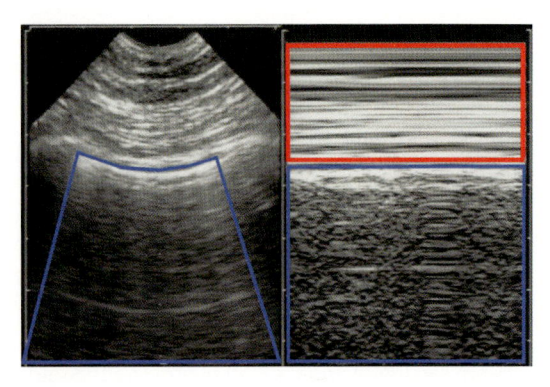

Fig. 8.3 Keye's and Merlin's space. To the left (real time), Merlin's space (*in blue*), framing what is below the pleural line (rib shadows excluded). To the right (M-mode), two spaces, separated by the pleural line, can be defined in any image of lung ultrasound. (1) An upper rectangle, Keye's space (*in red*), a virtual space, showing what is above the pleural line. (2) A lower rectangle, called for simplifying the MM-space, materializing what appears at and below the pleural line. Note this critical point: both images (*left and right*) are rigourously side by side. This will help in standardizing the field. Slightly premature now would be the description of the content of Merlin's space (an A-line); Keye's space (absence of dyspnea) and MM-space (lung sliding) are rich in data: the basis of the A-profile, schematically a normal lung surface

This notion, just introduced here, will have critical relevance when diagnosing pneumothorax in difficult settings. It will be developed in Chaps. 10 and mainly 14.

Standardizing Lung Ultrasound: The M-Mode-Merlin's Space

We have to define one more entity for clarifying the concept. Keye's space was defined as the upper square on the M-mode image. The lower square deserves a label. Since it corresponds to Merlin's space (real-time concept), we will label it the "M-Merlin's space." Any M-mode image in LUCI is built from two spaces, Keye's space above and the M-mode-Merlin's space below, both separated by the line materializing the pleural line (Fig. 8.3).

Reference

1. Lichtenstein D (2001) Lung ultrasound in the intensive care unit. Research Signpost Recent Res Devel Resp Critical Care Med 1:83–93

The A-Profile (Normal Lung Surface): 1) The A-Line

We now describe the 5th principle of LUCI. It should be understood that the A-profile is defined by both lung sliding and the A-line. Note that a lung sliding associated to one, or even 2 B-lines (described in Chap. 11), is still in the definition of an A-profile (3 B-lines would change it into a B-profile.

We do not use transversal scans. This would make lung ultrasound more difficult. Slight movements (of the physician or patient) would deeply change the image (see Fig. 1.2). See also some scary pitfalls in Chap. 14.

Our 5 MHz microconvex probe is perfect for this part of lung investigation.

The Artifact Which Defines the Normal Lung Surface: The A-line

Once a probe is applied on an intercostal space, only artifacts (from bones and lungs) are visible. These artifacts were always considered undesirable. Let us see them with more attention. For the sake of rapid communication, they were given short names using alphabetic classification (we describe 12 of them at the pleural line: A-, B-, C-, F-, I-, J-, N-, O-, P-, T-, X-, and Z-lines). This is simpler than seemingly at first view. Other artifacts are described above the pleural line (E-, S-, W-line), in other parts of the body (G-, M-, R-, V-, U-lines), or outside the body (H-, K-lines). Most are either horizontally or vertically oriented.

The normal artifact arising from the pleural line, i.e., displayed in Merlin's space, is the repetition of the pleural line, a roughly horizontal hyperechoic fine line parallel to the pleural line (Fig. 9.1). We coined this artifact the A-line, following the alphabetic logic in a nascent discipline. Air blocks the ultrasound beam, which comes back to the head, yielding this regular artifact. The distance between the pleural line and the A-line is equal to the skin-pleural line distance. Several equidistant A-lines can be visible. They can be called A1-lines, A2-lines, etc., according to the number of observed lines, with little clinical relevance. Of same relevance, horizontal artifacts are sometimes seen between two A-lines and called "sub-A-lines" and even "sub-sub-A-lines" (Pi-lines, see Fig. 40.4).

The A-line can be as long as the pleural line (slightly longer, given the sectorial image) but can be shorter or even not visible (Fig. 9.2). In this case, Merlin's space is homogeneous and darker than the pleural line. Slight Carmen maneuvers may make appear A-lines, but this is not a clinical problem, provided there is no visible B-line (see Fig. 11.1). This absence of any artifact is called O-line (O for non-A non-B) or again A° line, if one accepts to call the first visible A-line the "A1-line." In other words, to see the complete absence of any artifact arising from the pleural line has the clinical meaning of the A-line: just *gas*. The O-line concept allows to demonstrate the real tone of air: hydro-aeric

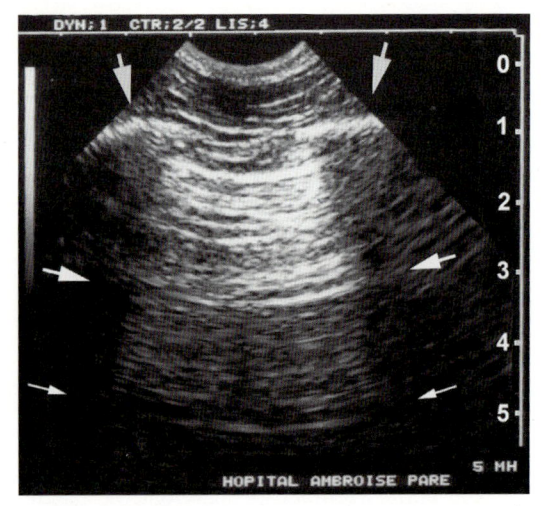

Fig. 9.1 The A-line. The normal lung surface. Continuation of Fig. 8.1, here featuring with a few *arrows*. The right vertical scale is centimetric. The pleural line is 1.75 cm deep, located half a cm below the rib line (*vertical arrows*, ribs). The *horizontal lines* visible at cm 3.4 and cm 5.2, in Merlin's space, are repetitions of the pleural line. These are the A-lines (*horizontal arrows*). They are located at standardized distances: the skin-pleural line distance, here 1.75 cm. The first A-line is large (*upper arrows*). The pleural line and the A-lines cannot be confused with other *horizontal lines* located above or below. Note that the center of gravity of the A-line is the head of the probe (the *top of the image*), as opposed to the one of the B-line, which is at the pleural line

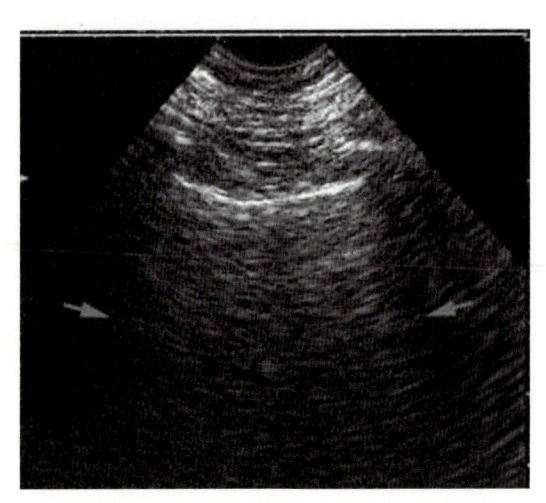

Fig. 9.2 The O-Line. Merlin's space is completely homogeneous here, without any anatomic nor artifactual image, horizontal (A-lines) or vertical (B-lines). The *arrows* delineate the expected location of real A-lines. This artifact, non-A non-B but having the value of A-lines, has been called O-line (don't search for any line; O is also for zero). As opposed to endless zoologic discussions about the zebra's coat, this figure proves that the natural tone of air is dark on ultrasound. Normal or pathologic gas (pneumothorax) can yield O-lines

artifacts (the B-lines) give hyperechoic patterns, up to a completely white diffuse Merlin's space (the Birolleau variant; see Fig. 12.6). We conclude that fluids, traditionally described as anechoic, yield hyperechoic tone, when they are minute and surrounded by gas. We also conclude that the natural tone of the pure air is, in the ultrasound world, the *dark*.

Note

The A-line is the normal artifact, yet it is also one of the signs of pneumothorax. What should be understood is that A-lines indicate air, either quasi-pure (normal lung surface) or pure (pneumothorax). The air of the ICU room, when the probe is on its stand, generates a kind of horizontal lines, the H-lines (see Fig. 40.2). Air yields horizontal lines.

Other Artifacts

The main other artifact is the vertical B-line. Its description raises a didactic issue: it is pathological but some locations are found at the normal lung. See Chap. 12, normal variants of the B-lines.

Some History

The first official mention of the label "A-lines" was made in 1997 [1].

Reference

1. Lichtenstein D. L'échographie pulmonaire: une méthode d'avenir en médecine d'urgence et de réanimation? Revue de Pneumologie Clinique. 1997;53:63–8.

The A-Profile (Normal Lung Surface): 2) Lung Sliding

10

In workshops, the lung sliding of healthy models is rather easy to study. In the critically ill, because either exacerbated but parasited by severe dyspneas or made too subtle by deep sedations, its study needs the consideration of adapted signs.

The normal lung surface is defined by the association of A-lines and lung sliding. At the anterior chest wall in a supine patient, this is the A-profile.

Detecting lung sliding is the first step of the BLUE protocol. Lung sliding is a physiological phenomenon that anyone can easily detect using appropriate tools. In the critically ill, because either dyspneic or ventilated, different phenomena occur. For describing them scientifically, several points must be specified, and this deserves a full chapter.

Like any vital organ, the lung moves from our birth to our death without interruption. Lung sliding is a kind of dynamic (sparkling, twinkling, glittering, shimmering, and "ant's walk" are suitable terms too) arising from the pleural line (Fig. 10.1, Video 10.1). The pleural line is built by two layers: the parietal pleura, always motionless, and the visceral pleura, only when the lung is at the chest wall, moving or not. The sliding of the visceral pleura against the parietal pleura creates this sparkling at the pleural line.

Lung sliding indicates that, first, the lung is at the chest wall and, second, this lung works.

"Lung sliding" is a euphonic locution; read Anecdotal note 1.

Our 5 MHz microconvex probe is ideal for this part of lung investigation. Using our technique (which can be summarized as withdrawing any kind of filter), it makes a work similar (if not superior) to the usual vascular probes advocated by some.

Lung Sliding: A New Sign, a New Entity in the Respiratory Semiology

Lung sliding indicates a physiological reality, the descent of the lung toward the abdomen. Is it a valuable sign? How to assess it? Not clinically of course; we don't benefit from any specific sign from the father of lung semiology [1]. So with what? Fluoroscopy? It is a too imperfect tool. Lung sliding should be considered as a new sign which speaks for itself and does not need any gold standard. Those who denied the reality of lung ultrasound were maybe in lack of a gold standard [2]. Some would have appreciated a tool allowing to better understand the lung physiology [3].

Electronic supplementary material The online version of this chapter (doi:10.1007/978-3-319-15371-1_10) contains supplementary material, which is available to authorized users.

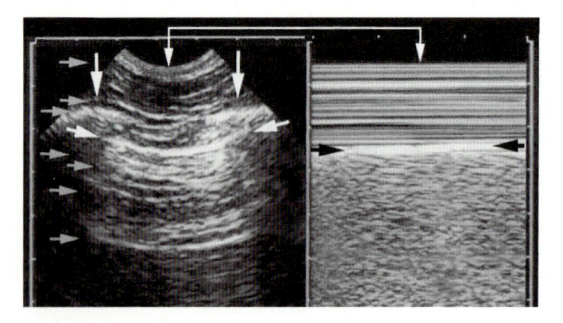

Fig. 10.1 The seashore sign. This figure is the continuation of Fig. 8.1 and Fig. 9.1, provided without any *arrow*. The present figure is crowded with *arrows*. *Left*, real-time image. The simple (isolated) *vertical arrows* show the ribs. The *white horizontal arrows* show the pleural line, clearly defined by the bat sign. Gray *horizontal arrows* show some of the numerous horizontal lines which should not be confused with the pleural line. They indicate, from *top to bottom*, the skin, some aponeuroses, a rib, minor air reflections below the pleural line called sub-A-lines (see Fig. 40.4), and (*lower gray arrow*) an A-line. Right: M-mode. A marked change appears between Keye's space, here "quiet" above the *black arrows*, and the space below, called M-Merlin's space or again MM-space. The *black arrows* indicate precisely the pleural line, with no space for confusion. Look at the upper coupled, vertical white arrows, indicating how finely real time and M-mode are tuned together: this allows immediate location of the pleural line in any circumstance, a critical point in extreme emergencies. Compare with Fig. 10.5. Keye's space displays something like quiet waves. The space below (MM-space) shows a homogeneous, sandy pattern, generated by the lung when sliding against the chest wall. This is the seashore sign. No need for video, this figure allows to identify a lung sliding without any confusion

Since when is ultrasound able to detect this fine movement? From our eyes, since at least 1982, but it is obvious that the antique, pantographic systems of the 1960s were able to demonstrate this dynamic, using M-mode.

Normal Lung Sliding in the Healthy Subject, a Relative Dynamic: The Seashore Sign

The lung works like a craniocaudal piston. Lung sliding is more easy to detect using longitudinal scans; this is one of the reasons why we advise them.

We now define lung sliding as a homogeneous sparkling of the whole of the Merlin's space, i.e., beginning at the very pleural line, not one mm above, not one mm below. This dynamic is relative, a critical notion since a diffuse dynamic of the whole image is unavoidable. First, the patient as well as the doctor are still alive, both generating minute movements. Second, there is a minute background noise. Yet these dynamics are diffuse, whereas lung sliding begins at the very pleural line. The M-mode appears to be insensitive to the background noise; this is why it displays a sandy pattern exactly at and below the pleural line. We called this pattern the seashore sign (Fig. 10.1). The use of the M-mode perfectly highlights the relativity between lung sliding and motionless wall.

The M-mode is useful for understanding lung sliding. The whole of Merlin's space twinkles, creating this seashore sign. The physicians able to interpret a posteriori a frozen M-mode image prove that they master lung ultrasound. They won't need videos. Yet one point is of prime importance: the operator's eye should recognize lung sliding through a real-time image *before using* M-mode. This must be a habit. One main reason is explained in the SESAME-protocol (cardiac arrest), where there is no time for starting the M-mode.

The M-mode is practical for data recording; it is easier to insert an image in a medical file. In the LUCIFLR project, one image is taken after any thoracic procedure and must show the bat sign at the left, the seashore sign at the right, and a mention where it was taken (e.g., upper BLUE-point, supine patient): this replaces (to advantage!) the chest radiography (Chap. 29).

Lung sliding is suppressed by many conditions (listed in Table 14.1). Apart from them, it is present in eupnea and dyspnea, in spontaneous as well as conventional mechanical ventilation. It is visible in skinny and bariatric patients (see Fig. 33.3). It is present in bronchial emphysema. In giant emphysema bulla, in our observations, a minute lung sliding (or equivalents, see below) is usually detected. Lung sliding is visible at any age, from the first second of extrauterine life to the dying breath.

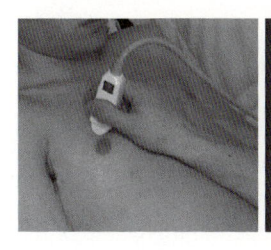

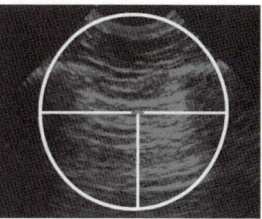

Fig. 10.2 Mastery of dynamics. As far as possible (setting permitting), the hand of the operator must be completely motionless and be able to wait for hours, without moving and without fatigue, like a *sniper*. Nonsteady hand is a key for failure. Only the patient is expected to move

Lung Sliding, Also a Subtle Sign Which Can Be Destroyed by Inappropriate Filters or So-Called Facilities. The Importance of Mastering Dynamics and Bypassing These Facilities

Simple clues will optimize the analysis of lung sliding. We face a dynamic feature. Therefore, the physician must control the dynamic dimension, i.e., suppressing, or understanding, all other dynamics.

1. A dynamic coming from the physician must be suppressed by any means.

    Only the patient is allowed to move. The operator's hand must be fully standstill (Fig. 10.2). Our small microconvex probe, easy to handle like a pen, favors this standstillness. Ecolight is a non-slippery product, and energy devoted for keeping the probe stable is spared. Once the operator gets the best image of the bat sign, he/she stops any movement and "quietly" watches at the pleural line, like a *sniper* (see again Fig. 1.1).

2. A dynamic impaired by filters must be recognized by any means, and these filters must be suppressed.

    All factors making lung ultrasound more difficult must be destroyed. The problem is simple: they have conceived sophisticated programs which slightly improve tissular imaging (a minor benefit for us) and deeply worsen lung imaging, the most critical. See the sections below, widely dealing with this issue.

3. A dynamic created by the critically ill patient, either exacerbated by dyspnea or decreased by mechanical ventilation.

    This dynamic cannot be suppressed; one must work with it. It will generate difficulties. These difficulties will be mastered. This also deserves a special section.

The Various Degrees of Lung Sliding, Considering Caricaturally Opposed States

Lung sliding is naturally weaker at the apex, a kind of starting block. Lung sliding is naturally weaker in quiet ventilation. We can therefore imagine two situations: Studying the lower BLUE-point of a hyperventilating, dyspneic patient will show a frank lung sliding but associated with parasite noise. Studying the upper BLUE-point of a deeply sedated patient will not show any parasite dynamic but will show an extremely weak lung sliding.

Note: one can be very dyspneic on mechanical ventilation.

For mastering lung sliding in these extreme, but daily, situations, we should master the real-time/M-mode harmony, as well as all filters. This proves highly useful when there is too much dynamic or not enough dynamic.

For making all this clear, we will ask a healthy volunteer to show us various degrees of breathing. These experiments will be done just for simplifying the concept, but the whole of the observations can be found in our critically ill patients.

Lung Sliding in the Dyspneic Patient. The Maximal Type. Critical Notions Regarding the Mastery of the B/M-Mode

A severe dyspnea generates uncontrolled movements of the patient, at the highest degree of anxiety. This patient tries to survive by any means, futile such as opening the window, useful such as recruiting the accessory respiratory muscles.

Observing the fine dynamic of lung sliding in such a "messy" environment may appear challenging, an equivalent of *shooting from a mobile point toward a mobile target*, obeying to the hectic rules of dogfights. All patients of the BLUE-protocol had a severe dyspnea, generating a parasite dynamic *above* the pleural line that we called muscular sliding on real time. Users may be unable to locate whether the dynamic comes from the pleural line or above. Here, the M-mode has a critical relevance. The rules of lung ultrasound make no space for approximation: a "sand" arising above the pleural line, even a few mm above, does not come from the lung. Any sandy phenomenon which arises above the pleural line cannot be labeled a "seashore sign."

Dyspnea and the Keyes' Sign

Take our healthy volunteer and lock him up in a confined room. You create a "pure" dyspnea (on healthy lungs) which gradually worsens (Technical note 1). Then analyze the lower BLUE-point or more caudal, where lung amplitude is maximal. Such a dyspnea will create two conflicting dynamics (apart from the body agitation due to uncontrolled anxiety).

A. The dyspnea creates an increase of the tidal volume. The amplitude of lung sliding is increased, resulting in a marked seashore sign.
B. The dyspnea recruits accessory muscles. This generates perturbations above the pleural line.

The real time (bat sign) locates the pleural line in any circumstances, allowing to define Keye's space on M-mode. A Keye space full of accidents instead of the regular stratified image has the meaning of a severe dyspnea and was coined Keye's sign (Fig. 10.3) (Video 10.2). Keyes' sign describes with no space for confusion these parasite dynamic phenomena occurring above the pleural line. And now, we have all elements for defining the seashore sign. The seashore must arise from the pleural line, always, i.e., the lower limit of Keye's space (defined using real time first, reminder).

For recognizing a lung sliding within Keye's sign and getting rid of any trouble, we use several successive approaches.

1. The first to do is to focus on the real-time image. Some patterns are disturbing when seen only on M-mode, especially when there is a permanent Keye's sand (we called them the Nogué-Armandariz sign, from spanish Ceurfers), but can be much easier to analyze on real time, allowing often to distinguish the muscular sliding from the lung sliding. Think "M like Moderate."
2. If the first approach does not work, sometimes muscular sliding and lung sliding are not perfectly synchronized. This makes transitory but sufficient instants where the seashore sign can be recognized, distinct from stratospheric pattern above (Fig. 10.3). These subtle signs remind how ventricular tachycardia is diagnosed (Anecdotal note 2).
3. If the first two approaches do not work, we use a sign not yet labeled (it is in actual fact the

Dyspnea and the Keyes' Sign

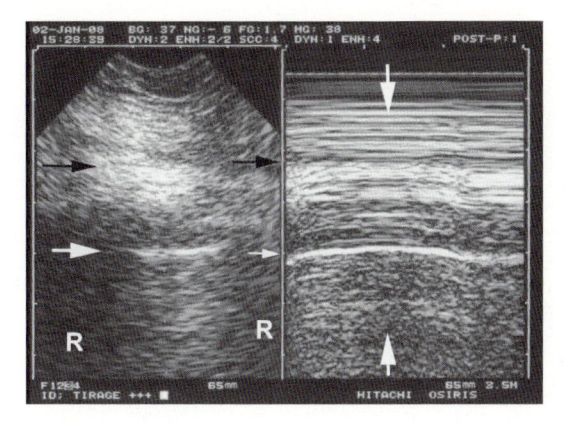

Fig. 10.3 Dyspnea and Keye's sign. *Left*, real time. The *black arrow* shows an intermuscular aponeurosis. The *white arrow* shows the pleural line. *R*, shadow of ribs. *Right*, M-mode. This image may appear as a stormy sea. The muscular contraction (indicating major dyspnea) has generated a sandy pattern beginning (*from top*) at the area of the *black horizontal arrow*, i.e., above the pleural line. Is this dyspnea due to a pneumothorax? The vertical white arrows (inserted at a distance of the event) clearly display an area of typical seashore sign with a short zone of preserved Keye's space. This is sufficient. The diagnosis of pneumothorax can be excluded. This 55-year-old lady suffered from a severe asthma. The location of the real-time and M-mode images at the same horizontal level makes easy the distinction between pleural line and muscular lines – in time-dependent settings. Would such an area not be displayed, subtle eyes may observe a fine change when the column of sand arising from the horizontal *black arrow* crosses the pleural line at the *horizontal white arrow*: this pattern is opposed to Avicenne's sign described in Chap. 14. Here, lung sliding has been identified as present

opposite of Avicenne's sign, described in Chap. 14 and demonstrating how an abolished lung sliding can anyway be detected). It requires full understanding of Keye's space. When the column of sand from above the pleural line (the dyspnea) undergoes a change, even slight, when crossing the pleural line, it is possible to affirm that lung sliding is present (Fig. 10.3).

Note (this can help) that the "sand" of the Keyes' sign is a bit different from the seashore sign of lung sliding. It is stretched, not as punctiform as the genuine seashore sign.

Confusing Configurations

We wrote in Chap. 8 that correctly designed machines locate the real-time and M-mode images exactly side by side. Not "side by side." *Exactly* side by side. Now an issue has to be known. Most laptop machines, from cheap to costly, display the M-mode with a lag when compared to the real-time image. This will prevent to locate immediately the pleural line with confidence in acute situations, when stress does not help.

We see two options. In one, the real-time image comes upstairs, small, with a large M-mode image downstairs; one must extrapolate, with haste, where the real pleural line is (Fig. 10.4). In another, both images are displayed apparently side by side, but not *exactly* side by side (Fig. 10.5). The perfect configuration we had in our 1982 ADR-4000 and our 1992 Hitachi 405, which both display both images exactly side by side, with no space for confusion, was not used again by the modern manufacturers, who, for incomprehensible reasons, display a gap, a lag. And nothing to rectify it. This lag corresponds roughly, bad luck, to the thickness of the intercostal muscle or more. The consequences are dealt with in Chap. 14. The operator must guess the pleural line location with extreme haste (when there is no time for guesses) or, worse, risks to believe that the right image corresponds to the left one. Therefore, the unexperienced operator will think that the

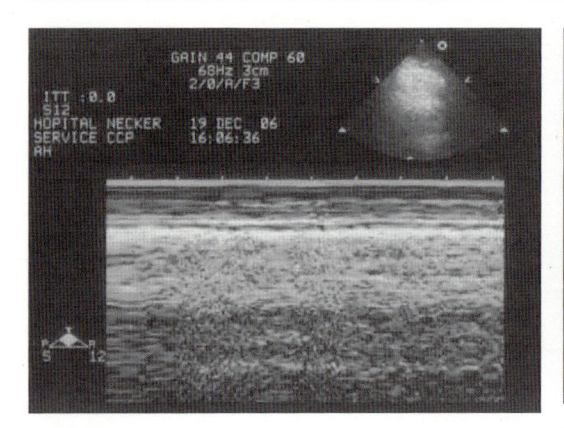

Fig. 10.4 One configuration of M-mode. Example of a nonsuitable setting for lung ultrasound. The image quality of the upper image prevents from locating the pleural line with accuracy (cardiac probe). Since the real-time image is not located at the left of the M-mode image, the pleural line cannot be rapidly and confidently located; the user must guess or extrapolate. The "seashore" pattern comes maybe from the pleural line, maybe from a more superficial structure. Please see Fig. 10.5, even more pernicious. Lung sliding in a ventilated neonate

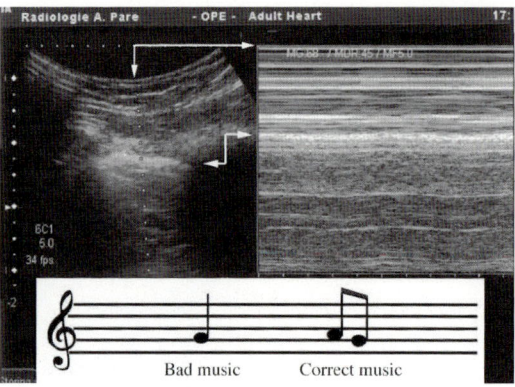

Fig. 10.5 M-mode and a wrong note. The *arrows* indicate the misconception. In very widespread machines, for unknown reasons, real time and M-mode are not exactly side by side (compare with Fig. 10.1). By bad providence, the lag corresponds to the intercostal muscle. In dyspneic patients, "sand" can be displayed from this level, i.e., above the pleural line. This will make more complex a diagnosis (pneumothorax) which asks to be, and is, simple – yet lung ultrasound does not need superimposed complexity. Here, more than in Fig. 10.1, young users can be fooled. At the bottom is a musical score. The left note is ill defined, and the composer's intentions are unclear. The notes at the right are perfectly defined; anyone can play them

M-mode pleural line is this line at the level of the real-time pleural line; confusing the pleura with an aponeurosis will confuse the sand arising above the pleural line with a lung sliding, conclude "lung sliding present," and miss the pneumothorax.

This configuration where both images are roughly but not exactly side by side is the worst.

These concepts are not suitable for optimal lung ultrasound. They have been built by manufacturers unaware of the existence of lung ultrasound. This adds complexity in a field which is simple but not that simple, so let's not add more. Look at the musical notes of Fig. 10.5.

This is not the last surprise. Some 2014 machines coming from self-proclaimed leaders in critical ultrasound display the M-mode at the detriment of the real time: once the M-mode is activated, the real-time image is frozen. The operator suddenly flies in the fog and loses control of lung ultrasound.

One last pitfall: beginning by M-mode (first mistake) and for no reason increasing the gain.

These wrong notes are easy to avoid (read Technical note 2).

Lung Sliding in the Ventilated Patient. The Minimal Type. Critical Notions Regarding the Mastery of the Filters

Take our healthy volunteer out of the confined room once the first demonstration is done, and now intubate him, sedate him deeply, curarize him, and apply a low tidal volume and a low frequency. You create a quiet bradypnea. Then analyze the upper BLUE-point (or more cephalad), where the lung sliding amplitude is naturally minimal.

In these pure conditions, Keye's space is absolutely homogeneous, without any sign of dyspnea, but lung sliding will appear very discrete and quite abolished. Lung ultrasound is a standardized field. For facing this apparent issue, we have to describe the variants of minimal lung sliding. First understand that *the slightest filter, in this setting, will completely obliterate a minimal lung sliding.*

The up-to-date, sophisticated machines are rich in facilities which can deeply impair the detection of minimal lung sliding. Some have disastrous effects on this subtle dynamics (Video 10.3). All filters must be disactivated. Take major care on this. Any filter attacking time is not compatible with critical ultrasound. The "instant response" technology was available in 1978. In most up-to-date machines, the computer works on the image before restoring it, hence an irreversible mode which creates a *time lag*, a destructive mode which is not compatible with a real-time discipline where every tenth of a second makes the difference for understanding the disease. Lung ultrasound requires natural images, showing the dynamic and the artifacts.

The less the filters, the easiest is lung ultrasound. The persistence filter, average filter, temporal averaging, dynamic noise filter, summation filter, etc., make lung ultrasound more difficult. Average filters give a soft image, nice to look at, at the very detriment of the dynamic (Video 10.3). Repeat: these filters yield flattering images, which mask the true content, like a makeup. Precisely, we want to see the wrinkles.

Compound, harmonics seem to be a powerful destructor of LUCI.

Now that this technical moment is over, we describe variants more or less intricated that we can also simplify in one sentence: "The slightest phenomenon arising at the pleural line and spreading below mean that the pleural line includes not only the parietal but also the visceral pleura."

Some maneuvers can help. Sometimes, decreasing the gain makes more visible a discrete lung sliding. Sometimes, lung sliding is more visible just near the ribs than at the middle of the pleural line (the Mezière sign).

Very importantly, there is an interdependency between lung sliding and lung artifacts: when Merlin's space displays B-lines (not yet

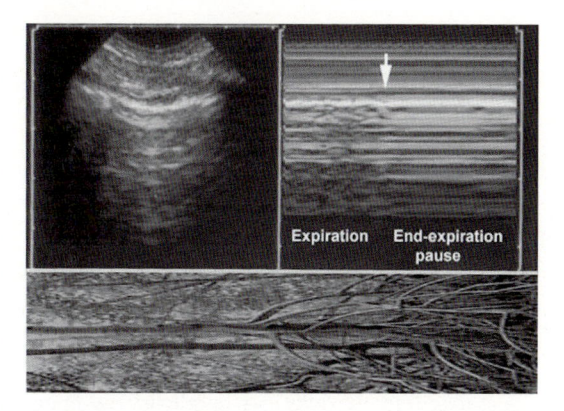

Fig. 10.6 The mangrove variant. *Left*, real time showing a pleural line with A-lines (example here of ill-defined A-lines). *Right*, M-mode showing a soft interruption of the sand yielding a regular horizontal pattern at the MM-space. This interruption is progressive (see Fig. 14.6 for comparison). This looks like aerial roots of mangrove trees (*bottom image*, horizontalized). The message is: don't press the M button if not necessary

described, hence a didactic challenge), those vertical artifacts move like pendulums, and this greatly helps in detecting a minimal lung sliding. When they are absent, replaced by A-lines, the challenge is to recognize the minimal lung sliding. A-lines and B-lines are a function of the underlying disease (pulmonary edema, COPD, etc.). Mainly, the mastery of the filters and wise use of the M-mode will demonstrate the extreme variants of minimal lung sliding.

Let us describe three kinds.

Variant 1: The Mangrove Variant
(Fig. 10.6)

The respiration is not a permanent dynamic; there are pauses. These physiological end-inspiratory and end-expiratory pauses are enhanced in sedated patients. These pauses generate a brief interruption (therefore, usually not seen in polypneic patients). On real time, the lung sliding quietly stops. On M-mode, the sandy pattern of lung sliding is transiently replaced by a regular horizontal pattern evoking a "stratosphere sign" (this makes a didactic challenge, since this pattern, evoking pneumothorax, will be detailed in the Chap. 14). This pattern, called mangrove variant (Anecdotal note 3), may be confused by young users with a lung point, i.e., a main sign of pneumothorax (Chap. 14 again). We must devote some lines for smashing this problem to smithereens.

1. First, the mangrove variant is a progressive phenomenon. Lung sliding is detected on real time. It quietly comes, stops, goes, stops, comes, etc. It does not suddenly disappear (like the lung point in pneumothorax). If beginning with the real time, there is no trouble. The mangrove variant is built by the use of M-mode. M-mode should not be used for *confirming* a lung sliding which has already been detected using the real time. This is one perverse effect of an immoderate use of the M-mode.
2. Second, the lung point should be sought for only if pneumothorax is suspected, i.e., in the case of anterior absence of lung sliding associated with exclusive A-lines (described as the A'-profile in Chap. 14). The mangrove variant occurs at the entire lung surface, including the anterior parasternal areas. In other words, the only confusion should be, if any, with a limited, parasternal, clinically insignificant pneumothorax. The visualization, more laterally and on the whole lung surface, of the strictly identical pattern avoids any confusion.

Variant 2: The Pseudo-A'-Profile

This label represents a daily reality seen on normal lungs (normal lung surface, better) in deeply sedated patients. It designates an apparently abolished lung sliding, which may, if associated with A-lines, suggest pneumothorax (Chap. 14). There is quite always one of these subtle signs, subtle but standardizable. We describe the lung pulse, the grain of sand variant, and the T-lines, which are roughly the same entity with some subtleties.

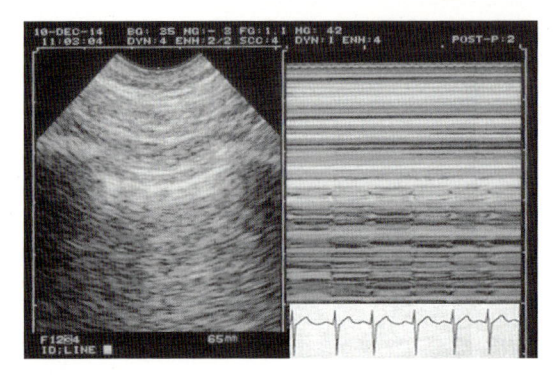

Fig. 10.7 The lung pulse. In this case of complete and recent atelectasis, lung sliding is abolished. Merlin's space displays O-lines (i.e., A-lines). Pneumothorax? Impossible: vibrations in rhythm with the heart activity are seen in real time, stopping at (or arising from) the pleural line. They can be recorded in M-mode (*q waves of ECG*). Patient probably on mechanical ventilation (quiet Keye's space in spite of this disorder)

The Lung Pulse

Take again our volunteer, still deeply sedated and curarized. Give him a normal tidal volume, a normal frequency, let us analyze the left lower BLUE-point, i.e., near the heart, all conditions for improving the detection of a lung sliding. There is a cardiac activity, but it is not visible as far as it is masked by the lung activity. Now, suddenly disconnect the endotracheal tube. We can observe an immediate abolition of lung sliding, which allows the heart to express its beatings through a motionless parenchymateous cushion. This generates a kind of vibration arising from (in actual fact, stopping at) the pleural line, in rhythm with heartbeats, visible in real time, recordable in M-mode: the lung pulse (Fig. 10.7, Video 10.4).

The lung pulse can be discrete. It is sometimes absent, maybe (not always) when the heart is too far (right lung) or if the heartbeats are too weak. Maybe the lung pulse is a sign of good cardiac function.

This variant of lung activity indicates a disease (loss of lung compliance, including atelectasis) but also an absence of disease (the visceral pleura is well attached, i.e., there is no pneumothorax).

The lung pulse rules out pneumothorax. In order to simplify medicine, we can avoid the

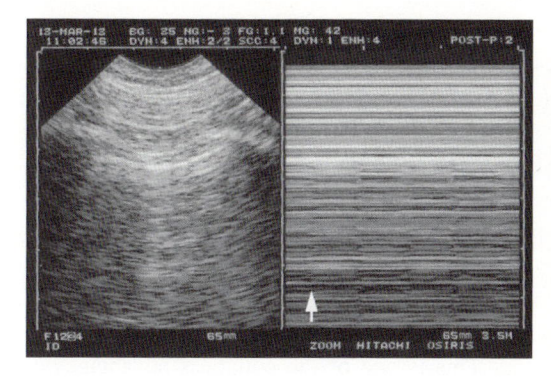

Lung Sliding in the Ventilated Patient. The Minimal Type. Critical Notions Regarding the Mastery   75

Fig. 10.8 An extreme variant of T-lines. An example of pseudo-A'-profile with the T-line. *To the left*, a short A-line. *To the right*, this very subtle lung activity, materialized by these T-lines (each looks like a "T"), stopping *exactly* at the pleural line. No pneumothorax here again. Just one arrow is inserted at the foot of the first T-line, for not spoiling this subtle image. Four T-lines are identified in the MM-space. This old patient had a large emphysematous bulla and respiratory discomfort, but the pneumothorax could be ruled out. Some antibiotics and physiotherapy solved the problem. Minor note, T-lines have nothing to do with B-lines (the T-line is an M-mode concept, the B-line a real-time image)

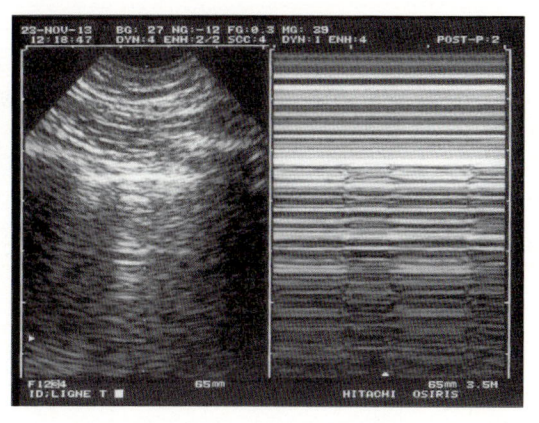

Fig. 10.9 A variant of lung sliding. This variant may be labeled the "bandoneon sign." The meaning is unchanged: no pneumothorax. Note to the left (real-time) a beautiful Z-line (see Chap. 11)

The T-Line

This is an extreme variant, shaping more or less the letter "T," starting exactly from the pleural line (Fig. 10.8). See also Fig. 8.3. Following the rule expressed above, the slightest T-line rules out pneumothorax. There are probably several ways for the T-lines to be displayed (Fig. 10.9).

Lung Sliding Abolished with One or Two B-Lines

These B-lines (see Chap. 11) are usually sufficient for demonstrating the presence of the visceral pleura against the parietal pleura. Note: with not one, not two, but three B-lines (or more), the pattern would be the "B'-profile"; see Chap. 13.

Variant 3: The A'-Profile

This profile, which is also the first main sign of pneumothorax, fully described in Chap. 14, combines complete abolition of lung sliding, complete absence of equivalents (lung pulse, T-line, etc.), and exclusive A-lines (which implies complete absence of B-line; see next chapters). Since medicine is medicine, in some cases, patients without pneumothorax can exhibit a genuine A'-profile (Video 10.5). We can explain it by considering an absence of lung expansion for any reason (see above) associated with complete

reading of long articles positioning the "lung pulse" at the end of long decision trees (lung sliding absent, then B-lines absent, then lung point absent, then lung pulse present = no pneumothorax). Please just consider that we can simply write: "lung sliding, or any equivalent such as the lung pulse" at the begin of the decision tree.

The impaired lung expansion is seen mainly in complete atelectasis (including one lung intubation, foreign body aspiration, lung exclusion in thoracic surgery, etc.), acute pleural symphysis (often seen in ARDS), chronic conditions (pleural sequelae), simple apnea, and expiratory pause, a.m.o. The lung pulse as a sign of atelectasis is detailed in the corresponding section in Chap. 35.

The Grain of Sand Variant

When lung sliding is extremely discrete, the seashore sign can be restricted to the visualization of some sand (we made previous comparisons with a termitarium). In these cases, detecting even a few grains of sand, provided they stop exactly at the pleural line, is enough for considering that the lung is at the chest wall.

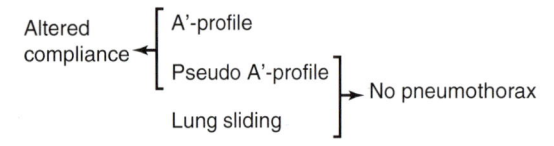

```
Altered      ┌ A'-profile        ┐
compliance ←─┤ Pseudo A'-profile ├─→ No pneumothorax
             └ Lung sliding      ┘
```

Fig. 10.10 Double dichotomy. The double dichotomy of lung sliding. Present or quite abolished, it rules out pneumothorax. Quite abolished or abolished, it indicates a major impairment of lung compliance

absence of interstitial syndrome or lung fissure and without any perception of heartbeats. One message: the A'-profile is not sufficient for the diagnosis of pneumothorax (See Table 14.1).

Lung Sliding: Three Degrees, but a Dichotomous Sign Anyway

Some users complain that the familiar dichotomy which defines lung ultrasound is not respected here.

It is. There are simply two levels of dichotomy (Fig. 10.10).

1. When the question is "pneumothorax," the completely abolished lung sliding is opposed to all other variants (normal lung sliding and all kinds of minimal lung sliding), which clearly rule out pneumothorax. Very discrete or abolished lung sliding makes a big clinical distinction.
2. When the question is "impaired lung compliance," an abolished or very discrete lung sliding is pathologic, as opposed to ample lung sliding. Very discrete or abolished lung sliding make no clinical difference. Lung sliding is decreased in several processes in the critically ill, mainly ARDS (See Table 14.1).

Can One Quantify Lung Sliding?

Absolutely, this is specified in Chap. 28.

Here and briefly, at the lower BLUE-point, a normal lung sliding covers the distance of the pleural line, i.e., roughly, 2 cm.

One word on the B-lines (next chapters). When they are present, using our probe and its sectorial image, they move like pendulums. This phenomenon amplifies the dynamics of lung sliding. This is one of the countless advantages of our microconvex probe.

At an advanced level, the user will identify "ample lung sliding," "weak lung sliding," and "absent lung sliding" – as easily as distinguishing an awake person, a sleeping person, and a corpse. The real A'-profile looks like a deadly standstillness.

How About Our Healthy Volunteer?

We have to thank him and apologize for the hard manipulations we made on him. After that, if you have difficulties to find a next enthusiastic one willing to undergo the same delights, don't worry: just ask any new volunteer to breathe deeper and deeper, up to recruiting accessory muscles (deep breathe through one nostril), then very slowly, then halt breathing. You reproduce all these patterns at will – and this should be done in all these workshops. Some academicians are sorry that the attendees of courses can feel a little frustrated not to see a lot of diseases there ("n'ont pas leur biscuit," according to the French words). Healthy models can express a lot of LUCI. See Chap. 38 on training.

Technical Notes

1. *Dyspnea and lung sliding*

    We created here a dyspnea on healthy lungs, for simplifying. Apart from pneumothorax, various diseases impair lung sliding (this is detailed through the textbook).

2. *Suboptimal control of the gain*

    If an operator for no reason increases the gain too much and looks at the M-mode before the real time (double mistake), the far field will be polluted by a background noise, looking from very far like a seashore sign. This pattern, called the Peyrouset phenomenon (our fellow, who witnessed it), is not a serious pitfall:

    a. The sand of the Peyrouset phenomenon is not punctiform like the seashore sign but rather micropunctiform.

    b. This sand progressively fades, whereas the sandy pattern of the seashore sign stops at the very location of the pleural line.

    c. The M-mode should not have a diagnostic interest except specific situations (objectifying minimal or maximal lung sliding). It should usually be used only for keeping a document showing on paper *what was actually seen on real time*. Lung sliding is detected using real time. In no case will the Peyrouset phenomenon give the illusion of a lung sliding in a patient with a pneumothorax if one cares among others in focusing on the real-time image.

    Figure 10.11 gives clues that allow easy distinction from a genuine seashore sign.

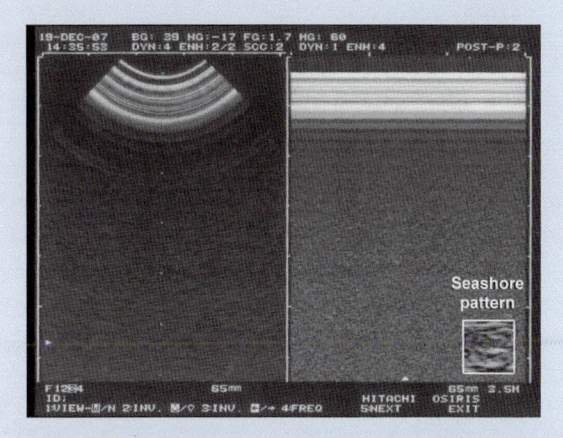

Fig. 10.11 The Peyrouset phenomenon, a side effect of excessive gain. *The left image* indicates the air of the ICU room – the probe is still on its stand. What is visible here is an air acoustic barrier. These roughly horizontal artifacts, called H-lines, are described in Chap. 40. To the right, on M-mode, the gain was (for no reason) too much increased, and a noise appears. We can see two major differences with the seashore sign. (1) The "sand" is microscopic (compare with standard seashore sign, in the white cartouche). (2) The sand density increases toward the bottom of the screen, progressively, without sudden change (whereas the seashore sign has a millimetric limit, precisely at the pleural line). To see displayed the (ill-defined) top of this parasite noise at the very level of the pleural line would really be bad luck. Don't press the M button if not necessary

Anecdotal Notes

1. *Euphonic note on lung sliding*

    Lung sliding, sliding lung, is easy to pronounce (and if we may allow, rather elegant). "Pleural sliding" and "pleural gliding" are more difficult (even for native English speakers) and longer, for no advantage. The "gliding sign," the worst, confuses with the pericardium, peritoneum, eyeball, and any muscle, all "gliding" structures. As to "seashore sign," the term "beach" sign, sometimes heard, is maybe a little short for such a precious application, with in addition the risk of ill-defined spelling generating more trite words.

2. *Note about ventricular tachycardia*

    The diagnosis is based on ECG on fleeting visualizations of fusion or capture complexes, quite exactly the same logic.

3. *The mangrove variant*

    The mangrove sign was conceived during a CEURF training program in a Pacific area full of mangrove (Neo Caledonia, 2004). The stretched aerial roots of these mangrove trees were reminder of the sand of the mangrove variant.

References

1. Laënnec RTH (1819) Traité de l'auscultation médiate, ou traité du diagnostic des maladies des poumons et du cœur. Paris/New York: J.A. Brosson & J.S. Chaudé/Hafner 1962, p. 127.
2. Weinberger SE, Drazen JM. Diagnostic procedures in respiratory diseases. In: Kasper DL, editor. Harrison's principles of internal medicine. 16th ed. New York: McGraw-Hill; 2005. p. 1505–8.
3. West BJ. Tests of pulmonary function. How respiratory physiology is applied to measure lung function. In: West BJ, editor. Respiratory physiology. The essentials. 9th ed. Philadelphia/Baltimore: Wolters Kluwer/Lippincott Williams & Wilkins; 2012. p. 159–72.

Interstitial Syndrome and the BLUE-Protocol: The B-Line

11

Nothing is banal with lung ultrasound in the critically ill. It requires the simplest machines, one ideal probe also suitable for the whole body, and only two signs for mastering the normal pattern of this organ which is the most voluminous and the most vital one. This is the paradox of lung ultrasound, again.

Interstitial syndrome does not escape this rule. If lung ultrasound is a raison d'être of critical ultrasound, the potential of interstitial syndrome is a raison d'être of lung ultrasound. Based on the artifacts' analysis, it changes the approach to the critically ill. The mastery of interstitial syndrome will be used in no less than 15 disciplines (Chap. 33).

One may wonder whether lung ultrasound is feasible and above all how infra-millimetric structures lost in all this gas could be detected. The artifacts are usually considered as undesirable [1, 2]. The potential of the diagnosis of interstitial syndrome, heralded since 1994 [3], more specified in 1997 [4], may surprise novice readers. One must very schematically see first *how* to detect it using ultrasound, then *why* to detect it. This chapter will simply describe the elementary note of this entity.

Our 5 MHz microconvex probe is perfect for this part of lung investigation.

A Preliminary Definition: What Should Be Understood by "Interstitial Syndrome"?

The radiologists often question the notion of ultrasound diagnosis of interstitial syndrome since this term involves many conditions and they are accustomed to high-resolution CT. Those who have heard about lung rockets argue that this sign is not specific, but they mean for distinguishing, for example, histiocytosis X from sarcoidosis. This is the typical misconception which can occur in medicine when a tool is not in the right hands. In the critically ill, the interstitial syndrome is limited to acute phenomena: nearly always pulmonary edema, either hemodynamic or permeability induced. Hemodynamic pulmonary edema includes fluid overload and cardiogenic pulmonary edema. Permeability-induced edema includes ARDS and any inflammatory syndromes surrounding infectious processes (bacterial, viral, etc.). Even in the rare cases of chronic interstitial syndrome seen in acute settings, the intensivist has tools for this diagnosis; see Chap. 35.

Electronic supplementary material The online version of this chapter (doi:10.1007/978-3-319-15371-1_11) contains supplementary material, which is available to authorized users.

The Usual Tools for Diagnosing Interstitial Syndrome

Before assessing the utility of interstitial syndrome, we must consider that this diagnosis is *not accessible* in acute situations using usual tools.

The auscultation? Two centuries old [5], it does not provide any sign of interstitial syndrome to our knowledge.

The bedside radiography? More than one century old [6], it rarely demonstrates interstitial changes in critical settings. It shows rough alveolar-interstitial patterns, but rarely the Kerley lines. Even in a good-quality radiograph taken in an ambulatory patient, this diagnosis is fragile: an imaging specialist can make different interpretations from one day to another [7].

CT? It has been available since the 1980s [8]. It can maybe describe interstitial patterns, but referring critically ill patients to this heavy technique for this diagnosis *alone* would be really questionable. What more is experience showed us that standard CT inconstantly demonstrates subtle interstitial changes.

Therefore, maybe for a lack of easy-to-access diagnosis, the intensivist has invested little for knowing whether this patient has, or not, interstitial syndrome: he or she never integrated this disorder in the medical thought process and got accustomed to do without, not aware of what could be done with, it.

Elementary Sign of Interstitial Syndrome, the B-Line

The B-line was coined using alphabetic order. It was even elegantly called "BLUE-line" by a colleague in Bangalore (Dr. Gana without mistake), which may result in a new term with the advantage of decreasing the effort of memory (BLUE speaks more than B – the very principle of SLAM (Anecdotal Note 1)).

The "BLUE-line" or, say for the moment, the B-line is a *hydro-aeric artifact*, indicating a mingling of fluid and air and whose definition has been updated from article to article (Anecdotal Note 2). The most recent definition is given in this book (this was one reason among others to build this new edition, paradoxically faster than trying to submit 1000 manuscripts).

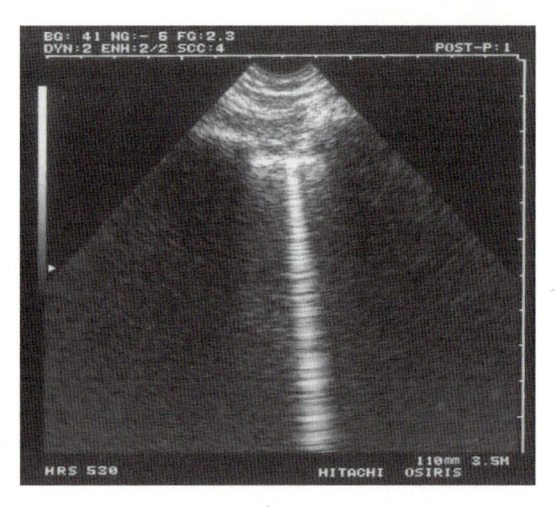

Fig. 11.1 An elementary B-line. We identify the ribs, the pleural line. From the pleural line arises a strong formation, having all criteria of the B-line (but the dynamic one, not displayed in this static view): comet-tail artifact, arising from the pleural line, well-defined, long, erasing A-lines, hyperechoic

The B-line is an artifact having seven characteristic features (Fig. 11.1). Three are constant and four almost constant.

Constant features:

1. This is a comet-tail artifact, always.
2. It arises from the pleural line, always.
3. It moves with lung sliding, always.

Almost constant features (93–97 %):

4. Almost always, it is well defined, laser-like.
5. Almost always, it is long, spreading out without fading to the edge of the screen.
6. Almost always, it obliterates the A-lines.
7. Almost always, it is hyperechoic.

This updated, standardized, comprehensive definition allows immediate distinction with any other artifact that can be seen in the human being, mainly E-lines and Z-lines (see below). The risk of confusion is decreased by a factor 10 (even more) for each added criterium (*read* Anecdotal Note 3). Here is how to understand this concept. A comet-tail artifact that arises from the pleural line can be a B-line or many others. If lung sliding is absent, the 3rd criterium does not work; the probability is, say, 90 % at worst. Now adding the well-defined criterium, it climbs up to 99 %; adding the long criterium, to 99.9 %; adding the dominant criterium, to 99.99 %; and adding the echoic criterium, to 99.999 %. In medicine, this precision appears as clinically sufficient.

The Seven Detailed Criteria of the B-Lines

1. *The B-line is a comet-tail artifact.* This sign is constant.

    But it is not *the* comet-tail artifact. The label "comet-tail artifact" was suggested long ago for describing shotgun pellets within a liver [9]. The point is that no study gave artifacts a precise meaning at the lung area. This generated confusion in the literature (some high-level experts still speak of "comet-tail" for designating the precious B-line). Some energy was necessary for making accepted the correct nomenclature. One may define the comet-tail artifact definitely as an artifact, definitely vertical (by definition), definitely echoic. The B-lines is a certain type of comet tail. When explaining the generation of the B-line, we will see that its "verticality" is a relative notion which may be debated; read below. Let us accept at this present step that the B-line is vertical.

2. *It arises from the pleural line.* This sign is constant.

    The longitudinal scans have only advantages, including the one to permanently show the lung surface (using the bat sign). Disrespecting this rule will make the user abused by comet-tail artifacts arising above the pleural line.

3. *It moves with lung sliding.* This sign is constant.

    It moves with lung sliding, provided there is a lung sliding. When lung sliding is abolished, the B-line appears standstill. Using the sectorial property of our probe and its long distance (17 cm), we can demonstrate the abolition of lung sliding by observing the lower end of the B-line, which does not move or quite not (its dynamic is amplified at this level (multiplied by 3 at a depth of 17 cm)).

    The four other signs are *almost* constant.

4. *It is well defined.*

    This makes the B-line immediately detected by beginners. B-lines are narrow (roughly, no more than one-tenth of the width of the pleural line).

    Rarely (less than 5 %), B-lines can be slightly ill defined.

    Rarely, the B-line can be large; this is the "squirrel variant" (see Fig. 12.3).

    Modern machines with too sophisticated facilities result in blurring the B-lines.

5. *It is long.*

    The B-line does not fade. Using our system, which provides a 17-cm depth, the B-line spreads up to this limit.

    In some occasions, B-lines can appear a little shorter, some 13–15 cm (i.e., anyway long). This distinguishes these lines from usual Z-lines. Slight probe angulations will make them reaching the edge of the screen if needed.

6. *It erases the A-lines.*

    This is of prime importance. The B-line dominates (obliterates) the A-line, so to speak.

    In rare instances, A-lines and B-lines are visible crossing (see Fig. 40.3). This pattern was coined X-lines (indicating the crossing of perpendicular lines). We still investigate this pattern, assuming that it may possibly indicate a mild degree of septal thickening.

7. *It is hyperechoic.*

    The B-line is as echoic as the pleural line. On occasion, it can be slightly less echoic.

Physiopathologic Meaning of the B-Lines

Defining the B-line independently from lung rockets is a didactic challenge. Our way of casting the lines, published in [4], can be done more academically from this point of view. Here, we try to isolate the very B-line.

The B-line indicates an anatomical element with a major acoustic impedance gradient with its surroundings [9], as are air and water. Air is an absolute barrier; fluids are facilitators for the ultrasound flow. Something must happen, a kind of uncontrolled explosion, when these two elements are too close from each other.

The fluid element should be small enough for not being directly detected by the ultrasound beam. The resolution of ultrasound is roughly 1 mm.

The edematous or thickened subpleural interlobular septum surrounded by aerated alveoli reproduces this situation. Fluids are present at such a small amount that they cannot be directly visualized using ultrasound (they are roughly 600 μm, for less than 300 for normal subpleural interlobular septa). These fluids are surrounded by air. This mingling seems the condition required to generate the ultrasound B-lines.

Since the B-line is present at the lung surface, all over the lung surface, is present (massively) in hemodynamic pulmonary edema, vanishes under therapy of pulmonary edema [10], and is seen also in any chronic interstitial syndrome, it can be assumed at first view that no element apart from the thickened subpleural interlobular septa (thickened by fluid, transudate or exudate, or by tissue disease) answers to so many criteria. The B-lines indicate diseased interlobular septa.

We spoke of didactic challenge because there is in fact one other structure having quite all these elements: the *lung fissure* (Fig. 11.2). These are fluid elements (cells) surrounded by gas, and we see quite always, in healthy subjects, an anterior B-line at a location expected to be the minor fissura. Since medicine is also done by unavoidable rarities ("always" and "never" are not medical words), we could see on exceptional occasion another disorder able to generate a minute fluid disorder surrounded by gas, described at Fig. 12.7. In massive pulmonary emphysema, the destroyed structures maybe no longer deserve the name of interlobular septa. They should however generate isolated B-lines. If readers have ideas of other structures with the same features, we should be glad to hear of them.

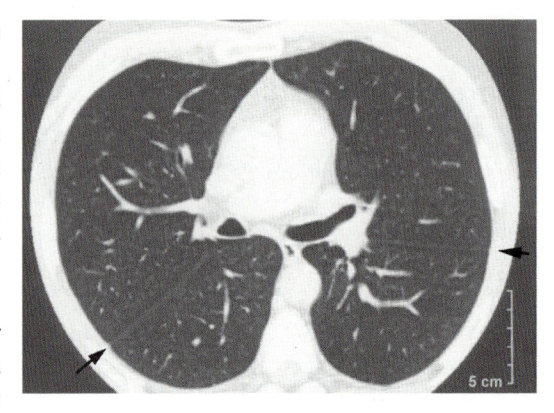

Fig. 11.2 Normal CT. This CT scan shows some fissures (*arrows*), generating fine structures abutting the pleural surface. Such structures are assumed to generate B-lines

Now, one point indicates that B-lines are the equivalent of diseased interlobular septa, when we consider that in diffuse interstitial syndromes (e.g., pulmonary edema), the B-lines are roughly 6 or 7 mm apart: this is the anatomical distance between two subpleural interlobular septa.

As a last proof, several B-lines are present at the last intercostal space in about one-quarter of normal subjects, such as the physiological Kerley lines (as proven in Chap. 12).

All these criteria precisely describe the subpleural thickened interlobular septa surrounded by air-filled subpleural alveoli. CT analysis showed that normal visible dense structures cease to be visible a few centimeters before the lung surface, whereas thickened interlobular septa reach the visceral pleura.

How Do We Explain the Generation of the B-Line? Is It Really "Vertical," Not a Bit Horizontal?

In every concept, one can see something or its opposite. This makes lawyers such a wealthy profession (Fig. 11.3). By carefully looking at a

How Do We Explain the Generation of the B-Line? 83

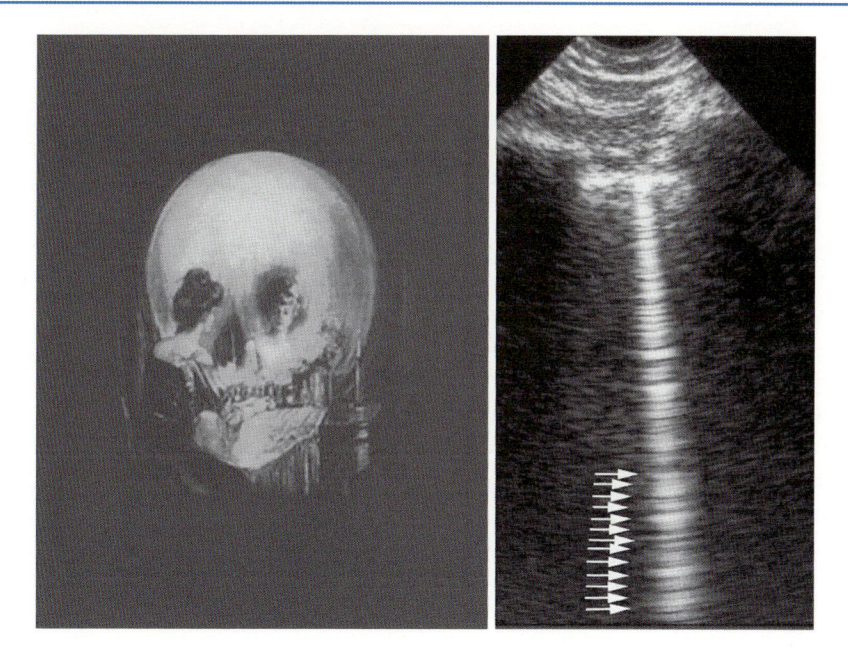

Fig. 11.3 J-lines. Lung ultrasound will have a future if we speak the same language and see the same things. The *left image* may appear scary at first view, but is rather peaceful if looking twice (or using a lens). The *right image* shows a typical B-line. It is in actual fact made of multiple horizontal lines, called the J-lines (*arrows*). We counted roughly 50 J-lines, but the real number is infinite by definition. They are superposed every 1.6 mm (data was calculated by dividing the length of the B-line (here 8 cm) by the number of J-lines). The upper J-line is roughly 3 mm large, the lower 13 mm large

B-line, this famous basic, vertical artifact, one can see that it is in actual fact horizontal. A high-level expert questioned our way to specify that the B-line is horizontal. The description of the *J-line* allows to understand how the B-line is generated. The ultrasound flow crosses the soft tissues, then reaches the lung surface. It should be normally fully rejected, but the microscopic fluid element located in the edematous subpleural interlobular septum allows the flow to *penetrate* the lung. Then, for a reason we still do not explain, the flow appears as trapped. The foot of the subpleural interlobular septum acts like a booby trap (a booby trap for ultrasound beam), trapped inside this structure and rejected between it and the visceral pleura. The beam tries to come back to the probe head but is trapped inside this structure and comes back toward the deep lung. This generates a pseudodistance, i.e., a small, *horizontal* line. This minute line has been called J-line, a tribute to Julie, a student who candidly saw first these B-lines as horizontal components. A to-and-fro dynamics is generated, in a kind of persistent phenomenon. We imagine that if a slow motion was made, it would show the generation of these multiple lines, superposed one after the other like a machine gun (or a ping-pong ball blocked between the racket and the table), spreading at the speed of 1,540 m/s to the bottom of the screen. The human eye instantaneously perceives this whacky dynamics as one, unique, and vertical structure.

We are sorry for this expert; the B-lines have a horizontal basis.

The J-line of Fig. 11.3 is roughly 2–3 mm wide at the beginning and roughly 1.5 mm separated from each other. One can count roughly 50 J-lines (this number depends on the chosen depth, since the B-line is unfailing).

For standardizing lung ultrasound and playing the same "music," it is critical that each physician has the same vision of the signs. The concept of the J-line avoids misconceptions.

Accuracy of the B-Line?

This way to speak makes little sense. The next chapter on lung rockets will answer this question with more pertinence for the diagnosis of interstitial syndrome (between 93 and 100 % in function of the gold standard); the chapter on pneumothorax shows how one single B-line usually rules out pneumothorax.

Comet-Tail Artifacts That May Mimic the B-Lines

Many comet-tail artifacts can on occasion be encountered. For saving energy, the reader can omit the reading of this section, provided the seven signs of the B-line are mastered.

The Z-Line

This frequent artifact should in no case be confused with a B-line. This is a comet-tail artifact, and it arises from the pleural line. The five last criteria are diametrically opposed to the B-line, making immediate distinction. It is ill defined. It is not hyperechoic. It is short, rapidly vanishing after 3–4 cm, usually. It does not erase the A-lines. Last, it is standstill, not synchronized with lung sliding (Fig. 11.4 and Video 11.1). This artifact has been called the Z-line, the last letter of the alphabet symbolizing the place it should take, since it seems for once to be a genuine parasite. Note that exceptional Z-lines can be long, and we called them perfid Z-lines. This label was witnessed by Gabriela in Milano (name not included in the absence of contact for authorization).

The E-Line

This artifact, again a comet tail, is well defined and spreads up to the edge of the screen without fading. However, it does not arise from the pleural line but from superficial layers and results in erasing the pleural line. The bat sign is no longer visible. This artifact has been called the E-line, E for emphysema (*see* Fig. 14.8). We will see that parietal emphysema (or rarely parietal shotgun pellets) can generate this artifact, which should never mislead the operator.

The A-Line

This is not a provocative heading. No A-line should ever mimic a B-line. Just some variants of narrow A-lines with numbers of sub-A-lines and sub-sub-A-lines may fool very ignorant users. The A-line is precisely one of the elements of distinction (see Fig. 40.4). For scientific minds

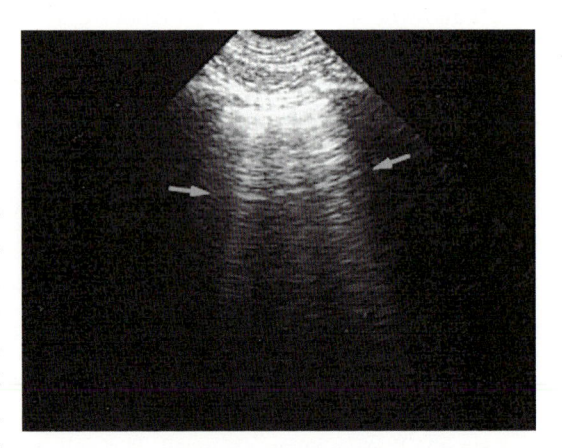

Fig. 11.4 Z-lines. This figure has relevance, since some colleagues still confuse B-lines with these parasite images. Three vertical comet-tail artifacts arising from the pleural line can be described, in actual fact. But they are ill-defined, fade after a few centimeters, do not erase the A-lines (*arrows*), and are *gray* at their onset with respect to the pleural line. These are Z-lines, typical parasites with no known meaning and which should never be confused with B-lines

who would appreciate clues to avoid any confusion, the A-lines have usually the width of the pleural line, the B-lines roughly one-tenth this width.

The I-, K-, M-, N-, R-, and S-Lines (See Fig. 40.3)

I-lines are a kind of B-lines but short (a few cm) and have no known meaning.

K-lines (Klingon) are parasites invading the whole screen, sometimes visible in our walls (electrical interferences?).

The M-line is a coarse pitfall; this artifact arises from the acoustic shadow of a rib.

N-lines are vertical artifacts that are black – i.e., far from hyperechoic. They were coined N-lines (N for Noir, i.e., black in French, and also for Neri, who witnessed this labeling). N-lines are maybe normal subpleural interlobular septa.

The R-lines, suggested by Roberta Capp, from Boston, have most patterns of the B-lines, but they arise from the pericardium-lung interface – often visible during TEE.

S-lines are sinuous vertical artifacts generated by large metallic structures (pacemakers).

The Sub-B-Lines

These artifacts have most patterns of the B-lines, but they arise from the lung line, i.e., below the pleural line, through a pleural effusion (see Fig. 16.3). Using the term "sub-B-line" indicates that the user has understood this subtlety. The detected disorder is pleural effusion, more severe than interstitial syndrome (especially on dependent locations). The BLUE-protocol favors the most severe disease. The "butterfly syndrome" is how we called this frequent mistake, when young colleagues see this brilliant line, where comet-tail artifacts arise, and which moves, a kind of hypnotic effect, hence the label (see Video 16.1).

Additional Features of the B-Lines

The Phenomenon of the Unstable B-Lines

In some occasions, the operator can detect B-lines at one moment, but cannot find them again some minutes (or seconds) after or the opposite. Three explanations are possible; the first two are obvious:

1. Probe placed again not at the B-line but just besides – a pitfall defused using the Carmen maneuver.
2. Off-plane effect when the septum does not strictly follow the ultrasound plane on respiration, a variant called the Blinder variant (from a French CEURFer)
3. One explanation has major interest; although it may appear frustrating at first view to see multiple B-lines, call your colleagues to see that together, and not finding them again. This property is detailed in Chap. 30 devoted on hemodynamics and should happen when the scanned patient has a pulmonary artery occlusion pressure turning around the value of 18 mmHg. This refers to the 2nd of the three critical pathophysiological notes to introduce the FALLS-protocol (Chap. 30).

Normal Locations of B-Lines

This basic point must be seen after the description of the lung rockets, for didactic reasons (Chap. 12). Briefly, isolated B-lines can be seen at the minor fissura; isolated or numerous B-lines (lung rockets) can be seen laterally, just above the liver or spleen.

> **Anecdotal Notes**
>
> 1. *The BLUE-line*
>
>   The SLAM was created with the simple idea that a letter does not speak a lot. The more letters are added, the more they speak. For instance, in the current literature, L would not mean a lot. LU for lung ultrasound is not really used. LUS is a really inaesthetical abbreviation. LUCI, for one added letter, expresses a completely distinct field (lung ultrasound, but devoted to the critically ill) and, to our personal opinion, sounds so more aesthetical.
>
> 2. *Updates*
>
>   The B-line was first described in 1994 as a comet-tail artifact arising from the pleural line, i.e., just two of the actual seven criteria [3]. Three more criteria were described in 1997: long, hyperechoic, and well defined [4]. In 1999, we specified that it had to move in concert with lung sliding [11]. In 2005, it was defined as obliterating the A-lines [12]. In 2014, we classify the seven criteria between three constant and four quite constant [13].
>
> 3. *B-lines and bad luck*
>
>   A patient with an actual pneumonia, who would happen to have none of the criteria 3–7 of the B-line, with precisely a confusing clinical presentation, would be so unlucky that we would expect him to have in addition, even with a correct diagnosis, rare complications (allergy to antibiotics, errors in doses, etc.). This is an extension of the Grotowski law.

References

1. Friedman PJ (1992) Diagnostic tests in respiratory diseases. In: Harrison TR (ed) Harrison's principles of internal medicine, 12th edn. McGraw-Hill, New York, p 104
2. Weinberger SE, Drazen JM (2001) Diagnostic tests in respiratory diseases. In: Harrison TR (ed) Harrison's principles of internal medicine, 14th edn. McGraw-Hill, New York, pp 1453–1456
3. Lichtenstein D (1994) Diagnostic échographique de l'œdème pulmonaire. Rev Im Med 6:561–562
4. Lichtenstein D, Mezière G, Biderman P, Gepner A, Barré O (1997) The comet-tail artifact: an ultrasound sign of alveolar-interstitial syndrome. Am J Respir Crit Care Med 156:1640–1646
5. Laënnec RTH (1819) Traité de l'auscultation médiate, ou traité du diagnostic des maladies des poumons et du cœur. J.A. Brosson & J.S. Chaudé, Paris
6. Williams FH (1986) A method for more fully determining the outline of the heart by means of the fluoroscope together with other uses of this instrument in medicine. Boston Med Surg J 135:335–337
7. Fraser RG, Paré JA (1988) Diagnoses of disease of the chest, 3rd edn. WB Saunders Company, Philadelphia
8. Hounsfield GN (1973) Computerized transverse axial scanning. Br J Radiol 46:1016–1022
9. Ziskin MC, Thickman DI, Goldenberg NJ, Lapayowker MS, Becker JM (1982) The comet-tail artifact. J Ultrasound Med 1:1–7
10. Volpicelli G, Caramello V, Cardinale L et al (2008) Bedside ultrasound of the lung for the monitoring of acute decompensated heart failure. Am J Emerg Med 26:585–591
11. Lichtenstein D, Mezière G, Biderman P, Gepner A (1999) The comet-tail artifact, an ultrasound sign ruling out pneumothorax. Intensive Care Med 25:383–388
12. Lichtenstein D, Mezière G, Lascols N, Biderman P, Courret JP, Gepner A, Goldstein I, Tenoudji-Cohen M (2005) Ultrasound diagnosis of occult pneumothorax. Crit Care Med 33:1231–1238
13. Lichtenstein D (2014) Lung ultrasound in the critically ill. Ann Intensive Care 4(1):1–12

Lung Rockets: The Ultrasound Sign of Interstitial Syndrome

It was first necessary to carefully define the B-line. Now, we can do one more step – the essential one: lung rockets. Several names were given; here is the latest update (see Anecdotal Note 1).

Our 5-MHz microconvex probe is ideal for assessing lung rockets.

Lung Rockets, Preliminary Definitions

Ultrasound interstitial syndrome is defined by the visualization of *three or more* B-lines simultaneously visible between two ribs, in a longitudinal scan (Fig. 12.1). Three or more B-lines were coined lung rockets, since the pattern is reminiscent of a rocket at liftoff. Said differently, lung rockets include *eight* features: they are comet-tail artifacts, arising from the pleural line, moving with lung sliding, usually long, usually well-defined, usually erasing A-lines, usually hyperechoic, and multiple in one longitudinal scan.

By definition, lung rockets are plural. Less than three B-lines are not consistent with interstitial syndrome. The b-line (lower case): It is defined by a single B-line between two ribs. It cannot be assimilated to interstitial syndrome nor any disease. Can be the sign of a minor fissura (see Fig. 11.2).

Isolated lung rockets (i.e., visible at only one focal area) define focalized interstitial syndrome, of minor importance in the BLUE-protocol. Lung rockets disseminated to the whole lung define diffuse interstitial syndrome, i.e., a characteristic of most disorders seen in the emergency.

The Data of Our Princeps Study and the Real Life

Our princeps study, assessing 121 cases of patients with diffuse alveolar-interstitial syndrome on radiography, and comparing them with 129 patients without any alveolar-interstitial pattern, showed a sensitivity of 93 % and a specificity of 93 % for the disseminated lung rockets [1]. When CT was used as a reference, the concordance was *complete* with interstitial syndrome.

These data mean that no disorder can yield lung rockets, if not interstitial syndrome. This was published in 1997, and we wanted to see how these data would age. With time, we never saw diffuse lung rockets in the countless healthy models we have insonated during workshops, which shows that time passing, ultrasound sensitivity would be 100 %. With time, a case of interstitial syndrome without lung rockets will maybe be described, but this will be an extreme rarity. Extremely rare cases of lung rockets not related to interstitial syndrome should now be described (read Peculiar Note 1).

Pathophysiological Explanation of Lung Rockets, Clinical Outcome

The average distance between two B-lines in the septal variant is roughly 6–7 mm. This corresponds to the average size of a lobule. The polyedric shape of these lobules explains that the 6-/7-mm distance is an average; it can be less, depending on the section. Between two ribs in an adult, 2 cm of pleural line is visible, i.e., space for three or four subpleural interlobular septa, let us keep in mind the minimal value of three.

The question whether one may miss deep interstitial syndrome (without superficial extension) is solved by looking any CT: the subpleural interlobular septal thickening is a representative sample of deeper changes.

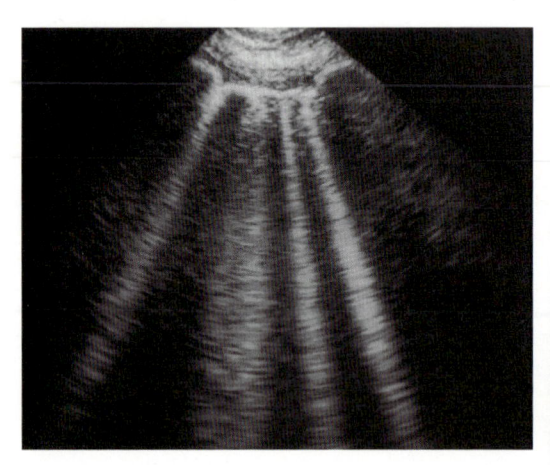

Fig. 12.1 Septal lung rockets. Patient with cardiogenic pulmonary edema. Four B-lines are identified in this longitudinal scan of the anterior chest wall. Reminiscent of a rocket at liftoff, this pattern has been called lung rockets. The B-lines are separated from each other by an average distance of 7 mm; this is the septal variant of the lung rockets, labeled *septal rockets*. Lung rockets indicate interstitial syndrome. Anterior disseminated lung rockets in the critically ill usually mean pulmonary edema. They have a basic place in the BLUE-protocol and FALLS-protocol

Characterization of the Lung Rockets in Function of Their Density: Morphological Patterns

There is a subtle gradation of the number of B-lines, with a dichotomy inside (Fig. 12.2). All data must be understood "between two ribs in longitudinal scans." To the left, all patterns which are not lung rockets are first the O-line (a variant of A-line), then the A-lines, then the isolated B-line, dubbed b-line (lower case), then two B-lines between two ribs, and dubbed bb-lines (lower case). To the right, there are three B-lines or more, i.e., lung rockets, i.e., interstitial syndrome. The label B-lines does not infer a specific number. Some B-lines can be large with a fusiform pattern; this does not mean, without mistake, a severe form of edema (Fig. 12.3).

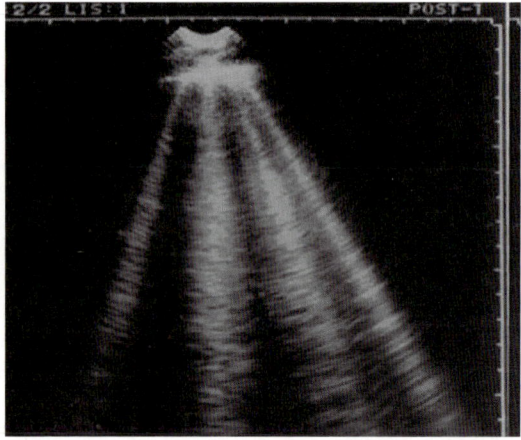

Fig. 12.3 Squirrel variant. These are typical (septal) lung rockets, with here two fusiform B-lines, at the center, reminiscent of a squirrel tail, the squirrel variant (unknown meaning, but no apparent link with the severity of the interstitial syndrome without mistake)

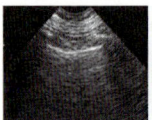

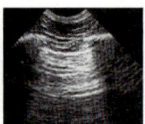

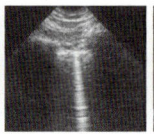

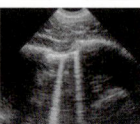

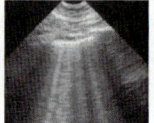

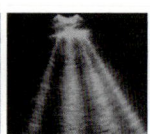

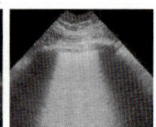

Fig. 12.2 From no B-line to countless B-lines, a continuum. This figure shows, from *left* to *right*, an O-line then an A-line, then a b-line then a bb-line. Then follow three types of lung rockets: septal rockets, ground-glass rockets, then the Birolleau variant (countless B-lines)

No Lung Rockets

O-lines mean A-lines.

One B-line means probably, when seen between the anterior BLUE-points, a minor fissura (*see* Fig. 11.2). For disseminated b-lines, an uncommon finding, we have not enough cases to conclude.

Two B-lines (labeled bb-lines) have no solid meaning yet. It is not enough for being assimilated to interstitial syndrome. This infrequent finding has still no pathological correlation.

Lung Rockets

Septal Rockets

This label specifies that B-lines are 6-/7-mm apart, i.e., space for three or four B-lines between two ribs. This is the anatomic distance between two subpleural interlobular septa in adults (Fig. 12.1). Septal rockets indicate thickened subpleural interlobular septa (probably a mild stage of edema). They appear as an ultrasound equivalent of the familiar Kerley B-lines [2] (Fig. 12.4).

Ground-Glass Rockets

This label indicates one more degree of severity. The B-lines are twice as numerous as septal rockets, i.e., separated by 3 mm from each other, i.e., space for 6–8 B-lines (Fig. 12.5). Ground-glass rockets indicate ground-glass areas on CT, a high-degree interstitial syndrome.

The Birolleau Variant

This is an extreme variant of ground-glass rockets. B-lines are so contiguous that no anechoic space is managed between the two, and the Merlin's space appears homogeneous and hyperechoic (Fig. 12.6). We suppose it corresponds to extremely severe edema. The correspondent disorder on CT is again a ground-glass lesion. This variant cannot be confused with an O-line (see Fig. 9.2), which also yields homogeneous Merlin's space: O-lines make a dark space, and the Birolleau variant makes a white space (the Storti's distinction).

The Clinical Relevance of the Lung Rockets in the Critically Ill, Some Illustrations

We have learned how to recognize the B-lines, lung rockets, their physiopathological basis. Now, the reader may ask: So what? Which change in my daily practice? A practical use of interstitial syndrome is not routine in our art; we have now to explain how it changes multiple thought processes.

Ultrasound Diagnosis of an Acute Respiratory Failure

This textbook is mainly devoted to the role of lung rockets in diagnosing hemodynamic pulmonary edema, exacerbation of COPD, acute asthma, pulmonary embolism, pneumonia, according to the presence or absence of B-lines, and the diffuse or unilateral distribution [3].

Diagnosis of Hemodynamic Pulmonary Edema

This is the main practical use of lung rockets, long heralded [4, 5].

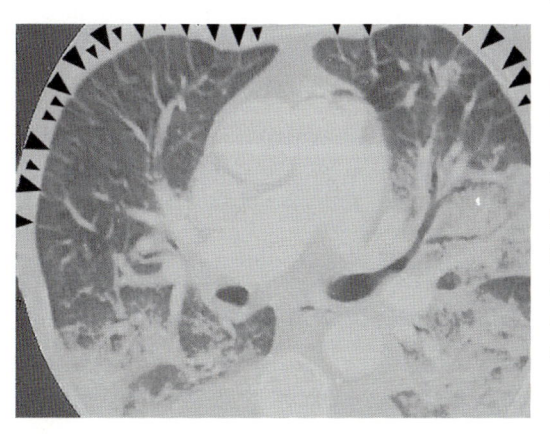

Fig. 12.4 CT correlating with septal rockets. CT scan of massive alveolar-interstitial syndrome. Thickened interlobular septa are visible touching the anterior surface (*arrows*). In a normal subject, no dense structure (apart from fissurae, see Fig. 11.2) is visible abutting the surface. This is the CT appearance of the Kerley lines

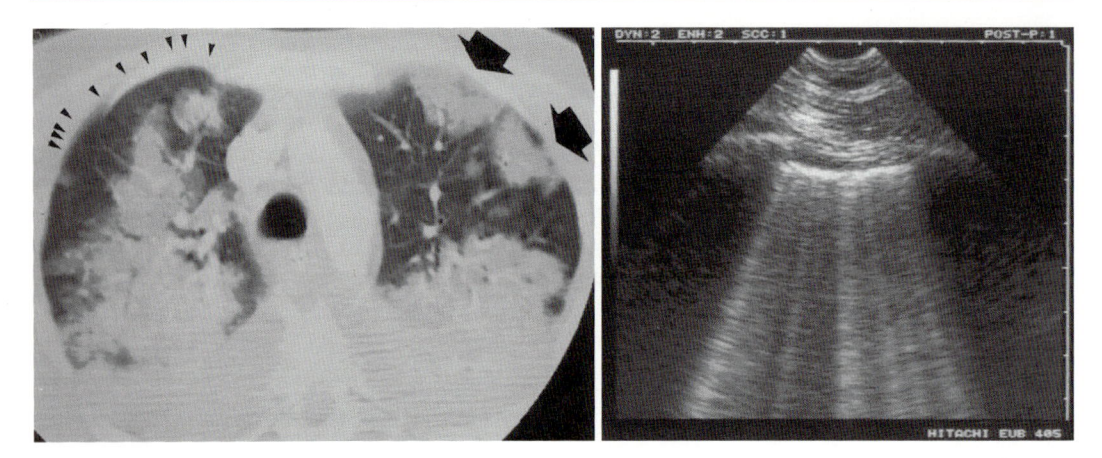

Fig. 12.5 Here, 6 or 7 comet-tail artifacts are visible. The distance between each B-line is roughly 3 mm. These lung rockets called *ground-glass rockets* correlate with CT ground-glass areas (arrows), i.e. severe stage of interstitial edema *Arrowheads*: thickened interlobular septa

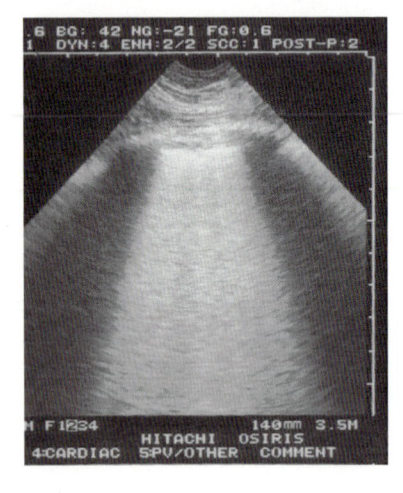

Fig. 12.6 Extreme case of pulmonary edema. The B-lines are so contiguous that they shape a homogeneous hyperechoic Merlin's space (Birolleau variant). The underlying CT pattern is a ground-glass disorder. The pleural line can be used as a reference tone. A lung consolidation would yield a less echoic pattern. An O-line would yield an anechoic Merlin's space. Here, in the Birolleau variant, the Merlin's space is as echoic as the pleural line (the Storti's distinction). This demonstrates that in this zebra, the native, natural tone is dark

Diagnosis of Asthma (and Differential Diagnosis from Cardiac Asthma)

Asthma involves bronchial disease. The bronchial tree is not accessible to ultrasound, and the main sign is indirect: absence of lung rockets in a dyspneic patient. Disseminated lung rockets are observed in no case of bronchial asthma and are the main pattern in cardiac asthma.

Diagnosis of Exacerbation of Chronic Obstructive Pulmonary Disease

Among patients seen by the intensivist (i.e., severe cases), diffuse lung rockets were observed in 8 % of cases of patients with exacerbation of COPD versus 100 % of patients with acute hemodynamic pulmonary edema [5]. In this situation, lung ultrasound offers a highly dichotomic test, with little place for intermediate situations (mild cases may raise different problems).

Diagnosis of Pneumothorax

The recognition of B-lines (even one B-line) immediately rules out complete pneumothorax [6]. This item is particularly relevant when lung sliding is absent, a common finding in ARDS.

Diagnosis of Pulmonary Embolism

The visualization of anterolateral lung rockets is uncommon [7].

Differential Diagnosis Between Hemodynamic and Permeability-Induced Pulmonary Edema in Patients with White Radiological Lungs

Asymmetric lung rockets (A-/B-profile), standstill lung rockets (B'-profile), association with minute anterior alveolar changes (C-profile), and absence of anterior lung rockets (A-no-V-PLAPS-profile) favor the diagnosis of permeability-induced pulmonary edema.

Managing Acute Circulatory Failure by Controlling Fluid Therapy Using Qualitative Estimation of Pulmonary Artery Occlusion Pressure

The application is detailed extensively in Chap. 30 on the FALLS-protocol. The absence of lung rockets basically indicates low PAOP. This gives, in a few seconds, clearance for initiating fluid therapy. Lung rockets appear when the PAOP comes above 18 mmHg [8].

Evaluation of Lung Expansion

The movement of the B-lines can be analyzed and measured. This can give an accurate index of the lung expansion, with clinical implications. The normal lung excursion is 20 mm at the bases in ventilated patients. It can be completely abolished in case of lung stiffness.

Assessing Diaphragmatic Function

A sectorial probe gives a pendular look of the B-lines, their distal (bottom) part moving more than their native part at the pleural line. This amplifies their movement. Using basic mathematical rules, this allows indirect assessment of the diaphragmatic dynamic.

Managing ARDS

This is dealt with in Chap. 28.

Diagnosis of Nonaerated Lung

The detection of lung rockets in a posterior approach of a supine patient is equivalent to ruling out lung consolidation, since 90 % of cases of consolidation reach the posterior pleura [9]. In these cases, the posterior aspect of the lung is interstitial, but not alveolar. Posterior lung rockets are quasi-physiological in chronically supine patients. Following this logic, if lung consolidation is detected in a dependent area, pleural effusion can be ruled out as well.

Airway Management

It is easy to demonstrate abolished lung sliding when B-lines are motionless (see above, lung expansion), making immediate diagnosis of correct intubation or the possibility of one lung intubation.

Weaning Ventilated Patients

It is probably not a good idea to wean a patient with massive lung rockets, meaning interstitial changes still present. Conversely, a pulmonary edema occuring during weaning can be detected (study in progress).

Managing Hyponatremia

The diagnosis of hyponatremia makes the distinction between the lucky doctors who master its physiopathologic mechanism and the others. For them (the others), we use the principle N°1 of lung ultrasound: simplicity. Depletion hyponatremia should yield low volemia and ultrasound A-lines. Dilution hyponatremia should increase the fluid volume and induce lung rockets, even before clinical respiratory signs.

Applications Outside Critical Settings

They are countless and regard more than 15 disciplines, such as anesthesiology, pediatrics, cardiology, emergency department, internal medicine, nephrology, neurology, thoracic surgery, obstetrics, pulmonology, radiology, functional explorations, ultrasound, and veterinary medicine, to cite only those. Just one example? The early diagnosis of chronic interstitial disease.

Normal Locations of B-Lines and Lung Rockets

One point should not confuse the reader: B-lines, even lung rockets, can be physiological. Probably each of us has one or some locations. These locations are, however, standardized:
1. One anterior B-line: it is usually seen around the lower BLUE-point and is possibly the expression of the minor fissura, which reproduces a minute fluid pattern trapped between two gas areas, i.e., the condition for generating the B-line.
2. Lateral B-lines or even lung rockets, at the last (or two last) intercostal space(s) above the abdomen: this is here the physiological interstitial syndrome long assessed by B. Felson in 1,000 healthy young men undergoing standard radiograph for the military duties [10]. Felson found 18 % of localized B-lines (we mean, *Kerley* B-lines) laterally just above the liver or spleen. Ultrasound obviously detects the same pattern. Its 27 % rate just indicates the slight superiority of ultrasound compared with radiography in detecting these very fine elements.
3. Posterior lung rockets. They are quite common in supine, ventilated patients. We guess someone sleeping all night long on the back without moving (after a good party, for instance) may have posterior lung rockets upon waking up. In supine patients, it possibly indicates that the lung water accumulates in the dependent areas. Analysis of CTs without lung disorders often shows these dependent changes. On the other hand, the absence of posterior lung rockets in a chronically supine patient may suggest substantial hypovolemia.

In normal subjects, the variant of ground-glass rockets has never yet been found.

Pathological Focalized Lung Rockets

Focalized interstitial syndrome can be the sign of a focal pneumonia, usually, or, rarely, focal interstitial scars (e.g., after breast radiotherapy).

Lateral lung rockets including more than two intercostal spaces above the diaphragm are not normal. The label used is "extensive lateral rockets." This is usually a redundant finding since anterior scanning usually shows anterior lung rockets and posterior scanning usually shows alveolar and/or pleural syndrome (PLAPS). Extensive lateral lung rockets without anterior lung rockets are rare and usually due to pneumonia in our experience. This may be also the sign of mild hemodynamic pulmonary edema, to be confirmed (it should more likely be a preclinical stage).

A Small Story of Lung Rockets to Conclude: Notes About Our Princeps Papers

We profit of this new edition for updating points of our work.

A preliminary note was published in 1994 [4], and then the serious work was done in the international literature. The title was "*The comet-tail artifact, an ultrasound sign of alveolar-interstitial syndrome*" [1].

The first part of the title is incorrect. Many comet-tail artifacts are not B-lines, particularly the Z-lines. This distinction was well specified through all our subsequent papers.

The second part of the title is incorrect. The B-lines are not a sign of *alveolar-interstitial* syndrome. They are correlated maybe with radiological alveolar-interstitial syndrome, but they clearly indicate the interstitial component, which is completely distinct from alveolar consolidation (as it was specified in the body of the article).

The section Results of the Abstract is incorrect. The sensitivity and specificity of the B-line are not really 93 and 93 % but, if CT correlations are taken into account, 100 and 100 %. This basic information was available, but no reviewer required to specify this in the Abstract section. In our previous edition, we asked the readers to kindly warn us 24/7/365, if they met diffuse lung rockets in patients with proven absence of interstitial syndrome, or their absence in patients with documented interstitial disease. In this updated edition, since we have described a new, extremely rare entity (in search for a label, temporarily the *gooey* sign), we still invite them to warn us, for assessing the frequency of this sign.

This manuscript (in the BLUE-journal) had been already rejected 1,000 times. We had the aim of at last publishing these findings – in order to be able to submit the subsequent ones (having in mind to rapidly submit the BLUE-protocol). Without arguing too much, we tightly followed the Reviewers requirements [11]. This was a mistake, because even today, nosologic confusions prevent lung ultrasound for being a fully homogeneous field, and some colleagues still speak without any discrimination of "comet-tail artifacts," "alveolar-interstitial syndrome" instead of "lung rockets," and "interstitial syndrome" (among many, many examples).

Peculiar Notes

1. Are lung rockets 100 % specific to interstitial syndrome? In two occasions (in 26 years), we saw bridges of apparently gooey substance (fibrin? pus?) coming from pneumothorax in ARDS patients and precisely separated like lung rockets in small areas (Fig. 12.7). The *gooey* sign, as we have temporarily labeled this entity, means an updated specificity less than 100 %, but clearly superior to 99 % (using extrapolations, we have calculated a 99.7 % specificity). This just indicates that situations where the "100 %" exist in medicine are exceptional. This is the case however – up to now – for the lung point, a sign of pneumothorax, and we still observed no case refuting its 100 % specificity. Regarding again the *gooey* sign, we wait our next case for assessing a sign which should theoretically make them distinct from B-lines. The usual problem with these extremely rare cases is that they must keep us cautious, but too much caution for such infrequent cases should show double sided (in addition, the gooey sign should possibly indicate a moderate pneumothorax, not far from the skin – to be confirmed). We will not use this highly specious argument: the gooey sign indicates that there is an (underlying, precisely, not attached to the wall) interstitial syndrome.

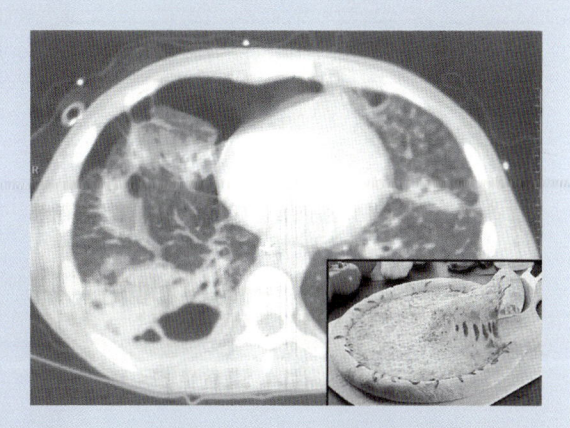

Fig. 12.7 Lung rockets not associated to interstitial syndrome. One can see a right pneumothorax, with three close bridges of (probably) exudative, gooey material which sticks more or less the lung to the wall. This geometry should generate an image of (standstill) lung rockets. This is an exceptional event, seen here in a patient with ARDS, just showing that nothing is 100 % sure in medicine. In the frame, a piece of cheese pizza with a similar phenomenon. This rare feature may be labeled with an explicit, suitable, and shorter label, the gooey sign. Just note that in this case, the lung is not far from the wall (meaning, possibly, that the gooey sign should be associated to moderate volumes of pneumothorax)

Anectodal Notes

1. Several names were successively given to the lung rockets and their declination. Discovering this pattern, in the early 1990s, we hesitated between the *sunset sign, the iridance, and the fan sign*, but these terms were too bucolic, somehow inappropriate (same remark about the "barcode sign"; see our Anecdotal Note at the end of Chap. 14). Then "lung rockets" came, answering to our requirements (short terms, not confusing, evoking some aggressive idea).

   The initial name of the septal rockets was the B7-lines, the ground-glass rockets B3-lines. David Curtelin, CEURFer from Canaries Islands, initiated this change. It was a bit logical, referring to the distance between two septa, but was inappropriate in children and neonates of course, since one can see three B-lines when they are B7-lines and seven B-lines when they are B3-lines. Much too confusing! The terms of septal and ground-glass rockets are independent from the age, therefore more universal. In addition, we try to spare the memorization work of the poor doctors. Septal edema: septal rockets. Ground-glass lesions: ground-glass rockets – we move more easily from a current knowledge to new terms.

References

1. Lichtenstein D, Mezière G, Biderman P, Gepner A, Barré O (1997) The comet-tail artifact: an ultrasound sign of alveolar-interstitial syndrome. Am J Respir Crit Care Med 156:1640–1646
2. Kerley P (1933) Radiology in heart disease. Br Med J 2:594
3. Lichtenstein D, Mezière G (2008) Relevance of lung ultrasound in the diagnosis of acute respiratory failure. The BLUE-protocol. Chest 134:117–125
4. Lichtenstein D (1994) Diagnostic échographique de l'œdème pulmonaire. Rev Im Med 6:561–562
5. Lichtenstein D, Mezière G (1998) A lung ultrasound sign allowing bedside distinction between pulmonary edema and COPD: the comet-tail artifact. Intensive Care Med 24:1331–1334
6. Lichtenstein D, Mezière G, Biderman P, Gepner A (1999) The comet-tail artifact, an ultrasound sign ruling out pneumothorax. Intensive Care Med 25:383–388
7. Lichtenstein D, Loubière Y (2003) Lung ultrasonography in pulmonary embolism. Chest 123:2154
8. Lichtenstein D, Mezière G, Lagoueyte JF, Biderman P, Goldstein I, Gepner A (2009) A-lines and B-lines: lung ultrasound as a bedside tool for predicting pulmonary artery occlusion pressure. Chest 136:1014–1020
9. Lichtenstein D, Lascols N, Mezière G, Gepner A (2004) Ultrasound diagnosis of alveolar consolidation in the critically ill. Intensive Care Med 30:276–281
10. Felson B (1973) Interstitial syndrome. In: Felson B (ed) Chest roentgenology, 1st edn. WB Saunders, Philadelphia, pp 244–245
11. Hoppin F (2002) How I, review an original scientific article. Am J Respir Crit Care Med 166:1019–1023

Interstitial Syndrome in the Critically Ill: The B-Profile and the B'-Profile

13

This chapter will probably be the shortest. It was necessary to understand quietly, step-by-step, the elementary sign (the B-line, Chap. 11), the developed sign (lung rockets, Chap. 12) of interstitial syndrome, and the phenomenon of lung sliding (Chap. 10).

Lung ultrasound is a dynamic tool investigating a dynamic organ, using a sign, lung sliding, with no equivalent using traditional tools (X-rays and CT mainly). This allows to define two opposing kinds of interstitial syndrome, the transudative and the exudative interstitial syndrome. In the BLUE-protocol, they were given short labels:

1. The detection in a *blue* patient, at the *anterior chest wall*, of *lung rockets* associated with *lung sliding* (each word is important) has been called the B-profile (Video 13.1).
2. The B'-profile is a B-profile with abolished lung sliding (Video 13.2).

This distinction follows the logic of the BLUE-protocol, by determining profiles using associations of signs [1]. When we write that lung sliding is "abolished" in the B'-profile, it can be completely, or quite completely abolished, with a 1-mm amplitude roughly. This distinction is of no relevance: both cases indicate a very impaired compliance. The question of pneumothorax makes no sense in the presence of any B-line. Note interestingly that videos are not mandatory if good quality M-mode data are provided (Fig. 13.1).

The B-profile and mostly the B'-profile are seen independently from the type of ventilation (spontaneous or mechanical).

The Ultrasound Transudative Interstitial Syndrome (B-Profile)

Briefly, hemodynamic pulmonary edema generates transudate, a kind of oil preventing the lung to burn during an all-life breathing. Usually, the B-profile will be seen in hemodynamic pulmonary edema.

The Ultrasound Exudative Interstitial Syndrome (B'-Profile)

Inflammatory diseases generate exudate, fibrin, and various viscous stuffs, which may stick the lung to the wall. The B'-profile will prove a highly specific sign of pneumonia/ARDS. The pathophysiology will be evoked in Chaps. 23 and 24, and detailed in the Chap. 35.

Electronic supplementary material The online version of this chapter (doi:10.1007/978-3-319-15371-1_13) contains supplementary material, which is available to authorized users.

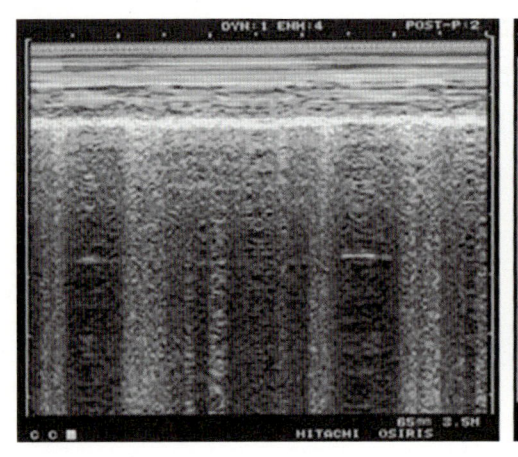

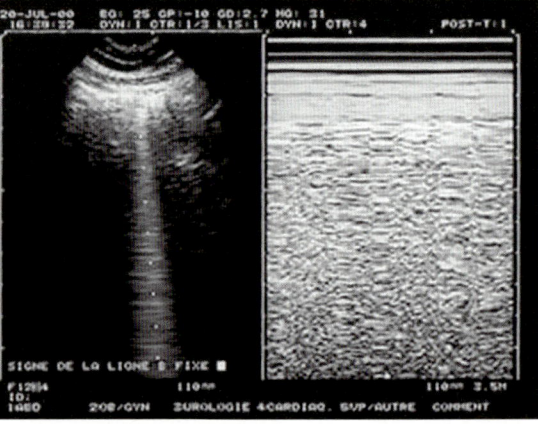

Fig. 13.1 This figure is devoted to show that static images can indicate dynamic phenomena. To the *left*, the alternation of vertical hyperechoic lines shows that B-lines come and go through the shooting line of the M-mode: lung sliding is present. Note also the marked dyspnea in the Keye's space: patient likely not intubated. To the *right*, the M-mode shows a homogeneous field below the Keye's space, indicating that the B-line taken by the shooting line is standstill

The Language of the BLUE-Protocol, Its Main Principle

The label "B-profile" should be understood, like in aviation language, where speed is life, and where most pieces of information must be said in a minimal time. Instead of "B-profile," one could have said: "the pattern with *ten* features, which is a comet-tail artifact, arising from the pleural line, moving with lung sliding, usually long, usually well-defined, usually erasing A-lines, usually hyperechoic, multiple (three or more) in one longitudinal scan, disseminated to the anterior bilateral chest wall, and moving with a preserved lung sliding," a little long for being adopted. Words are the principle of any language.

In usual conditions, the "B-profile" and the "B'-profile" are recognized in a few seconds or less. One of the immediate therapeutic outcomes is the suggestion of CPAP in the case of a B-profile and direct intubation in the case of a B'-profile, as seen in the detailed chapters.

Reference

1. Lichtenstein D, Mezière G (2008) Relevance of lung ultrasound in the diagnosis of acute respiratory failure. The BLUE-protocol. Chest 134:117–125

Pneumothorax and the A'-Profile

> A few seconds are sufficient to rule out pneumothorax, less than 1 min to rule it in, at the bedside. This justifies the length of the present chapter.

Chapter 27 will explain how the inclusion of this simple diagnosis can change the habits in several areas of medicine. The present chapter will be as technical and short as possible. Just imagine all situations where the diagnosis of pneumothorax is evoked, or routinely sought for. Just after the usual physical examination (or before, in the case of cardiac arrest), ultrasound will most of the time be the only used modality. Just imagine.

Referring to the air-fluid ratio, pneumothorax is pure air. In the gas-fluid ratio graph (*see* Fig. 5.2), it is on top. One may consider this diagnosis some sort of a "non-lung" diagnosis. The description of the interstitial syndrome had to be done previously. Note in the graph that the normal lung, which contains minute volumes of fluid, is placed between these two pathological conditions.

Our 5-MHz microconvex probe is ideal for the investigation of pneumothorax.

Electronic supplementary material The online version of this chapter (doi:10.1007/978-3-319-15371-1_14) contains supplementary material, which is available to authorized users.

Warning for the Reader

The diagnosis of pneumothorax – detecting air within air – appeared abstract, not to say fantasy for the experts, even experienced radiologists during decades. This is why even today, many emergency physicians know this potential but do not reach the next step, i.e., taking concrete decisions (chest tube insertion in extreme emergency). Using a methodical approach, the diagnosis can be fully standardized.

For being at ease and taking full profit of this chapter, we advise the readers a full control on Chaps. 8, 9, 10, 11, and 12. Each chapter is a basis for the following one.

Pneumothorax, How Many Signs?

The user will need *sequential thinking,* i.e., first searching for an A'-profile and then confirming the diagnosis using the lung point. This makes *two* signs.

The determination of an A'-profile includes two steps: abolished lung sliding, the A-line sign.

The first step, abolished lung sliding, will be studied in two settings: eupnea and dyspnea for simplifying what can be simplified. In Chap. 10, we studied three settings: normal breathing (where everything is easy), very quiet breathing, and dyspnea. We can here consider together two conditions: normal breathing together with very quiet breathing in mechanical ventilation (since none generates the Keye's sign), opposed to breathing exacerbated by acute dyspnea (with Keye's sign).

Determination of the A'-Profile

The detection at the anterior chest wall of abolished lung sliding with the A-line sign in a supine or semirecumbent patient defines the A'-profile. Lung ultrasound is an interactive field, with didactic challenges. Here, the challenge comes from the fact that the abolition of lung sliding, obvious in the case of coexisting B-lines, is more subtle to detect in their absence.

Where to apply the probe? The free pneumothorax is a light disorder (principle N°2). In supine patients, it collects at the less dependent area, near the sky [1]. All life-threatening, free cases involve *at least* the lower half of the anterior chest wall in a supine patient [2]. The probe should be applied at the point nearest to the sky. In extreme emergencies (cardiac arrest mainly), the patient is supine: the lower BLUE-point. In the semirecumbent patient: the upper BLUE-point. For diagnosing minute, apical cases, read Chap. 36.

Abolition of Lung Sliding

Abolition of Lung Sliding in Eupneic Patients: A Nice Basis

Pneumothorax should be learned "slowly." The abolition of lung sliding, a first step, should be first recognized on nondyspneic patients quietly. Idiopathic cases seen in the ER and cases occurring on mechanical ventilation do not generate dyspnea (nor do patients in cardiac arrest, but it is not the quiet place for learning). In these "pure" conditions, one can see, first on real time, that the pleural line is completely, strikingly standstill. The slightest sign of activity at the pleural line or Merlin's space should be considered (see again the variants of lung sliding in Chap. 10). *Here, nothing is moving.* This is definitely not normal at a vital organ, supposed to move all the time. The absence of parietal activity (severe dyspnea) makes the absence of lung sliding more obvious to detect. The absence of dyspnea is recognized on real time by simple observation (Video 14.1). Critical detail explained in Chap. 10: all filters should have been deactivated.

The M-mode analysis in LUCI shows two superimposed, rectangular areas: the upper Keye's space and the lower M-Merlin's space (MM-space). They are separated by the pleural line. In a pure pneumothorax, not dyspneic, the absence of motion from the chest wall makes a regular Keye's space (upper square), and the absence of lung motion makes a regular MM-space (lower square). Consequently, both spaces have exactly the same pattern, resulting in one M-mode stratified pattern, strikingly homogeneous, from top to bottom (the opposite of the usual seashore sign). Reminiscent of stratospheric condensation phenomena of B-17 flying fortresses squadrons in high altitude, this sign was called the stratosphere sign [3] (Fig. 14.1, Video 14.2). Those who really want by any means to call it the *barcode sign* should see the Fig. 14.2, read its caption (Fig. 14.2), and make their opinion.

We highly advise to take some time for fixing (in one's brain) the absence of lung sliding on real-time first. The M-mode helps for understanding the pathophysiology of pneumothorax and the difficult cases which will come soon or late. The control of the real-time pattern will be of major use for being operational in a few seconds, as requested in the first step of the SESAME-protocol (cardiac arrest).

Abolition of lung sliding, analyzed in a medical ICU with CT as reference, showed a sensitivity of 95 % [4]. The rules of reviewing are intangible [5]. Yet if rewritten today, the data would be 100 %; see Anecdotal Note 1. In other words, all cases of pneumothorax yield abolition of nondependent lung sliding. The negative predictive value is 100 % [4]. *A normal, nondependent lung sliding confidently rules out pneumothorax.*

Abolished lung sliding has a poor specificity: it is far from indicating pneumothorax (see Anecdotal Note 2). When ICU controls have no lung disease, ultrasound positive predictive value is 87 % [4]. This rate decreases to 56 % when the control population includes ARDS patients [6]. It falls to 27 % when patients in acute respiratory failure are selected [7]. In ARDS or extensive

Determination of the A′-Profile

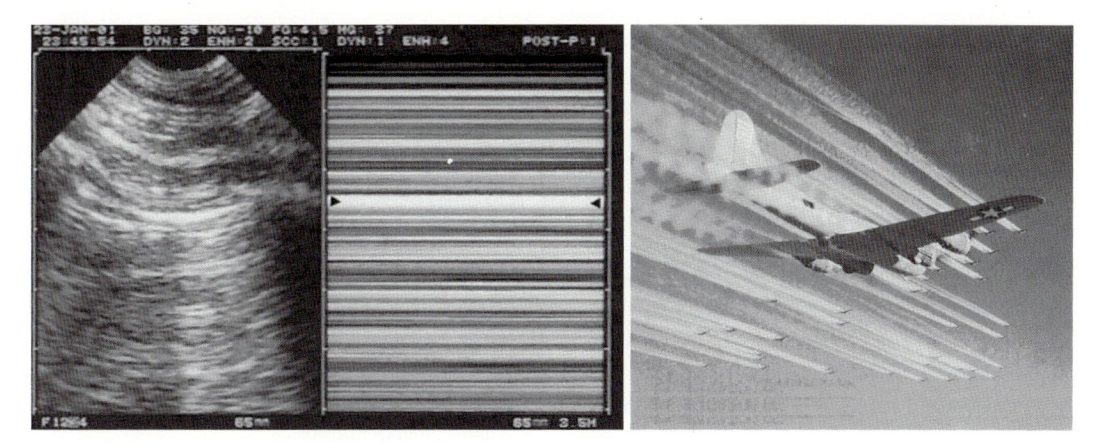

Fig. 14.1 The A′-profile, a basic sign of pneumothorax. The ultrasound diagnosis of pneumothorax. The *left image* shows an A-line. The complete abolition of lung sliding is perfectly demonstrated on the *middle image*, using the M-mode. This pattern made of exclusively stratified horizontal lines was called the stratosphere sign, an allusion to threatening stratospheric phenomena (*right figure*)

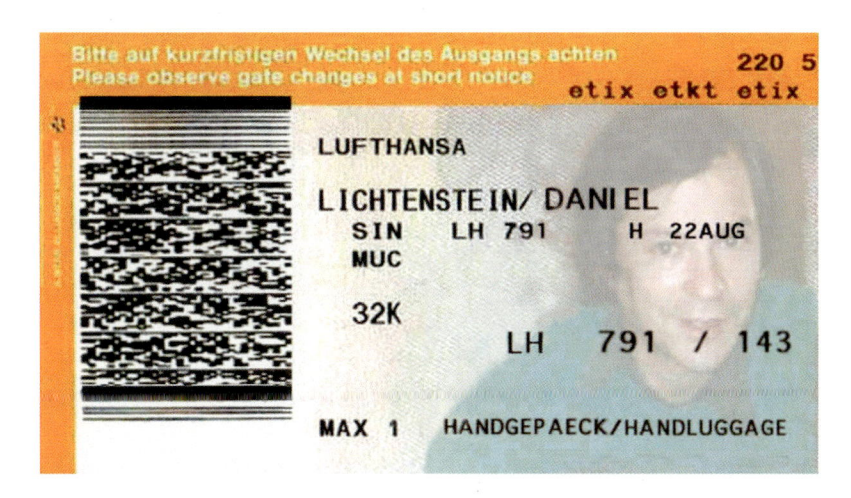

Fig. 14.2 Barcode sign? This smiling barcode shows that some expressions can confuse. A word should express an idea. Even if referring strictly to traditional barcodes, the image sounds like making nice shopping with the family in a supermarket on a sunny Saturday. The term of stratosphere suggests the threaten of imminent bombing – like pneumothorax, a deadly event. The suggested idea would create confusions when considering the modern barcodes, which actually display the seashore sign. Lastly, one can also just respect the chronology of publications and use the native term. "Barcode" is quicker? The locution "barcode sign" takes 1.40" versus 1.73" for "stratosphere sign," but the use of ultrasound (instead of radiography or CT) allows to save hours. For 0.33," we can use the original label – and avoid deadly confusions

pneumonia, lung sliding is abolished in more than one-third of cases. For some who believe that abolished lung sliding means pneumothorax, Table 14.1 is a list of many other causes.

How to complicate the procedure?
– If the hand of the operator is not standstill, the dynamic information is spoilt (see again Fig. 1.1).
– If the scan is transversal, just on a rib, this rib can show a standstill hyperechoic line (with sometimes this perfid pitfall: repetition lines called M-lines, looking like A-lines) (*see* Fig. 40.3).
– If the machine used is a digital unit especially from the first generations, the image resolution will be unsuitable (read Anecdotal Note 3).

– Unsuitable probes give unsuitable results. Most phased-array cardiac probes are not adequate to study lung sliding and the dyspnea at the superficial tissues. Linear probes in bariatric patients and abdominal probes in skinny patients make the same issues.

Abolition of Lung Sliding in Dyspneic Patients: A Higher Step in the Learning Process

The ultrasound diagnosis of pneumothorax is the science of standstillness. A dyspneic patient who tries to survive by recruiting the accessory muscles is not standstill at all. Examining the pleural line in such patients obeys in some sort to the rules of shooting from a mobile point to a mobile target (dogfight). A pneumothorax generates no movement, and a dyspnea generates hectic movements. This latter dynamics from superficial areas will parasite the characteristic standstill sign at the pleural line. The operator must detect a standstillness (at the pleural line) inside a hectic, moving area: an "absolute quandary?"

A standardized approach, using the M-mode and the concept of the Keye's space, gives the answer. The phenomenon observed on M-mode can be related to a column of sand. The top of this column is located *above* the pleural line, inside the Keye's space: this cannot be a seashore sign. A seashore sign would by definition begin at the very pleural line, not 1 mm above, not 1 mm below, spreading below homogeneously. Here, the dynamic comes from the contraction of the parietal muscles (pectoral, intercostal). The sand visible at the Keye's space, meaning severe dyspnea, is called the Keye's sign (see details in Chap. 10). Now, the whole of the sand column will be analyzed. In the case of pneumothorax, this sandy image will cross the pleural line without any change, even slight. This is the Avicenne sign (conceived in Avicenne Hospital) (Fig. 14.3, Video 14.3). The Avicenne sign demonstrates that, in spite of the diffuse movement coming from the muscular recruitment above the pleural line, lung sliding is definitely abolished.

Keep in mind that abolished lung sliding is not sufficient, but we are no longer blocked by a pat-

Table 14.1 Some of the situations creating abolition of lung sliding

1. Visceral pleura touching the parietal pleura but motionless
A history of pleurisy, with pleural adhesions
A history of pneumothorax, with efficient poudrage or pleurodesis
Acute pleural symphysis, a frequent complication of ARDS and massive pneumonia
Complete atelectasis
Massive fibrosis
Severe acute asthma
Apnea
Cardiorespiratory arrest
Esophageal intubation (bilateral abolition)
One lung intubation (usually left sided)
Jet ventilation
Severe abdominal compartment syndrome
2. Visceral pleural not touching parietal pleural
Pleural effusions of any volume
Pneumothorax
3. Visceral pleura absent
Pulmonectomy
4. Physical impediments
Parietal emphysema (by preventing clear analysis of the pleural line)
5. Technical insufficiencies
Machines, probes, filters (read text)

tern that would floor the youngests. The aim of CEURF is to insert "difficult" cases inside standardized rails.

Conversely, the slightest change when the column of "sand" has crossed the level of the pleural line would indicate the conservation of lung sliding or equivalents (Fig. 14.3, and see Fig. 10.3).

Now, the reader can understand why CEURF insists on having, on machines deserving the name of "critical ultrasound," both B and M images strictly at the same horizontal level (please, Anecdotal Note 4). Why complicate uselessly a field which is not that simple? For making this clear, just imagine, Switzerland, 1307. Mr. Wilhelm Tell is aiming at a certain apple. Using the sighting system of such laptop machines (i.e., quite all), the arrow would arrive directly in between the eyes, not really his purpose. Ultrasound should work like a gunsight. Not two

Determination of the A'-Profile

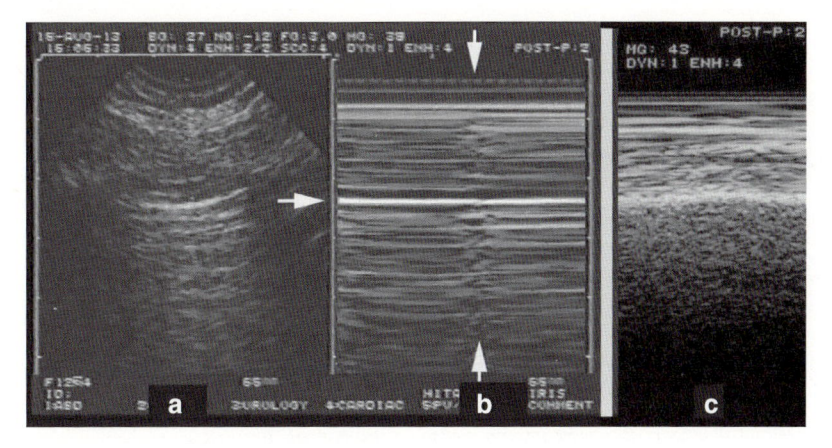

Fig. 14.3 The Avicenne sign. Which clinical elements can be extracted from these static views? First (*left image*, **a**), real time, this is lung ultrasound, with a bat sign. There is no B-line in the Merlin's space. Pneumothorax is not excluded. On the middle image (**b**), M-mode, a turbulence is seen (*arrows*), filling the Keye's space, *above* the pleural line. It descends without any change when crossing the level of the pleural line (the marked horizontal *white line*, at cm 2.2). This M-mode sign has been coined the Avicenne sign. It has the meaning of a muscular contraction due to severe dyspnea, but also *in fine*, of an abolished lung sliding. Pneumothorax is fully possible (to be confirmed using the lung point). On real time, this phenomenon can be difficult to see, and here, M-mode is of real help. The right image (**c**) shows for comparison a Keye's sign and a seashore sign: no pneumothorax

aligned metallic spots, but a serious, gyroscopic system. "In the battle," when stress does not help, the configuration of our old (updated 2008) Japanese unit makes the difference.

It is written again: the usual lag of most modern laptop machines corresponds to the thickness of the intercostal muscle, precisely. The Tell's apple. We are confident that the manufacturers will, one after the other, correct this detail.

In the unlikely event this approach does not work, here are nonacademic ones. First, we can ask the patient to control the breathing, relaxing accessory muscles, just for a few seconds (this is something that we never tried, maybe illusory). Figure 10.3 shows that a very brief moment of detected lung sliding is sufficient for ruling out pneumothorax. Second, the detection of a lung point, *if positive,* will clarify the problem (read below about the lung point). This is the logic of the Mocelin variant, i.e., an alternative to the "academic" (say, standardized) approach when there is no choice. For the cases where a massive subcutaneous emphysema prevents initially to detect the pleural line, see Video 14.5 and see another example in Fig. 8.2.

The A-Line Sign

Abolished lung sliding has a poor specificity. Yet it will be associated with another constant sign, the A-line sign. The A-line assumes that B-lines are sought for (using Carmen maneuver) and not found. This association makes the specificity deeply increasing. The term of "A-line sign" means a pattern of exclusive A-lines, a complete absence of B-line (Fig. 14.4). Chapter 12 showed that lung rockets indicate interstitial syndrome. To see a diseased lung also means to see the very lung – without air interposition between pleural line and lung.

B-lines were present in 60 % of controls (defined using CT) and in no case of complete pneumothorax; absence of B-line, in other words the A-line sign, had a sensitivity of 100 % and a specificity of 60 % for the diagnosis of pneumothorax; the negative predictive value was 100 %: B-lines allowed pneumothorax to be ruled out [8]. These data indicated that the parietal pleura alone was unable to generate any B-line. Lung artifacts were considered as a providential combination, since the patients who were the most at

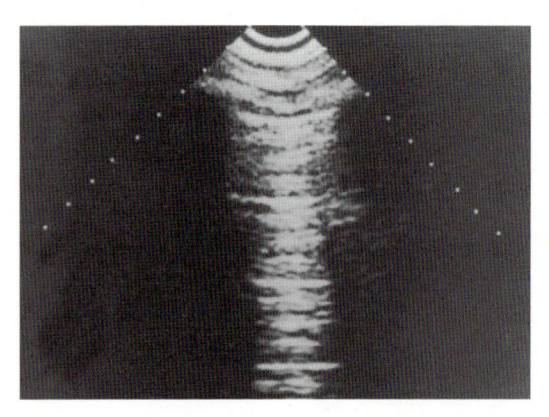

Fig. 14.4 Ultrasound diagnosis of pneumothorax since 1982. We show on purpose an image taken with the ADR-4000 (1982 technology) – with maybe a historical meaning, this was our first case (we left it free of any marking). Absence of lung sliding is visible in the contemporary Video 14.1. Three A-lines can be described and also all those intermediate horizontal lines, called sub-A and sub-sub A-lines, shaping the Pi-lines – see Chap. 40. An overall vertical artifact should not be imagined here. This characteristic absence of vertical B-line is called the A-line sign

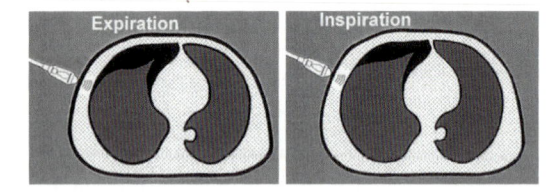

Fig. 14.5 Pathophysiology of the lung point. The probe is motionless. At the *left*, it faces the pneumothorax, on expiration. At the *right*, it faces the lung itself, on inspiration, which has slightly increased its volume

risk for pneumothorax, and the most at risk for not tolerating this pneumothorax, had usually these lung rockets: extensive pneumonia, ARDS. We saw meanwhile that the *gooey sign*, the "exception confirming the rule," was able to decrease this specificity at a level calculated just below 100 %, around 99.7 %. Read again this variant in Chap. 12 and Fig. 12.7. We hope such a rare event will not complicate the daily, basic rules of LUCI. We wait our next case (expected in several years) for making a manipulation which should, possibly, atomize this problem. LUCI is full of resources; we would not be surprised to find a clue here also.

Important note: any pneumothorax should generate a completely artifactual screen filling the Merlin's space. The A'-profile, as well as the A-profile, B-profile, and B'-profile is, first, a fully artifactual image.

Lung sliding or lung rockets identify a majority of patients who do not have pneumothorax. Specificity of abolished lung sliding plus the A-line sign is 96 % for the diagnosis of complete pneumothorax [8]. But we aim at the 100 %. Artifacts were usually considered indesirable parasites in the ultrasound textbooks [9]. Here is a nice use of them.

The Lung Point, a Sign Specific to Pneumothorax

Principle

The A'-profile can be seen in any lung with no freedom of movement (see the numerous causes in Table 14.1) and no interstitial syndrome. A 100 % specificity is here desirable since the consequence of diagnosing pneumothorax is to insert a needle in the thorax of a critically ill patient.

The lung, a vital organ, remains a dynamic organ. One must imagine that any lung inflates on inspiration: spontaneous as well as mechanical ventilation and normal as well as collapsed lungs. If the collapsed lung has a contact with the chest wall, a slight increase of contact will occur on inspiration, at a certain location: the boundary between the living air of the lung and the dead air of pneumothorax (Fig. 14.5). This generates a characteristic sign.

The Sign

When (and only when) the operator has detected an (anterior) A'-profile, the probe is shifted laterally or more, until the lung point is found: a sudden and fleeting pattern at a precise location of the chest wall, at a precise moment of the respiratory cycle, usually inspiration, with the probe

Additional Signs of Pneumothorax

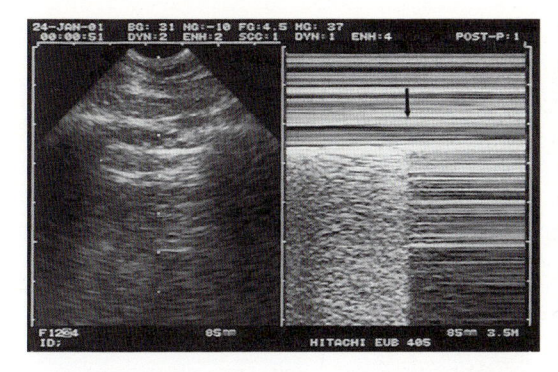

Fig. 14.6 The lung point. In real time (*left*), not featuring, a transient inspiratory movement was perceived at the pleural line along the posterior axillary line, in a young patient with suspected pneumothorax and an A'-profile. M-mode (*right*) shows that the appearance, or here disappearance of lung signs, is immediate, according to an all-or-nothing rule (*arrow*). The location indicates the volume (a lung point found at a PLAPS-point indicates substantial volume)

now strictly motionless. This pattern, which must mandatorily alternate with an A'-profile, is usually lung sliding or lung rockets (Fig. 14.6, Video 14.4). Exceptionally, at the anterior left wall, it may be the heart – the heart point [10]. This alternance is stable provided the size of the pneumothorax is stable. We speak of lung "point," but this is in actual fact a kind of roughly longitudinal line. However, one point (of this line) is sufficient, hence the current label. No other sign can mimic a lung point (read Anecdotal Note 5).

The Accuracy

Again in the ICU, when comparing pneumothorax and controls studied on CT, the lung point had a sensitivity of 66 % and a specificity of 100 % [6]. The lung point is pathognomonic of a pneumothorax, and we can write this still today, 15 years after the publication of the lung point. We have never observed a lung point in the countless patients we visited who had no pneumothorax. When the focus is done on radio-occult cases, sensitivity increases to 79 % [3]. Moderate cases, usually radio-occult, are anterior, explaining this high sensitivity [2].

Which Management in the Absence of a Lung Point?

A major pneumothorax with complete lung retraction will never touch the wall, explaining the low sensitivity of ultrasound for these cases. Without the lung point, the strategy must be adapted to the emergency. In noncritical settings, please ask for a traditional tool (chest radiographies should usually answer). In critical settings, please read the "Australian variant" in Chap. 27.

Slight Comments

The lung point demonstrates the high sensitivity of the all-or-nothing rule of lung sliding. It proves that a minimal, millimeter-scale pneumothorax is accurately detected. It confirms that the technique of search for lung sliding and the machine used (filters, probe, etc.) are correctly designed.

Abolished lung sliding with A-lines at one area, with lung sliding or B-lines at another area of the same lung, separated by ribs, for instance, but without lung point, is not sufficient; it can be explained by lobar atelectasis, focal adherences, among others. Only in extreme cases should this sign be considered of value.

A variant: the half lung point. The lung point can be frontal, i.e., touching the wall frontally (making a sudden change of pattern of the whole pleural line). It can be lateral, i.e., coming laterally on the screen, from one side to another side of the pleural line (creating a smoother sign that we call the half lung point, Video 14.4). Read Anecdotal Note 6.

Additional Signs of Pneumothorax

Other signs can sometimes be useful. The swirl sign, which has an equivalent at the abdominal level for the diagnosis of occlusion (see Figure 16.9 of our 2010 edition), indicates hydropneumothorax. The fluid collection is freely swirling in a depressurized pleural cavity.

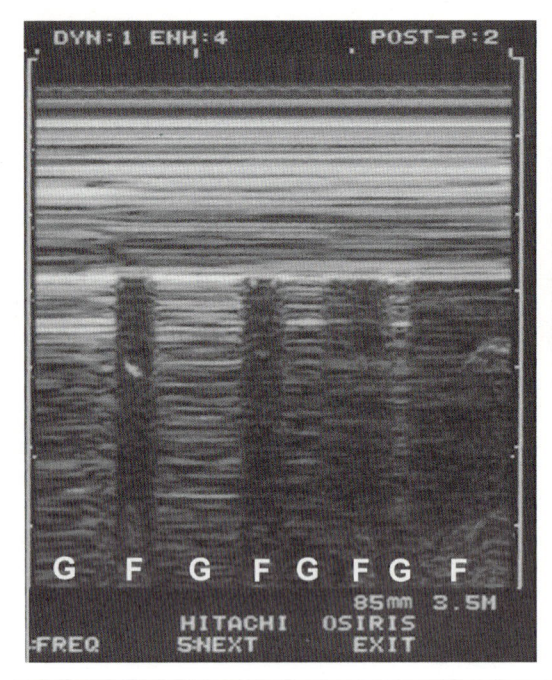

Fig. 14.7 The swirl sign of hydropneumothorax. On M-mode, a rapid succession of opposed patterns arising from the pleural line is visible. The globally *dark* ones (*F*) show fluid, a facilitator for ultrasound. The *brighter* ones (*G*) show the gas of pneumothorax, an absolute barrier for ultrasound. The rhythm, irregular and much faster than respiratory or cardiac activities, corresponds to the hectic swirl of the fluid in a depressurized cavity at atmospheric pressure

Consequently, when the probe is applied at bed level and when movements are gently transmitted to the patient, the fluid pleural effusion shakes in a characteristic manner (Fig. 14.7).

Evaluation and Evolution of the Size of Pneumothorax

This is dealt with in Chap. 28. We want to keep this chapter as short as possible.

Pitfalls and Limitations

There is no real pitfall, only some limitations. The reading of this long section allows users to take full advantage of ultrasound.

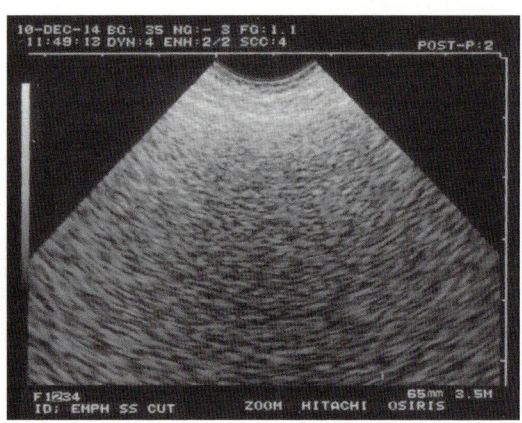

Fig. 14.8 Massive subcutaneous emphysema. This patient had a historical subcutaneous emphysema. Philippe Cornu witnessed it (hence the Cornu's sign); we could also have labeled it the Coluche sign, for the few who know him, because here, really, there is nothing to see. The probe was here unable to describe any anatomical pattern, in spite of a compression maneuver. Sometimes it works (see Video 14.5)

Parietal Emphysema

1. How it appears

It stops ultrasounds, preventing recognition of underlying structures. We can describe different patterns. Major cases create a remarkable image with no visible structure at all, which we called the Cornu's sign (Fig. 14.8). Less severe cases make comet-tail artifacts appear. They really look like B-lines, but one of the mandatory criteria is absent: they do *not* arise from the pleural line. The pleural line, deeper located, cannot be seen. They arise from parietal soft tissues. Small air collections can be randomly organized, generating W-lines since they shape a bit of a "W" (see Fig. 40.1). The gas collection can make a horizontal hyperechoic stripe between two parietal tissues, making aligned comet tails (Fig. 14.9). These comet-tail artifacts have been called E-lines (E for emphysema) since 2005 [3]. It will make a deadly pitfall for those who won't care at the basic bat sign. No bat sign? This is not lung ultrasound. The horizontal hyperechoic line is not the pleural line. This is one among many reasons why we advocate longitudinal scans, which display the bat sign.

Pitfalls and Limitations

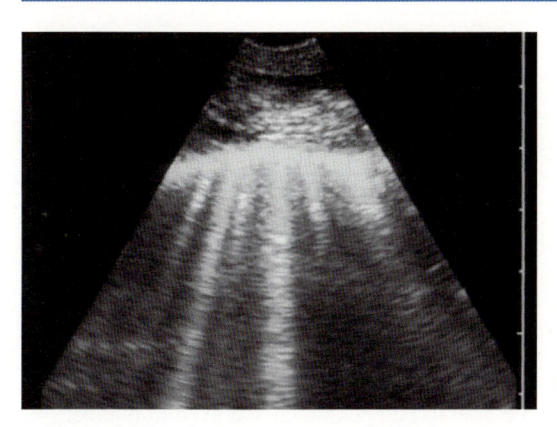

Fig. 14.9 E-lines, another presentation of subcutaneous emphysema. In this longitudinal scan of the chest wall, well-defined comet-tail artifacts are visible, some spreading up to the edge of the screen. They may give the illusion of lung rockets. However, no rib is identified: no bat sign. We are no longer in lung ultrasound. The hyperechoic horizontal line from which the comet tails arise is not the pleural line. Layer of parietal emphysema in a patient with traumatic pneumothorax. These lines were called E-lines (E for emphysema)

Note that E-lines and W-lines are motionless, a logical finding.

2. What to do then

   For simplifying, we can advise novices to switch off the machine and do with traditional tools, as done before, time permitting (and even not to switch on the machine when clinical emphysema exists).

   For more expert users: exploiting the small footprint of our probe, the advantage of the rigid rib cage, and the Carmen maneuver, we use the Compression Lung Ultrasound Examination, provided it will not create any pain (e.g., rib fracture). This maneuver sometimes results in hiding little by little the gas collections. And suddenly, the pleural line appears. One should not expect an academic bat sign, but rather the self-speaking sign of the "bat in the fog," so to speak (*see* Fig. 8.3). The rib shadows are the best landmarks here. Then, this blurred line, in between the rib shadows, is the pleural line. It is often possible to see a lung sliding or lung rockets, which answer the question (there is *no* pneumothorax) (Video 14.5). The A'-profile is more difficult to affirm, yet it is sometimes possible to detect a "beautiful" lung point – which answers the question (there *is* a pneumothorax). We succeeded to postpone many CTs using this protocol (read the LUCIFLR project, Chap. 29). Some extreme cases are an issue for all, experts included.

Subcutaneous Metallic Materials

Bullets and shrapnel fragments generate comet tails which are not B-lines since they arise *above* the pleural line, from soft tissues. This is fortunately rare in our setting but can be encountered in unstable areas on Earth. Metallic devices such as pacemakers create comet-tail artifacts with roughly an "S" shape, thus called "S-lines," of course above the pleural line (*see* Fig. 40.4).

Septated, Complex, Posterior Pneumothorax

Septated cases: they can locate everywhere. They occur within pleural symphysis, frequent in ARDS, with areas of motionless A-lines alternating with areas of motionless B-lines or A-lines (if there is no diffuse interstitial injury). Some cases have a really twisted, spiroid shape. This diagnosis is definitely subtle. Obviously, such cases cannot generate a regular lung point – one understands why it is required for confident diagnosis. This is time for a traditional X-ray, or even CT. Sudden changes in a routine daily ultrasound examination may be suggestive: disappearance of previous lung rockets from ARDS – those which are long to vanish – suggests pneumothorax.

Posterior cases: since we imagine that such a location plus clinical troubles is a rarity, one can probably speak of really exceptional events and keep this book as thin as possible. Here, an abolition of anterior lung sliding is expected. Why? We imagine that a posterior pneumothorax occurs only if there is a massive pleural symphysis. We *imagine* this sign because these locations are so rare; we did not see a lot of proven cases. Another logical sign should be the absence of posterior lung rockets, surprising after a long supine stage.

Similarly, anterior lung sliding should rule out posterior pneumothorax.

Apical cases: another rare location, which in addition occurs in a difficult area.

The mediastinal pneumothorax is rare; we will not describe subtle signs sometimes available.

Is the Tube Intraparenchymateous?

All the conditions are present for making this application a challenge: the dressing is at the worst location, subcutaneous emphysema is often present, and a lung that is not fully consolidated will never give satisfactory acoustic window for such a subtle diagnosis. It is worth trying, like always with ultrasound, anyway.

Dressings

Voluminous dressings (especially around chest tubes) are among our worst foes. Our solution is to "think ultrasound" and avoid too large dressings. Read Anecdotal Note 7.

Technical Errors

Using a technique other than longitudinal, focusing on dependent zones, an unsteady hand, confusion between B-, E-, and Z-lines, not aware of the mangrove variant, using inappropriate machine, inappropriate probe, and unsuitable filters (in *one* word: filters) are all errors erased using a correct teaching.

For the Users of Modern Laptop Machines

The machine must be ready to use. The obstacles should be displaced (e.g., ventilator). Full oxygen or more while the machine starts up. All filters should be disactivated. All buttons (Boeing cockpit-like) must be mastered. The user should now choose the probe. There is always a solution. Linear for skinny patients, abdominal for bariatric ones, and sometimes cardiac probes for the few of them which have the providential advantage to cover more or less superficial areas. If the probes have to be swapped during the test for a best result, they will. The lag between real time and M-mode should be perfectly integrated. If the real time is interrupted when the M-mode is activated, there is nothing to do but getting accustomed. All modern configurations can do the work; it is just more difficult than with the described equipment. Waiting for the perfect, simple equipment, these teams will be able to be operational and even to publish. We are confident that smart users will take the best of their machine and imagination. We just think that when the lack of room, the conditions (dyspnea, agitation) make additional difficulties, the machine should help, not confuse.

The Essential in a Few Words

A free pneumothorax locates anteriorly in supine patients. The first step is always the recognition of the bat sign, which locates the pleural line. The BLUE-points make the search effective in a few seconds by detecting an A'-profile (anterior abolished lung sliding plus A-lines). Lung sliding rules out pneumothorax, but is abolished by countless causes. B-lines rule out pneumothorax where they are observed. The lung point is a sign specific to pneumothorax (which indicates its size).

A cardiac probe is usually inadequate, a linear probe is limited for whole-body use, an abdominal probe is too large, yet each of them is far better than nothing.

Cases occurring on severe dyspnea require standardized analysis, and the equipment must be as simple as possible.

Ultrasound is superior to bedside chest radiographs for detecting pneumothorax.

An Endnote

This chapter was as structured as possible. The physician must remain humble and always prepared to see cases where difficulties will appear (and where the help of other modalities will be required). The more the unit, probe, and teaching will be simple and adapted, the less these situations should be encountered. The difficulties we found were always the opportunity to enrich the semiology of ultrasound (never the opposite), but our last refinement was rather recent, showing that it matters to remain careful. Medicine is the art of humbleness.

Anecdotal Notes for Nonhurried Readers

1. *Ninety five or hundred percent sensitivity?*

    Due to a basic misconception which escaped to the young authors as well as the expert reviewers, the exact sensitivity should be 100%, not 95%. Patients with parietal emphysema were wrongly considered as "false negatives," in the spirit that lung sliding could not be analyzed. False negative assumes present lung sliding. Either we exclude these patients for unfeasibility or we describe what is seen, i.e., characteristically, *no visible lung sliding*. Eventually, this misconception was maybe providential, because data priding on 100 %, in a discipline not supposed to exist, is not easily accepted.

2. *Lung sliding abolished*

    We had the pleasure to see, long after our first observations, that abolished lung sliding had been described as a sign of pneumothorax in the veterinarian domain [11]. We saw also some studies taking again this notion [12, 13]. Surprisingly, these works did not go more ahead in such an infinite domain.

3. *Laptops*

    The first laptop machines devoted for filling the ERs created a striking regression of image quality (see Fig. 2.2) – for no gain of space, on the contrary. They are now little by little slightly improving (they will hopingly reach our 1992 quality in a few years).

4. *An image*

    Teams working with a cardiac probe in a not standstill user's hand using a transversal scanning and dynamic filters on a first-generation digital screen, a non-instant response technology (time lag), and now, the confusion of a dynamic not coming from the pleural line, those ones will likely be rapidly discouraged of investing intellectual energy in lung ultrasound. This is what CEURF can avoid!

5. *The liver point*

    Some colleagues have written that the liver (or the spleen) respiratory dynamic simulates a lung point. There is no risk of confusion. First and above all, a living lung (lung sliding, lung rockets) alternates with a plain, anatomical tissular organ. The lung point alternates living lung with dead air. There is no comparison. Second, the wise user begins by the beginning: detecting an A'-profile, i.e., at the anterior BLUE-points (principle n°2 and 3 of lung ultrasound). Let us call the sign described by our colleagues the "liver point" if necessary.

6. *Half and double lung point*

    We used the term "half lung point" as a tribute to Roberto Copetti, who coined "double lung point" a finding seen in transient tachypnea of the newborn as a tribute to our label "lung point" [14]. The consensus conference found the term confusing (since it was reminiscent of pneumothorax); our proposal to label his sign the "Copetti's sign" was not accepted by the committee.

7. *Dressings*

    We recently talked with (university) thoracic surgeons who affirmed us that these postoperative dressings are not that mandatory.

References

1. Chiles C, Ravin CE (1986) Radiographic recognition of pneumothorax in the intensive care unit. Crit Care Med 14:677–680
2. Lichtenstein D, Holzapfel L, Frija J (2000) Projection cutanée des pneumothorax et impact sur leur diagnostic échographique. Réan Urg 9(Suppl 2):138
3. Lichtenstein D, Mezière G, Lascols N, Biderman P, Courret JP, Gepner A, Goldstein I, Tenoudji-Cohen M (2005) Ultrasound diagnosis of occult pneumothorax. Crit Care Med 33:1231–1238
4. Lichtenstein D, Menu Y (1995) A bedside ultrasound sign ruling out pneumothorax in the critically ill: lung sliding. Chest 108:1345–1348
5. Hoppin F (2002) How I, review an original scientific article. Am J Respir Crit Care Med 166:1019–1023
6. Lichtenstein D, Mezière G, Biderman P, Gepner A (2000) The lung point: an ultrasound sign specific to pneumothorax. Intensive Care Med 26:1434–1440
7. Lichtenstein D, Mezière G (2008) Relevance of lung ultrasound in the diagnosis of acute respiratory failure. The BLUE-pr laurenceotocol. Chest 134:117–125
8. Lichtenstein D, Mezière G, Biderman P, Gepner A (1999) The comet-tail artifact, an ultrasound sign ruling out pneumothorax. Intensive Care Med 25:383–388
9. Brügmann L (2007) Acoustic artifacts. In: Schmidt G (ed) Précis d'échographie. Maloine, Paris, pp 18–23
10. Stone MB, Chilstrom M, Chase K, Lichtenstein D (2010) The heart point sign: description of a new ultrasound finding suggesting pneumothorax. Acad Emerg Med 17(11):e149–e150
11. Rantanen NW (1986) Diseases of the thorax. Vet Clin North Am 2:49–66
12. Wernecke K, Galanski M, Peters PE, Hansen J (1989) Sonographic diagnosis of pneumothorax. ROFO Fortschr Geb Rontgenstr Nuklearmed 150:84–85
13. Targhetta R, Bourgeois JM, Balmes P (1992) Ultrasonographic approach to diagnosing hydropneumothorax. Chest 101:931–934
14. Copetti R, Cattarossi L (2007) The "double lung point": an ultrasound sign diagnostic of transient tachypnea of the newborn. Neonatology 91(3):203–209

LUCI and the Concept of the "PLAPS"

The pathophysiological basis of the BLUE-protocol shows that each acute condition able to generate a pleural effusion is also able to generate a lung consolidation (and vice versa, more logically). In acute pulmonary edema (hemodynamic and permeability induced), in pneumonia, and in pulmonary embolism, e.g., both disorders can exist together. In the aim of giving the most simple tool, we considered together effusion and consolidation. This simplification did not decrease the accuracy of the BLUE-protocol. Therefore, we present a new syndrome considering both disorders. The main outcome will be a faster training of the medical teams.

PLAPS (posterolateral alveolar and/or pleural syndrome) is a practical onomatopoeia (it can look like a splash), which figures out the image seen usually (Fig. 15.1). Let us analyze this term step by step.

Posterolateral

Anterior pleural effusion is uncommon (this would usually suggest a huge effusion). Anterior consolidations are, we will see, highly suggestive of pneumonia. The PLAPS is, by definition, lateral or posterior. The traditional site for searching a PLAPS is the PLAPS-point.

Alveolar

This disorder will be described in Chap. 17.

And/or

This highlights the fact that the detection of a consolidation, or an effusion, or both, has the same meaning: PLAPS (and the same diagnosis in the sequence of the BLUE-protocol: pneumonia).

Pleural Syndrome

This disorder will be described in Chap. 16.

The opposite of "PLAPS" is "absence of PLAPS," as far as lung ultrasound is a dichotomous discipline. In the absence of PLAPS, A-lines or B-lines can be seen (*see* Figs. 9.1 or 12.1). Since posterior interstitial syndrome can be due to gravity, and therefore of no significance, schematically, the visualization of A-lines, B-lines, or lung rockets does not require to be specified at the posterior lung. In other words, when the probe is positioned at the PLAPS-point, it can detect, either, a structural image (effusion or consolidation or both) or an artifactual image. This also means an optimized learning curve. This also means that even in difficult cases in challenging patients, an answer will be obtained: if the ribs then the pleural line can be detected, if the Merlin's space is too difficult for analysis, but if B-lines or A-lines are clearly seen, a lung consolidation (and a pleural effusion) is excluded.

In the BLUE-protocol, only the ten first signs of LUCI are used. The concept of PLAPS means that only seven signs are useful:

1. The pleural line
2. A-lines
3. Lung sliding
4. PLAPS (quad, sinusoid, shred, tissue-like signs)
5. Lung rockets
6. Abolished lung sliding
7. Lung point

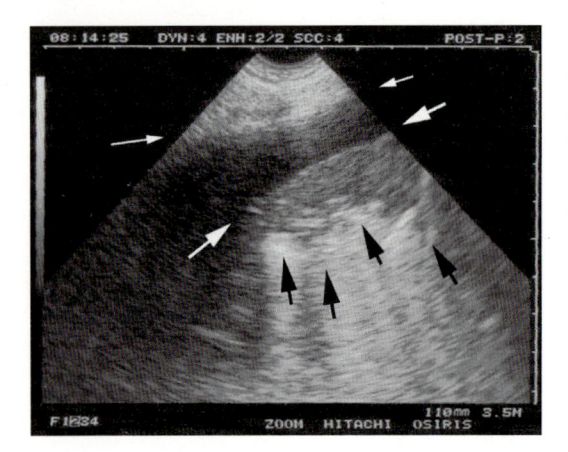

Fig. 15.1 Typical PLAPS. Both disorders are seen together. A pleural effusion, identified between the pleural line (*upper horizontal arrows*) and the regular lung line (*lower horizontal arrows*). A lung consolidation, identified between the lung line and the fractal line (*vertical arrows*)

The "PLAPS Code"

For relieving the memory, one can write PLAPS in infinite ways. As a suggestion, using upper and lower case, PLApS would mean consolidation and no pleural fluid. PLaPS would mean fluid but no consolidation detected. One can again write quantitative data, either in elementary style, i.e., $PLA^4P^{1.5}S$, or in a developed style, $PLA^{64}P^{600}S$. An informed reader would understand that this given patient has a lung consolidation at the PLAPS-point of 4 cm (or, roughly, 64 ml), and a pleural effusion of 1.5 cm (or, roughly, a corrected value according to the extent of the lung consolidation, of 600 ml). This language may appear complex at first view, but isn't medicine complex? The Chap. 28 will explain how to make rough volume estimations (i.e., hopingly suitable for clinically use).

One Major Interest of PLAPS

People skilled in geopolitics know what is England, Wales, Great Britain, etc. Those who are not skilled will always be right if speaking of "United Kingdom." The PLAPS are the UK of lung ultrasound. They expedite the learning curve of the BLUE-protocol.

PLAPS and Pleural Effusion

16

In the usual work of a physician, knowing how to detect a pleural effusion is a conclusion. The interest of the BLUE-protocol is to specify *what to do* with this information (redundant here, informative there) and how to link it to a cause.

The fast detection of pleural effusions is part of the BLUE-protocol, which simplifies the diagnosis by adding original approaches. This familiar application imagined by Dénier in 1946 and assessed by Joyner in 1967 has for many doctors summarized the interest of thoracic ultrasound [1, 2].

Why to use ultrasound in complement with other tools (physical examination and others) is detailed in Chap. 23.

Ultrasound evaluates the volume and the nature of an effusion and indicates the appropriate area for a thoracentesis, far better than radiography.

For this application, our 5 MHz microconvex probe is perfect.

The Technique of the BLUE-Protocol

From the old school and during decades, pleural effusions were detected during abdominal examinations, using abdominal probes and subcostal approaches. This route can mislead (Fig. 16.1). Our microconvex probe is perfect for direct analysis through the intercostal space. Therefore, new signs adapted to this direct approach will be described.

Pleural effusion collects in dependent areas (principle n°2 – fluid is heavier than air). Any free pleural effusion is therefore in contact with the bed in a supine patient. Rotating the patient laterally is sometimes difficult, and not satisfactory if the effusion moves to inaccessible dependent areas (Fig. 16.2). Scanning only the accessible, lateral wall will result in a loss of sensitivity. We insert the probe at the PLAPS-point, as far as we can (read again carefully the technique of the PLAPS-point in Chap. 5).

The principle of the PLAPS-point is simple: if only one "shot" is allowed for determining whether there is, or not, a pleural effusion, this location indicates immediately quite all free pleural effusions, either abundant or minute. Ultrasound can perfectly detect millimetric effusions (Fig. 16.3), provided the probe is applied at the correct spot.

The Signs of Pleural Effusion

Traditionally, the diagnosis is based on an anechoic image. CEURF does not use this criterion in the critically ill. Only anechoic effusions are anechoic. How about the others, which can have all degrees of echogenicity, especially the most life-threatening: hemothorax, pyothorax,

---

Electronic supplementary material The online version of this chapter (doi:10.1007/978-3-319-15371-1_16) contains supplementary material, which is available to authorized users.

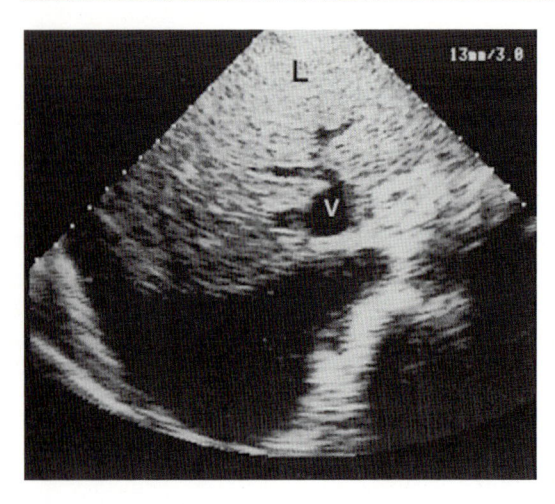

Fig. 16.1 Pleural effusion and traditional approach. This effusion appears during a transabdominal approach, through the liver (*L*), in a transversal scan. This does not provide a definite diagnosis with certain lower-lobe consolidations and also does not allow ultrasound-guided thoracentesis. Note that the effusion goes posterior to the inferior vena cava (*V*), a feature that distinguishes, if necessary, pleural from peritoneal effusion

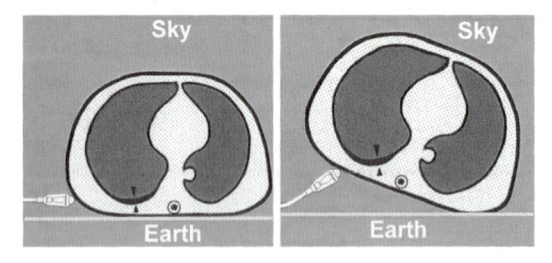

Fig. 16.2 PLAPS-point and Earth-sky axis. The lateralization maneuver. *Left:* the probe explores the lateral zone up to bed level. The bed prevents the probe from scanning further. Note the probe is far from perpendicular to the wall. Using this horizontal axis, the detection of the small effusion (*arrowheads*) is not obtained. *Right:* the back of the patient has been slightly raised (lateralization maneuver) (or the bed is soft enough for avoiding this maneuver). The probe gains precious centimeters of exploration and is now pointing to the sky, at a PLAPS-point, not far from perpendicular. Minimal effusion or posterior consolidation can be diagnosed. Note that the effusion has slightly moved toward the medial line (the *arrows* indicate the maximal thickness of the fluid, the circle the medial line), indicating that the maneuver of turning the patient should be minimal (a wider maneuver could result in locating this effusion at the mediastinal wall)

etc.? In addition, hard conditions (challenging patients) create parasite echoes with difficulties to affirm the anechoic pattern of the effusion. The CEURF definition has been made independent from the tone of the effusion. We first see a *structural* image (i.e., not an artifact) at the PLAPS-point. Structural images in the thorax, in critically ill patients, are of either pleural effusions or lung consolidations. What else? For defining the pleural effusion anyway and regardless of its volume, we use two signs of our own.

One Static Sign: The Quad Sign

This is the only static sign we use. A pleural effusion is limited by four regular borders shaping a quad (Fig. 16.3). These borders are the pleural line, from where it arises; the upper and lower shadows of the ribs, regular as any artifact; and the deep border, which is *always regular* and *roughly parallel to the pleural line* (15° more or less), as it represents the lung surface. We imagine that apart from irregular pleural tumors that we never yet see, the lung surface is always regular. This line was called the lung line, an ultrasound marker of the visceral pleura. The lung line is visible when the visceral pleura is separated from the parietal pleura by a structure that allows ultrasound transmission, i.e., a fluid effusion. In healthy subjects, the lung line is virtual, making the parietal and the visceral pleura one line (the pleural line).

From the lung line, only the lung must be visible. It can appear as normal, yielding horizontal artifacts. It can yield vertical artifacts, called the sub-B-lines (Fig. 16.3). It can yield lung consolidation (Fig. 16.4). If a heart happens to be seen in the depth, then only the question of a pseudopleural effusion and a real pericardial effusion may be raised. In 26 years, we never saw an effusion coming up to the lower extension of the PLAPS-point with a sharp angle and belonging to a pericardial sac.

Note: An aerated lung floats over the effusion. A consolidated lung floats within it (same density). The vision of the inferior part of the lung freely dancing within the effusion is reminder of alga, was coined the jellyfish sign, also "sirena tail" (suggested by Anne-Charlotte, from Tahiti 2005). Agnes Gepner gave a label which we could not assume. The jellyfish sign is just a variant of the sinusoid sign; see below (Fig. 16.5).

The Signs of Pleural Effusion

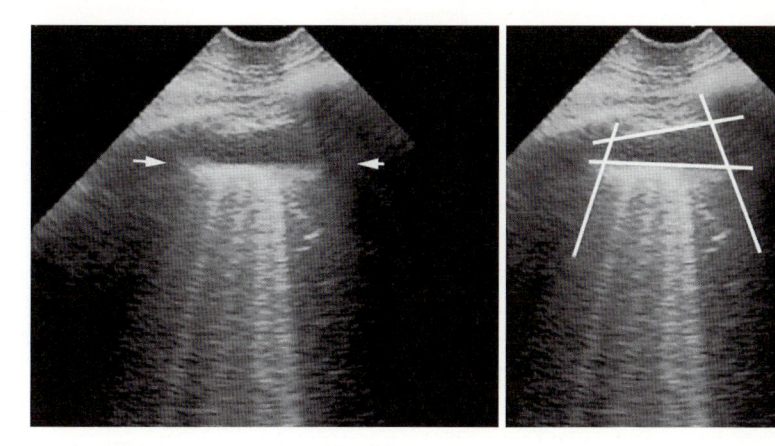

Fig. 16.3 Minimal pleural effusion. Longitudinal scan at the PLAPS-point. This figure indicates several pieces of information.
1. It shows the quad sign: the *dark image* is an effusion not because it is dark but because it is framed within four regular borders: the pleural line, the shadow of the ribs, and mostly the regular deep border (the lung line – *arrows*). The quad sign is drawn at the *right image*
2. It shows the absence of local lung consolidation, since the image beyond the lung line is artifactual
3. It indicates the volume of the effusion. The interpleural expiratory distance is 7 mm. This corresponds to a 20–40 ml effusion.
4. This effusion seems too thin for safe thoracentesis.
5. This figure allows to present the sub-B-lines (artifacts looking like B-lines, arising not from the pleural line but from the lung line, whose meaning is not the same, since only the pleural fluid must be on attention). This notion of sub-B-lines matters for those who want to know the volume of a pleural effusion; read more in Chap. 28

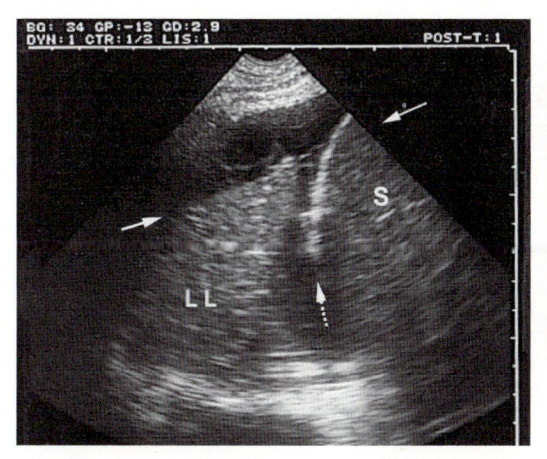

Fig. 16.4 Septated pleural effusion. Left PLAPS-point. The lung line (*plain arrows*, *right arrow* at a distance) demonstrates the pleural effusion. Septations are visible inside, indicating an infectious process. Deeper to the lung line, the lower lobe (*LL*) is consolidated. The cupola (*dotted arrows*) is completely motionless. The spleen (*S*) is far enough from the puncture site. Usual PLAPS: pleural and alveolar disorders in one same view

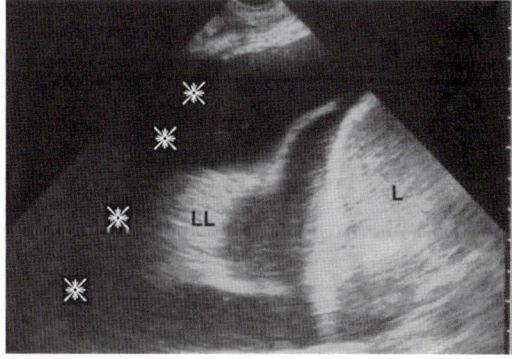

Fig. 16.5 Substantial pleural effusion. Intercostal route, longitudinal scan, PLAPS-point. The anechoic pattern just evokes the transudate but does not prove it. The lower lobe (*LL*) swims within the effusion in real time (yielding sinusoid sign). The BLUE-pleural index should be measured roughly at the lung line (i.e., here, 35 mm, indicating roughly 1,250–2,500 cc, slightly more if the lung consolidation is considered as having an index of 4, i.e., a correction factor of 1.2, i.e., 1,500–3,000 cc). No measurement should be done below the lung, since it should be meaningless, going up to the mediastinum with a fixed distance (here more than 9 cm). *L* liver. Slight trick, the pleural effusion and the shadow of the rib (*asterisks*) are both anechoic

Note: Sophisticated minds may ask how to distinguish a lung line from an A-line. First, the A-line is at a precise distance (the skin-pleural line distance). The A-line is strictly parallel to the pleural line. Just on a static image, a patient with a pleural effusion which would be located exactly at the same distance, and would be rigorously parallel to the pleural line, would be unlucky. In addition, the A-line is perfectly standstill, whereas the lung line usually has a dynamic: the sinusoid sign; see just below.

One Dynamic Sign: The Sinusoid Sign

A gas can modify its volume under pressure, not a fluid. This is a basic rule in medicine, used when managing a cardiac arrest (from a talk with Boussignac, as we understood him). A pleural effusion in a rigid thorax, surrounding an aerated organ which inflates, follows this rule. This generates a dynamic sign, the respiratory variation of the interpleural distance. On inspiration, this distance decreases: the lung line moves toward the pleural line (Fig. 16.6). This sign indicates the inspiratory increase of size of the lung, spreading the fluid collection. As the lung moves toward a "core-surface" axis, the pattern, on M-mode, is a sinusoid. This sign, also quite specific to pleural effusion, is therefore slightly redundant with the quad sign. It is mainly relevant in two cases:
1. In difficult examinations, when the quad sign is not easy to prove.
2. Mainly, the sinusoid sign indicates a low viscosity, as we will see in Chap. 35. In very viscous or septate effusion, the sinusoid sign is absent.

Minute effusions and the "butterfly syndrome": See Video 16.1.

Other Signs?

We heard on the spinal sign (showing the spine when there is an ultrasound window), a sign we don't use. We heard on signs allowing distinction between pericardial and pleural effusions (considering the location of the aorta), but don't feel the need when using our described technique. We do not conceive how a pleural effusion could be confused with something else.

Value of Ultrasound: The Data

The quad and sinusoid signs confirm the pleural effusion with a specificity of 97 % when the gold standard used is withdrawal of pleural fluid [3].

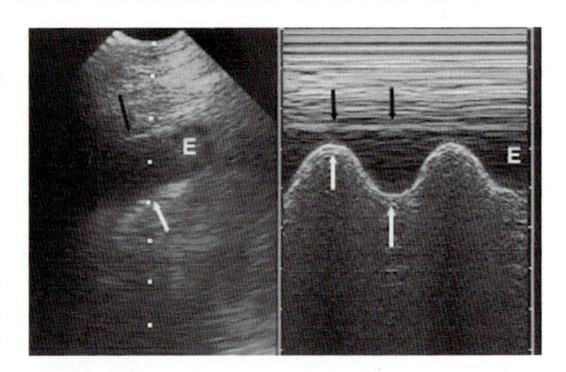

Fig. 16.6 The sinusoid sign. *Left* (real time). At the PLAPS-point, this collection's thickness (*E*) varies in rhythm with the respiratory cycle. The lung line, deeper border (*white arrows*) moves toward the motionless pleural line (*black arrow*) shaping a sinusoid. The sinusoid sign is specific to pleural effusion. *Right* (M-mode). This image shows the relative dynamic of the lung line (*white arrows*) and pleural line (*black arrows*)

Sensitivity and specificity are both 93 % with CT as gold standard [4]. Note that extremely small effusions generate the quad and sinusoid sign, those which can be missed on CT. This partly explains why our data are lower than 100 %, also raising the question of the pertinence of this gold standard.

Diagnosing Mixt Conditions (Fluid and Consolidation) and Diagnosing the Nature or the Volume of a Pleural Effusion: Interventional Ultrasound (Thoracentesis)

Complicated patterns can be seen, and we imagine that novices may find difficulties in distinguishing echoic fluids from anechoic, necrotizing lung consolidations. Here one can open to expert approaches [5], but the principle of the BLUE-protocol is first, not to pay attention to this distinction, i.e., call it a PLAPS. Foremost, the puncture will tell which antibiotic should be given, either the needle comes in the pleural cavity or within a very consolidated lung. Using this philosophy gives to the present chapter a reasonable thickness (*see* Chap. 35 for developed details such as the ways to know the nature of a pleural effusion, including direct thoracentesis).

Regarding the assessment of the volume, for making this chapter short, this information is in Chap. 28. Just note at this step that the slightest

Additional Notes on Pleural Effusions

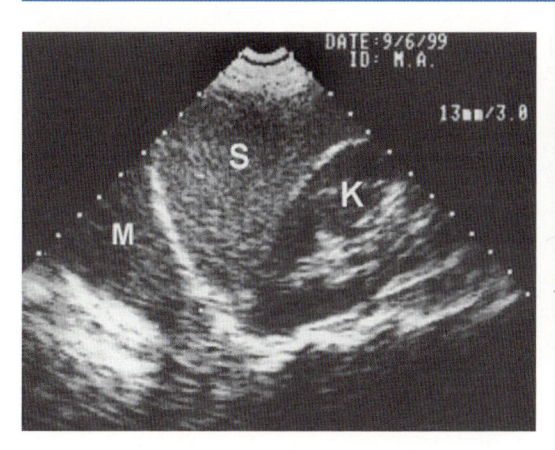

Fig. 16.7 A ghost. On this longitudinal subcostal scan, the left kidney (*K*), the spleen (*S*), the hemidiaphragm, and then an area (*M*) evoking pleural effusion can be observed. This mass *M* has a structure a bit too close to the spleen. This can be a ghost generated by the spleen reflected by the diaphragm, a concave structure. Direct intercostal scans make these ghosts vanish

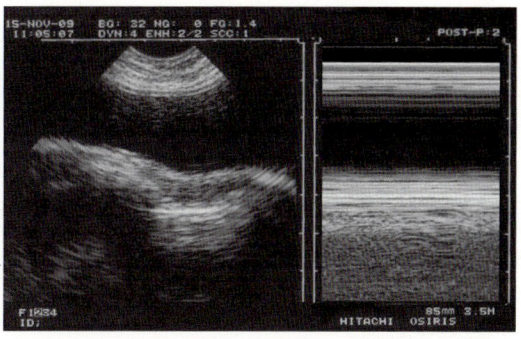

Fig. 16.8 An odd pleural effusion? A charming confusion. Hasty users, when diagnosing here a pleural effusion, would violate at least two principles of lung ultrasound. Principle N°2: a pleural effusion would not be sought for anteriorly (apart from rarities). Principle N°4: always begin by the bat sign, for not being abused by this silicone breast here. The pleural line is clearly visible below the "effusion," with in addition a marked lung sliding at the right on M-mode (seashore sign)

pleural effusion is taken into consideration, defining a positive PLAPS (see Chaps. 20 and 23).

Chap. 23 explains why a pleural effusion has the meaning of a pneumonia in the sequence of the BLUE-protocol.

Pseudo-pitfalls

We don't know any real pitfall.

An image appearing through the diaphragm during an abdominal approach can be due to pleural fluid but also compact alveolar consolidation or the ghost of subphrenic organs (spleen, liver). Like all concave structures, the diaphragm can reflect (reverberate) underlying structures at the upper location (generating genuine ghosts) (Fig. 16.7). The solution for avoiding this pitfall is to forget this abdominal technique.

By carefully detecting the quad sign, the user avoids to perpetrate a major error: diagnosing "pleural effusion" (meaning, by the way, inserting a needle in it) when fluid is seen. A stomach full of fluid and touching the wall, below the cupola (not far from the PLAPS-point), or, much worse, an ectopic stomach within the thorax create "fluid" collections. These collections, as a rule heterogeneous, may evoke the empyema. Here, there is *no* lung line. The deep boundary is scalloped (the gastric wall). In addition, when there is an air-fluid level, a typical "swirl sign" can be generated (see Fig. 14.7). The swirl sign shows the freedom of this air-fluid collection at atmospheric pressure, whereas a pleural effusion is the prisoner of the pleural pressure (apart from pneumothorax, etc.).

A picturesque pseudo-pitfall is the anechoic collection of silicone that we can find within certain breasts. Read Fig. 16.8 caption for knowing, if needed, the tricks for not falling under the charm of this troubling confusion (Fig. 16.8).

Additional Notes on Pleural Effusions

Abundant effusions allow analysis of deep structures (lung, mediastinum, descending aorta). One must take advantage of this effusion to explore them before evacuation: a ruptured descending aortic aneurism can be detected.

Does a pleural effusion abolish lung sliding? Of course it does, even a millimetric effusion.

Pleural Effusion: Some Main Points

Our 5-MHz microconvex probe is perfect in the adult (12 MHz in the newborn). One should forget the subcostal route. Search for small effusions first at the PLAPS-point. The main sign: regular deep limit (the quad sign). Slightly more accessory sign: the lung line moves toward the pleural line on inspiration (sinusoid sign). The echogenicity is *usually* dark (anechoic), but echoic effusions are straightforward detected using these universal signs.

References

1. Dénier A (1946) Les ultrasons, leur application au diagnostic. Presse Med 22:307–308
2. Joyner CR, Herman RJ, Reid JM (1967) Reflected ultrasound in the detection and localization of pleural effusion. JAMA 200:399–402
3. Lichtenstein D, Hulot JS, Rabiller A, Tostivint T, Mezière G (1999) Feasibility and safety of ultrasound-aided thoracentesis in mechanically ventilated patients. Intensive Care Med 25:955–958
4. Lichtenstein D, Goldstein I, Mourgeon E, Cluzel P, Grenier P, Rouby JJ (2004) Comparative diagnostic performances of auscultation, chest radiography and lung ultrasonography in acute respiratory distress syndrome. Anesthesiology 100:9–15
5. Mathis G, Blank W, Reißig A, Lechleitner P, Reuß J, Schuler A, Beckh S (2005) Thoracic ultrasound for diagnosing pulmonary embolism. A prospective multicenter study of 352 patients. Chest 128:1531–1538

17

PLAPS and Lung Consolidation (Usually Alveolar Syndrome) and the C-profile

The lung consolidation is a fluid disorder, therefore easily traversed by the ultrasound each time the consolidation is subpleural, which is the case in acute settings in 98.5 % of cases [1] (Fig. 17.1). The fluid fills an alveola. Countless alveoli are contiguously filled, up to a macroscopic, visible volume. This fluid can be transudate, exudate, pus, blood, sweet or saline water, or any saline solution. The BLUE-protocol will allow to determine the kind of fluid involved.

As early as 1946, the father of medical ultrasound evoked the potential of detecting lung consolidations [2]. Some works arose [3–5]. Aiming at simplifying lung (and critical) ultrasound, we present here signs from CEURF which aim at being standardized.

Our 5-MHz microconvex probe is perfect for this investigation, neonate apart.

Some Terminologic Concepts

Numerous terms are used in current practice: alveolar syndrome, condensation, density, infiltrate, parenchymatous opacity, pneumonia, bronchopneumonia, pulmonary edema, atelectasis, etc. The word atelectasis in particular is often used facing any consolidation. The ill-defined radiologic term "alveolar-interstitial" just demonstrates an inability for experts (radiologists) to separate each disorder. We explain this profusion of words by the fact that "traditional" intensivists do not care too much and will not initiate a particular therapy; therefore words have less importance.

With the advent of lung ultrasound, words have much more sense. "Hepatization" is a nice ultrasound word, since the lung and the liver have similar patterns. The term "alveolar filling" implies a nonretractile cause. The term we long used, "alveolar consolidation," has the advantage of remaining neutral, not involving a particular etiology (infectious, mechanical, hydrostatic). From Angelika Reissig' talks, we now use the word "lung consolidation," more logical, since the alveoli and interlobular septa are together concerned by the pathological process. By the way, the term "alveolar-interstitial syndrome" should be really reserved to these lung consolidations (see Anecdotal Note 1).

Please, the word "consolidation" does not mean "pneumonia." Hemodynamic pulmonary edema, ARDS, pneumonia, pulmonary embolism, tumor, and even pneumothorax are causes of lung consolidation. In the BLUE-protocol (in dyspneic patients), posterior consolidations are sought for only when there is no anterior interstitial syndrome, no anterior consolidations, no abolished lung sliding, and no deep venous thrombosis. Only at this step, they indicate pneumonia.

In the BLUE-protocol, lung consolidations are not used for the diagnosis of pulmonary embolism.

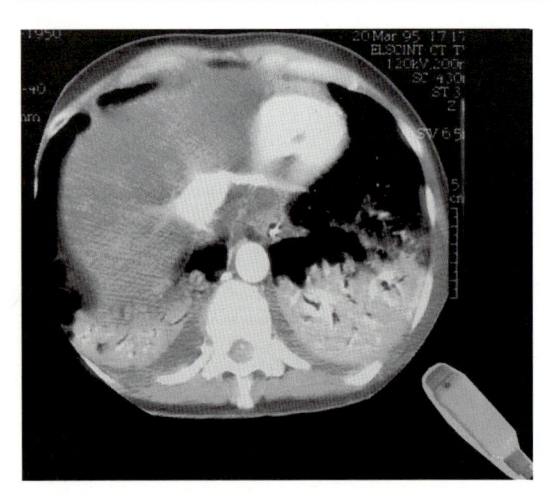

Fig. 17.1 Shred sign on CT. This CT scan of a lung consolidation shows a large pleural contact at the posterior aspect of the left lung, a condition usual but necessary to make it accessible to ultrasound. Such a consolidation cannot be missed, even if only the PLAPS-point is investigated (note the longitudinal orientation of the microconvex probe). This consolidation is non-translobar and has the expected fractal, shredded border with the black aerated lung

Why Care at Diagnosing a Lung Consolidation, Whereas the Concept of "PLAPS" Allows Energy Saving?

It is true, in the BLUE-protocol, once a structural image is detected at the posterior thoracic area, it cannot be but a PLAPS? What else?

This is why our approach is aimed at simplifying as far as possible the sole diagnosis of lung consolidations, by providing as few signs as possible: two signs, namely, the shred sign and the tissue-like sign.

One Ultrasound Peculiarity of Lung Consolidations: Their Locations

Whereas pleural effusion, pneumothorax, and interstitial edema benefit from extensive location and therefore from standardized points of search (the BLUE-points), lung consolidations can be located in various sites and have various sizes. Where to apply the probe raises an issue.

Applying it at the PLAPS-point detects most cases (90 %) [1] and makes ultrasound already superior to bedside radiography in terms of diagnostic accuracy. We saw in Chap. 6 that if the PLAPS-point is negative, one should expect to see small or very small consolidations at the extended PLAPS-points.

Whole-lung consolidations (massive atelectasis, massive pneumonia) are visible everywhere (including the PLAPS-point).

Random consolidations should be sought for where they are. This can be apical, axillary, juxta-rachidian, trans-scapular (yet see the nice Fig. 28.3), or on anterior areas not scanned by the BLUE-points. Those who wish to increase the 90 % rate are condemned to make comprehensive, time-consuming, and chancy scanning. This option is acceptable for assessing ARDS but is questionable in critical settings; in actual fact deeply linked to the clinical question: dependent consolidations in ventilated patients after a few days (Pink-protocol) are pathologic but not surprising. Anterior (even small) consolidations, i.e., C-profile, in a patient with acute dyspnea, or a young lady with chest pain, have major relevance.

Rough correlations between BLUE-points and lobes were seen in Chap. 5 rapidly: upper BLUE-point and upper lobe, lower BLUE-point and middle lobe, and PLAPS-point at the lower lobe.

Ultrasound Diagnosis of a Lung Consolidation

Considering translobar from non-translobar forms allows deep simplification of the teaching part. Obviously, in many cases of translobar cases, the same patient can display areas of non-translobar consolidations.

Non-translobar Consolidations: The Shred (or Fractal) Sign

We use a biological fact: almost all consolidations seen in the critically ill have irregular boundaries with the underlying aerated lung (Fig. 17.1). In a

Ultrasound Diagnosis of a Lung Consolidation

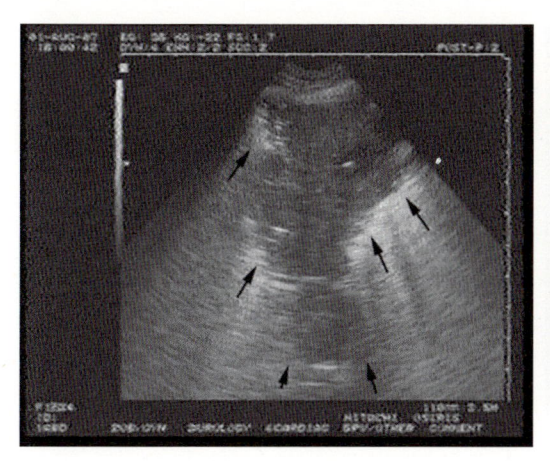

Fig. 17.2 The ultrasound shred sign. Typical non-translobar lung consolidation. First, instead of an acoustic barrier (with A- or B-lines), an anatomic, structural image is detected, arising from the pleural line. Note its tissue-like pattern but, above all, the highly irregular, shredded border (*arrows*), since the consolidation is in contact with the aerated lung: the shred sign. In spite of the ill-defined image (see the letters, showing major loss of definition), the image is self-speaking. Quantitative data: the arrow is 6.5 cm, indicating a BLUE-consolidation index of 275 ml

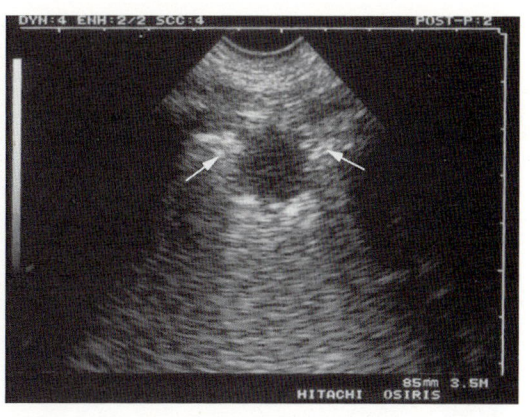

Fig. 17.3 The C-line. The pleural line is interrupted by a centimeter-scale image, concave in depth. This is a C-line, a sign of very distal (and small) alveolar syndrome. It seems round. One dimension is 1.25 mm, showing a BLUE-consolidation index of roughly 2 ml (confirming if needed its small volume). The shred sign is not caricatural here. It is in practice replaced by an equivalent: the transition radius is concave (*arrows*), impossible with a pleural effusion, even encysted

longitudinal view, the upper, superficial border is the pleural line or, in the case of associated pleural effusion, the lung line (see Fig. 15.1). The deep border is almost always shredded, displaying the shred line or fractal line (Fig. 17.2) [6] (read Anecdotal Note 2). This sign usually allows immediate diagnosis, within fractions of seconds, regardless of the size (just before the step it becomes translobar; see below). Figure 17.3 is an example of a small (i.e., for sure non-translobar) consolidation. It is also distinguished from a pleural effusion with a lung line. Figure 17.4 is an extreme example of alveolar syndrome, quite alveolar miasma.

Translobar Consolidations: The Tissue-Like Sign

In these voluminous cases, the beam crosses a huge volume of alveoli, and the multiple reflections on the interlobular septa make possible to see the tissue-like pattern more easily (see Fig. 5.3 and corresponding caption). This alveolar-interstitial mass is reminiscent of a liver

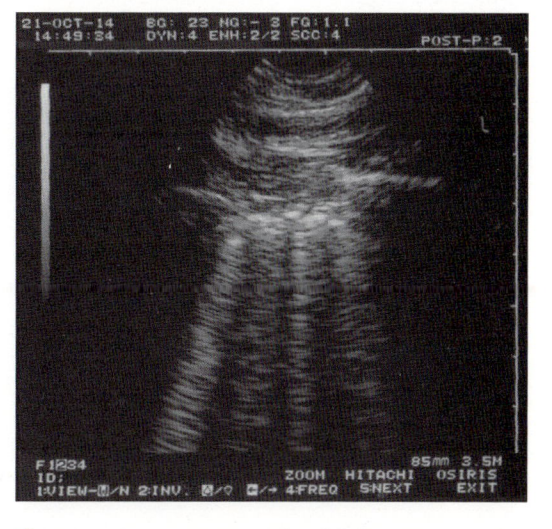

Fig. 17.4 An extreme example of C-line. Some readers may see here lung rockets, but the BLUE-protocol first notes this irregular pleural line, somehow dotted. This is an extreme example of small lung consolidation. At the anterior chest wall, it concludes the BLUE-protocol as a "C-profile." Seen at the PLAPS-point, it would be an extreme equivalent of a PLAPS. The "thickened, irregular pleural line" of the Italian literature is called "C-profile" or "PLAPS" in the terms of the BLUE-protocol

(Fig. 17.5). We should add an *ill* liver, like in mesenteric infarction, since small gas collections are possibly present. In massive, translobar

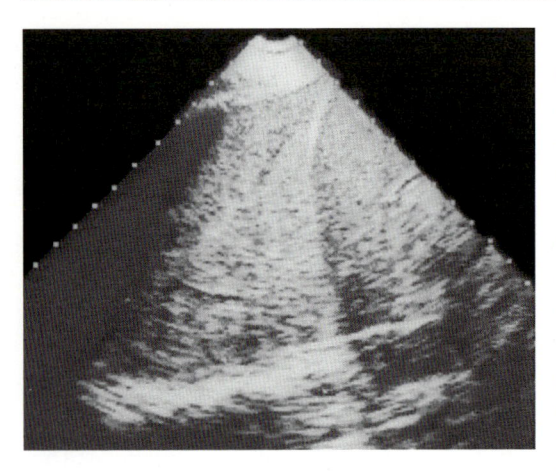

Fig. 17.5 Massive, translobar consolidation of the lower left lobe. The basic sign is here the tissue-like pattern (quite paradoxical for a fluid lesion). The homogeneous pattern indicates absence of necrotizing complication. Pleural effusion and air bronchogram are not visible in this pure case. Longitudinal scan of the left base, lateral approach. Quantitative consideration: the longest measurement is 9.5 cm (a maximum, since the consolidation is translobar), making a simplified consolidation index of 875 cc, i.e., a huge consolidation

The label tissue-like sign assumes a tissular behavior of the mass, which keeps constant dimensions during breathing, consequently not generating any sinusoid sign. But it is not tissue.

Young operators (or sharp minds) may ask why this regular line seen in the depth is not a lung line, with an echoic pleural effusion. Apart from the complete absence of fluid dynamic (plankton's sign of pleural effusion, sinusoid sign), the simplest clue is to measure the dimension of this image, caring at being as perpendicular as possible to the chest wall. The distance between the pleural line and the regular deep limit is 9–11 cm (in adults), i.e., the translobar size of the lung. This size may appear small, but see Fig. 17.6. A pleural effusion cannot reach this dimension (5 or 6 cm is an extreme limit). In other words, the deep border can be called the "mediastinal line," or the "heart line," for clarifying the concept. In the neonate, the same rule applies (see Chap. 32).

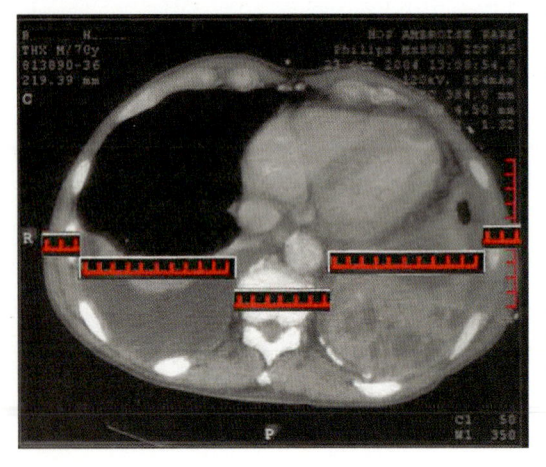

Fig. 17.6 Thoracic dimensions. This is the thoracic CT of a normal size adult. One can see that the laterolateral width of this thorax is roughly 30 cm, and each laterolateral lung width is not greater than 10 cm

consolidations, the deep border is the opposed visceral pleura. It is regular, since it outlines the mediastinum (whole-lung consolidation) or the heart (lingula consolidation). No aerated lung tissue, i.e., no shred sign, is visible.

Other Signs Not Required for the Diagnosis of Lung Consolidation in the BLUE-Protocol but Useful for Its Characterization

Among countless signs, some are of interest for giving more to the patient. Some can help, just in difficult cases. Others will help in the causal diagnosis. *None* of these signs changes the basic BLUE-diagnosis of "pneumonia." They will be detailed in the extended BLUE-protocol (Chap. 35):

Abscess or necrotizing pneumonia.
Air bronchograms. If yes, static air bronchogram or dynamic air bronchogram. Note: air bronchograms are *not* considered as a sign of consolidation (because of redundancy).
Lung sliding amplitude or (redundant) diaphragm dynamics.
Volume of the consolidation (read Chap. 28 devoted to ARDS). Reminder, a very small consolidation is a consolidation in the BLUE-protocol.

Association with interstitial patterns in the surroundings.

Association with pleural effusion.

Signs of loss of lung volume (elevated motionless cupola, shifted heart etc.).

The *coffee sign*. If the user is able to detect a lung line, followed by any structural (not artifactual) image below, the diagnosis of lung consolidation (associated with a pleural effusion) is made, following this logic: we see something below a pleural effusion. What can it be, if not a lung consolidation? *What else*? And the field of ultrasound is again simplified. See Figs. 15.1, 16.4, and 16.5.

Accuracy of the Fractal and Tissue-Like Signs

When the definition of the lung consolidation includes both signs, the specificity of ultrasound is 98 % with CT as the gold standard [1]. The sensitivity of 90 % can be easily increased if the operator makes comprehensive, time-consuming scanning. In the study where this data is extracted, the operator missed consolidations that were small or in unusual locations. The interest of detecting a small consolidation is a function of the setting (see below).

The C-Profile and the PLAPS

The C-profile defines, basically, any detection of *anterior* lung consolidations – regardless of number and size. In the BLUE-protocol, irregular, thickened pleural lines are the C-profile.

The PLAPS is the term which concludes the A-no-V-PLAPS-profile, a profile which considers *posterolateral* lung consolidations or just isolated effusions.

Pseudo-Pitfalls

1. The distinction between complex pleural effusion and alveolar consolidation

    First note that for the diagnosis of an acute respiratory failure, in the BLUE-protocol, the PLAPS concept does not require subtle distinction. If needed, the sinusoid sign, the shred sign, and air bronchograms, especially when dynamic, usually make the difference. See Chap. 35 for refinements.

2. Abdominal fat

    It may really mimic alveolar consolidation, with long explanations for proving it is not (see Fig. 6.3). For making rid of this issue, one just needs to follow the BLUE-points: using them, the operator will be *above* this embarrassing abdominal fat. Apart from this, the diaphragm is usually recognized, separating the thorax from the abdomen. In exceptional cases of unfrequent morphotypes, we see areas of abdominal fat around the lower BLUE-point. Here is, if really needed, one very small indication for Doppler which should, supposedly, show colors in some consolidations and no color in fat.

3. Liver and spleen

    Same remark with that of abdominal fat: use the BLUE-points and locate the diaphragm.

4. The F-lines

    These parasites are shortly considered in Chap. 40. They don't generate a big deal.

Lung Consolidation, Briefly

Our 5-MHz microconvex probe is perfect in the adult (12 MHz in the newborn). Most cases locate at the PLAPS-point in the critically ill. A shredded deep border, the detection of the mediastinal line (10 cm distance in the adult), and a tissue-like pattern are our main standardized signs. A lung consolidation can be found in patients with hemodynamic pulmonary edema, pneumonia, ARDS, pulmonary embolism, atelectasis, and even pneumothorax. The BLUE-protocol associates a consolidation to its cause.

For advanced iconography, see also Chaps. 15, 16, 28, 32, and 35.

Anecdotal Notes

1. Alveolar-interstitial syndrome.

    We sometimes hear that ground-glass rockets are advocated as being linked with the alveolar-interstitial syndrome. Ground-glass areas on CT are a sign of interstitial syndrome (personal talks with world specialists of imaging).

2. Benoît Mandelbrot wished to see his concept used by as many disciplines as possible. Geometry, geography, and even politics and philosophy used it, and we regret that he left us too quickly (in 2010) to see that even medicine took a part of his elegant concept [6].

References

1. Lichtenstein D, Lascols N, Mezière G, Gepner A (2004) Ultrasound diagnosis of alveolar consolidation in the critically ill. Intensive Care Med 30:276–281
2. Dénier A (1946) Les ultrasons, leur application au diagnostic. Presse Med 22:307–308
3. Weinberg B, Diakoumakis EE, Kass EG, Seife B, Zvi ZB (1986) The air bronchogram: sonographic demonstration. Am J Roentgenol 147:593–595
4. Dorne HL (1986) Differentiation of pulmonary parenchymal consolidation from pleural disease using the sonographic fluid bronchogram. Radiology 158:41–42
5. Targhetta R, Chavagneux R, Bourgeois JM, Dauzat M, Balmes P, Pourcelot L (1992) Sonographic approach to diagnosing pulmonary consolidation. J Ultrasound Med 11:667–672
6. Mandelbrot B (1975) Les objets fractals. Forme, hasard et dimension. Champs Sciences, Paris

The BLUE-Protocol, Venous Part: Deep Venous Thrombosis in the Critically Ill. Technique and Results for the Diagnosis of Acute Pulmonary Embolism

18

> A long chapter, but an easy, reasonable procedure, provided some clues are followed.

> Vascular probes are not fully suitable for vascular assessment in the critically ill.

Why Is This Chapter Long and Apparently Complicated?

Why is this chapter so long (22 pages), whereas the practical achievement is so short? In practice, the venous step of the BLUE-protocol takes 2 min or less. Half the cases of deep venous thrombosis (DVT) are detected within the first seconds, and the average timing is 55 s (Accessory Note 1).

This contrast is explained mainly because we have to explain what we do not do, more than what we do. Also because, it is true, the venous network is extensive, and nearly each area has some peculiarities. The principle of the BLUE-protocol, i.e., a sequential scanning of the most frequently involved areas, expedites the procedure.

Electronic supplementary material The online version of this chapter (doi:10.1007/978-3-319-15371-1_18) contains supplementary material, which is available to authorized users.

Our contact product also enables a really fast protocol.

Our 5 MHz microconvex probe is ideal for assessing almost all deep veins (popliteal, calf, subclavian, including the caval veins - i.e, the superior caval too - a.m.o.).

For the Very Hurried Readers: What Is Seen from the Outside at the Venous Step of the BLUE-Protocol?

The operator applies the probe at the common femoral vein, looks, and then compresses. If this area is thrombosed, the BLUE-protocol is concluded. If not, the superficial femoral vein just above the knee is scanned. If this area is normal, a calf analysis is done. If normal, jugular internal and subclavian veins are scanned. If normal, the operator comes back to the lower extremity: one shot at the midfemoral area, one at the popliteal vein. This sequence, which replaces the laconic term "venous analysis" of the decision tree, results in a larger decision tree, but eventually expedites the venous step.

When to Make Use of Venous Ultrasound in the BLUE-Protocol

The venous assessment is the critical step in the BLUE-protocol, when diagnosing pulmonary embolism. Venous ultrasound is also done in the

ICU first (routine assessment in stable patients, cause of a fever in a long-staying patient (Fever-protocol), evaluation of volemia using mainly the caval veins (FALLS-protocol) and first step for venous line insertions) and many other settings (e.g., geriatric dept).

The BLUE-protocol offers a 99 % specificity for the diagnosis of pulmonary embolism in those patients who have a normal anterior lung surface associated with a deep venous thrombosis (DVT). This highlights the importance of the present chapter.

A DVT is able to create sudden death, acute respiratory failure, but also simple fever, multiple so-called pneumoniae delaying the weaning of our ICU patients. Ultrasound can assess the venous network at the bedside, noninvasively, and almost all this network is accessible. Our 5 MHz microconvex probe is perfect for the search for DVT at all areas. In the BLUE-protocol, this is a requirement, since it will be used for any vein and the lung (plus the heart) without any delay.

The decision tree shows that the venous investigation is decided by the *BLUE-protocol* in the case of an A-profile, i.e., normality of the anterior chest wall in a severely dyspneic patient. We remind the main property of the BLUE-protocol, written in its label: it is only a protocol, not designed for exempting doctors to think. The doctor pilots this protocol, and his/her expertise tells him/her when to go beyond. Once this is understood, the BLUE-protocol gives its best.

Of critical importance (it will be reminded in the text), the BLUE-protocol takes into account only positive findings. In the spirit of the LUCIFLR, it will already allow 80 % of having shorter management with less radiations.

To Who Can This Chapter Provide New Information?

The traditional venous ultrasound did not consider the critically ill, mainly. Little by little since our underground use (1985), we saw that our empiric approach was different from the usual teaching we saw here and there. The differences are substantial and we suspect in actual fact that the same experts who proclaimed that lung ultrasound was unfeasible had developed, in their way, vascular ultrasound.

Here are our ten main differences:
1. We do not use vascular probes.
2. We do not use Doppler.
3. We do not use longitudinal approaches.
4. We do not use compression – when it is not necessary.
5. We do not use tough compression – when it is decided.
6. We use a new sign (the escape sign).
7. We do not restrict to "two-points" compression.
8. We pay little attention to the popliteal veins.
9. We pay special attention to the calf level.
10. The BLUE-protocol invites the first-line physician to provide this service immediately, 24/7/365, since 1989. This allows to bypass the traditional landscape where the expert (the radiologist) is not present on night. Or, if present, not immediately. Or, if immediately present, not accustomed to this kind of patient. Or, if accustomed, not always fully aware of some specific developments (here detailed). This makes many limitations.

We have the satisfaction to see that, in 2015, the point N°10 seems acquired: the tool is now in the right hands. A whole community of clinicians is at last convinced that ultrasound venous scanning is part of *their* discipline. We still believe, however, that the "rights hands" did not benefit up to now from the "right tool," hence this long chapter. Let us now, precisely, detail the 9 other points.

1. Vascular Probes Are Not Used

We are not quite sure if "vascular" probes deserve this label. We prefer to call them "linear," what they are for sure. Yet are *we* linear? We are not. Critical areas of interest are really not linear, such as the subclavian vein, the superior caval vein, and all veins when various materials surrounding the critically ill (catheters, devices, mechanical ventilation, tracheostomy, renal replacement catheters, any tubes and drains, etc.) prevent traditional approach with large footprint linear probes. The cutaneous availability is highly limited – the ergonomy of vascular probes makes a serious hindrance. Were we snakes, i.e., the most linear living creature, long axis would be fine, but in the short axis, due to the curvature, the probe contact to the skin would be suboptimal. The label "vascular" is not appropriate for probes which are unable to scan nonlinear areas (subclavian, skinny patients), which are unable to scan deep veins (caval vein), and which are condemned to follow anatomic constraints, for example, a short axis of the internal jugular vein if the patient has a short neck.

In other words, we consider that vascular probes are not suitable for studying vessels (we are not studying ambulatory chronic venous insufficiency).

Reminder, the necessity to change probes makes a loss of time, a failure of critical ultrasound, which the BLUE-protocol does not know.

We use a Japanese 5 MHz microconvex probe which makes a universal assessment: all veins in all orientations from all areas, linear or not, superficial and deep (Anecdotal Note 1). This smart probe can be inserted anywhere, at nonlinear areas (subclavian, popliteal, superior caval vein) as well as very linear ones (abdomen for inferior caval vein) and in areas of limited access (devices etc.), everywhere briefly. It can be rotated in long or short axis without increasing the skin contact. With a range from *0.6 to 17 cm*, it exposes all the veins we need to see (Fig. 18.1). Of course, some veins can be seen very well with linear probes, but the principle of the BLUE-protocol is to use the same probe for the veins (all), the lungs, and the heart, a.m.o., without losing one second (nor one dollar).

Third interest of the microconvex probe, its limited skin contact allows less energy for the compression, focused on the vein.

Colleagues who advocate vascular probes are happy to see nice images (in passing, not so spectacular if low-quality laptop equipment is used), but must acknowledge its limited value (scanning only superficial veins, only linear areas, no choice for orientation between short and long axis). The principle of the optimal compromise shows why our probe is the winning choice (see Chap. 3 devoted on the concept of the optimal compromise).

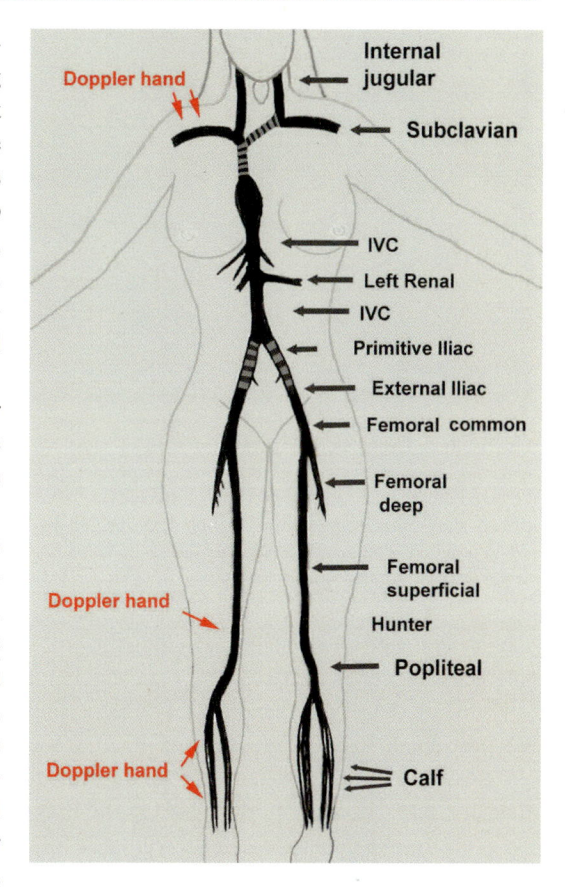

Fig. 18.1 The venous network, anatomical reminder. This figure shows the deep venous axes accessible to ultrasound. The superior caval vein, brachiocephalic trunk, and the primitive iliac veins, inconstantly exposed, are in gray or dotted. The areas where the second hand ("Doppler hand") is necessary are indicated

2. Doppler Is Not Used: What Does the BLUE-Protocol Instead

We promise to buy a Doppler equipment (and throw our Hitachi-405 to the garbage) at the very minute where we will feel blocked – a point not yet reached after our 26/30 years of clinical use. Read Anecdotal Note 2. Increasingly, clinicians admit that Doppler is not that mandatory for assessing the content of a vein [1–5]. Gray-scale ultrasound is a gold standard – a powerful bedside gold standard. The usual craze for Doppler appears ill defined to us; read Anecdotal Note 3.

Let us apply our probe on this patient we care to. Let us apply it correctly, i.e., like a fountain pen, at zero pressure. Just enough pressure for

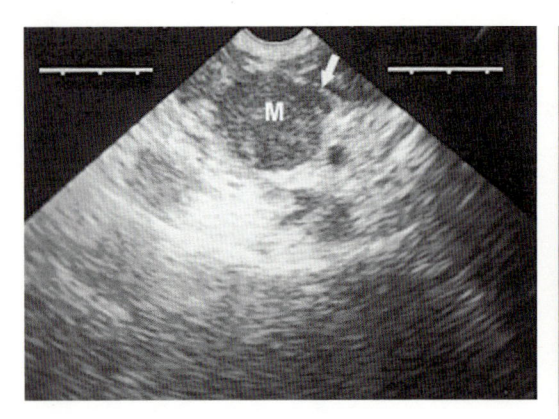

Fig. 18.2 A lymph node. Transverse scan of the neck. This "M" may be a venous thrombosis, a tissue-like mass detected outside the artery. The Carmen maneuver immediately shows this is an enlarged lymph node, egg shaped when scanned. The *arrow* designates the shifted and flattened internal jugular vein

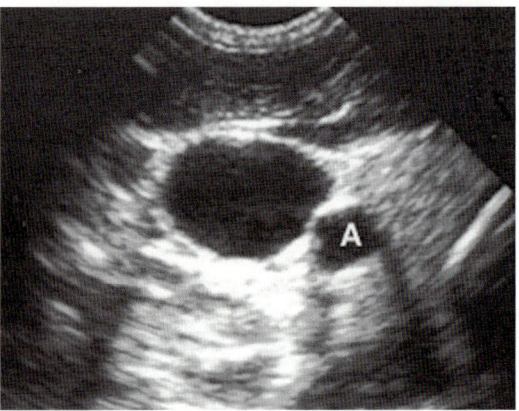

Fig. 18.3 Normal right internal jugular vein. Cross-sectional scan. The vein is located outside the artery (*A*) and has a round shape, a caliper of 13 × 20 mm, and an anechoic content. Note the vagus nerve behind the angle between the two vessels. It is difficult for us to understand what a vascular probe would add in terms of resolution, when compared to our universal microconvex probe

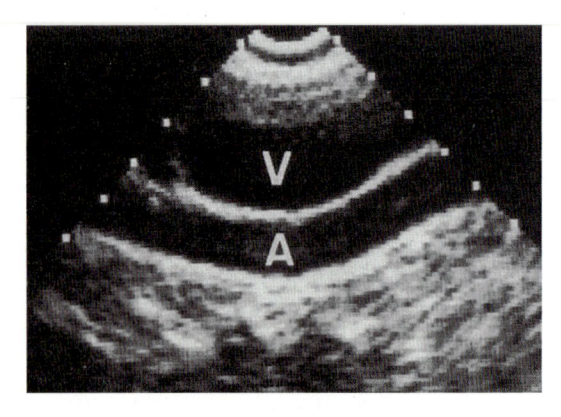

Fig. 18.4 Normal jugular internal vein, long axis. In this scan, the vein lies anterior to the artery (*A*), a rare (not exceptional) finding. Note this 1982 technology, taken here on purpose for showing that even this system was fully suitable at the bedside

having an image on the screen. Holding the probe another way would compress the vein, making it invisible on the screen (see Fig. 1.1). Decreasing the pressure up to the "zero pressure" level would progressively show the collapsed vein. Remember that an external operator must be able to withdraw the probe from the operator's hand without effort.

Let us apply the probe in the short axis of the vessels (this makes their detection immediate; see next section). Let us first rule out all what is not vascular. Round images can be vessels, but also cysts, lymph nodes, and hematomas (Fig. 18.2). No need for Doppler: just a Carmen maneuver shows that a lymph node has a beginning and an end, whereas a vessel has no end. Now we know we are scanning vessels. Muscles (sternocleidomastoidian for the internal jugular vein) are usually flat, not tubular.

Then the vascular pair is identified. Apart from rarities (brain, saphenous veins, etc.), there is one vein per artery (Figs. 18.3 and 18.4). Cross-sectional scans immediately show this pair. If the pair is not well seen, the Carmen maneuver is done until the image quality is optimized. Then the probe is held standstill. For keeping ultrasound a simple discipline, we advise to position the probe always perpendicular to the skin, above the area of interest, avoiding these sophisticated oblique approaches (see Fig. 1.1).

So now, which tube is the vein? A few of the following criteria is sufficient for immediate recognition. This is really easy for central veins, more subtle at distal veins, yet not an issue (read).
1. Central veins (jugular, subclavian, caval veins)
    (i) The vein is the one which is at the anatomical location of a vein (see again your anatomic lessons).
    (ii) The vein is the one not perfectly round in cross-section: it is more or less ovoid,

even concave and sometimes collapsed, whereas the artery is always round (aneurism apart).
- (iii) The vein is the one, in long axis, with walls quite never fully parallel, as opposed to the artery.
- (iv) The vein is the one with ample, respiratory movements – or no movement – whereas the artery has pulsatile systolic variations, visible on real time. On occasion, the vein has a complete inspiratory collapse. On occasion, we see superimposed cardiac-rhythm variations in large veins, especially in the case of tricuspid regurgitation, but these variations are not the abrupt systolic expansion seen in the arteries. The vein flattens on spontaneous inspiration and enlarges on mechanical inspiration.
- (v) The vein is the largest of both, since 2/3 of the blood volume is stocked in the venous compartment.
- (vi) The vein may contain fine valves (see Fig. 12.4 of our 2010 Edition), and the artery may contain coarse calcifications, never the opposite.
- (vii) The normal vein content is rather less echoic than the artery.
- (viii) A particular flow can on occasion be seen in a vein, never in an artery.
- (ix) When all these clues fail, a compression can then be attempted; only a free vein should collapse (see above).

2. Distal veins (femoral to calf veins) (iliac often)

At these areas, the features from 2 to 8 are increasingly more subtle. In practice, the compression step is more readily done. If one vessel begins to collapse, this vessel tells us it is the vein. If none of the vessels collapses, we know that one of them is a thrombosed vein, the other an artery (read Sophisticated Note 1). No matter which is the vein, the BLUE-protocol is positive. For those willing absolutely to know which one is the vein, a comparison with the other side shows the venous location (provided there is no exceptional bilateral venous thrombosis, of course). The few who will not be convinced will use the Doppler function, i.e., buy a Doppler machine.

3. Long-Axis Scans Are Not Performed

They make ultrasound more difficult. A slight rotation upsets the pattern in a long-axis view, whereas it does not affect a short-axis one (see Fig. 1.2). Let us remind that the words "longitudinal" and "transversal" are anatomical, body landmarks, whereas long axis and short axis regard only a given vessel.

For subclavian vein cannulation, we advocate a long axis (but this is no longer the BLUE-protocol).

We always use the Carmen maneuver, which allows, once a short-axis view of the vein is displayed, to see a centimetric bit of its distal and proximal aspect in a few seconds. In other words, we are short axis and long axis simultaneously in some sort.

4. Compression Is Not Performed: Not Systematically

Teachers have accustomed us to compress the veins for checking if they are thrombosed. This rather popular habit means skipping the first step of the BLUE-protocol, i.e., first observing the vein. This also maybe means that the usual "vascular" probes do not provide such a perfect image resolution. Using our 1982 technology, we are accustomed to see venous thromboses directly (Fig. 18.5). In the BLUE-protocol, "controlled compression" means slight compression, or no compression at all. When a static analysis has detected a DVT, this answered the question, and the compression technique is of no interest, possibly dangerous for no benefit.

We often see that when young doctors assess a vein, they compress it suddenly, at the moment they see it, without a breath, without a time for observation. The vein will not suddenly jump somewhere else. We must take time to locate it in the gunsight, aim, and then shoot without

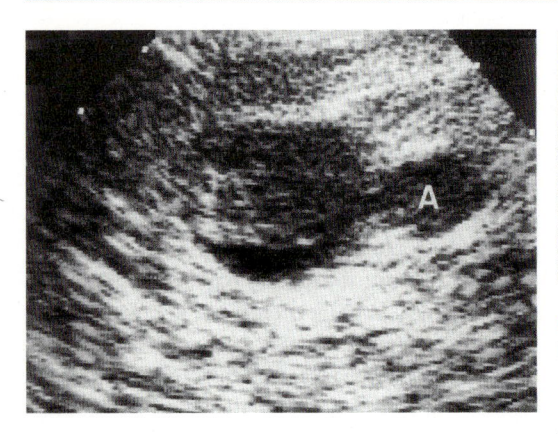

Fig. 18.5 Subocclusive thrombosis. Echoic image indicating a thrombosis of the jugular internal vein. The free lumen is reduced to an anechoic moon shape. A slight compression maneuver should make disappear this free lumen; an increased compression should initiate an escape sign. Cross-sectional scan of the cervical vessels (*A*, artery)

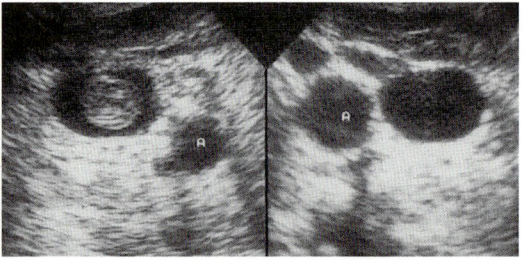

Fig. 18.6 Jugular internal vein floating thrombosis. Blatant thrombosis and comparative look. There is no video but such thrombosis, surrounded by the bloodstream, is by definition floating. This figure exploits the concept of the best compromise: this is the reprint of a reprint (original long lost), but in spite of the degradation, this image clearly demonstrates the disease. These patterns were observable at the bedside since 1992. Ultrasound is really a gold standard

exaggerated haste (please, just identify the enemy before shooting!).

A normal, free vein appears homogeneous. Sometimes anechoic, sometimes just hypoechoic, mostly depending on the local acoustic conditions, but it appears always homogeneous – apart from ghosts, easily spotted. Like some microclimates, some areas quite always have a favorable surrounding: jugular internal vein in particular. In these cases, the static approach can be considered a gold standard: "black means free." The compression here is really redundant. Subclavian and femoropopliteal veins are usually black gray.

A visible DVT yields static and dynamic signs. The dynamic signs are striking and would convince any reluctant academician, yet they are redundant to our opinion.

Static Sign: The Anatomical Image

Once we have chosen the correct unit, the correct probe, the correct probe holding, the correct axis (short axis), and the correct pressure, at the chosen location, we can now see the ultrasound image and interpret it. A thrombosis can be nonocclusive or occlusive. When it is nonocclusive, the eye of the operator immediately detects two anomalies:
- There is a contrast between the anechoic (or hypoechoic) tone of the circulating fluid, and the more echoic tone of the thrombosis.
- The shape of this supposed thrombosis is well defined and convex, with well-defined borders: a shape of cumulus or cauliflower.

This allows an immediate recognition (Figs. 18.5 and 18.6).

When the thrombosis is occlusive, these two patterns are no longer available, but it is sometimes possible to see a tissue-like, heterogeneous, irregular pattern, standstill, striking in Fig. 18.7, and see Fig. 28.8. This semiology is striking when the caliper of the vein is large, increasingly more subtle when this caliper shrinks. Each time this pattern is not easily detected, the compression will confirm the diagnosis.

Simple, real-time ultrasound informs that such thromboses are more or less occlusive (Fig. 18.7), more or less extensive (Fig. 18.7), more or less floating (Fig. 28.10 and Video 28.1), and more or less infected (see Fig. 28.11). Extensive, floating, infected cases are probably more severe than others. Really, ultrasound has the power of a gold standard.

Some signs of ours:
- The sequel sign: the image of (suspected) thrombosis is prolonged downstream (or upstream) by an image clearly identified as the patent vein.
- The echoic flow. In some machines (at least, the old ADR-4000), it was possible to see echoic flows through the veins (see Fig. 13.14 of our 2010 Edition). This informed on the flow (not a big deal in our duties), a possible

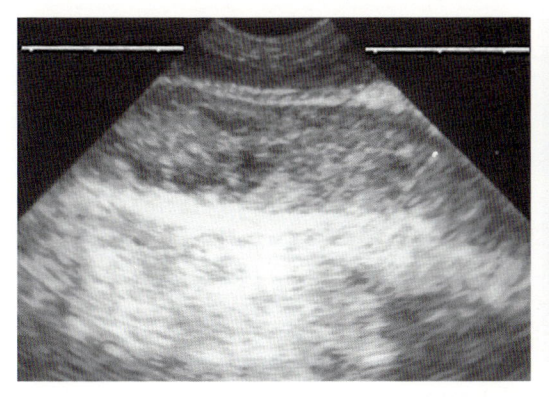

Fig. 18.7 Occlusive and extensive jugular internal venous thrombosis. Long axis. We can measure at least a 6 cm extension. Note the echoic, tissue-like standstill echogenicity, making the diagnosis of thrombosis

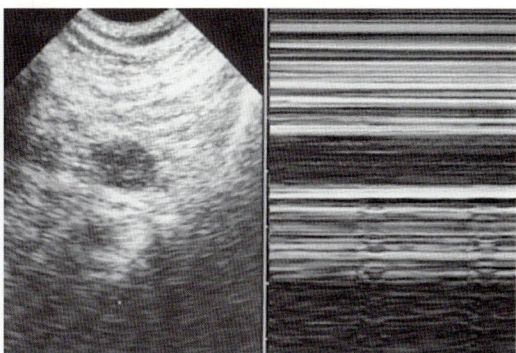

Fig. 18.8 Occlusive thrombosis of the subclavian vein. Short axis. The vein is incompressible. The *right figure*, in M-mode, depicts a sensitive sign of occlusive thrombosis: complete absence of respiratory dynamics of the vein

tricuspid regurgitation (sudden inversion of flow in rhythm with respiration), and mostly the venous patency.

Dynamic Signs
The Floating Thrombosis
The floating character of a DVT, although spectacular, does not add a lot to the diagnosis of DVT; it is rather a prognosis indicator. A blue patient with a floating DVT is, clearly, at the highest risk of sudden death. In the BLUE-protocol, floating patterns are rarely seen. They were likely present just before the sudden drama (i.e., patients we don't see). They are much more often seen in the ICU, within the CLOT-protocol, presented in Chap. 28, where a video is available (Video 28.1).

For floating DVTs, ultrasound appears to us as a gold standard, making venography fully obsolete, without long descriptions.

The Adynamic Vein
A more subtle dynamic sign is the absence of dynamics. Free upper veins (internal jugular, subclavian) have usually ample movements in spontaneous breathing (negative inspiratory pressure). A standstill upper vein suggests thrombosis (Fig. 18.8).

Some Particular Images of Thrombosis
Incipient Thrombosis
Between blood and clot, there is a short transient step. The vein is soft; we are quite sure such a vein can be flattened by the probe pressure, but

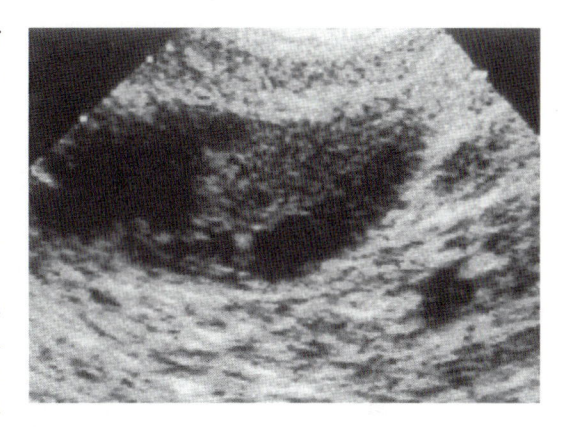

Fig. 18.9 Incipiens thrombosis. Diaphanous curls are floating, dancing likes wreaths, in the lumen of this internal jugular vein. A part is fixed against the wall. This pattern appears as the first step of a rising venous thrombosis. This figure was taken in a night shift in 1989 with the ADR-4000. Just by looking at this potential, we had the feeling that bedside ultrasound was a giant, just (deeply) sleepy

we never tried (we hesitate to compress). A kind of diaphanous image is visible within the venous lumen, partly fixed against the wall, partly freely floating, and nearly dancing (Fig. 18.9). A day later, a complete thrombosis is usually present.

Thrombophlebitis
It is dealt with in the CLOT-protocol, Chap. 28.

Images Which Are Not Thrombosis
We will not come again on the lymph nodes, cysts, and hematomas, but on ghost artifacts. The BLUE-protocol believes in ghosts. They exist,

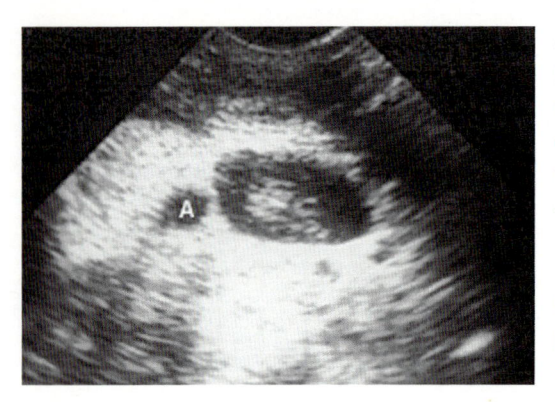

Fig. 18.10 A ghost. Ghost artifact. This echoic image, in the lumen of the left internal jugular vein, has hyperechoic pattern and regular shape. It appears fully motionless on video. A very soft pressure of the probe pushes this image outside and completely collapses the lumen, proving its artifactual nature (*A*, left carotid artery). Note the oblique course of this artifact (created by strongly reflecting surrounding structures)

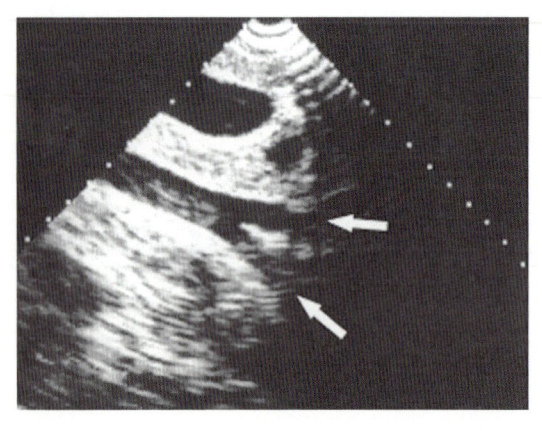

Fig. 18.11 Another ghost (at the aortic bifurcation). This vessel is nicely exposed using our 1982-tech ADR-4000 (*arrows*, primitive iliac vessels). The ghost is rather parallel to the long axis, there is a strongly hyperechoic structure (fat) just surrounding the aorta (in addition to a slight acoustic enhancement). Seen within a vein, this pattern should not scare. It would be completely motionless. It would vanish if using a perpendicular scan

and one task is to recognize them and respect them. They are usually created by hyperechoic surrounding structures. No need for ghost detectors: these artifacts are regular, hyperechoic, and geometric (usually horizontal/vertical, sometimes following the surrounding structures, like in Fig. 18.10 and 18.11): the ghost looks like a cirrhus (i.e., rather linear) and never anatomic like a cumulus. It is motionless. In case of persistent doubt, a slight compression will compress the vein, and the ghost will quietly disappear, without any escape sign (see below), yielding complete collapse of the vein.

5. Compression *(If Performed)* Is Controlled

Controlled compression means either no compression, as seen, or *mild* compression. A mild compression is fully sufficient for collapsing a normal vein. A strong pressure would crash a thrombosed vein (and conclude to a normal test). A strong pressure may dislodge an unstable thrombosis [6]. A strong pressure may result in collapsing an artery (especially if the blood pressure is low).

The physiology has taught us that the venous pressure is low. Therefore, a very slight pressure is more than sufficient for collapsing a normal vein in most cases (some cases of extreme venous hypertension excluded). It is not only sufficient but also mandatory. We fear the effects of a tough compression on a fresh, floating thrombosis, which may create a sign which we called the *sudden death sign*. At best a simple chest pain, which may be it is true highly suggestive of pulmonary embolism, but not, it is true too, a fully elegant sign. If schools teach to compress, but don't specify how, we must be ready to face from time to time this "sudden death sign."

When Do We Eventually Perform a Compression?

In these distal areas where the venous content is often a bit echoic, occlusive thromboses are less obvious to diagnose. The compression maneuver will be done more rapidly.

How Do We Perform Soft Compression

Let us take a breath and make a slow motion of a compression maneuver. What happens? When a normal vein is softly and slowly compressed, the

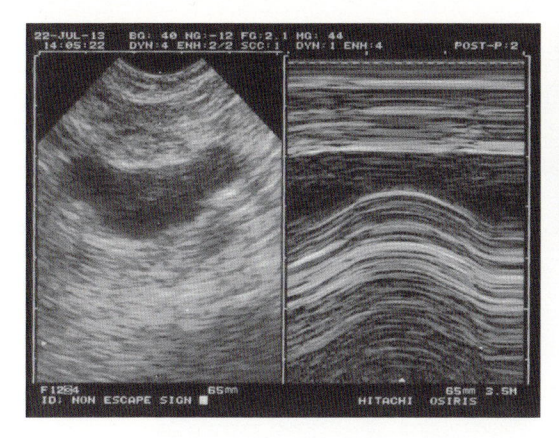

To Who Can This Chapter Provide New Information?

Fig. 18.12 Non-escape sign – normal compressibility. The shrinking sign. This patent common femoral vein is here slightly compressed. M-mode clearly indicates that the distal wall moves toward the proximal wall, which seems standstill. This is the expected dynamic in a normal compression maneuver. The whole of the underlying soft tissues begin to shrink in concert with the venous lumen (in this incomplete compression)

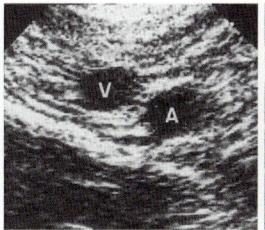

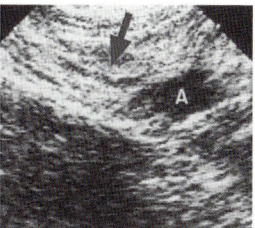

Fig. 18.13 Fully compressible subclavian vein. The left image shows how the subclavian couple immediately appears on a longitudinal scan below the clavicle. The right image shows the complete collapse of this vein when pressure is exerted by a probe (*arrowhead*), helped if needed by the Doppler hand. Cross-sectional scan of the subclavian vein (*V*), with the satellite artery (*A*)

walls are seen getting nearer to each other. More exactly, one can see the *distal* wall coming toward the *proximal* wall, which seems apparently standstill. We slightly increase the pressure, quietly. The more the pressure, the more the distal wall moves toward the proximal wall (Fig. 18.12). Eventually, the distal wall reaches the proximal wall, resulting in a complete collapse of the vein using mild pressure. Both the venous lumen and the soft tissues surrounding the vein are seen shrinking; we may call this sign the *shrinking sign*. There is a kind of acceleration at the end; both walls seem to attract and slap against each other. The normal compression maneuver should reach this 100 % result, i.e., a complete (not 95 %) collapse of the vein (Fig. 18.13). Small footprint probes, i.e., our microconvex one, have the perfect design for making this dynamic pattern easy to observe. The operator should be accustomed to feel the necessary pressure to obtain this result (Anecdotal Note 4).

Exceptionally, for external reasons (body habitus, soft tissue edemas), the necessary pressure is higher than usual. Just a bilateral analysis will help here, showing that the effort for compressing is symmetrical.

Rule No. 1 in critical ultrasound, the probe is perpendicular, exactly at the zenith of the vein before compressing. It must stay in this axis when compressing.

How many hands? When there is a bone behind the vein, one hand is sufficient. In three strategic areas (Fig. 18.1), the absence of bone needs the use of the "Doppler hand" (see below about the lower femoral vein). This is why we permanently need our two hands (and why we feel fully comfortable with machines on carts and are a bit embarrassed when using, in hospital settings, pocket machines which monopolize one hand, among several points; read Anecdotal Note 5). Do not forget that the described technique in this chapter is mainly useful in the SESAME-protocol, i.e., cardiac arrest.

6. A Sign Absent from the Textbooks: The Escape Sign

Instead of "savagely" compressing the vein with haste, immediately once seen, let us again do it softly, in a kind of slow motion.

A compression maneuver affects not only the vein, but all surrounding tissues. When a vein is fully thrombosed, under compression, the whole vein is seen moving, both proximal and distal walls keeping the same distance, whereas the soft tissues are seen shrinking. This contrast is what we call an uncompressible vein: no shrinking

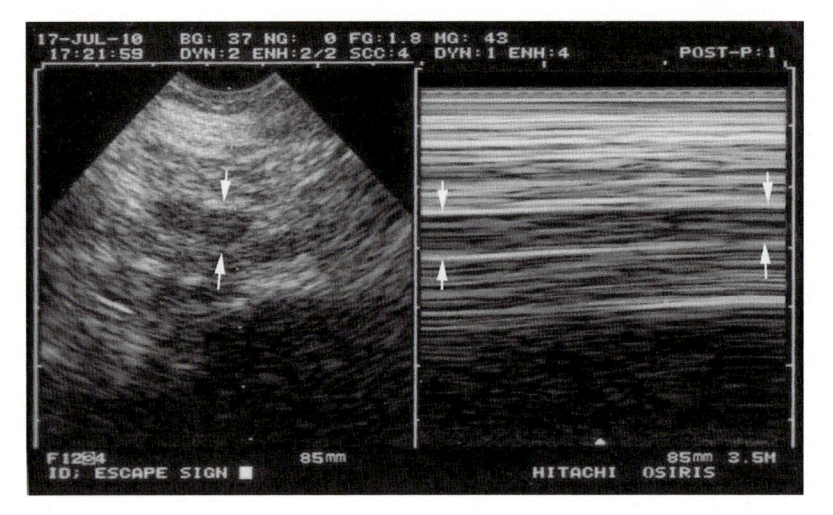

Fig. 18.14 The escape sign. *Left*, the vein (*arrows*). Then the compression is made. The *right figure* illustrates the phenomenon of the escape sign. In spite of a probe pressure sufficient for shrinking the soft tissues, and moving the vein in one go, the walls of the vein remain parallel, without initiating any collapse. Slight detail, the walls in M-mode (*arrows*) remain strictly parallel and flat. If one does this on an artery, one would see eventual systolic expansions, recordable in M-mode

sign. The thrombosed vein behaves like a sausage (a blood sausage so to speak).

Around the vein, the soft tissues shrink, under the pressure. This results in the feeling that the thrombosed vein escapes. In the BLUE-protocol, this contrast between the shrinking of the soft tissue and the non-collapsibility of the vein has been labeled the escape sign.

The pressure of the probe succeeds in displacing the vein (relatively to surrounding tissues), but not in collapsing it.

The escape sign can be standardized: by locating in the image a deep and a superficial structure well visible (any aponeuroses), we estimate that a 20 % (approximately) shrinking of these soft tissues with no change of the venous caliper is an escape sign (Fig. 18.14 and Video 18.1).

When a normal vein is compressed, its volume decreases, but its pressure remains unchanged, until it is completely collapsed. When a thrombosed vein is compressed, the pressure immediately increases (which can lead to the previously described "sudden death sign").

This is critical, since in many instances (agitated patient, focal tension of the soft tissues, some morphotypes), the soft tissues do not shrink well. In these situations only, we are authorized to apply a higher compression.

A slight probe pressure is sufficient for initiating the escape sign. With experience, this is sufficient for the diagnosis. The escape sign makes us interrupt the compression maneuver. Any additional pressure intensifies and confirms the escape sign, but increases the risk of dislodgement. In a partial occlusion, the slight compression maneuver easily collapses the free lumen (Fig. 18.5) and then initiates an escape sign. It should be emphasized and repeated that a moderate probe pressure is necessary and sufficient to collapse a normal vein.

7. The BLUE-Protocol Does Not Restrict to Two-Point Protocols

Now the question is: where shall we apply our probe?

We heard of these protocols, called "four points," that we call "two points": one of the common femoral vein and one at the popliteal vein make two. These protocols are popular in emergency rooms; they work when the patient has local trouble. Such protocols are providential in the overcrowded ER where the main goal is to relieve this chronic pressure. This does not work in the BLUE-protocol where the patient is in acute respiratory failure and the question is rather to find where is, if any, the *remaining* thrombosis. This makes a philosophy opposed to the traditional ER protocols.

The perspective of scanning the whole venous network may scare. The BLUE-protocol answers this issue by proposing a *sequential* scanning based on a 26-year analysis of files, answering the question asked above. Once a DVT has been seen, the BLUE-protocol is over.

Obviously, the venous analysis should follow the clinical point of interest (painful leg); we assume for schematizing that there is no clinical sign of DVT.

The decision tree follows the most frequent locations and may appear hectic, because it assesses some points at the lower extremity and then jumps on the upper axes and then, if negative, comes back to other points of the lower extremities. This is just a way to expedite the BLUE-protocol. One can scan more, but this does not affect the initial therapy.

This is the sequential order of the BLUE-protocol (readers can adapt it at will; some can make step 5 before 4; we just optimized the speed):

1. Common femoral vein
2. Lower part of the femoral vein, just above the knee
3. Calf vein (at mid leg)
4. Jugular internal and subclavian veins
5. If all is negative, jump to the middle femoral vein
6. Popliteal vein for concluding

This allows for a really fast protocol, 3 min or less as published [7]. On the 3 min of the BLUE-protocol, 2 min is devoted to the veins (when they have to be assessed), making this assessment the longest part. It is the longest, but anyway provides a diagnosis in 3 min or less. We again remind that the BLUE-protocol aims at an overall

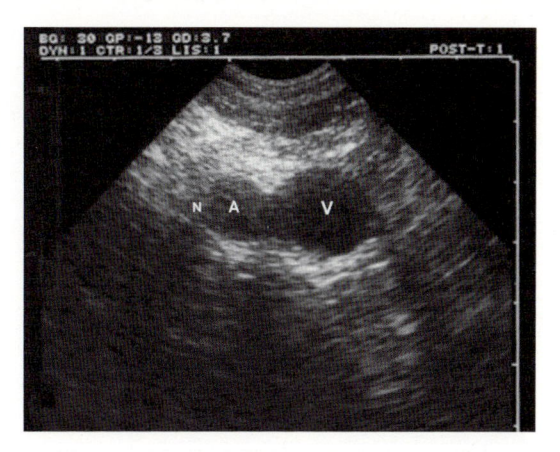

Fig. 18.15 A common figure: the common femoral vein. Cross-sectional scan at the groin. The absence of apparent separation between artery (*A*) and vein (*V*) is due to a tangency artifact, hence this peanut pattern. We heard about a Mickey Mouse sign in the near area, an image which would be of interest for very young students. For those interested in nerve blockade, the nerve (*N*) is featured

90.5 % of accuracy, and the physician is free to use more time for making better.

Let us see these locations, *in the sequence of the BLUE-protocol*.

Common Femoral Vein

There is little to say; this area is *now* familiar to an increasing number of physicians. For the laggards, this vein lies inside the femoral pulse (Fig. 18.15). The deep femoral vein leaves the main axis and goes toward the femur, whereas the superficial femoral vein (a strange name for a deep vein) descends, vertical, inside the femur, up to the knee. On occasion, the femoral superficial vein is duplicated, yielding two venous channels surrounding the artery.

The static approach is rarely contributive. There is not enough space for floating patterns apart from rare cases. The compression is useful here.

This area is found to be positive in one-quarter of our patients. With a 99 % specificity, this unpublished data means that *one-quarter of all patients with massive pulmonary embolism generating acute respiratory failure and admission to the ICU will be diagnosed after one venous shot*. If this area is free, we resume.

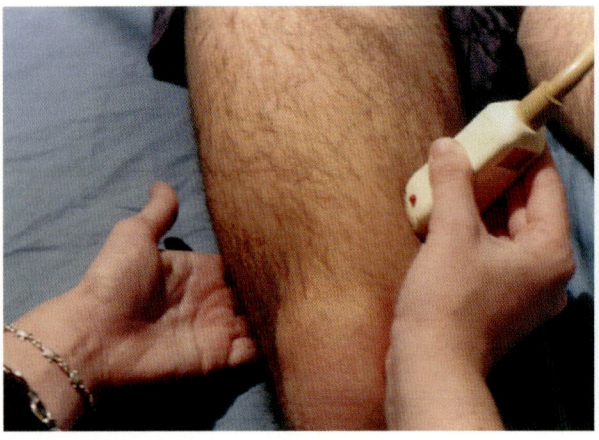

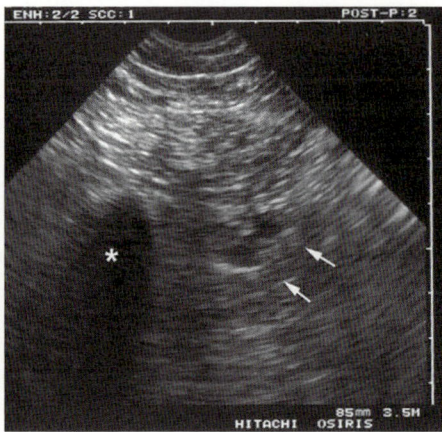

Fig. 18.16 The Doppler hand at the V-point. This figure shows how easily the lower femoral vein is studied using a two-hand compression, making Doppler useless. The microconvex probe has the ideal shape for this use. See how it can be applied everywhere, in any incidence. Note how the right hand gently holds the probe while firmly lying on the leg. At the right, the ultrasound image (transversal scan of lower thigh). The femur generates frank shadow (*star*). The femoral vessels are seen within the femur (*arrows*). Which one is the vein? The compression will tell (among other signs)

Lower Femoral Vein: The "V-Point"

Shortly, critically ill patients are supine, and this is an easy-to-access area. The manufacturers will probably tell you: "We are sorry, but here, you assess a segment which cannot be compressed. You really *need* Doppler, Sir." And the radiologists will solemnly approve: "He is right, this is an uncompressible area." This belief has made the delight of those who sold Doppler equipments. Considering that we have two hands, we will just use our unoccupied hand as a counterpressure, to be applied opposed to the probe. By the way, critical ultrasound is permanently practiced using both hands, which constantly interact, like in any physical examination.

A minimal expertise is needed at the beginning for understanding how to make an efficient V-point maneuver. Several attempts should be done (usually, the hand is not at the exact level of the probe, usually the free hand is too deep), but, once the user has found the correct point, it smells like a small victory, hence the "V" ("V" for victory against the Doppler philosophy). The probe is in a transversal scan, roughly located one patella above the patella, scanning the short axis of the vein (Fig. 18.16). The free hand is positioned exactly on the other side than the probe. The fingers should surround the biceps, and then compress. The probe and the free hand make a simultaneous rapprochement, 3/4 from the free hand, 1/4 from the probe hand (Video 18.1). A very soft pressure from the fingers of the free hand is sufficient for easily collapsing a normal vein. Another reason for using Doppler is pulverized. This maneuver, called facetiously the "Doppler hand" by Marcio and Bianca Rodriguez (from Porto Alegre), is achieved in a few seconds.

Advantage: it seems to us and most users much easier, and more accessible, than the popliteal veins. It is a good compromise between the common femoral vein, easy but not very sensitive (only one-quarter), and the calf vein, more difficult technically.

A positive V-point (i.e., a DVT at the Hunter canal) is frequent, and the association "common femoral" plus "V-point" is positive in half the cases. This means that, at this step, *half of the patients have a positive BLUE-protocol for pulmonary embolism.*

The Calf Veins

This deserves a specific section (see below). It will just allow *two-thirds* of the patients to benefit from extremely fast diagnosis of pulmonary embolism.

The Jugular Internal Vein and Subclavian Vein

The technique for the jugular internal vein has no peculiarity. This location is extremely frequent in the intensive care unit. See about the CLOT-protocol in Chap. 28. For the subclavian vein, the "Doppler hand" is used, inserted above the clavicle, compressing softly with the finger tips while the probe is held below the clavicle. With roughly 4 % of positive findings, this fast analysis is of interest (Fig. 18.8).

The Midfemoral Vein

We exceptionally (roughly 2 %) see such locations, i.e., surrounded by free upper and lower segments.

The Popliteal Vein

This area is assessed in 20 % of cases (all those with negative previous steps) and seems useful in less than 1 % of cases, yet by adding and adding small numbers, we reach the roughly 80 % overall sensitivity. With the usual equipments (long and large linear probes), we find this approach technically feasible but more complicated than the others. The patient that does not help (too tired) will not take the prone positioning. In supine patients, each centimeter of length saved makes the test easier. See Fig. 18.17.

Is It Enough? How About the Other Veins? Iliocaval Veins? Others?

The interest of this sequence is that, in an extended series (on submission), the rate of DVT finding (81 % in the native article) stabilizes at 78/79 %. This rate will maybe now slightly increase if we fully include the right pulmonary artery in our protocol (see this approach of interest in Step 2 of the SESAME-protocol, Chap. 31).

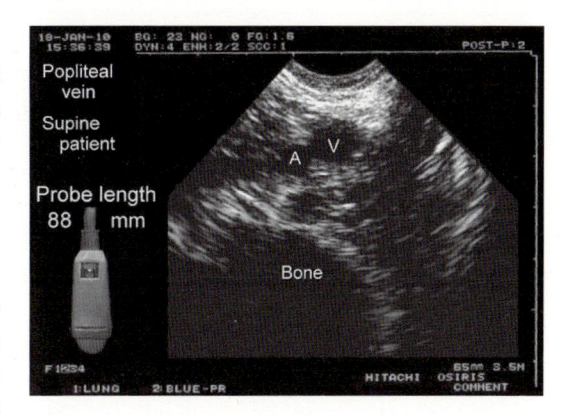

Fig. 18.17 Popliteal vein using our microconvex probe. Posterior cross-sectional approach of the popliteal fossa, showing the vein (*V*), generally single, and the artery (*A*). In the cartouche, our 88 mm-long probe

The caval vein is not included in the BLUE-protocol. We really think that just before a massive pulmonary embolism, an iliocaval thrombosis is probably very frequent, but rarely after. Caval or iliac thromboses, isolated, i.e., with free common femoral vein, were not seen in patients of the BLUE-protocol with massive pulmonary embolism. Since these locations are slightly more difficult (iliac mainly) and disappointing because of body habitus (disturbing gas are seen in not far from half cases), this decision, of no consequence in our data, expedites the learning curve.

We hypothesize that when a patient develops a DVT, the calves are first involved, and then the DVT quietly invades the popliteal and femoral areas, before quietly propagating to iliac and then caval veins. These veins are large, and we assume that iliocaval thromboses are always floating there. Then the accident occurs, suddenly making iliocaval veins free from DVT. This is why we do not advise to spend too much energy in these areas. In the CLOT-protocol, which is an anticipating test (learn about it in Chap. 28), they are under extreme care.

The inferior caval vein is dealt with in the section on CLOT-protocol of Chap. 28. The superior caval vein was, for simplifying, withdrawn from this chapter. See its analysis in Chap. 30 devoted to hemodynamic assessment. The left brachicephalic vein is sometimes visible anterior to the aortic cross using a suprasternal route and the microconvex probe. This segment is skipped for keeping this chapter simple.

Note: users not fully accustomed to anatomy can simply detect one vein, and follow step by step where this vein runs through other territories, since all the vascular network is connected.

8. Calf Veins: The "Forbidden Zone"

A calf DVT is a major finding.

Why does the BLUE-protocol pay major attention to the calf veins? Because it searches for pulmonary embolism, and the test is concluded once a DVT, even at the calf (especially at the calf), has been found. The patients of the BLUE-protocol are critically ill. Our manuscript was rejected several times for the allotted reason that a calf thrombosis is not a major problem and does not embolize, which is true [8]. Read, if not hurried, Anecdotal Note 6. We are sure that no doctor is worried by isolated calf vein thromboses. Even if though, the more the number of segments are free, the lower the probability of deadly surprises according to the Grotowski law (read Anecdotal Note 7). Our reviewers think, rightly, that death does not come from isolated calf thrombosis [9–13] but from iliofemoral extensions [14–17]. We respect them; they just forgot that here, we see a patient who has *already* embolized. And the more the patient is critically ill, the more the possibility of detecting only a distal remaining thrombosis (if any) is high. We do not treat this small DVT, we treat the severe pulmonary embolism. Comprising this area in the protocol allows to count 20 % more patients as positive.

Why is this area a "forbidden area"? Indeed, these 18 vessels (two per artery, three arteries per leg) make a small world. But we think that the community has increased this "difficulty." By using the posterior approach, vascular probes, long-axis views, and Doppler and, mostly, by confiding ultrasound to radiologists, who have been educated to making comprehensive examinations and would be reluctant not to provide a 100 % confidence test to the first-line physician, the community has superadded all difficulties.

How do we proceed? By erasing these difficulties one by one. For this, we made the opposite of the traditional protocols.

First, not radiologists, we can assume a non-"100 %" result in these cases. Having all other data in mind (i.e., making an extended BLUE-protocol even unaware of this), we can accept this limitation. A critically important reminder is that the BLUE-protocol takes into account only the positive findings.

The (critically ill) patient is kept supine.
The microconvex probe is used.
It is inserted anteriorly.
It is applied in the transversal axis of the leg.

Venous Detection

And now, we can standardize landmarks (Fig. 18.18): the leg bones, the interosseous membrane, and the posterior tibial muscle are sequentially seen. We skip the tibial anterior group for simplifying (Accessory Note 2). Now, the exact location of the (posterior) veins is standardized: they are applied just posterior to the posterior tibial muscle. Identifying these vascular groups is the critical step. These veins in the short axis appear as holes. These "holes" are small and can be millimetric, but in the same manner that we will detect a *fly* in our soup, we will pay attention to these structures. Their names? Fibular group near the fibula and posterior tibial group near the tibia. Each group is one artery and two veins. This makes six holes in the short axis (Fig. 18.18). The six are sometimes so near to each other that this looks like the long axis of a vessel, but it is not (this very pattern may even deserve a label; we will search for one). The Carmen maneuver is the point which makes the venous location easy.

Static Analysis?

We have now reached the step where the vein has been located. From this observational step, can a

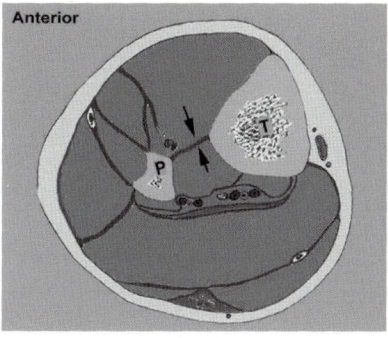

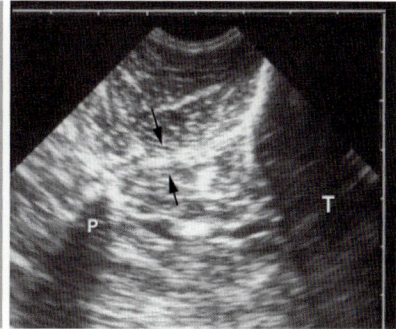

Fig. 18.18 Topographic and ultrasound anatomy of the calf veins. *Left*, a transversal section of a calf, showing the location of the three vascular groups. One anterior to the interosseous membrane, near the fibula (*P*), two posterior to the posterior tibial muscle. Bones, interosseous membrane, and tibial muscle make strong landmarks. *T* tibia. *Right*: ultrasound correlation, same landmarks, anterior approach. About 2 cm posterior, through the posterior tibial muscle, the tibial posterior and fibular veins are visible, inside the location of the letters P and T: *P*, shadow of the fibula. *T*, shadow of the tibia. Anterior group slightly visible between fibula and *upper arrow*

DVT be detected? Here a place for a static approach would be too fragile. Usually, thrombosed veins are larger than normal ones, but we regularly see large cross-sections which get perfectly compressible. Thrombosed veins are more echoic than normal ones, but again, this sign is too fragile. This step is usually not sufficient.

Dynamic Analysis (the Step of Compression)

The veins are so small that one should operate like a sniper, with the eye fixed at these vascular targets. Now, the Doppler hand (free hand) comes posterior to the calf, and its thumb searches for the other thumb, while the eye is fixed at the screen (if not, these small targets risk to be lost). Importantly, the Doppler hand must just touch the skin, quite a "negative compression": even a simple touch can begin to shrink normal veins. The free hand softly catches the posterior calf with zero pressure and softly initiates the compression. Normally, it results in a shrinking of the soft tissues, with a progressive and complete collapse of the veins, i.e., four targets. Two targets remain open: the arteries. The number "four" should not be an obsession, even a partial vision of these four veins is sufficient in some difficult cases; read below. If the "Doppler hand" completes the compression at higher degree, the small arteries become pulsatile. This change is a way, not developed in this textbook, of showing the absence of arterial obstruction without, once again, using Doppler. A calf DVT shows (usually) large, gray tubules which above all do not compress, associated with the escape sign, and a contralateral normality. All these points are gathered in Videos 18.1 and 18.2.

Is It Always That Easy?

In 80 % of cases, it is. Simplicity was optimized at each step. Three ways are possible:

1. The venous groups are identified. They are compressible. A compression at one point is done in a few seconds and rules out local calf thrombosis. The probability of thrombosis decreases with the number of measurements. A comprehensive analysis would be time-consuming, with the risk of not reaching the 100 % of volume scanned, and here, we agree for making reasonable one-, two- or three-point protocols. The ultrasound report will describe a calf venous system free in one, two, or three points.

2. A pathological structure is identified: tubular, noncompressible, echoic, enlarged, and yielding an escape sign (Fig. 18.19) and a sequel sign. Calf thrombosis is quasi-certain.

3. No tubular group is easily identified. The operator fails in locating the venous targets. This happens in 20 % of cases. Read next section.

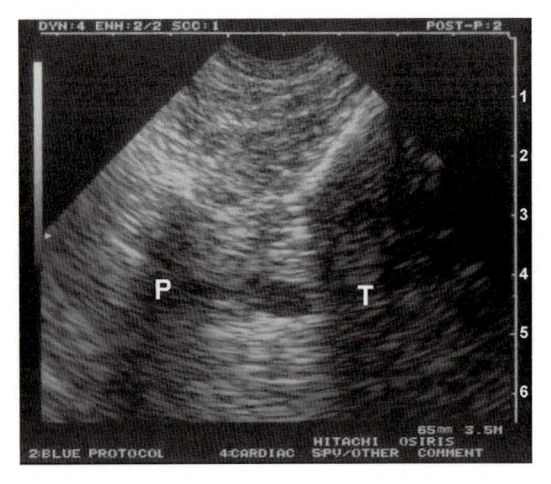

Fig. 18.19 A calf venous thrombosis. In this transverse anterior scan, an enlarged structure is visible, at the normal place of a posterior tibial vein. This structure is tubular on dynamic scanning, and not compressible using the Doppler hand, as opposed to the contralateral one. The letters labeling the bone shadows (*P* fibula, *T* tibia) are located at the level of the veins (at roughly 4 cm)

What to Do in Those Difficult Cases

Several factors explain the difficulty, some being accessible to simple maneuvers:

1. Because the calf veins are saccular. What is not seen at one level may be more easily seen 1 mm above or below. The solution is therefore a (very slight) Carmen maneuver.
2. Because of insufficient filling of the veins (hypovolemia?). For filling them, one can use fluid therapy, or this maneuver: a tourniquet applied above the patella, at the V-point (by definition free of thrombosis). It stops venous return, which usually enlarges the venous cross-section. Pulmonary embolism, by increasing the venous pressure, should enlarge the veins, but we see often small or collapsed veins, including the IVC (we will carefully assess this point).
3. Because of an iso-echoic thrombosis (iso-echoic to the surrounding structures). This is up to now a pitfall, but this would also result in an isolated artery: a fully unusual event. A Carmen maneuver would possibly show a tubule satellite to the artery. Devoid of traditional gold standard, we cannot conclude.
4. One can try the "Mocelin variant" (a term designed when the approach begins by the conclusion, i.e., not academic, sometimes very helpful). We compress, without knowing where the veins are. If we happen to see small structures touching each other under compression, they prove to be veins – normal veins. To be used when really nothing works.
5. One can still try lateral approaches, posterior to the tibia, or sometimes to the fibula (Fig. 18.18). It is more difficult because we failed up to now to find a standardized way to detect these veins.
6. Users with Doppler equipment can still use Doppler.
7. Intrinsic body habitus. Here is not a lot to do. Let us remind, again, that the BLUE-protocol works only when a DVT is identified. If not, but if the suspicion of embolism is high (using those familiar pre-test probabilities), it is always time to turn to usual tools. When there is an A-profile with no visible DVT, the BLUE-protocol requires to come back to the lungs. It concludes either to a pneumonia (if PLAPS) or COPD/asthma (in their absence), but the user is a "pilot" and must know when to go beyond this simple protocol when common sense asks for more. For decreasing the irradiation (by asking scintigraphy instead of helical CT), see Chap. 29.

9. The Patients in the BLUE-Protocol Are Critically Ill: They Don't Like to Be Turned in the Prone Positioning; How About Popliteal Analysis?

This area, familiar in the ER, is not prioritized in the BLUE-protocol, as explained above. It comes last. The vein is posterior in a patient who cannot be easily turned (Fig. 18.17). The BLUE-protocol proposes instead the V-point, much easier, and the calf analysis, much more sensitive.

In addition, the knee is a zone of *flexion*, one of the most mobile parts in the human body. We consider (personal opinion based upon physiology) that, similar to a metallic wire, repeated flexions and extensions should result in weakening the DVT at this point. Applying the probe at an area of such instability does not appear as a perfect idea, not fully logical, and we prefer to consider the calf veins, an area appearing much more "stable."

There is also a debate between those who argue they can scan the popliteal vein in all supine patients and others who find it difficult. Prone positioning, Valsalva maneuvers, etc., are irrelevant in the critically ill patient.

In spite of these limitations, the users will once again appreciate the holistic power of the BLUE-protocol: we just have to slightly bend the knee, and insert our 88 mm-long microconvex probe.

10. The BLUE-protocol Is Done by the First-Line Physician

No comment, read at the beginning of this chapter.

An Eleventh Point?

Definitely. The venous BLUE-protocol can be used in multiple settings, without any adaptation. It also works in cardiac arrest (Step 2 of the SESAME-protocol, Chap. 31). From cardiac arrest to a simple medical airborne transportation (ULTIMAT-protocol, Chap. 33) or the visit at your grandmother who has a slight complaint at the leg (DVT? Simple arthrosis?), the protocol will be applied the same. In between, all these settings, the emergency room, with leg pain or all those kinds of troubles, the intensive care unit, routine scan of standstill patients, the ward or geriatric department… can make use of the BLUE-protocol.

We can here evoke the daily question, in the ER, of the management of a non-critically ill patient suspected with mild pulmonary embolism and with negative venous ultrasound scanning. In order to make a homogeneous textbook, this situation is detailed in Chap. 36.

The Developed BLUE-protocol

All this chapter generates a change in the decision tree. As said initially, the short term "venous analysis" is replaced by the current sequence, which results in making the protocol much simpler (Fig. 18.20).

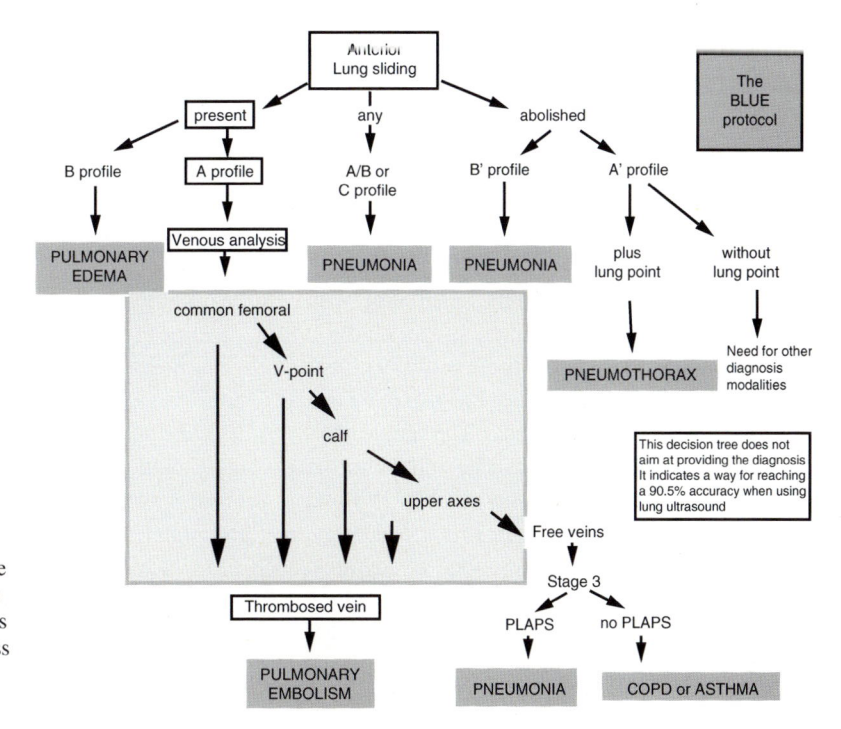

Fig. 18.20 The BLUE-protocol, extension of the venous branch. This figure shows the developed item "venous thrombosis." This makes more items, but less time spent than a comprehensive scanning

Limitations of Venous Ultrasound (Reminder)

Natural limitations
  Abdominal gas for iliocaval veins.
  Fat (plethoric patients) for deep veins.
  Natural echogenicity. Some patients are more difficult to scan than others.
  Chronic thromboses (see in text, calf veins).
Pathological limitations
  Hypovolemia, when it makes the venous section smaller.
Artificial limitations
  Dressing (of catheters).
  Tracheostomy cord (but see CLOT-protocol in Chap. 28).
  Orthopedic materials (plaster cast at the legs, cervical collar at the neck).
  The more the probe has small footprint, the less these obstacles.
Confusions with other structures
  Real structures:
    Lymph nodes, cysts, and hematomas.
  Ghosts.
Limitations in the interpretation
  A nonthrombosed vein can mean a no longer thrombosed vein.
Other hindrances
  A compression on a painful area. Here, on occasion, Doppler may be of interest.

Some Main Points for Concluding

The search in extreme emergency of a venous thrombosis is a raison d'être of the BLUE-protocol. The described equipment (one small unit with immediate switch-on, one unique probe) allows a 3 min scanning. Our multipurpose probe is probably the most precious tool, since it can explore any area (lung, heart, vein, belly, etc.). The simple analysis of the venous content can be sufficient; the compression is done if there is no visible DVT and with minimal pressure. Doppler is not mandatory. Simple approaches can be described at any area, including popliteal, calf, and superior caval vein.

Large venous thromboses are easily detected, until the moment they are suddenly no longer visible. Finding a small distal DVT has major relevance when massive pulmonary embolism is suspected.

Simple venous ultrasound should be recognized the gold standard.

Accessory Notes
1. Timing
    This average timing of 55 s comes from these data:
      10 s necessary for 1/4 of patients (positive examination at common femoral vein)
      25 s for 1/4 (V-point)
      65 s for 1/5 (calf)
      85 s in roughly 5 % (jugular/subclavian)
      95 s in roughly 2 % (middle femur)
      115 s in roughly 1 % (poplitea)
      120 s in 1/5 of patients with negative venous test
2. Anterior tibial veins
    The BLUE-protocol simplifies by not considering the anterior group (supposedly not emboligenic by the way), although usually easy to detect, just anterior to the interosseous membrane and just smaller (see Video 18.2).

Sophisticated Notes
1. Vein or artery?
We open to a theoretical situation, which may be seen from time to time in a carrier. When examining a patient with a pulmonary embolism plus a shock plus a thrombosed low femoral vein, the compression maneuver may collapse the artery (if the pressure is superior to the arterial pressure) and not the vein. Stricto sensu, this may make a false-negative. Apart from a subtle sign (the collapsed artery will show systolic saccades) and hoping that the patient will not, precisely, have a bilateral, symmetrical pattern, the simplest clue is a comparative view, allowing to locate the vein (if a left low femoral vein is outside, the right low femoral vein will also be outside).

Anecdotal Notes

1. How to transform a microconvex probe in superficial, "vascular" probe

   See Fig. 31.4 which shows, from the 6 mm to 17 cm range of our probe, how to see even the first 6 mm, for one dollar (cheaper than buying a vascular probe).

2. Perverse effects of Doppler

   The non use of Doppler *today*, when quite all machines are equipped, may appear futile. There is a section in Chap. 37 explaining in which perverse way Doppler was, indirectly, responsible for deaths. In a few words: a high cost, preventing the purchase of machines which, simpler, would have made simple life-saving diagnoses, at a period where doctors were not informed of the power of simple ultrasound.

3. Craze for Doppler

   When we ask physicians why they need Doppler, we are surprised by the number of reasons, different from physician to physician. One of the most popular, "it helps for recognizing the vein from the artery." This distinction is of high simplicity. It is nearly as immediate as recognizing a cat from a small dog (see Fig. 3.2).

4. Scientific assessment of the pressure during compression

   We used utensils for calculating pressures and estimated wisely (and sufficiently) to limit pressure to the reasonable value of 0.5–1 kg/cm^2 for keeping ultrasound a noninvasive tool.

5. Smiling ads for the pocket machines

   We often see advertisements of some pocket machines, with a group of enthusiastic young doctors showing a large smile, one hand holding the probe, the other holding the screen. We agree, it is good to have a positive mind and to be always enthusiastic, but we consider that the instrument "critical ultrasound" should be "played" seriously with two hands.

6. Why this textbook

   Instead of trying to publish 1000 details, i.e., 5000 submissions, and one success per year, we prefer to write one unique book. Not peer reviewed, just our 26-year observations.

7. The Grotowski law

   This law speculates that a non-critically ill patient who has a slight suspicion of embolism, and no thrombosis detected using our simple method, including the calf area in *at least* one point, is *not* at risk of sudden death. See all details in Chap. 36, section on pulmonary embolism.

References

1. Davidson BL, Elliott CG, Lensing AW (1992) Low accuracy of color Doppler ultrasound in the detection of proximal leg vein thrombosis in asymptomatic high-risk patients. The RD Heparin Arthroplasty Group. Ann Intern Med 117(9):735–738
2. Cronan JJ (1993) Venous thromboembolic disease: the role of ultrasound, state of the art. Radiology 186:619–630
3. Lichtenstein D, Jardin F (1997) Diagnosis of internal jugular vein thrombosis. Intensive Care Med 23:1188–1190
4. Lensing AWA, Doris CI, McGrath FP et al (1997) A comparison of compression ultrasound with color Doppler ultrasound for the diagnosis of symptomless postoperative deep vein thrombosis. Arch Intern Med 157:765–768
5. Bernardi E, Camporese G, Bueller H, Siragusa S, Imberti D, Berchio A et al (2008) Serial two-point ultrasonography plus D-dimer vs whole-leg color-coded Doppler ultrasonography for diagnosing suspected symptomatic deep vein thrombosis. A randomized controlled trial. JAMA 300(14):1653–1659
6. Perlin SJ (1992) Pulmonary embolism during compression ultrasound of the lower extremity. Radiology 184:165–166
7. Lichtenstein D, Mezière G (2008) Relevance of lung ultrasound in the diagnosis of acute respiratory failure. The BLUE-protocol. Chest 134:117–125

8. Alpert JS, Smith R, Carlson J, Ockene IS, Dexter L, Dalen JE (1976) Mortality in patients treated for pulmonary embolism. JAMA 236:1477–1480
9. Moser KM, LeMoine JR (1981) Is embolic risk conditioned by location of deep venous thrombosis? Ann Intern Med 94:439–444
10. Appelman PT, De Jong TE, Lampmann LE (1987) Deep venous thrombosis of the leg: ultrasound findings. Radiology 163:743–746
11. Cronan JJ, Dorfman GS, Grusmark J (1988) Lower-extremity deep venous thrombosis: further experience with and refinements of ultrasound assessment. Radiology 168:101–107
12. Meibers DJ, Baldridge ED, Ruoff BA, Karkow WS, Cranley JJ (1988) The significance of calf muscle venous thrombosis. J Vasc Surg 12:143–149
13. Philbrick JT, Becker DM (1988) Calf deep venous thrombosis: a wolf in sheep's clothing? Arch Intern Med 148:2131–2138
14. Browse NL, Thomas ML (1974) Source of non-lethal pulmonary emboli. Lancet 1(7851):258–259
15. De Weese JA (1978) Ilio-femoral venous thrombectomy. In: Bergan JJ, Yao ST (eds) Venous problems. Mosby Year Book, St. Louis, pp 423–433
16. Mavor GE, Galloway JMD (1969) Iliofemoral venous thrombosis: pathological considerations and surgical management. Br J Surg 56:45–59
17. Yucel EK, Fisher JS, Egglin TK, Geller SC, Waltman AC (1991) Isolated calf venous thrombosis: diagnosis with compression ultrasound. Radiology 179:443–446

Simple Emergency Cardiac Sonography: A New Application Integrating Lung Ultrasound

19

The heart, this organ that prevents us to examine the lung.... Ph. Biderman
(December 26, 2007)

We use the best of our 1992 Edition, Chap. 20 (the heart), born from the privilege of having been working in echocardiography in a pioneering institution [1], a typical spirit of intensive care, a discipline aiming at reaching its autonomy.

Even if they have the feeling to master the heart, readers would find interest in understanding the spirit of this chapter. The heart is a perfect example for holistic ultrasound. Simple signs, a simple technique and, mostly, its association with LUCI define a new field, fully distinct from traditional echocardiography (even the one devoted to the critically ill). The consideration of the BLUE-protocol and the FALLS-protocol will allow to position our simple emergency cardiac sonography between the traditional basic and expert echocardiography, aiming at making this traditional separation less necessary. Without lung ultrasound, the simple emergency cardiac sonography as defined would be insufficient. Therefore, this chapter will be fully understood only if integrated in the following chapters.

Obviously, prestigious works on expert echocardiography Doppler are numerous. They come from cardiologic fields [2], pioneering intensive care fields [1], many honorable sources [3], recent trends [4, 5], and so many sources that we can cite just a few, humbly apologizing for our lack of space [6–11]. This chapter will be poor in references, many hemodynamic references being inserted in Chap. 30 on the FALLS-protocol.

We use the simple emergency cardiac sonography since 1985/1989 and wrote the devoted chapter in 1992 (with no need for acronym; it was not a fashion in 1992, nor necessary). The basic echocardiography was popularized under several names, some rather elegant (the dynamic RACE of McLean, the FEER [12], FATE [13], etc., all now obsolete in the name of the recent FOCUS) [14]. This shows that, beyond the war of acronyms, the community took interest in this concept.

For taking the best of our approach, experts must understand that we deal with the very first minutes of management, when critical actions have to be done.

The term "sonography" on the title was chosen on purpose: for most, "Echo" means traditional Doppler echocardiography, while "ultrasound" (please note the lowercase) means traditional abdominal examination by a radiologist. Cardiology and radiology are two different worlds. Critical care is a completely distinct world, with its own logic.

The main protocols of LUCI (BLUE-protocol, FALLS-protocol, and SESAME-protocol) are fully cardiac centered. This is obvious for the FALLS-protocol, which begins by the heart, and the SESAME-protocol by essence (cardiac arrest). The BLUE-protocol aims at helping precisely when cardiac windows are lacking, another mark of interest. We just consider the heart as a vital organ like another, and this respect must be shared with other vital organs.

Our concept evolves as far as our main articles were published. We aim at providing a textbook increasingly complementary to the echocardiography textbooks. Consequently, from edition to edition (1992, 2002, 2005, 2010, etc.), the place of the heart, rather long in our first one (26 figures), is now limited to its essentials.

Daily concerns in critical care are mainly acute respiratory failure, acute circulatory failure, and cardiac arrest. The habit of looking at the heart in case of lung disease can be questioned: a lung approach is more direct. In the case of a circulatory failure, the FALLS-protocol shows that when one bases all of one's calculations on the analysis of only one actor (the heart), this approach is direct only when the cause of shock is cardiac (what in passing the BLUE-protocol also detects using the lung approach). Adding the lung allows to keep the best of the simple heart. The amount of information "lost" in terms of Doppler or transesophageal echocardiography will possibly be compensated using precious data that lung ultrasound provides, mainly a *direct* parameter of clinical volemia.

So Still No Doppler in The Present Edition?

Dealing with echocardiography without mentioning Doppler or transesophageal approaches may appear bold today. Having accrued experience in a pioneering institution in echocardiography in the ICU since 1989 [1], the authors came to the temptive conclusion that therapeutic procedures can be deduced from the observation of simple phenomena. The integration of the lung gives birth to a new, holistic approach. The reader will therefore not take offense if TEE and Doppler do not feature.

Sophisticated echocardiography has a huge place in more quiet settings. Topics and terms such as Doppler physics, measurements of stroke volume and cardiac output, assessment of LV and RV function, measurement of filling pressures and of diastolic function, evaluation of valve function, determination of preload sensitivity and of intracardiac pressures, and identification of adverse subtle flow interactions, none of these terms is dealt with at the CEURF courses: LUCI allows to simplify echocardiography and provide a simple unit, easy to purchase everywhere, using the same single probe; this is, again, holistic ultrasound.

The reader must understand that during as long as necessary, the DIAFORA approach will be used. Here, a variant of DIAFORA will be used, "from inside," i.e., by regular members of the ICU trained to echocardiography. We write and will repeat at the end that the ideal combination in any modern ICU is a comprehensive unit able of all cardiologic measurements and, beside, our simple unit as defined. This unit can be complementary in many settings to the usual cardiological approaches (read quietly Chaps. 20 and 30).

Do not forget that the expert echocardiographic approach is not an option for most patients on Earth.

Most figures come from a 1982 technology (ADR-4000®). Most figures of our previous editions have been deleted (see our 2010 Edition, or any classical echocardiography textbook).

The life-saving diagnoses made using the simple cardiac sonography can be made without compromise using our 5-MHz microconvex probe and our slim gray-scale machine.

At the Onset, Two Basic Questions

We raise two questions about cardiac sonography.
1. *How to see the heart* is modestly described in this chapter (we don't aim to teach a lot to experts). Today, the critical care physicians know where the right ventricle is, what is a dilated right ventricle, etc.
2. *Why do we want to see the heart* is a more critical question, which should be answered in light of the emergence of lung ultrasound. As regards respiratory failure, this basic question will receive an answer in the BLUE-protocol (next chapter), showing that the diagnosis of

pulmonary edema pertains to lung ultrasound. Facing circulatory failure, Chap. 30 will show that the look to the heart is indirect each time the cause is not cardiac. In the FALLS-protocol, after a simplified cardiac approach, lung ultrasound provides a direct parameter for fluid therapy. As regards cardiac arrest, the heart will come fifth in the SESAME-protocol (Chap. 31).

The Signs of Simple Emergency Cardiac Sonography Used in the BLUE-Protocol: What Is Required?

Nothing, since the BLUE-protocol uses lung and venous data. Echocardiographic data are associated to it, not included. LUCI provides a 97% sensitivity for diagnosing hemodynamic pulmonary edema. The Extended BLUE-protocol adds points using *simple* cardiac data.

The Signs of Simple Emergency Cardiac Sonography Used in the FALLS-Protocol: What Is Required?

The acute circulatory failure benefits first from a clinical examination, which usually provides a correct diagnosis. When no cause appears, the FALLS-protocol is initiated. It begins by the heart. This exploration is limited to two items: pericardial effusion and dilated right ventricle.

We therefore need to know which machine to use, which probe, where to apply the probe, how to understand the structures, and how to recognize the anomalies. The CEURF spirit will be used for simplifying this part.

Which Machine?

We use the same gray-scale unit used for the lungs, veins, abdomen, optic nerve, etc., a 1992 technology described in Chap. 2.

Which Probe?

We use the same probe used for the lungs, veins, abdomen, optic nerve, etc., a 1992 Japanese technology described in Chap. 2.

Where to Apply the Probe?

Traditional windows (parasternal, apical, subcostal, etc.) have been carefully defined. It is assumed today that intensivists, emergency physicians, etc., control these windows (see Appendix 1). Holistic ultrasound integrates them, but proposes an immediate, pragmatic solution when the windows are not perfect. The readers will see that the SESAME-protocol (Chap. 31) begins by the lung for the main reason that the fear not to find correct windows is absent from this first step.

As a critical detail, we do not spend high energy for having perfect cardiac windows, because we are not cardiologists, especially those working for other physicians (or even sonographists, who master this art). In the same way that you recognize a familiar face at first sight even if not strictly face/profile, you recognize the cardiac chambers. This critical detail makes simple cardiac sonography fully different to traditional echocardiography. The subcostal approach, very appreciated by intensivists in ventilated patients since often the only available, follows this philosophy: it offers a cardiac view of major interest even if truncated (Fig. 19.1).

The apical approach gives at last the feeling that the heart, a complex organ, has a simple anatomy, since the ventricles are anterior (the auricles posterior) and the left chambers are at the right (the right chambers at the left). For once, things seem symmetrical (Fig. 19.2).

Countless details can help when windows are lacking. Wait for end-expiration to have a brief look to the heart. In the subcostal route, taking some liver tissue can increase cardiac image quality. The right parasternal route can show dilated right structures. When nothing works, the lung will answer many questions.

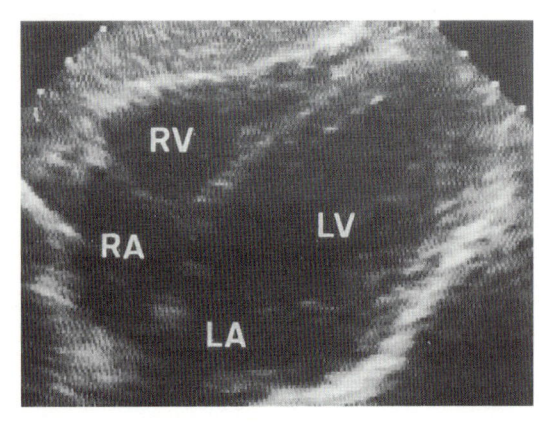

Fig. 19.1 Subcostal view of the heart. This approach is a classic in the intensive care unit. It is a truncated equivalent of the four-chamber apical view of Fig. 19.2. *RV* right ventricle, *RA* right auricle, *LV* left ventricle, *LA* left auricle. The operator should move the probe from top to bottom (Carmen maneuver in fact) to acquire a correct three-dimensional representation of the volumes. The pericardium is virtual here

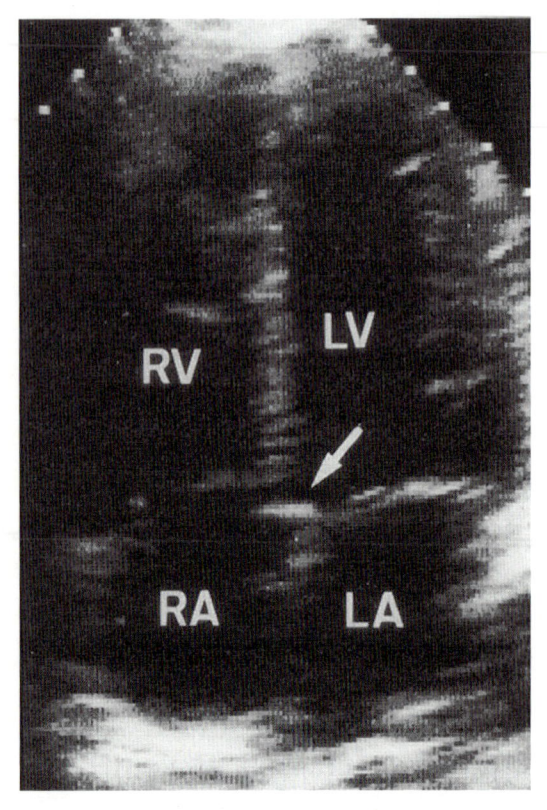

Fig. 19.2 Four-chamber view, apical window. Here, the heart seems to be a symmetric structure. *LV* left ventricle, *LA* left auricle, *RV* right ventricle, *RA* right auricle. This incidence allows immediate comparison of the volume and dynamics of each chamber. Note that the plane of the tricuspid valve is more anterior than the plane of the mitral valve. Right auricle and left ventricle are in contact (*arrow*), a detail which allows correct orientation

How to Understand the Structures?

The anatomy of the heart is complex. Those who will compare it to the rather simple ultrasound of the anatomy of the lung (just *two signs*) will make a step toward holistic ultrasound (the next step is to learn how far lung ultrasound answers to "cardiac questions"). Any echocardiographic textbook or costly simulators will show the cardiac structures. Ultrasound is a good way to understand, noninvasively, this anatomy.

Normal cardiac anatomy in 20 lines. The left ventricle is ovoid shaped, with a thick muscle and a long axis pointing leftward, downward, and forward. It has a base (where the aorta and, deeper, the left auricle are inserted), an apex, and four walls: inferior, lateral, anterior, and septal. The right ventricle has a more complex anatomy and is wounded around the left ventricle, with a thin free wall and a thick septal wall. Its volume assessment is subtle (due to its complex shape, novices taking a wrong plane will imagine enlargement where there is no enlargement). Its apex covers the septum; its base (infundibulum) covers the initial aorta. The main intracavitary structures are the valves and the left ventricular pillars. The auricles are visible behind the ventricles, yet, since we are not cardiologists, they are rarely of interest. The cardiac muscle is echoic. The chambers are anechoic. The pericardium is virtual.

Which Measurements?

In the spirit of simple emergency cardiac sonography, measurements are not of prime relevance. In addition, most intensivists have now been trained and know them. Read Appendix 2. Simple cardiac sonography is based on visual medicine.

How to Identify Cardiac Anomalies Pertaining to the FALLS-Protocol?

Pericardial Fluid

This is one of the most basic applications of critical ultrasound. It is life-threatening, easy to diagnose, and easy to treat. A circumferential

The Signs of Simple Emergency Cardiac Sonography Used in the FALLS-Protocol: What Is Required?

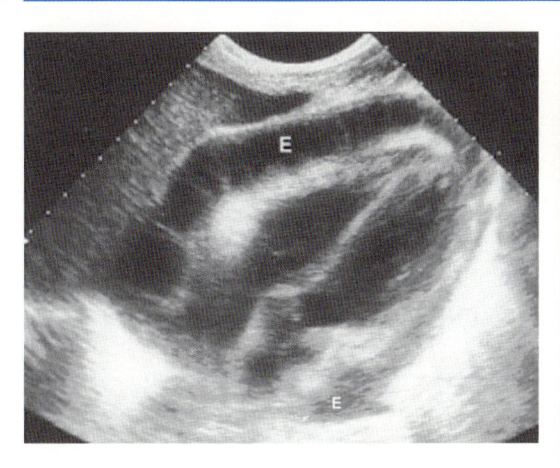

Fig. 19.3 Fluid collection in the pericardial space. The septations indicate an infectious cause. Note that the effusion (*E*) surrounds the entire heart: it is visible anterior to the left ventricle in this subcostal approach (*smaller E*). Pleuropericarditis due to pneumococcus

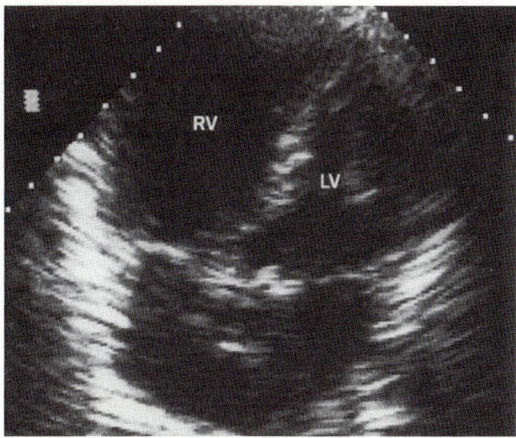

Fig. 19.4 Massive pulmonary embolism. Major dilatation of the right ventricle (*RV*) in a four-chamber view using the apical route. *LV*, left ventricle

pericardial effusion is detected when the external border of the heart is outlined by another, larger, external border, it is really simple to assess (Fig. 19.3). An equivalent of the sinusoid sign is found between the parietal and visceral layers of the pericardial sac during cardiac contractions. Usually anechoic, fluids can be echoic, septated (hemopericardium, purulent pericarditis) (Fig. 19.3), etc., and we avoid to define a pericardial effusion as an anechoic space, exactly like pleural effusions in the BLUE-protocol.

In exceptional cases, usually postoperative, loculated effusions can threaten the circulation if located on strategic areas. Pericardial fat is usually limited anteriorly, echoic, and devoid of sinusoid dynamics.

The FALLS-protocol defines as pericardial tamponade any substantial pericardial fluid seen in a patient with an acute circulatory failure. The real-time analysis of the right cavities, showing chamber collapsus, dramatically increases this likeliness. The sign of the dancing heart, not used in the FALLS-protocol, is easy to diagnose. For other signs, see Appendix 3 and Video 31.1.

Our personal technique of pericardiocentesis is dealt with in Chap. 31.

Right Ventricle (RV) Volume

There are two reasons to look at the RV in the FALLS-protocol.

Mainly, for Detecting an Enlargement

The RV normally works under a low-pressure system. Any hindrance to RV ejection, as seen in severe pulmonary embolism, but also severe asthma, ARDS, extensive pneumonia will promptly generate its dilatation [15]. Acute right heart failure associates early RV dilatation (Fig. 19.4), a displacement of the septum to the left, a tricuspid regurgitation (see Video 30.2).

The apical four-chamber view provides the most objective way to detect an RV dilatation, defined when its volume is the same as in the left ventricle or more.

When cardiac windows are poor, one can use instead either a transesophageal approach or the BLUE-protocol: the combination of an A-profile with a venous thrombosis in a patient seen for acute respiratory failure has a 99 % specificity for the diagnosis of pulmonary embolism [16]. It will be seen that the BLUE-protocol works for blue patients; patients with ARDS are not blue (under full oxygen, sedation etc.), and different rules apply; see the CLOT-protocol in Chap. 28.

Pulmonary embolism is a field where everything has been said [17, 18]. TEE sometimes provides a direct sign (clot in the pulmonary artery). However, the CEURF protocols have developed a way of optimizing this approach; read this section in Chap. 31.

Note that the place of Doppler (major here for years) gradually decreases, since the severity of pulmonary embolism was correlated with the degree of obstruction, a data little correlated with pulmonary arterial pressure (not always elevated in severe cases of embolism) but better correlated with the RV volume (and the left/right ratio), i.e., a simple cardiac sonography [19].

More Occasionally for Detecting a Volume Decrease

More occasionally, for these reasons:
- A small RV seen in hypovolemia would be redundant in the FALLS-protocol with the A-profile.
- A small RV within a substantial pericardial effusion, in a shocked patient, is quite redundant for the diagnosis of pericardial tamponade.

Yet since this is not the most difficult part of echocardiography, holistic ultrasound is fully opened to include this analysis.

The Signs of Simple Emergency Cardiac Sonography Used in Cardiac Arrest (the SESAME-Protocol)

In the first seconds, tension pneumothorax (lung), pulmonary embolism (lung and veins), hypovolemia (abdomen, pleural cavity, etc.), then a pericardial tamponade (see above) are sought for. The heart comes 5th. Diagnoses of ventricular fibrillation, auriculoventricular block, etc., are sometimes obvious and sometimes subtle. Asystole is a rather easy diagnosis, although of limited interest. See Chap. 31.

Signs of Simple Emergency Cardiac Sonography Not Used in the BLUE-Protocol, FALLS-Protocol, Nor SESAME-Protocol

Chapter 30 (hemodynamic assessment of shock) does not insert basic signs such as the left ventricle contractility in the decision tree, but we admit it should be really strange not to use these basic, easy-to-learn signs.

Left Ventricle (LV) Overall Contractility

How to measure it: the ejection fraction is the most academic and is not described here. The shortening fraction, a basic measurement easy to obtain, is sufficient for having a diagnosis in critical settings. With a little experience, one can classify without any measurement a hypocontractile, normocontractile, and hypercontractile LV, what we do since 1990 and what was fortunately recently admitted. The diagnosis of a LV hypocontractility is done by detecting a decrease in the amplitude of muscle shortening (Appendix 2)

Why to measure it: LV hypocontractility in a shocked patient is due to cardiogenic shock, basically, and can be seen in septic shock (recent data suggest that all patients in septic shock develop the septic cardiomyopathy, more or less occult, depending on post-charge and other parameters) [20]. The first condition invites to inotropic support; the second suggests it with a call for confirmation. An exaggerated contractility suggests that an inotropic option is not useful and that, according to the principle of the communicating vessels, the probability increases for the remaining options: vasopressors or fluids (in the FALLS-protocol, these options will be answered before the LV analysis, but the physician is free to do the opposite).

Echocardiography integrated within the BLUE-protocol will open to multiple subtleties. For instance, an acute respiratory failure with no B-profile indicates a suffering of the right, not left, heart, with the theoretical exception (to be confirmed) of a major septal interference, impairing the left heart function.

The echocardiographic science has recently been complicated/enriched by the notion of diastolic dysfunction, which should be responsible for half of the cases of left heart failure (until new articles balance these data). Read below.

Hypovolemic Shock

It typically shows hypercontractile LV, small end-diastolic cavity, and sometimes virtual end-systolic volume (Fig. 19.5). This approach is not

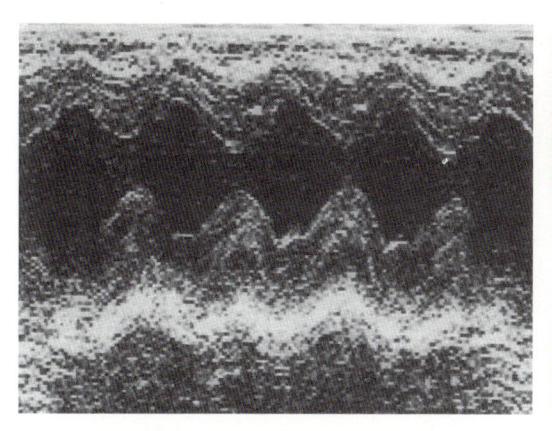

Fig. 19.5 Profile of possible hypovolemia. Hypercontractile pattern of the left ventricle. M-mode acquisition in a short-axis parasternal view. Small diastolic chamber. Quasi-virtual systolic chamber. Tachycardia. This shocked patient had abdominal sepsis. The hypovolemia is probable since the further images improved (contractility, size, frequency) – in a patient who had by the way the A-profile

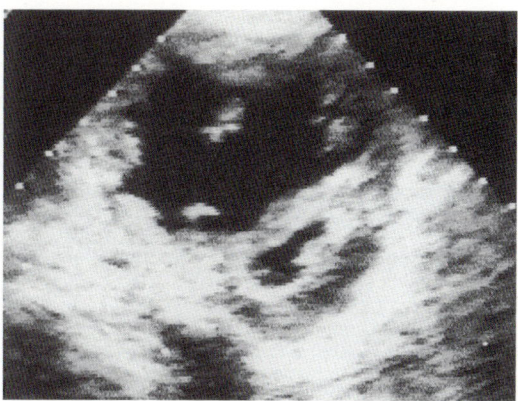

Fig. 19.6 Exacerbation of chronic right heart failure. Major right ventricle dilatation. Note the squashed left ventricle, and the substantial thickening of the free wall of the right ventricle. Short-axis parasternal view

used in the CEURF protocols (read Chap. 30 or a summary in Anecdotal Note 1).

Dilated Cardiomyopathy

One just has to appreciate the size of the chambers.

Hypertrophic Cardiomyopathy

One just has to appreciate the thickness of the walls.

Chronic Right Heart Insufficiency

One has just to measure the free wall of the RV, thickened in the case of a chronic obstacle, as seen in COPD (Fig. 19.6).

A Preview of More Complex Cardiac Applications Which Are Not Used in Our Protocols and Rarely in Our Daily Clinical Practice

This is just a preview, unless this section would (a bit) look like any echocardiographic textbook.

Diastolic Ventricular Dysfunction

We will not pretend to have the slightest expertise in this field. Just an observation from a distance allows us to see, as usual, two opinions. Some tell it is an easy field, well mastered [21]; others consider it as a whole science of illimited complications (private talks with Michèle Desruennes). Its frequency is variable according to the schools. The philosophy of simple emergency cardiac sonography uses a simple, accessible data, the hypertrophy of the LV walls (Fig. 19.7), and asks the question: doesn't it provide already an interesting piece of information (not arguing to solve the problem from A to Z)? A thickened LV, even with a preserved contraction, or an enlarged left auricle should alert for a diastolic anomaly (free talks from Drs McLean and Voga).

We will mostly use the help of lung ultrasound, because it would show early signs of left heart dysfunction (whatever the cause: systolic, diastolic). The BLUE-protocol begins by searching signs of pulmonary edema, i.e., the B-profile. No B-profile? No LV diastolic dysfunction.

Myocardial Infarction

Ultrasound must be a tool, not a disease. ECG data allow usual diagnoses, although some advocate that ultrasound anomalies are visible early, thus modifying immediate management [22]. The

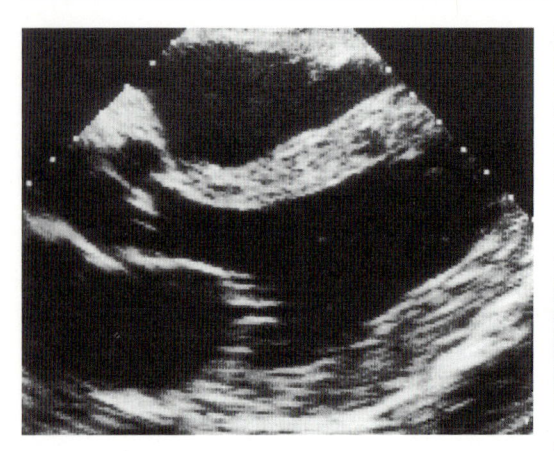

Fig. 19.7 LV hypertrophy. The parietal LV thickness is 16 mm. A parietal shock was perceived, synchronized with the auricle systole, probably indicating a sudden increase in pressure in a chamber whose volume could not increase. Long-axis parasternal view. Note the image quality of this 1982 portable technology. Note: we took the liberty of using radiological conventions, i.e., head to the left, feet to the right. This is probably the only detail we borrowed from the radiological culture

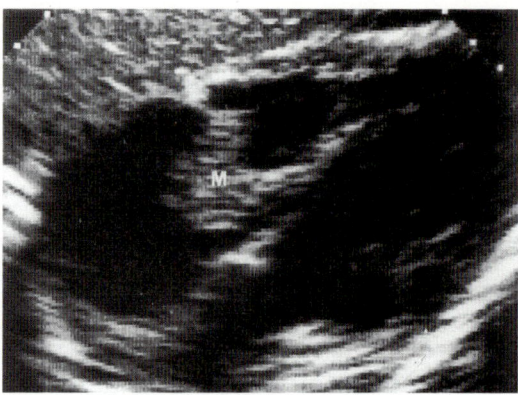

Fig. 19.8 Endocarditis. Tissue-like mass depending on the tricuspid valve. A diagnosis of endocarditis in a young drug addict was immediately made using this subcostal ultrasound view, quickly confirmed by positive blood cultures (staphylococcus). *M* vegetation

subtle diagnosis of segmental anomalies requires expertise. Right ventricle dilatation suggests right ventricle infarction. One advantage of critical ultrasound is to immediately rule out other diagnoses of thoracic pain (pericarditis, pneumothorax, pneumonia, aortic dissection, etc.).

Endocarditis

Some words about this diagnosis.

First, its rarity is a typical indication to our opinion for the DIAFORA approach, while several blood cultures are performed. There is no space for arguing that TEE should be the gold standard. This also regards cases on metallic valves. However, our experience showed that in many cases, real-time imaging with a good resolution probe (such as our microconvex one) shows "something." This change is usually clear enough (Fig. 19.8). Instead of the regular, thin valvular pattern, a pathological image is seen, thicker, irregular, with hectic dynamics, echoic like a tissue, and larger at the end of the valve. A calcification is recognized through its hyperechoic superficial pattern and its anechoic acoustic shadow.

Valvular Diseases

Valvular diseases, issues with mechanical valves, some mechanical complications of myocardial infarction, septal rupture, and hypertrophic asymmetric cardiomyopathies would be beyond the scope of this book. Specialized techniques such as transesophageal Doppler echocardiography, used by specialists, will here provide the best approach [23].

Like endocarditis, in very echoic patients, overt mitral valve anomalies can be detected (mitral valve prolapse, valvular thickening, etc., diagnosed for cheap without Doppler).

Intracavitary Thrombosis, Tumor, and Device

Intracardiac thromboses (Fig. 19.9) show scary images of echoic patterns, sometimes mobile, of high specificity. For the sensitivity, transesophageal approach should give better results (if a simple approach did not answer). Right ventricle normal structures (e.g., papillary muscle) are not thromboses.

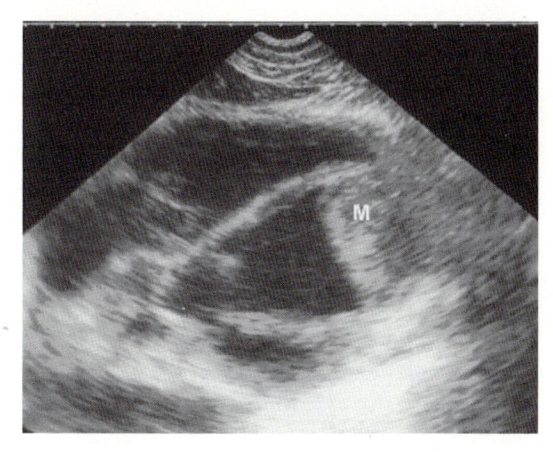

Fig. 19.9 Left ventricular thrombosis. Substantial thrombosis (*M*) at the apex of the left ventricle. Subcostal view

Tumors are so rare that we do not develop this field: make DIAFORA instead.

A too long distal end of a catheter should be searched for in the right chambers, acoustic window permitting. Interesting was the ability to check, in real time, the progression of the Swan-Ganz catheter through the vena cava, auricle, ventricle, pulmonary artery, etc.. See Figure 22.23 of our 2010 Edition. One operator inserted the material; the other guided the distal end of the catheter using the subcostal approach. Asepsis could be efficiently controlled. This was around 1991–1993, then we asked, why have an ultrasound probe in hand and perform anyway a cardiac catheterization?

The position of a electrosystolic probe can be checked in the right ventricle.

Gas Tamponade

This is typical. When cardiac chambers are collapsed by massive gas under tension, instead of spending energy for trying to have the cardiac windows (quite always not accessible), our approach is to see rather the lungs, detecting immediately the (sometimes bilateral) pneumothorax. We will see that in shock (FALLS-protocol), this search comes third and, in cardiac arrest, it comes first.

Gas Embolism

It yields large, hyperechoic echoes, highly dynamic, with posterior shadow (see Fig. 22.20 of our 2010 Edition). In a supine patient, these gas bubbles transiently collect at the anterior part of the right ventricle and travel little by little in the pulmonary artery – unless the patient is promptly turned to the left lateral position. Gas embolism complicating the central venous line insertion can be predicted (see Chap. 34).

Anecdotal Diagnoses

Many can be described here, but their exhaustive description would overburden this book. Let us just cite this severe shock with pulmonary edema due to an esophageal abscess squashing the left auricle, making the conditions for septic shock plus cardiogenic shock by compromised pulmonary venous return (see Fig. 22.25 in our 2010 Edition). This young lady had the correct diagnosis, mostly thanks to TEE.

Before Concluding: How to Practice Emergency Echocardiography When There Is No Cardiac Window

One aim of this textbook is to develop solutions, to be considered in extreme emergencies.

The BLUE-protocol was designed for assessing the origin of a respiratory failure.

The FALLS-protocol can be used [24], since the first step (cardiac) can be simplified: pericardial tamponade usually provides windows, and pulmonary embolism can be detected most of the time using the BLUE-protocol.

How to assess the cardiac overall contractility may be solved using, once again, lung ultrasound: the lung pulse, detailed in Chaps. 10 and 35, may be a sign of good contractility (to be confirmed using carefully designed studies).

Repeated as Previously Announced, Our Take-Home Message

We have no willingness to replace traditional TTE or TEE. This would not be scientific at all. What we advocate, in any current ICU equipped with the up-to-date Doppler echocardiographic unit which makes "all," is, *besides*, a modest black-and-white unit with a single probe, easy to buy, for making "the rest." Our vision of the "rest" is modestly defined in this textbook. What we bet is that at the beginning, the simple machine will be used from time to time (e.g., check for empty bladder). Then, increasingly, control coming, the simple unit will be used for hundred daily tasks (e.g., subclavian vein cannulation). Time running, the simple unit will then make shy attempts in echocardiography (e.g., checking for absence of pericardial tamponade), then with more assurance (e.g., associating hypercontractile left heart with an A-profile for suggesting a clearance for fluid therapy). At one more step of evolution, the simple unit will be used as often as the comprehensive, cardiac one (a victory of holistic ultrasound).

Appendix

1. Heart Routes

The left parasternal route is, as labelled, the left parasternal area (2010 Ed, Fig. 22.1). The apical route corresponds to the systolic shock. The left positioning is not easy in a ventilated patient. Mechanical ventilation often creates a hindrance to the transthoracic approach of the heart, and the subcostal route has been widely used in sedated supine patients. This is an abdominal approach, with the probe applied just to the xiphoid, body of the probe applied almost parallel the abdominal wall.

2. Measurements

Only rough estimates (some possibly obsolete) will be given. In a short axis at the pillar level, the LV walls (septal or posterior) are 6–11 mm thick in diastole. The LV chamber caliper is 38–56 mm. The RV free wall is less than 5 mm thick. A precise measurement of the RV volume should include subtle criteria, since its shape is complex.

An M-mode image through the LV small axis can measure (2010 Ed, Fig. 22.8) the LV chamber dimension in diastole, which indicates a dilatation, and this dimension in systole, which defines contractility. The difference of these two values, divided by the diastolic dimension, defines the LV shortening fraction, a parameter of the ventricular systolic function. It is normally 28–38 %.

The parietal thickening fraction (the ratio of the difference of diastolic and systolic thickening over diastolic thickening, normal range from 50 to 100 %) is less useful in our day (and above all night) routine.

3. Pericardial Tamponade

Some signs in concert with cardiac and respiratory cycles can be observed, in spontaneously breathing patients. Inspiration facilitates venous return, and the right ventricle dilates at the expense of the septum, which is more compliant than the free wall. The septum is shifted to the left and compresses the left ventricular chamber. Diastole creates a decrease in intracavitary pressures, whereas intrapericardial pressure remains constant. The right chambers are thus collapsed by the surrounding pressure. The right auricle wall collapses first, then the right ventricle.

The description of signs using Doppler would have a beneficial effect: showing physiopathologic patterns. It may also complicate the design, if time is wasted, if too sophisticated units are used, and if the operator is not trained enough.

> **Anecdotal Note**
>
> 1. Hypovolemia
>
> Traditionally, for diagnosing hypovolemia in a shocked patient, the heart is the main target (with Doppler and TEE). This textbook focuses at the lung – especially in extreme emergency and/or if no cardiac window is available. In the FALLS-protocol and SESAME-protocol, hypovolemia is defined by an A-profile (associated if possible with the ultrasound detection of massive free fluid).

References

1. Jardin F, Farcot JC, Boisante L, Curien N, Margairaz A, Bourdarias JP (1981) Influence of positive end-expiratory pressure on left ventricle performance. N Engl J Med 304(7):387–392
2. Braunwald E (1992) Heart disease. Saunders, Philadelphia
3. Benjamin E, Oropello JM, Stein JS (1996) Transesophageal echocardiography in the management of the critically ill patient. Curr Surg 53:137–141
4. Vignon P, Goarin JP (2002) Echocardiographie-Doppler en réanimation, anesthésie et médecine d'urgence. Elsevier, Amsterdam
5. Diebold B (1990) Intérêt de l'échocardiographie Doppler en réanimation. Réan Soins Int Med Urg 6:501–507
6. Vieillard-Baron A, Charron C, Jardin F (2006) Lung "recruitment" or lung overinflation maneuvers? Intensive Care Med 32:177–178
7. Price S, Nicol E, Gibson DG, Evans TW (2006) Echocardiography in the critically ill: current and potential roles. Intensive Care Med 32:48–59
8. Vieillard-Baron A, Slama M, Cholley B, Janvier G, Vignon P (2008) Echocardiography in the intensive care unit : from evolution to revolution ? Intensive Care Med 34(2):243–249, Epub 2007 Nov 9. Review
9. Vieillard-Baron A (2009) Assessment of right ventricular function. Curr Opin Crit Care 15(3):254–260. doi:10.1097/MCC.0b013e32832b70c9, Review
10. Jardin F, Vieillard-Baron A (2009) Acute cor pulmonale. Curr Opin Crit Care 15(1):67–70, Review
11. Vieillard-Baron A (2009) Is right ventricular function the one that matters in ARDS patients ? Definitely yes. Intensive Care Med 35(1):4–6
12. Breitkreutz R, Walcher F, Seeger FH (2007) Focused echocardiographic evaluation in resuscitation management: concept of an advanced life support-conformed algorithm. Crit Care Med 35:S150–S161
13. Sloth E (2006) Echocardiography in the ICU. Intensive Care Med 32:1283
14. Via G, Hussain A, Wells M, Reardon R, ElBarbary M, Noble V, Tsung JW, Neskovic AN, Price S et al (2014) International evidence-based recommendations for focused cardiac ultrasound. J Am Soc Echocardiogr 27(7):683.e1–683.e33. doi:10.1016/j.echo.2014.05.001
15. Jardin F, Dubourg O (1986) L'exploration échocardiographique en médecine d'urgence. Masson, Paris
16. Lichtenstein D, Mezière G (2008) Relevance of lung ultrasound in the diagnosis of acute respiratory failure. The BLUE-protocol. Chest 134:117–125
17. Goldhaber SZ (2002) Echocardiography in the management of pulmonary embolism. Ann Intern Med 136:691–700
18. Schmidt GA (1998) Pulmonary embolic disorders. In: Hall JB, Schmidt GA, Wood LDH (eds) Principles of critical care, 2nd edn. McGraw Hill, New York, pp 427–449
19. Jardin F (2009) Acute cor pulmonale. Curr Opin Crit Care 15(1)
20. Vieillard-Baron A, Cecconi M (2014) Understanding cardiac failure in sepsis. Intensive Care Med 40(10):1560–1563
21. Saleh M, Vieillard-Baron A (2012) On the role of left ventricular diastolic function in the critically ill patient (Editorial). Intensive Care Med 38:189–191
22. Horowitz RS, Morganroth J, Parrotto C, Chen CC, Soffer J, Pauletto FJ (1982) Immediate diagnosis of acute myocardial infarction by two-dimensional echocardiography. Circulation 65:323
23. Vignon P, Mentec H, Terré S, Gastinne H, Guéret P, Lemaire F (1994) Diagnostic accuracy and therapeutic impact of transthoracic and transesophageal echocardiography in mechanically ventilated patients in the ICU. Chest 106:1829–1834
24. Lichtenstein D (2013) FALLS-protocol: lung ultrasound in hemodynamic assessment of shock. Heart Lung Vessel 5(3):142–147

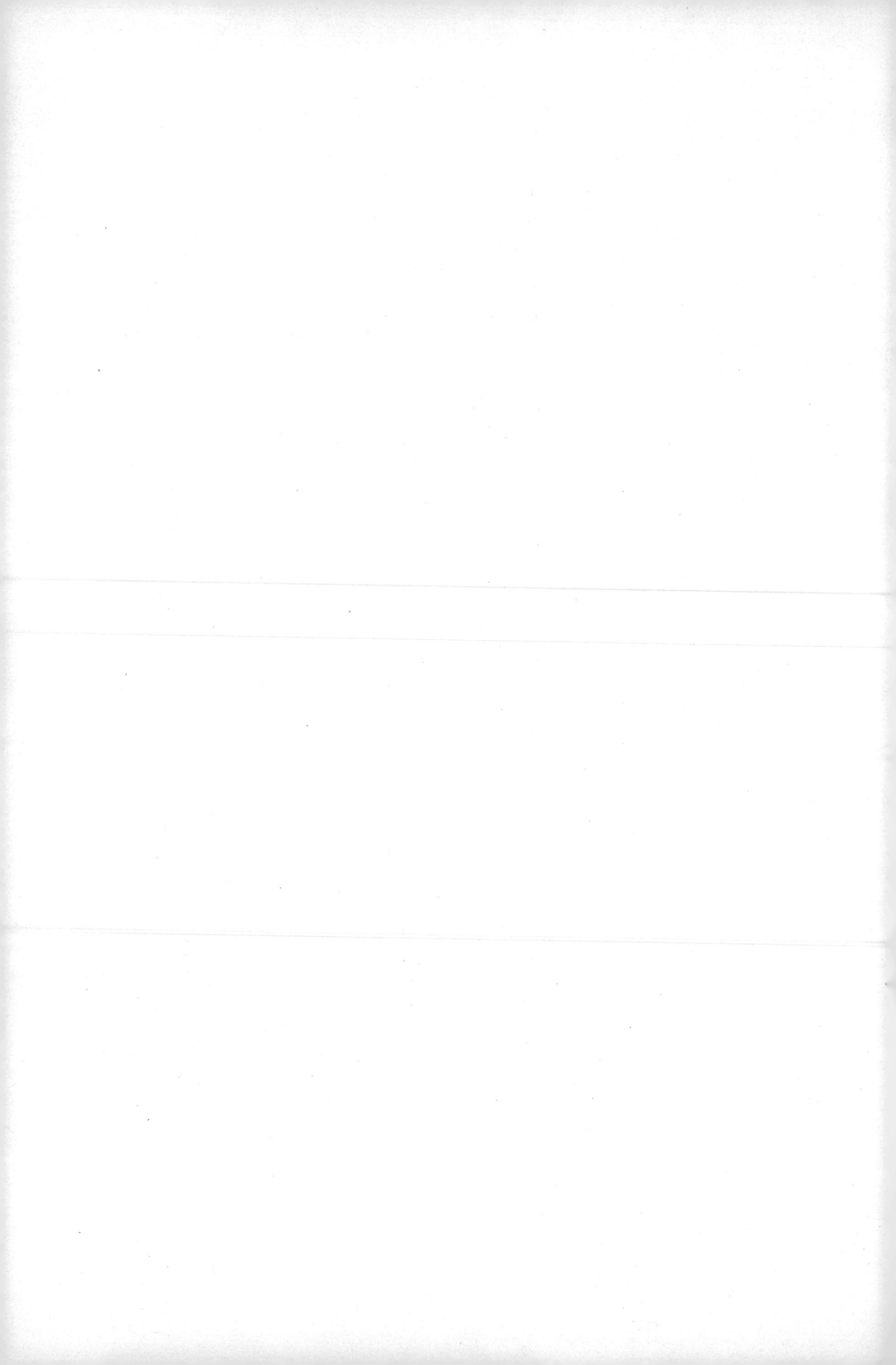

Part II
The BLUE-Protocol in Clinical Use

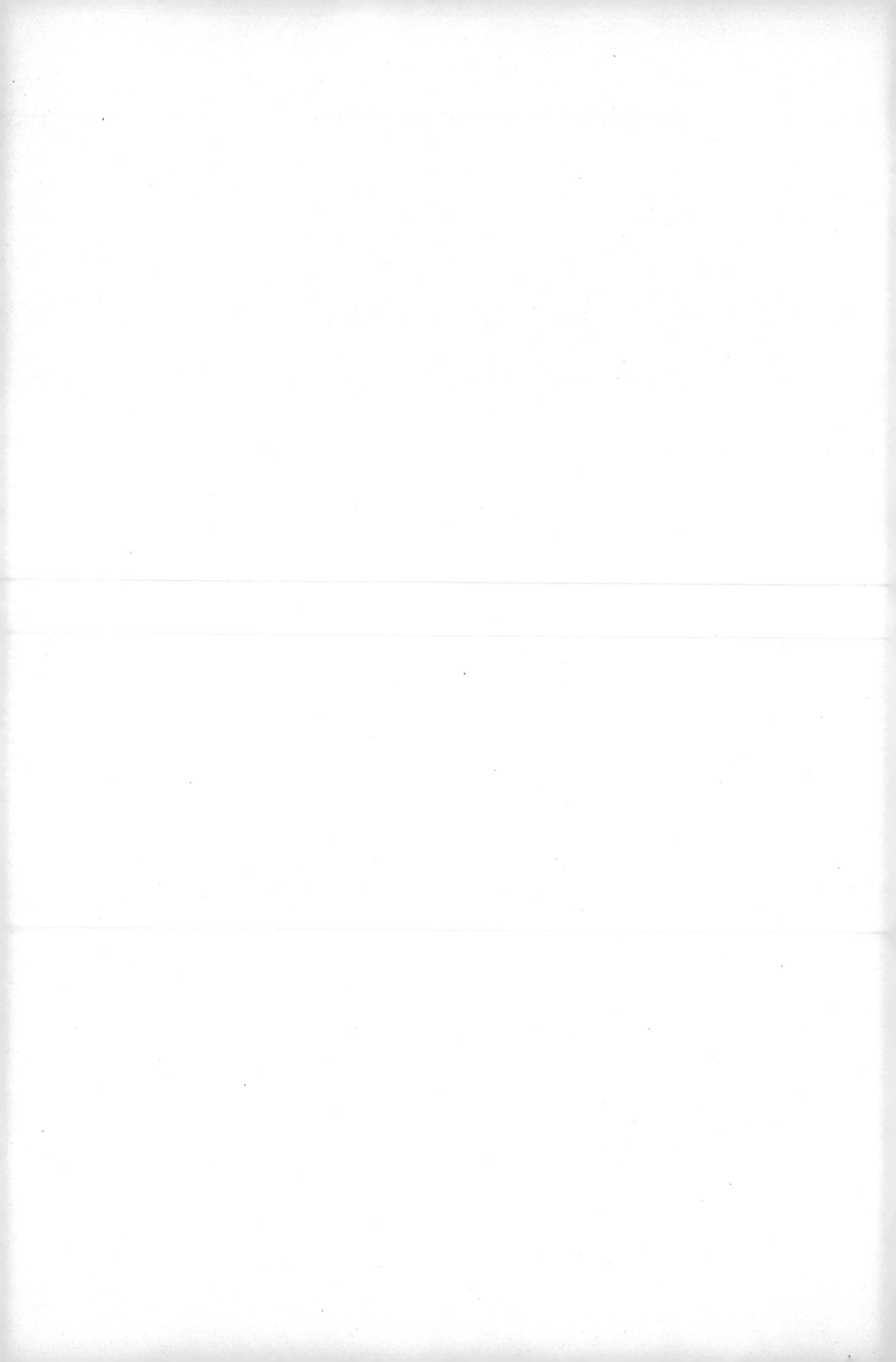

The Ultrasound Approach of an Acute Respiratory Failure: The BLUE-Protocol

20

> Severe dyspnea is one of the most distressing situations for a patient. Aiming at a therapy based on immediate diagnosis is a legitimate target.

The acute incapacity to breathe is one of the most distressing situations one can live [1]. The BLUE-protocol concentrates 18 years of efforts (mainly repeated submissions) aiming at promptly relieving these patients.

The idea of performing an ultrasound examination in time-dependent patients was not far from a *blaspheme* in 1985, definitely not envisageable according to the rules. Our approach possibly intrigued some doctors and nurses in the ERs of our institutions. During the management of these critical situations, time was not for quiet explanations. What the emergency doctors (who had to rush to the next patient in the overcrowded ER and eventually rushed after duty for a deserved nap, end of the story) did not fully see was that, after a few minutes, we were able to give to the nurse therapeutic options, while organizing the transfer to the ICU. And what they did not see at all (occupied by 1,000 other tasks, medical, administrative, familial, etc.: this was not time for international guidelines on lung ultrasound) was that these options were in accordance with the final diagnosis.

In the emergency setting, we use familiar tools since decades and centuries, mainly physical examination [2] and radiography [3], two basic tools, yet increasingly known for having limited precision. The crowded emergency room is not the ideal place for serene work, an acknowledged issue [4–8]. One-quarter of the patients of the BLUE-protocol in the first hour of management received erroneous or uncertain initial diagnoses, and many more received inappropriate therapy. The online document of *Chest* 134:117–125 details these 26 % of wrong diagnoses. CT seems a solution, but Chap. 29 will demonstrate its heavy drawbacks. One day, the community will maybe find this tool definitely too much irradiating [9].

We initiated this long work using an ADR-4000 (from 1982) then shifted for our Hitachi-405 (from 1992, last update 2008). Their 3 MHz sectorial probe and 5 MHz microconvex probe were perfectly suitable.

The Spirit of the BLUE-Protocol

Basically, the BLUE-protocol is a protocol. Yet it was designed for being a flexible one. Some protocols are possibly built for exempting doctors to think, but this one requires to keep on being a doctor. It is permanently "piloted." In some situations, it will just confirm an obvious diagnosis. In others, it will confidently invalidate a diagnosis which looked the likely one.

For being perfectly understood (and anticipating remarks), the BLUE-protocol should be considered as an "intellectual exercise," a tool just designed for using the minimal bunch of data for the maximal accuracy, when used alone. Countless articles are now using lung ultrasound, and many propose various algorithms including echocardiography and other items, advocating a "multiorgan approach." This is not the spirit of our protocol: it associates these various items but does not *include* them (the difference is substantial). Comparing these studies with our approach would therefore make little sense. Regarding, for instance, the heart, see at the end of this chapter and at the end of Chap. 24 that we did not "forget" it (it is known that searchers may sometimes be absent minded, but up to forgetting the heart, there is a substantial step!); we just deleted it from our data. The accuracy of "BLUE-protocol plus echocardiography" is anyway featuring at end of this chapter, and we invite the readers to make an opinion.

Same remark for all clinical signs. Some academicians reproached to the BLUE-protocol to forget these precious signs [10] (don't miss the discussion at the end of Ref. [10]). The clinical signs are, ironically, in the center of the Extended BLUE-protocol, for an improved accuracy (Chap. 35). The BLUE-profiles are here, available, up to this respected physician to integrate his favorite clinical data at will in his clinical approach.

The Design of the BLUE-Protocol

The BLUE-protocol was conceived in an observational study in a Parisian university-affiliated teaching hospital. We performed ultrasonography on admission, in the climax of dyspnea, on serial patients with acute respiratory failure. Acute respiratory failure was defined based on clinical criteria requiring admission to the ICU.

The gold standard was the final diagnosis considered in the hospitalization report, made by a medical ICU team (expert panel) who did not take into account the lung ultrasound data and used traditional approaches. Uncertain diagnoses, multiple diagnoses, and rare causes (frequency <3 %) were excluded (see Chap. 21).

After years necessary for the publication of the preliminary background (mostly lung terminology), we were able to propose the analysis of *three* items at the lung area – with dichotomous answer, collected at standardized points (upper and lower BLUE-points, PLAPS-point).

1. Abolished anterior lung sliding (yes or no)
2. Lung rockets at the anterior wall (present or absent)
3. Alveolar and/or pleural syndrome (called PLAPS if posterior or/and lateral) (yes or no)

We added an adapted venous analysis (indicated in 54 % of cases). Note that the venous analysis takes the major time (2 min of a 3 min examination), which is nonetheless short, since we use a simple machine with fast start-up, the same microconvex probe, time-saving maneuvers, only one setting, and a contact product which allows major time savings. This will be repeated again, intentionally.

The BLUE-Profiles: How Many in the BLUE-Protocol?

A work of a "profiler," based on analysis of hundreds of pre-data, was done during 7 years. From this observational work, the profiles of the BLUE-protocol were defined (Fig. 20.1).

There are eight profiles. The anterior analysis, which initiates the BLUE-protocol, can describe six situations. Five of them conclude the protocol: the B-, B'-, A/B-, C-, and A'-profile. One of them is the A-profile (Video 10.1). The A-profile designates an anterior chest wall with predominant A-lines and lung sliding. The A-profile opens to three more profiles (A-DVT, A-no-V-PLAPS, and nude profile).

Here are the profiles, which were assimilated to specific diseases. The term "profile" assumes an association of signs (two), plus a location (Fig. 20.2).

1. *The A-profile plus DVT* was assimilated to pulmonary embolism. The term "DVT" or "no DVT" was fully detailed in Chap. 18, because it is integrated in a specific, adapted protocol.
2. *The A-no-V-PLAPS* profile is a temporary label which designates an A-profile with no

The BLUE-Profiles: How Many in the BLUE-Protocol?

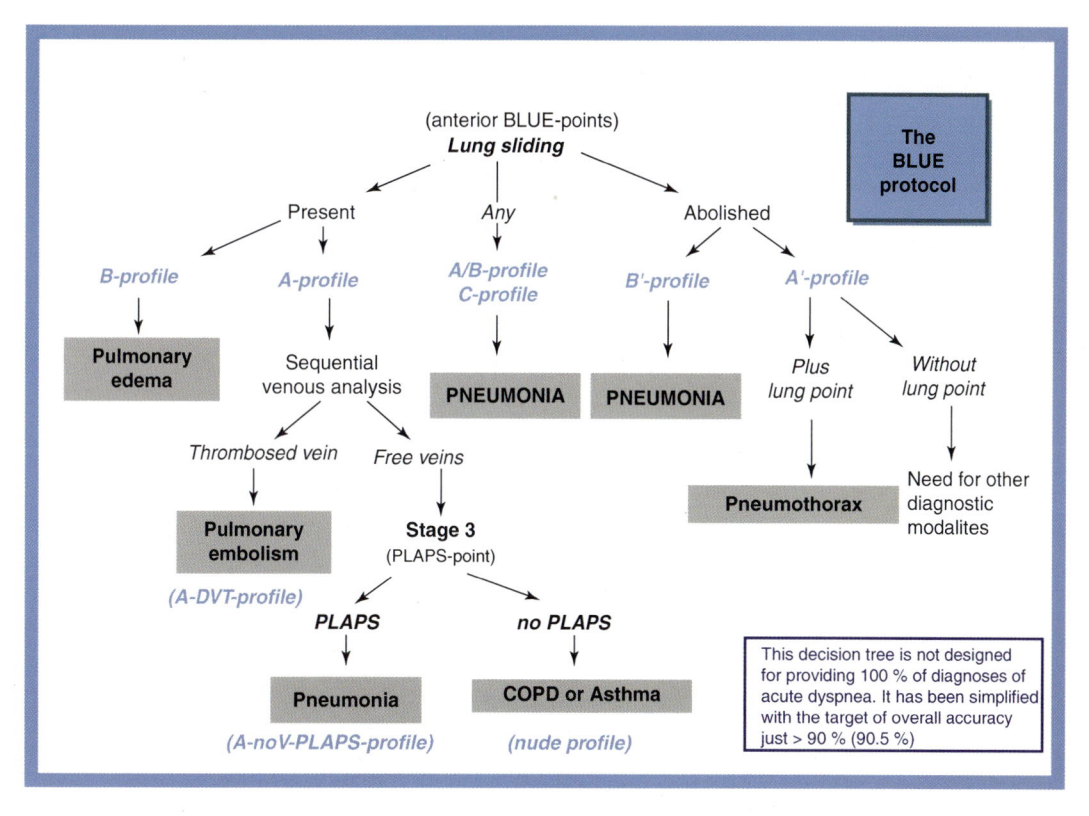

Fig. 20.1 The decision tree of the BLUE-protocol. A decision tree using lung and venous ultrasound to guide the diagnosis of acute respiratory failure: the BLUE-protocol (Adapted from Lichtenstein and Mezière [11], with the authorization of Chest)

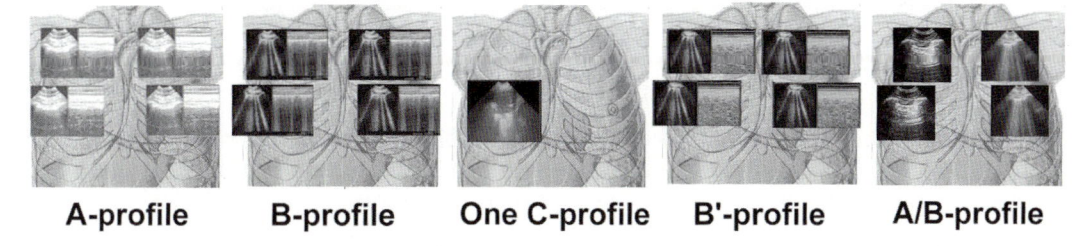

Fig. 20.2 Regular distributions. The main regular profiles of the BLUE-protocol. Note that this figure uses a particular representation of the B-profile and the B′-profile in static images: on M-mode, lung sliding is materialized by this succession of vertical white and black stripes (it reminds real-time images done with vascular probes), since the B-lines come and go through the shooting line of the M-mode. Abolished lung sliding generates a homogeneous MM-space in M-mode: hyperechoic if the shooting line strings a B-line (like here) and hypoechoic if done between two B-lines. Note for the C-profile than only one point is required. The A′-profile does not feature for space management (already dealt with)

DVT and with a PLAPS (uni- or bilateral). Called in some of our articles the A-V-PLAPS-profile, it is now slightly longer but more logical, thus hopingly easier to remember. When "A-no-V-PLAPS" is spelled slowly, we can understand "A," i.e., no pneumothorax and no pulmonary edema; then "no V," i.e., schematically, pulmonary embolism unlikely; and then "PLAPS," making at this step COPD/asthma unlikely. The A-no-V-PLAPS profile was assimilated to pneumonia.

3. *The nude profile* is a normal profile, i.e., A-profile with no DVT and no PLAPS. It was assimilated to asthma or COPD, two bronchial

diseases put together because of a same origin (bronchial obstruction), a roughly same therapy, and a same pathophysiological absence of interstitial, alveolar, pleural, or venous signs.
4. *The B-profile* designates anterior predominant bilateral lung rockets associated with lung sliding (Video 13.1). It was assimilated to hemodynamic pulmonary edema.
5. *The B'-profile* is a B-profile with abolished lung sliding (Video 13.2). It was assimilated to pneumonia.
6. *The A-/B-profile* designates anterior predominant lung rockets at one side and predominant A-lines at the other. It was assimilated to pneumonia.
7. *The C-profile* designates anterior lung consolidation, regardless of size and number. The C-profile was assimilated to pneumonia.
8. *The A'-profile* is an A-profile with abolished lung sliding (Video 14.2). When a lung point was associated, it was assimilated to pneumothorax.

Once these profiles were predefined as written, the study could begin. We then assessed the concordance between profiles and diseases.

Some Terminology Rules

We specify the precise language used in the BLUE-protocol for enabling other teams to reproduce our results.

When the first of the four anterior BLUE-points shows lung sliding with A-lines, labeling it a "quarter of A-profile" indicates that the user has understood that the "A-profile" is defined on the four anterior points. We prefer to read that a given patient had "four quarters of B-profile" (i.e., a B-profile, clearly expressed).

One of the four anterior points with a lung consolidation, even minute (C-line), makes a C-profile.

One isolated B-line visible at all four anterior BLUE-points: this is such a rare pattern that we do not know its clinical relevance. We should temporarily consider this profile as an A-profile.

Some profiles should not generate too much troubles (Fig. 20.3).

A quarter of B-profile visible on three of the four anterior BLUE-points makes sensu stricto "three-quarters of a B-profile." It should probably be linked to a B-profile.

A quarter of B-profile at the right upper BLUE-point with a quarter of B-profile at the left lower BLUE-point and a quarter of B-profile at the right upper BLUE-point with a quarter of B-profile at the left upper BLUE-point are rare profiles, rare enough for not having been seen in the BLUE-protocol. We think wise and logical to link such profiles to an irregular A/B-profile (much more than a B-profile) – suggesting pneumonia/ARDS.

Two-quarters of B-profile at the two lower BLUE-points: this profile, seen in 5 % of cases of hemodynamic pulmonary edema, should probably be considered as an irregular B-profile

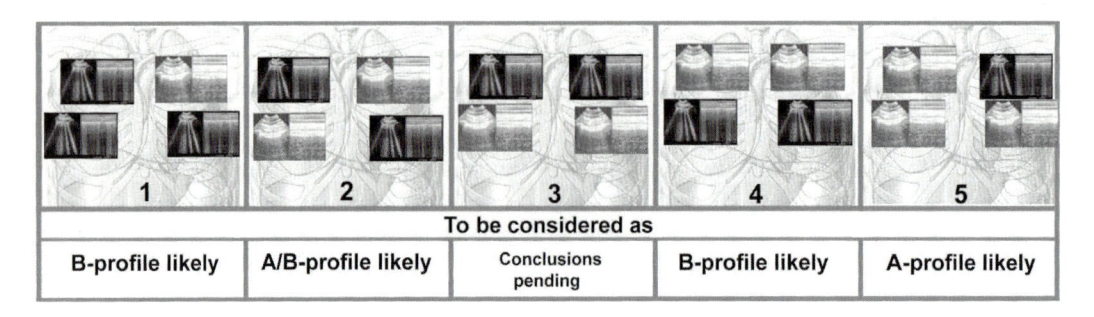

1	2	3	4	5
		To be considered as		
B-profile likely	A/B-profile likely	Conclusions pending	B-profile likely	A-profile likely

Fig. 20.3 Atypical distributions. Some atypical distributions of anterior lung rockets

(patient under beginning of depletive therapy?).

Three-quarters of A-profile with one-quarter of B-profile must be assimilated to an A-profile. This is usually a pneumonia, which will be recognized using the long sequence of the BLUE-protocol: no venous thrombosis and a PLAPS usually present: "A"-no-V-PLAPS-profile.

The Results

At the submission of the manuscript, 302 patients were analyzed. After exclusion of 16 patients for unknown diagnosis, 16 for double diagnosis, and 9 for rare diagnosis, 260 dyspneic patients with one definite diagnosis were considered. The main causes of acute respiratory failure seen in our walls were pneumonia (31 %), pulmonary edema (24 %), decompensated COPD without cause (18 %), severe asthma (12 %), pulmonary embolism (8 %), and pneumothorax (3 %). Table 20.1 details our results.

In this population, the BLUE-protocol *alone* provided the correct diagnosis in 90.5 % of cases [11]. Each of the BLUE-profiles warranted a specificity for the considered disease greater than 90 %.

Table 20.1 details the accuracy of ultrasound for each diagnosis. All these major causes of acute respiratory failure in the adult have characteristic patterns.

Acute hemodynamic pulmonary edema: nearly all cases, i.e., 62 of 64, yielded bilateral disseminated anterior lung rockets, a pattern always associated to lung sliding: the B-profile. PLAPS were present in 56 of 62 cases.

Pneumonia: of 83 cases, 74 had one of four characteristic profiles. The A-no-V-PLAPS-profile was seen in 35 cases, the C-profile in 18, the A/B profile in 12, and the B′-profile in 9. Each of these four profiles was infrequent, but the sum made an 89 % sensitivity, and these patterns were 94 % specific to pneumonia.

Exacerbated COPD, severe asthma: patients had usually a normal pattern (nude profile). Of 49 cases of COPD, 7 had pathologic patterns. These results will be commented below ("missed" cases of the BLUE-protocol).

Pulmonary embolism: patients had nearly always (20 of 21) an anterior normal surface (A-profile). None had anterior lung rockets (in the B, A/B, or B′ variant). Eighty-one percent had visible deep venous thrombosis. Half of the cases had PLAPS.

Table 20.1 Accuracy of the BLUE-protocol

Mechanism of dyspnea	Profiles of BLUE-protocol	Sensitivity	Specificity	Positive predictive value	Negative predictive value
Acute hemodynamic pulmonary edema	B-profile	97 % (62/64)	95 % (187/196)	87 % (62/71)	99 % (187/189)
Exacerbated COPD or severe asthma	Nude profile (A-profile with no DVT and no PLAPS)	89 % (74/83)	97 % (172/177)	93 % (74/79)	95 % (172/181)
Pulmonary embolism	A-profile with deep venous thrombosis	81 % (17/21)	99 % (238/239)	94 % (17/18)	98 % (238/242)
Pneumothorax	A′-profile (with lung point)	88 % (8/9)	100 % (251/251)	100 % (8/8)	99 % (251/252)
Pneumonia	1. B′-profile	11 % (9/83)	100 % (177/177)	100 % (9/9)	70 % (177/251)
	2. A/B-profile	14.5 % (12/83)	100 % (177/177)	100 % (12/12)	71.5 % (177/248)
	3. C-profile	21.5 % (18/83)	99 % (175/177)	90 % (18/20)	73 % (175/240)
	4. A-no-V-PLAPS profile	42 % (35/83)	96 % (170/177)	83 % (35/42)	78 % (170/218)
	The four profiles	89 % (74/83)	94 % (167/177)	88 % (74/84)	95 % (167/176)

Adapted from Lichtenstein and Mezière [11]
Brackets: No. of patients

Pneumothorax: all had abolition of anterior lung sliding with the A-line sign (A′-profile). Eight of nine had a lung point.

These profiles and results will be sharply explained, detailed, and commented in the following chapters.

Pathophysiological Basis of the BLUE-Protocol

The pathophysiology fully explains the scientific basis of the BLUE-protocol and the results. It is detailed in devoted chapters, one per disease (see Chaps. 23, 24, 25, 26, and 27).

A-lines indicate air, which can be physiological (normal lung surface seen in COPD, asthma, pulmonary embolism, and anterior wall of posterior pneumonia) or pathological (pneumothorax).

Lung rockets indicate interstitial syndrome. Hemodynamic pulmonary edema and some cases of pneumonia display anterior and symmetric lung rockets.

Alveolar and pleural changes are usually posterior (defining PLAPS) and are common to pulmonary edema, pneumonia, and pulmonary embolism (even pneumothorax), therefore not of major discriminating potential if used alone. Anterior consolidations are typical of pneumonia. PLAPS not associated with anterior interstitial changes are seen in pneumonia and pulmonary embolism. PLAPS have a discriminative value only in patients with A-profile and without venous thrombosis: this provides a BLUE diagnosis of pneumonia, likely.

Lung sliding is seen in hemodynamic pulmonary edema, a disease which creates a transudate. Transudate is a kind of oil, allowing us to breathe from birth to death without burning. Lung sliding is also seen in pulmonary embolism, COPD, and some pneumonia. It is present in asthma, although of limited amplitude in very severe cases.

Abolished lung sliding is seen in many cases of pneumonia, a group of diseases which create exudate. Exudate acts like glue, sticking the lung to the wall. Pneumothorax always abolishes lung sliding.

The Decision Tree of the BLUE-Protocol (Fig. 20.1)

To get a 90.5 % accuracy in a few minutes, we first check for anterior lung sliding. Its presence discounts pneumothorax. Anterior B-lines are then sought. The *B-profile* calls for pulmonary edema. *B-′*, *A/B-*, and *C-profile* call for pneumonia. The *A-profile* prompts a search for venous thrombosis. If present, the BLUE-diagnosis is pulmonary embolism. If absent, PLAPS are sought. Their presence (*A-no-V-PLAPS-profile*) calls for pneumonia and their absence (*nude profile*) for COPD or asthma. To get a far higher accuracy, read Chap. 35.

The Missed Patients of the BLUE-Protocol. What Should One Think? An Introduction to the Extended BLUE-Protocol

These critical points are developed through the textbook. The BLUE-protocol was designed for using the simplest decision tree for reaching the highest accuracy. The target to reach was the value of "90 %" (it was, actually, 90.5 %). Wanting to reach 91, 92 %, etc., would have complicated this decision tree, and so on, up to the theoretical value of 100 %. Reminder, the BLUE-protocol is only a protocol. It should be considered as a tool, permanently *piloted* by the physician. Using basic clinical data, some simple tests (ECG, D-dimers, etc.), the common sense (a precious tool), and some more developed ultrasound tools (in one sentence, performing an Extended BLUE-protocol), the accuracy climbs substantially. Please consider the BLUE-protocol as an initial approach (with already an overall 90.5 % accuracy, just used alone).

In 9.5 % of included patients, the BLUE-protocol yielded a profile which was not in agreement with the official diagnosis. We must consider two groups.

1. Some are real limitations (4 %).
   Pulmonary embolism without visible venous thrombosis (19 %) is a typical limitation of the BLUE-protocol. Pneumonia with the

B-profile (7 %) looks like hemodynamic pulmonary edema. Piloting the BLUE-protocol would correct this kind of limitation. Just a short example, in a pneumonia with a B-profile, considering simple signs (history, fever, white cells, etc.) and simple emergency cardiac sonography, the physician enters into the Extended BLUE-protocol and usually corrects the error. See Chap. 22, and don't forget to read, once basic data are integrated, Chap. 35.
2. Other cases (5.5 %) possibly indicate a failure of the gold standard.
   When a patient has standardized ultrasound signs of lung consolidation and receives the official diagnosis of exacerbated COPD, there is likely a failure in the traditional tools. This patient has likely a superadded diagnosis (radio-occult pneumonia, pulmonary embolism). Patients with the B-profile but officially considered COPD are other possible mistakes. Patients without the B-profile but considered pulmonary edema are again possible mistakes. These cases are detailed in Chaps. 24 and 25.
   All in all, while accepting the final diagnosis as a gold standard, we consider that the 90.5 % rate of correct diagnoses is below the reality. We may calculate an *officious* rate of 90.5 + 5.5 %, i.e., 96 % (−1 % for the science, say 95 %), yet this kind of calculation would violate the rules of scientific publications. In any honest study, the gold standard cannot be always perfect, but how to prove it, when it is the gold standard? Just common sense can alert. Commercial pilots make mistakes; we assume doctors are not exempt from some mistakes too.

When Is the BLUE-Protocol Performed

The raison d'être of the BLUE-protocol, which uses ultrasound *alone*, is to be inserted in the first stages of the usual management of an acute dyspnea. In this traditional management, one can describe three steps (Fig. 20.4):
1. *Step 1*: The physician receives the patient and, time permitting, learns the history and makes the physical examination. This step is decisive. A young dyspneic patient with fever has not the same disease with an apyretic old cardiopathic one, e.g.

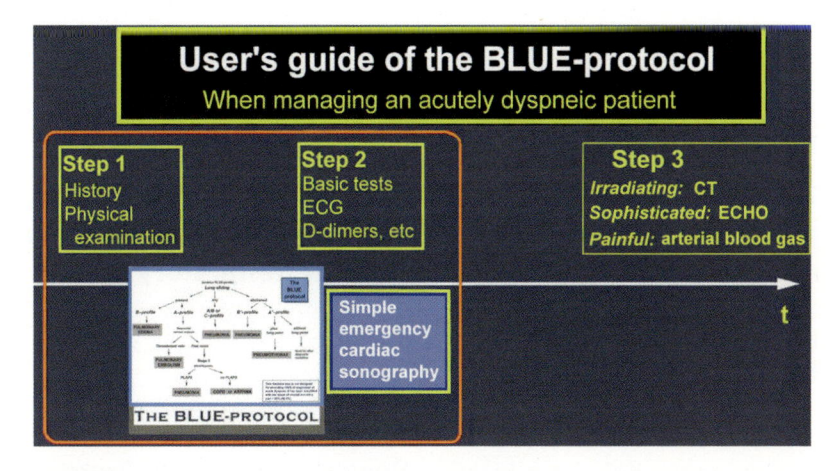

Fig. 20.4 Integration of the BLUE-protocol in the traditional management. This figure illustrates the usual steps of management of an acute respiratory failure, and the place that the BLUE-protocol and the simple emergency cardiac sonography can take, between the clinical examination and the first paraclinical tests. One main aim of the BLUE-protocol is to relief the patient before – or in substitution to – the usual late tests (*Step 3*). We aim at making the simple clinical examination, the BLUE-protocol, the simple cardiac sonography, and the initial current basic tests the *fab four* in acute respiratory failure management. The integration of the BLUE-protocol within these three other major tools is part of the definition of the Extended BLUE-protocol

2. *Step 2*: Simple tests are done, like ECG, D-dimers, and basic *venous* blood tests (see below).
3. *Step 3*: With all these elements in hand, the doctor decides whether sophisticated examinations will be ordered. This is usually time for asking a CT scan or a sophisticated echocardiography.

The BLUE-protocol aims at being inserted between Step 1 and Step 2. Its 90.5 % official rate of accuracy will be dramatically enhanced using basic data, making the need for the traditional Step 3 less mandatory (see below), for reaching the LUCIFLR spirit (Chap. 29).

The Timing: How Is the BLUE-Protocol Practically Used

The BLUE-protocol is usually done in Stage 1′ (semirecumbent patient). We apply the probe on the right upper BLUE-point (1″). We identify the bat sign (2″). Then we search for lung sliding. With experience, two seconds are enough to recognize lung sliding (2″). Pneumothorax is instantaneously ruled out. Then we analyze the Merlin's space. A-lines should be rapidly identified (2″). A pulmonary edema is ruled out. A routine Carmen's maneuver indicates that no B-line is visible. This takes 3″. The lower BLUE-point is then analyzed (10 more seconds). The left lung analysis adds 20″. Facing a B-profile, an A/B-profile, a C-profile (one point is enough, in terms of specificity), or a B′-profile, the protocol is over. The rest of the lung will of course be analyzed but outside the protocol (searching for PLAPS after detecting a B′-, C-, or A/B-profile is redundant), same remark for the venous network. The A-profile calls, using the same probe, for a venous analysis. If no venous thrombosis is detected (2 min), the diagnosis of pulmonary embolism is not ruled out of course, but the user comes back to the lung posteriorly. Stage 3 is performed (6″ for setting the patient) and the PLAPS-point is analyzed, searching either air artifacts or PLAPS (7″). This step prioritizes the diagnosis of pneumonia if PLAPS are present or COPD/asthma if PLAPS are absent. Facing an A′-profile, a lung point is sought for, laterally, posteriorly, etc. (a matter of half a minute). Once the BLUE-protocol is over, the physician decides if this information is in agreement with the Steps 1 (history, etc.) and 2 (basic tests, ECG, etc.), making a part of Extended BLUE-protocol, and initiates active therapy or goes up to Step 3 (CT, etc.) if necessary.

All in all, scanning the patient in the longest sequence takes 3 min and 6 s. This is done in the case of asthma/COPD (the longest sequence). In the case of the A′-, B′-, C-, and A/B-profiles, the test takes a few seconds.

As one example of how to pilot the BLUE-protocol, a patient with the B-profile will have a priority diagnosis of hemodynamic pulmonary edema. If meanwhile, the simple history learns that this patient is followed for a chronic interstitial disease, the diagnosis will of course be shifted to the profit of exacerbated chronic interstitial disease, statistically 16 times less frequent [11]. The Extended BLUE-protocol uses this history, some echocardiographic data (showing here rather right heart anomalies), and studies the PLAPS-point, which is not required in the native BLUE-protocol but will here provide basic data: PLAPS favors the diagnosis of a chronic interstitial disease complicated by something (edema, embolism, pneumonia, etc.); absence of PLAPS will suggest a simple exacerbation with no visible factor of complication (read Chap. 35).

We routinely make a comprehensive venous analysis in patients without A-profile, but this is done outside the protocol, again.

The BLUE-Protocol and Rare Causes of Acute Respiratory Failure

They are dealt with mainly in Chaps. 21 and 35.

Frequently Asked Questions Regarding the BLUE-Protocol

All these questions are answered in the specific sections through the book. Here are some:
Why isn't the heart featuring in the BLUE-protocol?
Why just three points and no lateral analysis?

What should one think of the "missed" patients of the BLUE-protocol?

Didn't the exclusion of patients create a bias limiting the value of the BLUE-protocol?

Challenging patients?

What about the mildly dyspneic patients (simply managed in the emergency room)?

What happens when the BLUE-protocol is performed on *non-blue* patients?

What is the interest of the PLAPS concept?

Can the BLUE-protocol allow a distinction between hemodynamic and permeability-induced (ARDS) pulmonary edema?

How about patients with severe pulmonary embolism and no visible venous thrombosis?

What about pulmonary edema complicating a chronic interstitial disease?

Will the BLUE-protocol work everywhere?

Will multicentric studies be launched for validating the BLUE-protocol on huge numbers?

Are 3 min really possible?

Is the BLUE-protocol only accessible to an elite?

By the way, why "BLUE" protocol?

A Whole 300-Page Textbook Based on 300 Patients

It may be one more FAQ. Any honest physician knows that huge numbers do not change a reality. Using 3,000 or 30,000 patients would have made only slight changes. The countless patients we managed once the study was submitted (years and years from the printing of this textbook) and the countless patients we could "pilot" from our world laboratory, i.e., all the information we received from hundreds of physicians through the planet, just confirmed the value of this series, based on logic. Our aim is to see this method aging well and see it used by increasing critical care physicians – and all other fields concerned.

How Will the BLUE-Protocol Impact Traditional Managements?

Three main fields should be affected:
1. If the *lung* is admitted in the court of ultrasound, the *heart* will be the definite winner. Combining our lung and (adapted) venous approaches should result in considering the simple emergency cardiac sonography as a new, valuable entity.
2. Less irradiation will be provided. Physical examination, BLUE-protocol, simple cardiac sonography, and basic tests (without arterial puncture) should summarize the investigation of most patients (Fig. 20.4). The decrease of requirement for Step 3 examinations (mainly CT) is one of our major satisfactions. Chapter 29 will show the drawbacks of CT.

   The traditional *arterial puncture* was placed among these targets. The simple perspective of decreasing this test would have fully awarded our 18-year research. This test is painful: patients remember it. We guess that these blue patients are hypoxic. So the question becomes: "Why do we need blood gases?" Searching to know the CO_2 level for making a diagnosis indicates how blind we are (without ultrasound) facing acute dyspnea. We keep this test in the ICU, on an arterial line, for monitoring circulatory status in sedated patients.

   As to expert echocardiography Doppler, we see no drawback to see this test performed, provided the team is already equipped and trained, in a patient who already received the initial therapy and in the countries where this option is envisageable.
3. We appreciate this possibility to immediately relieve the acutely dyspneic patient by providing appropriate therapy (full O_2, e.g.). The rate of deaths which are the immediate or remote consequence of initial errors should decrease – not to speak of the comfort of the patients and the satisfaction to see simplicity winning in this demanding field of medicine.

A Small Story of the BLUE-Protocol

Read if there's time the introduction of this textbook, describing when, where, and how the real work began.

Having had the privilege of working in a pioneering ICU developing echocardiography in the critically ill since 1989, we had easy access to the heart. We integrated elements from pleural, lung, and venous ultrasound, allowing to propose the use of ultrasound in acute dyspnea since 1991 [12].

Our first mention of a decision tree for managing acute respiratory failure was available in 1995 [13]. It was rather comprehensive at this time, including the heart, inferior caval vein. The inferior caval vein was quickly withdrawn, for no added value. Three cardiac items were featuring up to the years 2000–2003: left heart contractility, right heart enlargement, and pericardial effusion [14]. Withdrawing the heart was not our initial intention. One day in the corridor, we were advised to remain far from this area which was reserved to specialists. Desirous to keep it scientific, we did not answer first and took one whole week (24/7) for deeply reviewing all our data, and three sequential features appeared to us.

First, withdrawing the pericardial item was not an issue. A pericarditis creates pain more than respiratory failure and is not on focus here.

Second, we observed that each blue patient without a B-profile had a disease able to generate right heart enlargement (embolism, pneumonia, COPD, etc.) and had usually (*usually*) no visible left heart anomaly. We could therefore withdraw the right heart analysis without damage.

The third regarded the left heart analysis, the last item which remained in our decision tree [15]. Read in Chap. 24 how withdrawing the left heart data resulted in *improving* the performances of the BLUE-protocol.

For being able to submit the BLUE-protocol, we had to publish the whole of the nomenclature allowing standardized analysis, i.e., basic articles about pneumothorax, pleural effusion (adding criteria for an application which was not so much standardized), lung consolidation, interstitial syndrome, etc. This resulted in endless rejections, making the story last between 1990 and 2008. We deliberately sacrificed countless other findings (meanwhile published by other teams) and the opportunity of taking any leadership (idem). The manuscript of the BLUE-protocol was rejected by several international journals. These factors explain why we were able to share our approach in the peer-review literature only 13 years after its first public mention and 18 years after the onset of our clinical use.

References

1. Irwin RS, Rippe JM (2008) Intensive care medicine, 6th edn. Lippincott Williams & Wilkins, Philadelphia, pp 491–496
2. Laënnec RTH (1819) Traité de l'auscultation médiate, ou traité du diagnostic des maladies des poumons et du cœur. J.A. Brosson & J.S. Chaudé, Paris. Hafner, New York, 1962, pp 455–456
3. Roentgen WC (1895) Ueber eine neue Art von Strahlen. Vorläufige Mittheilung. Sitzungsberichte der Wurzburger Physik-mediz Gesellschaft, 28 Dec 1895, pp 132–141
4. Wasserman K (1982) Dyspnea on exertion: is it the heart or the lungs? JAMA 248:2039–2043
5. Greenbaum DM, Marschall KE (1982) The value of routine daily chest X-rays in intubated patients in the medical intensive care unit. Crit Care Med 10:29–30
6. Aronchick J, Epstein D, Gefter WB et al (1985) Evaluation of the chest radiograph in the emergency department patient. Emerg Med Clin North Am 3:491–501
7. Lichtenstein D, Goldstein G, Mourgeon E, Cluzel P, Grenier P, Rouby JJ (2004) Comparative diagnostic performances of auscultation, chest radiography and lung ultrasonography in acute respiratory distress syndrome. Anesthesiology 100:9–15
8. Ray P, Birolleau S, Lefort Y, Becquemin MH, Beigelman C, Isnard R, Teixeira A, Arthaud M, Riou B, Boddaert J (2006) Acute respiratory failure in the elderly: etiology, emergency diagnosis and prognosis. Crit Care 10(3):R82
9. Brenner DJ, Hall EJ (2007) Computed tomography. An increasing source of radiation exposure. N Engl J Med 357:2277–2284
10. Lichtenstein D (2007) L'échographie "corps entier", une approche visuelle du patient en état critique. Bulletin officiel de l'Académie Nationale de Médecine, Paris Tome 191, mars N°3:495–517
11. Lichtenstein D, Mezière G (2008) Relevance of lung ultrasound in the diagnosis of acute respiratory failure. the BLUE-protocol. Chest 134:117–125
12. Lichtenstein D, Axler O (1993) Intensive use of general ultrasound in the intensive care unit, a prospective study of 150 consecutive patients. Intensive Care Med 19:353–355
13. Lichtenstein D (1995) Echographie pulmonaire. Diplôme Inter-Universitaire National d'Echographie, Paris VI, Dec 1995
14. Lichtenstein D, Mezière G (2003) Ultrasound diagnosis of an acute dyspnea. Crit Care 7(suppl 2):S93
15. Lichtenstein D (2005) Analytic study of frequent and/or severe situations. In: General ultrasound in the critically ill. Springer, Berlin, pp 177–183

The Excluded Patients of the BLUE-Protocol: Who Are They? Did Their Exclusion Limit Its Value?

21

The letters to the editor generated by the native article well go beyond the 2,500 word limit [1–10]. We had the honor to answer five letters, i.e., 5×500 more words, an honorable providence for specifying with more details what the BLUE-protocol is (before the production of this textbook where each detail is thoroughly described).

Let us analyze an apparently significant issue: how about the excluded patients?

The Exclusion of Rare Causes: An Issue?

These rare patients were advocated by some to be the most difficult, so their exclusion was advocated as creating a bias [1]. Why? Why is the exclusion of these patients not an issue? Simply because "rare diagnoses" does not mean "difficult" diagnoses. Massive pleural effusion is the best example. No need for multicentric randomized studies for understanding the interest of ultrasound there. No need for BLUE-protocol. The diagnosis is easy using usual tools, including traditional ultrasound.

The BLUE-protocol has incorporated 97 % of the patients seen in the ER (or pre-hospital medicine) and eventually admitted to the ICU of our parisian hospital. The multiple diagnoses of the 3 % remaining patients were not considered, in order to keep our protocol simple, fit for use: daily problems were prioritized. Those daily patients had pneumonia, pulmonary edema, COPD, asthma, pulmonary embolism, and pneumothorax. The 3 % remaining causes were [11]:

- Exacerbation of chronic interstitial disease (1.4 %)
- Massive pleural effusion as causing agent (1 %)
- Complete atelectasis, foreign body aspiration (0.3 %)
- Tracheal stenosis (0.3 %)
- Fat embolism (0.3 %)

If the protocol includes not 300 but 3,000 or 30,000 patients, the list would be enriched by countless but rare diseases: acute gastric dilatation, pneumoniae linked to drugs, sterile aspiration pneumonia, phrenic palsy, Guillain-Barré syndrome, extended causes of chronic interstitial disease (histiocytosis X, sarcoïdosis and other alveolar proteinosis, etc.), acute hypovolemia, metabolic dyspnea, etc. Ask to experts for a comprehensive list. Most of these diseases will be accessible to the Extended BLUE-protocol (Chap. 35). For assessing ultrasound for one given rarity, years of large-scale multicentric studies will be necessary for gathering enough patients. The BLUE-protocol favors the real life.

Interestingly, each of the rare diagnoses had a profile among the eight of the BLUE-protocol. Let us see these main rare causes.

Regarding chronic interstitial diseases, the B-profile is linked to a lung disease using various tools. The simplest is disease history, when the disease is known (most of the cases). During the first episode (an occurrence far lower than 1.4 %), simple tools from the Extended-BLUE-protocol, mainly the simple cardiac sonography, will find right heart anomalies together with the left heart normality, immediately linking this interstitial syndrome to a pulmonary origin.

Massive atelectasis yields numerous standardized signs, as discussed in Chap. 35.

Tracheal stenosis had a nude profile, following the logic: this is the main profile of asthma and COPD, i.e., obstruction (as is tracheal stenosis). The characteristic clinical signs should make ultrasound of lesser relevance, although an anterior location of granuloma (usual location) can be found using ultrasound.

We can consider infinite combinations, such as hemodynamic pulmonary edema due to myocarditis complicating an infectious pneumonia. These patients will likely have the appropriate B-profile.

Thoracic disorders occurring in children and neonates are detailed in Chap. 32.

The case of the diaphragm. The BLUE-protocol was reproached not to include it [9]. First, the diaphragm is included: *detecting an abolished lung sliding means a motionless cupola*. Second, we wanted to keep our decision tree as simple as can be. Bilateral causes, although having originated the birth of intensive care in 1954, are now an extinct cause. Would it even be seen, the therapy is purely symptomatic. Read Anecdotal Note 1 which explains why the diaphragm was not included. Read also the section on diaphragm in the chapter dealing with non-critical ultrasound (Chap. 36).

To say it differently, the BLUE-protocol works always, even when it is not used. When rare diagnoses are suspected by the initial approach, the Extended-BLUE-protocol will be used, with increased ultrasound potential. The native BLUE-protocol makes nothing but adding decisive points to the usual management. Used this way, we are accustomed to work with the correct diagnosis.

Patients Excluded for More Than One Diagnosis: An Issue?

Five percent of the patients had more than one diagnosis. Their exclusion was advocated as creating a bias [1]. Pulmonary edema and pneumonia were the most frequent. This raises an interesting methodological issue. When two diseases are suggested, does each mechanism generate exactly 50 % of the cause of respiratory failure? Of course not. This rate may be 51 % versus 49 %, which remains fine, but it can be as well 99 % versus 1 %, etc. The issue is that no gold standard is able, at a given time, to assess this ratio. The BLUE-protocol gave one of the two incriminated diagnoses with quite the same accuracy than in the regular population that had one diagnosis: 87.5 % (quite the 90.5 % accuracy of the BLUE-protocol). Therefore, the BLUE-protocol was not misleading.

Note that the BLUE-protocol was designed to provide *one* profile, yielding *one* ultrasound diagnosis, subsequently correlated with *one* final diagnosis, which we retained as the gold standard. For this first methodological reason, patients with several diagnoses could not be included.

The Extended-BLUE-protocol considers these double diagnoses (see Chap. 35).

Patients Excluded for Absence of Final Diagnosis: An Opportunity for the BLUE-Protocol

Five percent of the patients never received a definite diagnosis using traditional tools. Their exclusion was advocated as creating a bias [1]. The BLUE-protocol was designed to suggest a diagnosis, subsequently correlated with the final diagnosis. It was methodologically impossible to include patients who did not benefit from a final diagnosis. However, of major interest, *all these patients* had a precise BLUE-profile, among the eight defined profiles. We bet that when it will be widely used and followed by therapeutic decisions, the BLUE-protocol will be *precisely* a tool allowing to highly decrease this rate of patients without final diagnosis.

> **Anecdotal Notes**
> 1. Diaphragm
>
>   Isolated phrenic palsy is not listed as cause of acute respiratory failure [12]. It must be associated to a comorbid state for yielding troubles [13].
>
>   In addition, phrenic palsy is an exceptional event – seen in none of the patients in the BLUE-protocol. Independently of its exceptional participation as an associated cause of respiratory failure, and even if the comorbid disorder is accessible to ultrasound, this association should be a mix cause, by definition excluded from the BLUE-protocol, like rare causes (even if easy to diagnose) [10].
>
>   Even if a phrenic palsy is diagnosed in acute respiratory failure, this finding would be of minor relevance, since there is no specific routine therapy.
>
>   Note that if a patient has been intubated and sedated, the mechanical ventilation generates passive phrenic movements, and the diagnosis at this step is impossible.
>
>   What we see in the current thinking is a confusion between *palsy* and *akinesis*. Akinetic cupola in severe pneumonia is a common feature, seen in 27 % of cases [11]. These patients have abolished lung sliding. Akinetic cupola in a severe pneumonia is usually linked to adhesions and not phrenic palsy. When such patients are intubated and sedated, it is easy to see that the disorder (abolished lung sliding, akinetic cupola) remains (proving the adhesions, infirming the phrenic palsy).

> The phrenic analysis is part indeed of our systematic ultrasound examinations, using our polyvalent microconvex probe, but we have not included it in our decision tree [14].

References

1. Khosla R (2009) Utility of lung sonography in acute respiratory failure. Chest 135:884
2. Lichtenstein D, Mezière G (2009) Response to Khosla R. "Utility of lung sonography in acute respiratory failure". Chest 135:884
3. Reissig A, Kroegel C (2009) Relevance of subpleural consolidations in chest ultrasound. Chest 136:1706
4. Lichtenstein D, Mezière G (2009) Response to "Relevance of subpleural consolidations in chest ultrasound" (Reissig A & Kroegel C). Chest 136:1706–1707
5. Volpicelli G, Cardinale L, Mussa A, Caramello V (2009) Diagnosis of cardiogenic pulmonary edema by sonography limited to the anterior lung. Chest 135:883
6. Lichtenstein D, Mezière G (2009) Response to "Diagnosis of cardiogenic pulmonary edema by sonography limited to the anterior lung" (Volpicelli G et al.). Chest 135:883–884
7. Mathis G (2010) Why look for artifacts alone when the original is visible? Chest 137:233
8. Lichtenstein D, Mezière G (2010) Response to "Why look for artifacts alone when the original is visible?" (Mathis G). Chest 137:233
9. Khosla R (2010) BLUE-protocol: a suggestion to modify. Chest 137:1487
10. Lichtenstein D, Mezière G (2010) Response to "BLUE-protocol: a suggestion to modify" (Khosla R). Chest 137:1487–1488
11. Lichtenstein D, Mezière G (2008) Relevance of lung ultrasound in the diagnosis of acute respiratory failure. The BLUE-protocol. Chest 134:117–125
12. Offenstadt G et al (2001) Réanimation Médicale. Collège National des Enseignants de Réanimation Médicale, Masson/Paris
13. Aldrich TK, Tso R (2004) The lung and neuromuscular diseases. In: Murray & Nadel's textbook of respiratory medicine, 4th edn. Elsevier Saunders, New York, pp 2287–2290
14. Lichtenstein D (2010) Analytic study of severe and/or frequent situations in the critically ill. In: Whole body ultrasonography in the critically ill. Springer, Heidelberg, pp 277–289

Frequently Asked Questions Regarding the BLUE-Protocol

22

Pretending to help in expediting the causal diagnosis of a respiratory disorder using a method which was not supposed to exist and advocating data >90 % probably deserve some explanations. It generated multiple questions. From the most recurrent, here is a selection (plus some anticipated ones).

Why Isn't the Heart Featuring in the BLUE-Protocol?

This is the most FAQ.

We may expedite the answer this way: the BLUE-protocol was devoted for patients *without* suitable cardiac windows. This doing, we saw that the performances had an overall 90.5 % accuracy. This accuracy is independent also from the clinical data. When they are added, when echocardiography is added, i.e., when the BLUE-protocol is expanded to the Extended BLUE-protocol, the accuracy will jump far beyond this 90.5 %.

The heart is associated to the BLUE-protocol, not integrated (it is fully integrated in the Extended BLUE-protocol; see Chap. 35). Yet users may be disappointed to see that the consideration of this expert science will only slightly increase the value of the BLUE-protocol (clinical data and simple lab tests will increase it much better). This is explained first because the lung data allow to predict the cardiac status and, second, because the cardiac data can sometimes be misleading. This explains why the withdrawal of cardiac information resulted in a slight improvement of the accuracy (from 90.3 to 90.5 %; see the small story at the end of Chap. 24). The third and main reason is that the lung analysis is a *direct* approach in a patient suffering from the respiratory function. Showing an absence of B-profile demonstrates that the left heart function is normal (or not the actual problem). The BLUE-protocol does not search for a left heart anomaly but for the consequence of this anomaly: pulmonary edema. The detection of the B-profile has shown high accuracy for the diagnosis of hemodynamic pulmonary edema (with rare cases of pneumonia and exceptional cases of chronic interstitial disease). The detection of a non-B-profile was correlated with the absence of pulmonary edema.

We will see in Chap. 35 that the Extended BLUE-protocol takes carefully into account not only simple items from Step 1 (history, age, temperature, physical examination, etc.) and Step 2 (white cells, CRP, etc.) but also the simple emergency cardiac sonography. The B-profile in a young patient with fever, no cardiac history, and a well-contracting left ventricle will be immediately suspected as a "failure" of the BLUE-protocol (brackets because it pretends only at a 90.5 % accuracy with the simplest tools).

We therefore advise to begin the analysis of a blue patient (with no clear clinical orientation) with the lung, confirming or not edema, then simple cardiac sonography. This inversion of priorities means gain of time, since lung ultrasound needs shorter training; has less operator dependencies, less patient dependencies, and less risk of poor windows; and is cheaper. In the same time, the physician is free to initiate a training in traditional echocardiography, which will allow to better understand and manage situations where more information is required. It will indicate for instance the need for emergency valvular repair, but these are not frequent scenarios (and we rarely need to repair a valvular disease in the night).

In fact, the therapeutic management is usually decided at the end of the BLUE-protocol, with a slight subtlety. The moment when the nurse prepares the therapy (heparin, fibrinolytics, inotropics, diuretics, beta-agonists, antibiotics, low- or high-flow oxygen, CPAP or endotracheal tube, etc.) is the time for initiating our simple emergency cardiac sonography – enhanced by the lung approach. Apart from exceptional cases, an acute respiratory failure with a hypokinetic left ventricle but with an A-profile will be considered as a *pulmonary* dyspnea (occurring in a patient who it is true has a quiescent chronic left heart disease). In actual fact, the sequence is lung–veins–nurse–heart.

> **Sophisticated Note**
> For optimizing the cost savings, the nurse is trained to break the costly ampullae (fibrinolytics) *last*. If the cardiac sonography happens to find, for instance, a pericardial effusion, it is still time to stop the action of the nurse – time for rebuilding a story of, for example, here, pulmonary embolism complicating a history of neoplasia responsible for hemorrhagic pericardial effusion. Using this way, not many costly fibrinolytic ampullae will be broken for nothing.
>
> Not only the BLUE-protocol but also the FALLS-protocol favors the lung, making it equal to the heart. The absence of B-profile indicates a pulmonary artery occlusion pressure <18 mmHg, with direct consequences on hemodynamic management [1]. See Chap. 30.
>
> Nonscientific reasons why the heart was deleted from the BLUE-protocol can be consulted in the last section of the Chap. 20.

Are Three Minutes Really Possible?

Some colleagues were intrigued by such a timing [2]. These 3 min (let us concede "less than four" for simplifying) were done by experienced users, precisely in the aim of not interfering with the traditional management. Of course, novice doctors are free to take more time. Three-minute examination was an average timing, allowed when using the fast protocol we defined since 1992: one smart machine, one universal (microconvex) probe, one setting, no Doppler, and our substitute to gel. The lung is superficial. Time for finding windows (unlike "ECHO") is null. Detection of A-lines or B-lines is immediate. The timing is shortened each time the BLUE-protocol does not require venous analysis or posterolateral lung analysis: B-, B′-, A/B-, or C-profile occurs in 46 % of cases and makes a BLUE-protocol duration inferior to 1 min.

We use the same fast protocol for searching for deep venous thrombosis, using the same probe, the same settings, cross-sectional scan, Carmen maneuver, etc.

Using our contact product makes the time between two regions of interest (e.g., lung and calf veins) <2 s. We keep our soaked compress near our scanned field and can do flash scanning. No time is lost for taking the traditional gel bottle, squeezing it, and applying the gel to areas distant from each other and wiping after.

Why Is the Lateral Chest Wall Not Considered?

This is part of the spirit of the BLUE-protocol, a minimal bunch of data for a maximal accuracy. Quite always, the lateral analysis gives redundant pieces of information, as an example, the lateral lung rockets.
- If associated with the (anterior) B-profile, they are redundant for a diagnosis already done (hemodynamic pulmonary edema).
- If associated with B′-, C-, or A/B-profiles, they were redundant for a diagnosis already done (pneumonia).

- If associated with an (anterior) A-profile, they will be redundant with PLAPS for a diagnosis of pneumonia (3.5 times more often than pulmonary edema in the unpublished data of the BLUE-protocol).

Didn't the Exclusion of Patients Create a Bias Limiting the Value of the BLUE-Protocol?

This question appeared critical for some, and we took full consideration of it [2]. We devoted the whole Chap. 21 for showing how these exclusions could not decrease the performances of the BLUE-protocol.

Is the BLUE-Protocol Only Accessible to an Elite?

The development of the BLUE-protocol may appear complex, but the final use is simple. Many details make a training curve efficient for a large-scale training. The BLUE-points are accessible to any student. The venous analysis is possibly longer to master, although each step is elementary.

Note that intensive care medicine is a discipline for an elite. Inside this exacting discipline, fields such as TEE are mastered. *Even if complicated*, the BLUE-protocol should be mastered by such an elite.

Also note a critical point that most doctors have forgotten from their remote medical studies. For understanding a (simple) pulmonary edema, they have mastered a huge amount of information, beginning by the anatomy and physiology of the lung, then the clinical approach, then the mastery of reading a radiograph, interpreting blood gases or ECG, etc., up to the understanding of the pathophysiology. Compared to this wide culture required for making traditional medicine, the BLUE-protocol can appear as a slight adjunct. Apart from those who like complicated disciplines, a whole rebuilding of medical studies integrating ultrasound would not increase their duration, since huge simplifications of complex fields will occur.

Can the BLUE-Protocol Allow a Distinction Between Hemodynamic (HPE) and Permeability-Induced (PIPE) Pulmonary Edema?

It definitely can solve this daily problem. Here are basic elements.

Roughly, the B-profile is present in 97 % of cases of HPE and only 14 % of cases of PIPE.

Roughly, the four profiles of pneumonia are present in 86 % of cases of PIPE and 3 % of HPE.

Roughly, following the seven principles of lung ultrasound, HPE creates pressurized transudate, i.e., lung rockets with no impairment of lung sliding. PIPE creates nonpressurized exudate, i.e., impaired lung sliding with irregular anterior lung rockets, and random areas of consolidation.

Read more in Chap. 35.

How About Patients with Severe Pulmonary Embolism and No Visible Venous Thrombosis?

See Chaps. 26 and 35.

Why Look for Artifacts Alone When the Original Is Visible?

These authors referred to these lung consolidations [3]. We answered that the "original" was not so original: lung consolidations can be seen in a wide range of diseases, whereas the sequence used in the BLUE-protocol allows to link some with the diagnosis of pneumonia, others with the diagnosis of pulmonary edema, pulmonary embolism, etc. [4].

What About Pulmonary Edema Complicating a Chronic Interstitial Lung Disease (CILD)?

This was argued as a possible limitation [2]. The B-profile indicates usually pulmonary edema, rarely pneumonia, exceptionally CILD. Considering pulmonary edema complicating an exceptional disease means a really exceptional condition. Concluding on these cases would therefore imply years of international multicentric studies. Meanwhile, in a known CILD patient, left ventricle hypocontractility should suggest additional left heart decompensation. Another point, PLAPS are not supposed to be present in simple CILD. Their presence would be an argument for a complication: edema, pneumonia, embolism, or rare causes (tumor). Similarly, a C-profile would indicate a pneumonia, the absence of lung rockets a likely pneumothorax.

What About the Mildly Dyspneic Patients (Simply Managed in the Emergency Room)?

These patients are not in the scope of the BLUE-protocol. Their case is dealt with in Chap. 36.

Challenging (Plethoric) Patients?

See this case in the corresponding section of Chap. 33.

What Happens When the BLUE-Protocol Is Performed on *Non-Blue* Patients?

The BLUE-protocol is designed for severely dyspneic patients.

A healthy subject will have a BLUE-diagnosis of asthma or a COPD.

A postoperative patient with simple basal atelectases has an A-no-V-PLAPS profile, i.e., a BLUE-profile of pneumonia.

An "uncomplicated" ARDS patient (i.e., pink, under pure oxygen) has B-, B'-, A/B-, and C-profiles, sometimes A-no-V-PLAPS profile.

An acute pulmonary edema becoming pink (and eupneic) under appropriate therapy will have, at one precise moment, no anterior lung rockets, only bilateral lateral extensive lung rockets, and usually PLAPS, i.e., a profile of pneumonia. The next step – after healing – will show only PLAPS, i.e., again a profile of pneumonia, until the thorax is completely dry, making a profile of COPD/asthma.

Will the BLUE-Protocol Work Everywhere?

We assume not. In many parts of the world, there will be more pneumonia, such as tuberculosis. There again, time lacks for many deprived people for reaching the age for developing modern chronic diseases (COPD, coronary obstructions, etc.). In areas with no care but low exposure to modern life and pollution, such as Amazonian areas, maybe the rate of infectious diseases is paradoxically lower. Our next edition should clarify these basic points.

One additional but critical aim of the BLUE-protocol is to provide to physicians who have no access to radiographies and basic tests a cost-effective tool of high accuracy.

Will Multicentric Studies Be Launched for Validating the BLUE-Protocol?

We actively work on this, trying to bypass some issues:
Training teams will be the least.
Having an appropriate, intelligent equipment may be another problem.
We attract the attention on studies emerging from the emergency rooms. The BLUE-protocol suffered from a methodological problem; i.e., in spite of an optimized gold standard (university-affiliated medical intensivists' reports), there were overt gaps which resulted in "only" a 90.5 % accuracy. We guess that the conditions for making the correct diagnosis in the ER will not make better. Those studies will have unavoidable methodological issues.
But the main problem will be ethical: how shall we order randomized studies, i.e., not taking profit of the information of the BLUE-protocol (built from published papers, using evidence-based medicine) in the management of asphyxic patients?

What Is the Interest of the PLAPS Concept?

The label PLAPS is first an onomatopoeia which aims at suggesting a splash, what actually is this image of fluid and tissue-like pattern with shred border, instead of the rigid barrier of air artifacts. A frank consolidation with an uncertain image of effusion, an effusion with ill-defined consolidation, or both will have the same meaning: an acoustic window for ultrasound. Finely differentiating alveolar from pleural disorder does not influence our decision tree.

Said differently, the concept of PLAPS makes of four signs one sign, which is "absence of artifactual pattern," decreasing the number of lung signs from ten to seven. This concept allows shorter training for the interested teams.

By the Way, Why "BLUE"-Protocol?

The blue is the dominant tone of these patients.

The blue is the color of the veins, pointing that the venous analysis is on the frontline.

We carefully checked that there was no space for confusion and found that the term "BLUE-protocol" did not refer to any particular known setting. Our wish was to create a term indicating at a glance that the clinician:

- Uses a fast protocol fully adapted to the extreme emergency
- Needs nothing but a very simple unit, without Doppler, switching on in 7 s, and a unique probe
- Analyzes the lung (which was supposed to be immune to ultrasound)
- Uses a few standardized points (the BLUE-points)
- Uses only ten signs at the lung area
- Uses no more than eight profiles for six main diseases
- Gives an adapted vision of the veins, using the same probe
- Uses a contact product without gel allowing fast examination (<3 min)
- Permanently integrates this approach to the clinical context in order to increase its overall 90.5 % efficiency

The acceptance of the BLUE-protocol initiated the creation of the SLAM [5] (*see* Chap. 37 for knowing if "BLUE" is an acronym or not).

References

1. Lichtenstein D, Mezière G, Lagoueyte JF, Biderman P, Goldstein I, Gepner A (2009) A-lines and B-lines: lung ultrasound as a bedside tool for predicting pulmonary artery occlusion pressure in the critically ill. Chest 136:1014–1020
2. Khosla R (2009) Utility of lung sonography in acute respiratory failure. Chest 135:884
3. Mathis G (2010) Why look for artifacts alone when the original is visible? Chest 137:233
4. Lichtenstein D, Mezière G (2010) Response to "why look for artifacts alone when the original is visible?" (Mathis G). Chest 137:233
5. SLAM – Section pour la Limitation des Acronymes en Médecine (2009) Déclaration 1609. 1er avril 2008. Journal Officiel de la République Française, 26 avril 2008 (N° 17):2009

The BLUE-Protocol and the Diagnosis of Pneumonia

Pathophysiological Reminder of the Disease

Pneumonia creates an inflammation of the lung tissue. The edema enlarges the interstitial tissue, the exudate fills the alveoli, the inflammation crosses the visceral pleura, and fluid invades the pleural cavity. Some germs come from the airways, others from blood. The homogeneity of the distribution of the disorders partly depends on this.

The Usual Ways of Diagnosis

Usually, fever is the main first sign. Fever with clinical respiratory signs (cough, dyspnea) evokes the pneumonia. Physical examination basically (apart from subtleties) searches for sounds suggestive of consolidation (rales mainly) and pleural effusion (loss of pleural murmur). It is usual to ask for a chest radiograph, which shows dense areas (and possibly indicates that the physical examination is not a sufficient step). CT is done sometimes for knowing more, but it is done also in countless occurrences when other diagnoses are suspected (helical CT usually). Blood gas shows hypoxia and hypocapnia. CRP and other inflammatory tests are elevated.

The diagnosis of "pneumonia" (not to deal with its origin) raises probably little problem at this step.

When Is the BLUE-Protocol Performed? Which Signs? Which Accuracy?

When the clinical presentation and basic tests are self-speaking, the diagnosis of pneumonia is done. The question of which microbe, although crucial, is not yet evoked at this step. When the physical examination is difficult, the patient has complex comorbidities, complex disorders, and factors decreasing the response to aggression, antibiotics taken earlier and masking some signs, or when the radiograph does not perfectly answer the question, or systematically, ultrasound is performed. Just note as regards pleural effusion that bedside radiographs miss up to 525 ml [1, 2]. One-third of pleural effusions in ventilated patients, which were substantial enough for a safe thoracentesis were radioccult [3].

Pneumonia generates four profiles: the B′-profile (11 % sensitive, 100 % specific), the C-profile (21 % sensitive, 99 % specific), the A/B-profile (14 % sensitive, 100 % specific), and the A-no-V-PLAPS-profile (42 % sensitive, 96 % specific). The overall accuracy is a 89 % sensitivity and a 94 % specificity. As seen, each profile is not frequent (low sensitivity), but the summation of the four profiles makes an acceptable sensitivity. Regarding the rates of 100 %, seen twice, please read Anecdotal Note 1.

For being able to compare the BLUE-protocol with the current literature, just consider that the C-profile includes consolidations of every size.

The C-line is a centimetric consolidation. Smaller, it results in a thickened pleural line (Fig. 17.4). An anterior thickened, irregular pleural line is called a "C-profile" in the BLUE-protocol. Just also consider that the A/B-profile can be understood, not only as a difference between both lungs, but also within one lung, areas with lung rockets, areas with A-lines (sometimes called spared areas in the literature).

Another point to be understood. The BLUE-diagnosis of pneumonia is done when there are interstitial signs (B'-profile, A/B-profile), alveolar signs (C-profile, PLAPS), and pleural signs (PLAPS). A pleural effusion, even small and isolated, in the sequence of the BLUE-protocol, evokes pneumonia, although the diagnoses of pneumothorax, pulmonary edema, and pulmonary embolism can all generate pleural effusions, but they were previously excluded. Searching for internal echoes is not required by the BLUE-protocol since the diagnosis of pneumonia has been done, but it can be done in the Extended BLUE-protocol for deciding the best therapy (Chap. 35).

Value of the BLUE-Protocol for Ruling Out Other Diseases

Usually, pneumonia cannot be confused with pneumothorax, COPD, or asthma.

Acute hemodynamic pulmonary edema is rarely a concern, see notes about this issue in Chap. 22, but mostly in Chap. 35.

Confusions will be raised exceptionally with pulmonary embolism. An enlarged right heart is expected in both cases. A thoracentesis would in both cases find exudate. Using "strictly" the BLUE-protocol, in the case of a pneumonia mimicking an embolism, the patient will be protected of the confusion because the DVT will be missing. An embolism looking like a pneumonia can be seen, in the unlikely event where these conditions will be met together: embolism without DVT (20 %) *and* with anterior small consolidation (5 %), i.e., mathematically speaking, 1 % of cases. The principle of the BLUE-protocol is to be permanently piloted by the clinical notions. If now these clinical notions are included, a misdiagnosis should occur in far less than 1 % (Grotowski's law).

Ultrasound Pathophysiology of Pneumonia

While there is only one pulmonary edema, one pulmonary embolism, one asthma, and one pneumothorax, there are hundreds of microbes responsible for pneumonia. Providentially, they generate only four profiles.

The inflammation creates an alveolar exudation. The alveoli get filled of fluid, from exudate to frank pus. Therefore, lung consolidation is a fluid disorder. The edema of the interstitial tissue creates an interstitial syndrome. This part is either frankly visible at the lung surface when there is no alveolar filling between two edematous subpleural interlobular septa, or mixed with the filled alveoli, resulting in this tissue-like pattern of lung consolidation. When there is lung consolidation, there is often pleural effusion.

The B'-profile: we explain the abolition of lung sliding (*B'-profile*) by inflammatory adherences due to exudate, generating acute pleural symphysis. This disorder was long described [4]. It seems frequent in massive pneumonia and ARDS. Whereas the transudate is a lubricant which does not impair lung sliding, exudate is a biologic glue. We assume that each exudative B-line acts as a *nail*. Since B-lines are numerous, these multiple nails should appear sufficient for sticking the lung to the wall. Some privileged cases (for the science) allowed us to demonstrate inflammatory adherences. An acute pleural symphysis should logically impair lung expansion and generate acute restrictive disorder in ARDS. Note that abolished lung sliding shows low specificity for pneumothorax (27 % positive predictive value here). In patients with pneumonia, 30 % of cases had abolished lung sliding.

The C-profile: it indicates anterior lung consolidations. As opposed to the alveolar syndrome of hemodynamic pulmonary edema which is generated by gravity, the lung consolidation of pneumonia can be found everywhere, including anteriorly, and especially in the case of bronchial dissemination, which does not follow gravity – explaining anterior patterns in supine patients.

Diffuse C-lines are usually found in severe pneumonia with hematogenous extension in our experience.

The A/B-profile: Pneumonia can be found in a wide variety of locations, making asymmetry a major feature: latero-lateral asymmetry (A/B profile) and anteroposterior asymmetry (A/PLAPS profile). Anterior consolidation is again highly specific to infectious phenomena.

The A-no-V-PLAPS-profile: it is explained by posterior infections which do not generate anterior interstitial involvement (hence an A-profile) and of course no venous thrombosis. Here, a lung consolidation, even minute, strongly suggests the diagnosis of pneumonia. Often, a pneumonia able to generate a lung consolidation also generates an exudative pleural effusion (read again the concept of PLAPS). If the consolidation is too small, or not superficial, or an unusual place, the presence of a pleural effusion is a providence, since it will be much less chancy to detect: always or quite, at the PLAPS-point.

How are the profiles dispatched in function of the microbes? We expect in the next decades to succeed to publish three, maybe four, original articles (renouncing to the paternity of hundreds which are still waiting in our archives). The answer to the question "can we infer a microbe in function of a profile" would possibly be part of these few expectations. Meanwhile, for not frustrating the reader, we consider that it is possible to devote limited time for answering this question: each time a pleural effusion allows thoracentesis, this expedites the etiologic diagnosis.

Why Not 100 % Accuracy? The Limitations of the BLUE-Protocol. How Can They Be Reduced?

The C-profile, almost specific, can be seen, exceptionally, in pulmonary embolism. See equivalent section in Chap. 26.

The A-no-V-PLAPS-profile can be seen in some cases of pulmonary embolism.

Some interstitial pneumonias display the B-profile, which can be interpreted maybe as an early step where the lung can still move, before the B′-profile. How to distinguish between hemodynamic pulmonary edema and ARDS is answered in Chap. 22 and mostly in Chap. 35.

For reducing the limitations of the BLUE-protocol, the extended BLUE-protocol invites to several actions, including large policy of diagnostic thoracentesis, and even more; see Chap. 35.

Miscellaneous

The BLUE-protocol has this advantage: a patient with BLUE-profiles of pneumonia will benefit not only from antibiotics but also from prompt intubation, since we expect exudate to remain (noninvasive alternatives, CPAP, are rather for hemodynamic pulmonary edema, since transudate vanishes more easily).

Anecdotal Notes

1. *The 100 % accuracies*

    The B′-profile and the A/B-profile were 100 % specific. This value is unusual in medicine, and we simply precise that these profiles are infrequent. The limited number of our patients explains this accuracy. Studies including thousands of B′-profile will find results <100 %. Just because no gold standard is 100 % solid, this is expected. Again, although usually simple, medicine can sometimes be very complicated. The "art" of the doctor is to detect, among all visited patients, the one who comes with a rarity.

References

1. Müller NL (1993) Imaging the pleura. State of the art. Radiology 186:297–309
2. Collins JD, Burwell D, Furmanski S, Lorber P, Steckel RJ (1972) Minimal detectable pleural effusions. Radiology 105:51–53
3. Lichtenstein D, Hulot JS, Rabiller A, Tostivint T, Mezière G (1999) Feasibility and safety of ultrasound-aided thoracentesis in mechanically ventilated patients. Intensive Care Med 25:955–958
4. Laënnec RTH (1819) Traité de l'auscultation médiate, ou traité du diagnostic des maladies des poumons et du cœur. J.A. Brosson & J.S. Chaudé, Paris. Hafner, New York. 1962, pp 455–456

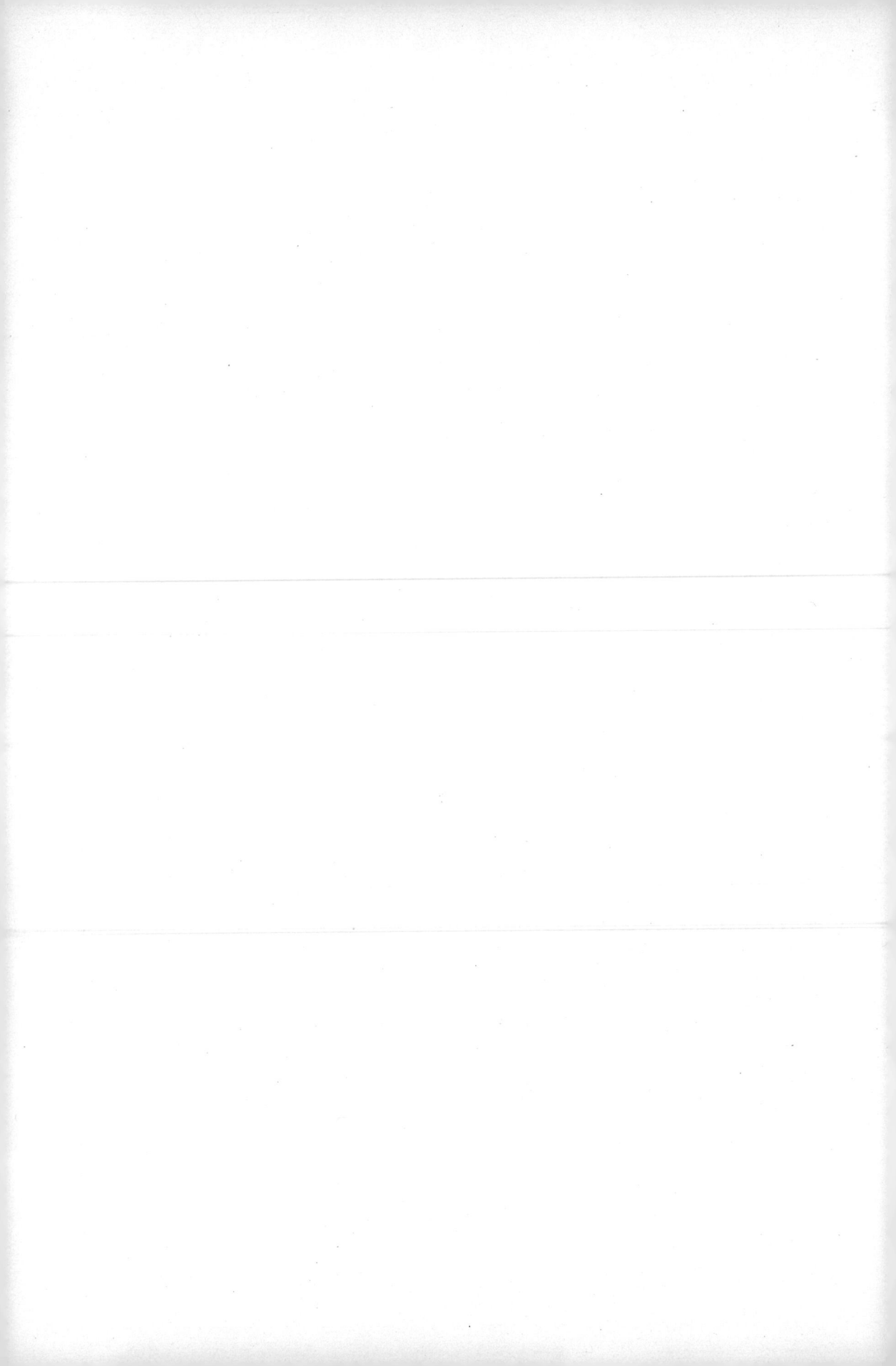

BLUE-Protocol and Acute Hemodynamic Pulmonary Edema

Pathophysiological Reminder of the Disease

Acute hemodynamic pulmonary edema, referred to as AHPE, is usually a disease of the left heart (here called acute cardiogenic pulmonary edema) and sometimes the consequence of a fluid overload, hence the general term AHPE.

The Usual Ways of Diagnosis

The dyspnea usually begins with a feeling of tightness of the thorax, which seems heavy. The dyspnea is relieved by sitting. A history of cardiac disease is often present. Auscultation shows the main sign, rales. Bedside radiograph typically shows bilateral, symmetric signs of congestion. Blood gases show hypoxia and hypocapnia. BNP is elevated in cardiac causes.

The signs of the underlying cause are numerous (clinical, ECG, biological, etc.).

Each of these signs can be absent and difficult to assess (e.g., rales in bariatric patients). Radiography provides its dose of radiation, is not always present through the world, and can be difficult to read in challenging or any patients, up to a normal initial pattern. Arterial blood gases are painful procedures and provide rather limited information.

So Why Ultrasound?

Imaging tests would not be so useful if the clinical examination answered perfectly the question. Rales can be absent at an early stage [1] or replaced by wheezing, yielding the cardiac asthma. Fine auscultation is illusory in ventilated patients or in point-of-care medicine, airplane, crowded ER, etc.

As regards imaging, we simplify our last edition, gathering in the same paragraph all situations where the radiographic diagnosis is tricky (subnormal radiograph, because it is made too early, but also in genuine severe cases of pulmonary edema [2, 3]), difficult (ill-defined), not immediately available (extreme emergency), or not available at all (extra-hospital settings mainly, poor countries). We assume that the radiologic signs speak only in advanced stages. A radiograph taken in optimal conditions can be difficult to interpret [4]. Taken in an emergency, at the bedside it cannot be but worse. Signs like vascular redistribution do not work in supine patients. X-ray sensitivity in detecting interstitial edema can range between 45 and 18 % [5, 6]. Kerley B-lines can be observed in exacerbation of COPD [7].

When Is the BLUE-Protocol Applied? Which Signs? Which Accuracy?

AHPE provides the B-profile, which theoretically concludes the BLUE-protocol, with a 97 % sensitivity and a 95 % specificity.

PLAPS are seen in 88 % of cases. Echocardiography can show simple signs (global left ventricle hypocontractility) or more subtle signs, requiring Doppler. Please consult reference textbooks for this, since the aim of the BLUE-protocol is to provide a diagnosis, which is pulmonary edema. Where does it come from is another (basic) question. The inferior caval vein is not seen in all cases, far from this. When it is seen, a dilatation is far from the rule (we currently see again all our cases).

Lung ultrasound for diagnosing interstitial syndrome is increasingly used, we quote only a very few from the first works [8–11].

Value of the BLUE-Protocol for Ruling Out Other Diseases

The B-profile rules out pneumothorax, simple COPD (even severe), and simple asthma (even severe).

The B-profile makes the diagnosis of pulmonary embolism unlikely. Apart from ICU-acquired embolism, the B-profile was not seen in patients with embolism in the BLUE-protocol and makes 2 % of patients in a larger series (under submission). These cases of pulmonary embolism with diffuse interstitial syndrome may be explained by severe right ventricle dilatation and paradoxical septum (generating elevated left pressures), which means that a simple emergency cardiac sonography would immediately (in patients with a cardiac window) correct the diagnosis (an enlarged right ventricle with a small left ventricle and a septal shift). This cardiac sonography, part of the Extended BLUE-protocol, is done always, after the BLUE-protocol. Note that we are surprised not to see more B-profiles in our series of severe pulmonary embolism, which may mean that our explanation (septal interference generating elevation of PAOP) is not the best one.

Pneumonia is a main differential diagnosis, since some show the B-profile. The physician is warned by some clinical elements (fever, mainly). We devoted the answer in Chap. 22 for a small part and the larger part in Chap. 35. Here, the physician is invited to extend the BLUE-protocol to part or whole of these targets: shifting the B-profile to a C-profile, searching for non-decreased left heart function, measuring volume of PLAPS, puncturing a pleural effusion (read the section on thoracentesis in Chap. 35), etc.

Patients without the B-profile and considered as severe pulmonary edema (3 % in our series) should also raise the question of a possible error from the managing team.

Diseases outside the BLUE-protocol: chronic interstitial diseases make the main group. They are part of the 3 % of patients excluded for rarity and account for one-third of them, i.e., 1 % of the patients, seen in the conditions of the BLUE-protocol 24 times less often than hemodynamic pulmonary edema (read Chap. 35).

Ultrasound Pathophysiology of Acute Hemodynamic Pulmonary Edema (AHPE)

Lung Rockets

AHPE creates a pressurized transudate. It invades all interlobular septa up to the anterior wall, against gravity. The edema of the interlobular septa is a constant feature [12, 13]. Similarly, lung rockets are consistently present, usually disseminated, making an immediate diagnosis wherever the probe is applied at the anterolateral chest wall. Like hair when you have the gooseflesh and like soldiers standing at attention, all interlobular septa of a wide given area (lateral, anterior) are involved the same. We don't see any scientific reason (apart from possible focal emphysema bullae) for observing one septum thickened by edema and not its immediate neighbor. This explains the symmetric, diffuse interstitial patterns. This is the first level of dichotomy of LUCI in AHPE.

There is a second level of dichotomy in the B-profile. First the lung surface generates A *or* B-lines, with no space to our knowledge for intermediate artifacts. This demonstrates that the transformation from A-lines to B-lines follows an all-or-nothing rule, when a critical amount of fluid has enlarged the interlobular septum. This subpleural septal enlargement is a representative sample of the deeper interstitial compartment (not accessible to ultrasound), as all CT observations show [14].

We must distinguish anterior, lateral from posterior ultrasound interstitial syndrome. Anterior lung rockets correspond to anterior Kerley lines, which are almost never visible on a front radiograph but are the most clinically relevant. Lateral interstitial syndrome was not considered in our algorithm for reason of redundancy (see Chap. 35). Posterior interstitial syndrome was not sought for, since gravitational interstitial changes can be physiological [15].

Lung Sliding

Transudate is a lubricant. We have minimal amounts of physiological transudate around the lungs, allowing to breathe from birth to death without burning. In AHPE, the transudate allows the lung to slide over the chest wall, explaining the conserved lung sliding (see below).

PLAPS

PLAPS were usual. Their search was not required since it did not change our decision tree. On the other hand, anterior areas of consolidations were not observed in hemodynamic pulmonary edema. This finding should mean complete alveolar filling from the posterior to the anterior areas according to the principle N°2 (Earth-Sky axis), a disorder not compatible with life in our hypothesis (Fig. 24.1).

We detail the distinction between hydrostatic and permeability-induced pulmonary edema in devoted chapters (Chaps. 22 and 35) in order to avoid repetitions (see below).

Chronological Considerations

The B-profile is assumed to be an early change. In a familial dinner, a grandpa is about to be victim of

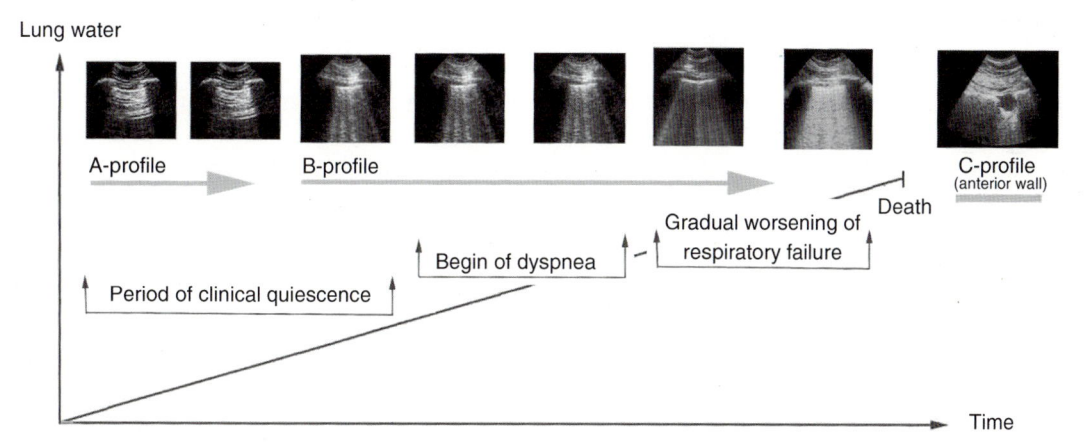

Fig. 24.1 Ultrasound dynamic of pulmonary edema. This figure shows the relative independency between clinical status and ultrasound changes. With worsening of the disease, the lung ultrasound artifacts make sudden changes whereas the clinical worsening makes regular changes. In this figure, the first clinical signs appear once a B-profile is present. In other words, ultrasound allows to anticipate the clinical signs of edema. Mostly, this figure shows that patients with the same ultrasound profile (the B-profile) can have a wide range of clinical presentations, from quiescence to acute respiratory failure. This diagram also highlights the hypothesis that the C-profile is unlikely in hemodynamic pulmonary edema and should occur only at a very late stage (if occurring)

a hemodynamic pulmonary edema. We assume he has a normal lung surface. The dinner is delightful; dietetic advices have been forgotten for a while. Then he quietly digests his seafood on the armchair, watching TV. The excess salt is extracted from the GI tract and little by little penetrates the circulating compartment, increasing its volume. When the heart function reaches the inflexion point of the Frank-Starling curve, the end-diastolic left ventricle pressure increases, increasing on return the capillary pressure. The transudate quietly invades the interstitial compartment. The physiopathology of pulmonary edema indicates that the interstitial edema is an early phenomenon, which precedes alveolar edema [12, 13]. Inside this early, interstitial phenomenon, the portion initially drowned is the interlobular septum [15]. This segment is not involved in the gas exchanges, which occur at the alveolocapillary membrane. The interlobular septa are called "puisards," the French term [15]. Since the fluids are under pressure, the interlobular septa are massively filled, including their subpleural part, including the anterior, nondependent ones – a feature which will explain the B-profile. Our patient is still watching his favorite TV series. Possibly, his anterior lung surface is already invaded by "silent" lung rockets. At one moment, the whole interstitial compartment is saturated, and the lymphatic resorption is insufficient. The transudate now invades the alveolar space. We assume this is the moment where the papy feels the first discomfort. His wife calls the doctor in an emergency. When the doctor visits the patient, still mildly dyspneic initially, we assume that the B-profile is present. We also assume that later stages, on blue patients, will always have the B-profile (Fig. 24.1).

So to speak, the anterior interstitial compartment initiates a race with the posterior alveolar compartment, according to the Earth-Sky axis. The question is: does the excess fluid first reach the anterior interstitial tissue (subpleural septa), or does it begin to pour into the posterior alveoli before the anterior septa are saturated? In the first hypothesis (our hypothesis), lung ultrasound will detect pulmonary edema before the clinical, alveolar stage. The second hypothesis could explain mild cases of clinical edema without B-profile (see below). Figure 24.1 shows that the clinical course evolves gradually, whereas the ultrasound profiles change suddenly – pointing out that possibly patients with the B-profile may have no clinical sign of pulmonary edema. Look at Fig. 11.2. In a standard thorax, the postero-anterior column is roughly 18 cm. An 18-mmHg PAOP is equivalent to a 24 cmH$_2$O high column of pressure, decreased by some impedance gradient. Again, the zero hydrostatic reference is not at the posterior wall but at the heart level. In other words, an 18-mmHg capillary pressure (threshold for interstitial and not yet alveolar edema) would easily create anterior septal thickening, against gravity. One should imagine a 24-cm high geyser (pressurized by definition).

Why Not 100 % Accuracy? The Limitations of the BLUE-Protocol

The sensitivity is only 97 %. Can one imagine cases of genuine AHPE without diffuse interstitial syndrome? Some works describe the absence of B-profile in hemodynamic pulmonary edema [16]. To answer to some concerns of this kind, it must be clearly stated that, first, the diagnosis of edema is the good one. The methodology of the BLUE-protocol aimed at optimizing this critical point (see this section in Chap. 20). We assume that in the emergency room, the conditions for diagnosis (of mild cases by definition) will be *less* optimal. We also assume that the patient is seen at the climax of the respiratory failure, like all patients in the BLUE-protocol, not after the start of relief: lung rockets disappear rapidly after appropriate therapy. We assume that the very mild cases and even the preclinical presentations display already diffuse lung rockets (see above). Yet for scientifically answering the issue, and remaining ethical (and *not* bothering animals), we should visit at home, by surprise, countless grandpas and grandmas, "hoping" to see among them one case in the preclinical stage of hemodynamic pulmonary edema. Some patients we were able to scan at preclinical stages of pulmonary edema showed in actual fact the B-profile.

This being said, the only situations without B-profile we can imagine are patients with giant anterior bullae (rarefying the parenchyma).

The specificity is only 95 %. This means that some cases of pneumonia appear with a genuine B-profile (not B′, not C, not A/B, not A-no-V-PLAPS), meaning pure interstitial syndrome and preserved lung compliance. The BLUE-protocol is designed for dyspneic, not shocked, patients. In real life, patients can combine respiratory and circulatory suffering at various degrees, yet this limitation is reduced when there is a pure respiratory failure. If a shock is associated to the dyspnea, the left heart contractility can be either normal or impaired. A normal contractility should favor the diagnosis of lung sepsis (associated with history, clinical signs etc.).

A Small Story of the BLUE-Diagnosis of Hemodynamic Pulmonary Edema in the BLUE-Protocol

At the time we designed the BLUE-protocol, the pericardium then the right ventricle were withdrawn (see Chap. 20). The next step regarded the left heart analysis, which only remained in our decision tree [17]. This was definitely the most delicate step. Aware of this challenge we had to face (read if having time the small history of the BLUE-protocol in Chap. 20), but wanting to combine simplicity and efficiency, we carefully analyzed all files. In 2.64 % of cases, the left ventricle analysis proved contributive, showing correct contractility with the B-profile and a final diagnosis of pneumonia. In 2.98 % of cases, the left ventricle analysis provided misleading information, i.e., impaired contractility in patients whose final diagnosis was not pulmonary edema – none of them having a B-profile. More information was gained in terms of "pulmonary edema versus non-pulmonary edema" than lost in terms of challenge in "hemodynamic versus permeability-induced pulmonary edema." Withdrawing the left heart was not only possible, simplifying our decision tree, but also slightly *improving* the accuracy of the BLUE-protocol (90.3 % if including the left heart, 90.5 % if not considering it at all). Detailed results are featured in the online data from *Chest* 134:117–125 [18]. This demonstration is central to the concept of the BLUE-protocol: when a direct lung analysis shows absence of pulmonary edema, the need for a sophisticated heart examination should not generate exaggerated energy at the time of admission.

With population aging, hypocontractile left ventricle is seen with increasing frequency, but is not always the cause of the dyspnea. In patients without B-profile, left heart anomaly is not expected unless there is a previous chronic disease that ironically does not participate to the acute failure. In other words, detecting a non-B-profile immediately informs on the *systolic left ventricular function*, the *diastolic ventricular function*, as well as the *mitral and aortic valve function*. None of them is impaired. Even if impaired, the cause of the respiratory distress should be somewhere else.

References

1. Braunwald E (1984) Heart disease. W.B. Saunders Company, Philadelphia, p 173
2. Stapczynski JS (1992) Congestive heart failure and pulmonary edema. In: Tintinalli JE, Krome RL, Ruiz E (eds) Emergency medicine: a comprehensive study guide. Mc Graw-Hill, New York, pp 216–219
3. Bedock B, Fraisse F, Marcon JL, Jay S, Blanc PL (1995) Œdème aigu du poumon cardiogénique aux urgences : analyse critique des éléments diagnostiques et d'orientation. Actualités en réanimation et urgences. Arnette, Paris, pp 419–448
4. Fraser RG, Paré JA (1988) Diagnoses of disease of the chest, 3rd edn. WB Saunders Company, Philadelphia, p 296
5. Badgett RG, Mulrow CD, Otto PM, Ramirez G (1996) How well can the chest radiograph diagnose left ventricular dysfunction? J Gen Intern Med 11:625–634
6. Rigler LG (1950) Rœntgen examination of the chest: its limitation in the diagnosis of disease. JAMA 142:773
7. Costanso WE, Fein SA (1988) The role of the chest X-ray in the evaluation of chronic severe heart failure: things are not always as they appear. Clin Cardiol 11: 486–488
8. Reissig A, Kroegel C (2003) Transthoracic sonography of diffuse parenchymal lung disease: the role of comet tail artifacts. J Ultrasound Med 22:173–180
9. Jambrik Z, Monti S, Coppola V, Agricola E, Mottola G, Miniati M, Picano E (2004) Usefulness of ultrasound lung comets as a nonradiologic sign of extravascular lung water. Am J Cardiol 93(10):1265–1270

10. Volpicelli G, Mussa A, Garofalo G, Cardinale L, Casoli G, Perotto F, Fava C, Frascisco M (2006) Bedside lung ultrasound in the assessment of alveolar-interstitial syndrome. Am J Emerg Med 24:689–696
11. Fagenholz PJ, Gutman JA, Murray AF, Noble VE, Thomas SH, Harris NS (2007) Chest ultrasonography for the diagnosis and monitoring of high-altitude pulmonary edema. Chest 131:1013–1018
12. Staub NC (1974) Pulmonary edema. Physiol Rev 54:678–811
13. Safran D, Journois D (1995) Circulation pulmonaire. In: Samii K (ed) Anesthésie Réanimation Chirurgicale, 2nd edn. Flammarion, Paris, pp 31–38
14. Lichtenstein D, Mezière G, Biderman P, Gepner A, Barré O (1997) The comet-tail artifact, an ultrasound sign of alveolar-interstitial syndrome. Am J Respir Crit Care Med 156:1640–1646
15. Rémy-Jardin M, Rémy J (1995) Œdème interstitiel. In: Rémy-Jardin M, Rémy J (eds) Imagerie nouvelle de la pathologie thoracique quotidienne. Springer, Paris, pp 137–143
16. Volpicelli G, Cardinale L, Mussa A, Caramello V (2009) Diagnosis of cardiogenic pulmonary edema by sonography limited to the anterior lung. Chest 135:883
17. Lichtenstein D (2005) Analytic study of frequent and/or severe situations. In: General ultrasound in the critically ill. Springer, Berlin, pp 177–183
18. Lichtenstein D, Mezière G (2008) Relevance of lung ultrasound in the diagnosis of acute respiratory failure. The BLUE-protocol. Chest 134:117–125

BLUE-Protocol and Bronchial Diseases: Acute Exacerbation of COPD (AECOPD) and Severe Asthma

Pathophysiological Reminder of the Disease

These two diseases were put together for the sake of simplicity, since both are bronchial diseases where the respiratory hindrance comes from acute or chronic obstruction of the lumen, due to inflammatory, mechanical, or muscular actions.

The Usual Ways of Diagnosis

The dyspnea is classically more expiratory than inspiratory. Auscultation shows a major sign, *wheezing*. A stethoscope is usually required. Radiography shows distended lungs. Blood gases show classically hypocapnia in severe asthma and hypercapnia in EACOPD.

How Does the BLUE-Protocol Proceed? Which Signs? Which Accuracy?

The BLUE-protocol provides a basic piece of information: the patients have usually the A-profile (89 %). The A-profile calls for a venous investigation, which will be, by definition, negative. A DVT found in such patients would clearly indicate that the bronchial crisis, even if genuine, has maybe been generated by a genuine pulmonary embolism. When the venous network is free, the examiner comes back to the lungs, at the PLAPS-point. These locations will be, by definition, negative (if positive, the bronchial crisis is due to an external factor, likely a pneumonia). The whole profile (A-profile, no DVT, no PLAPS) is called the nude profile.

Asthma and COPD were analyzed separately. For asthma, the nude profile (A-profile, no DVT, no PLAPS) was seen in 94 % of cases. For COPD, the same nude profile was seen in 77.5 % of cases, PLAPS were present in 10 %, the B-profile in 6 %, and the C-profile in 2 %. We saw in Chap. 20 that such rates are maybe due to frequent diagnostic issues in COPD.

Value of the BLUE-Protocol for Ruling Out Other Diseases

Pneumothorax is definitely ruled out.

Pulmonary edema is ruled out, especially if an extension shows absence of lateral and all the more posterior lung rockets.

A pneumonia able to generate acute respiratory failure with no visible alveolar or interstitial patterns should be a rare event (at this time, we have no such observation).

Pulmonary embolism. In roughly 20 % of cases of proven embolism, no DVT is found. In roughly half of the cases, PLAPS are not found. The theoretical percentage of massive cases of pulmonary embolism generating a nude profile is therefore roughly 10 %. A "nude" pulmonary embolism should therefore occur every *40 cases* of COPD/asthma. In these cases, the physician, who *pilots* the BLUE-protocol, and can extend it at will (the Extended BLUE-protocol) will recognize suggestive clinical signs: a complete absence of history of COPD or asthma, a history favoring embolism (contraceptive pill, e.g.), chest pain, hemoptysis, ECG troubles, positive D-dimers, etc. The physician will then suspect a pulmonary embolism. This is for the rare patients who have a pulmonary embolism with the nude profile and a clinical suspicion that the BLUE-protocol opens to more (scintigraphy, rather than the more irradiating CT, and once pregnancy is absent).

In the Extended BLUE-protocol, one tool, not new (1819), not sophisticated, has a critical importance: our beloved stethoscope, which has here, at this step of the BLUE-protocol, a clear relevance. It was designed for hearing sounds such as wheezing [1]. The bronchi are the only structures (with vessels) not visible using ultrasound (when they are surrounded only by gas), making the stethoscope a first-line tool today, a major element for distinguishing bronchial diseases, i.e., asthma, from pulmonary embolism (distinction made by Gilbert Mezière).

Ultrasound Pathophysiology of AECOPD or Asthma

The bronchi (surrounded by air) are inaccessible to current noninvasive ultrasound. The main sign is indirect: absence of lung rockets in a dyspneic patient – present lung sliding. Another structure is not accessible: the pulmonary artery, this is why the search for venous thrombosis should be done and should be negative. Similarly, a severe but simple COPD or asthma exacerbation would have no reason to develop a PLAPS.

Why Not 100 % Accuracy? The Limitations of the BLUE-Protocol

The BLUE-protocol described wrong diagnoses: Ten percent of patients labelled "decompensated COPDs" in our study had lung consolidations. Six percent of patients were considered as COPD in spite of having a B-profile. These are wrong diagnoses of the BLUE-protocol when accepting the final diagnoses. Yet during this study and much more with time, we wonder how and why COPD or asthma in crisis, simple (even severe), would generate PLAPS or interstitial syndrome.

Miscellaneous

Technical note: in very severe asthma, lung sliding can be very weak. Using a simple technology, lung sliding or its equivalents (sometimes pseudo-A′-profiles) are easily seen.

Other signs can be seen: the distension is likely when more than two down extensions of the PLAPS-point are necessary for having the abdomen on the screen. The distension can show other signs: enlarged intercostal spaces, flat or even reversed diaphragmatic cupola.

Reference

1. Laënnec RTH (1819) Traité de l'auscultation médiate, ou traité du diagnostic des maladies des poumons et du cœur. J.A. Brosson & J.S. Chaudé, Paris; Hafner, New York, 1962

BLUE-Protocol and Pulmonary Embolism

Pulmonary embolism has a special place in most minds, probably because of the risk of sudden death if the diagnosis is not immediate. Atypical cases, generating delays in the therapy, are the most dangerous. Any help should be studied with interest, especially if noninvasive.

This disease was the guest star of our previous edition, featuring in six chapters (DVT, pleural effusion, alveolar syndrome, interstitial syndrome, echocardiography, all acute situations). It benefits here from a synthesis.

The BLUE-protocol aims at expediting the diagnosis. We no longer ask whether ultrasound examination should be ordered or not. We just do it routine. It allows most of the time to avoid transportation of unstable patients to the CT room. Or worse, to initiate blind heparin therapy or blind thrombolysis in this shocked patient without major proof. Finding here evidence of embolism, or there differential diagnoses (pneumonia, pulmonary edema, abdominal disorders with thoracic pain, etc.), our simple approach should find interest to the intensivist.

Pathophysiological Reminder of the Disease

For various reasons, a thrombosis is formed in the venous network. This thrombosis extends, is dislodged, and creates an embolism when the cross section of the vessel prevents further migration. Very large clots are stopped at main branches of the pulmonary arteries, creating massive circulatory disorders. Transversal roads avoid distal ischemia. If very small clots migrate up to the deep areas of the lung, hemodynamic disorders are minimal (unless the clots are very small but numerous), but the distal circulation is altered, resulting in local areas of infarction, hemorrhage, etc. Lung vessel occlusion is not supposed to be accessible using transthoracic ultrasound. Pulmonary embolism does not yield interstitial change.

The Usual Ways of Diagnosis

Obvious cases raise minor issues, when, e.g., a patient with risk factors (contraceptive pill, e.g.) has chest pain, dyspnea, painful leg, etc. In other instances, the diagnosis is more subtle. Sometimes, pulmonary embolism generates an acute circulatory failure, sometimes mimicking septic shock. Cardiac arrest is another familiar presentation.

We don't know any direct and specific clinical sign of embolism. The radiograph is traditionally and schematically normal, of importance for the logic of the BLUE-protocol. Subtle signs are in actual fact often present (plane atelectasis, elevated cupola, among others). The ECG can show the signs of the series of Stein [1]. Blood gases show hypoxia and hypocapnia. D-dimers are positive. The pulmonary artery angiography has long been replaced by the angio-CT, which shows the

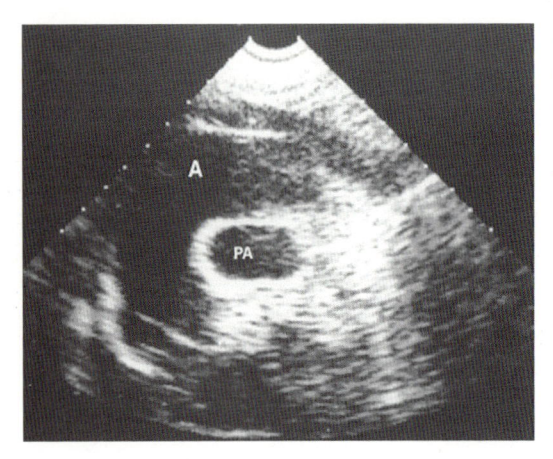

Fig. 26.1 The right pulmonary artery. This artery (*PA*) is seen through its short axis, surrounded by the aortic arch (*A*). Suprasternal scan (only short footprints, and inconstantly, can achieve this route). Floating tissular patterns can here directly demonstrate acute pulmonary embolism in an extreme emergency. The conjunction of a chancy window and a rare pattern using external route makes a rather rare sign – which should deserve however to be routinely sought for

clots within the branches of the pulmonary arteries. Traditional echocardiography shows signs of acute right failure. Transesophageal echocardiography can rarely show the embolus within a branch of the pulmonary artery [2]. This is a direct sign. In exceptional, privileged cases, simple ultrasound with the microconvex probe can expose the main pulmonary arteries and demonstrate the clot (Fig. 26.1). The most direct way should probably be endovascular ultrasound [3] that could possibly be done at the bedside (read Anecdotal Note 1).

For this daily concern, many issues are raised. The clinical data have notorious insufficiencies [4, 5], an issue when the risk of death from undiagnosed cases is 40% [1, 6]. The usual diagnostic tools were, and still are, risky [6]. Their accuracy can be debated [7]. D-dimers raise increasing reluctance. Helical CT, the gold standard, is not perfect [8]. It misses very distal clots, a real issue if they are numerous (and generate circulatory troubles). Giving inappropriate therapy has an 11% risk of major bleeding and a lethal risk between 0.7% and 1.8% [9–11]. The abundance of current protocols indicates the importance of the issues generated by this disease in the physicians' minds.

When to Proceed to the BLUE-Protocol? Which Signs? Which Accuracy?

In the BLUE-protocol, the diagnosis of pulmonary embolism is prioritized (compared to COPD, asthma, posterior pneumonia), because these critically ill patients are at high risk of suddenly worsening.

The A-Profile

Massive pulmonary embolism typically generates an A-profile, found in 95% of cases with acute respiratory failure. Sensitivity is 95 % [12].

Venous Thrombosis

It was found in 81 % of cases in the BLUE-protocol (i.e., an 81 % sensitivity [12]). This number stabilizes around 78 % with large number of cases (under submission). These data were acquired using a specific tool and a specific method.

The location of the DVT is usually correlated with the severity of embolism. We never saw caval thrombosis at the time of diagnosis. In data under submission, common femoral location is present in 1/4 of cases, low femoral location in 1/2 of cases, and calf location in 2/3 of cases. The more severe the embolism, the more distal the remaining thrombosis.

The A-Profile and Deep Venous Thrombosis

The association of A-profile plus DVT has a 99 % specificity [12].

Lung Consolidations

Posterolateral locations are found in half of the cases (52 % precisely), often located against the diaphragm, usually of small volume, often associated with small pleural effusions [12]. Note that a posterolateral analysis is not required in the BLUE-protocol once an A-profile and a DVT have been found, since the diagnosis is done, with or without PLAPS. Anterior locations of lung consolidation were 5 % [12].

Echocardiographic Signs

We remind that they are not included in the BLUE-protocol. They were long standardized [2]. The dilatation of the right ventricle is of major relevance in acute circulatory failure (the relevance is more moderate in acute respiratory distress, where several causes can create it). The BLUE-protocol has demonstrated that a patient with acute respiratory failure and an A-profile (the usual presentation of pulmonary embolism) has no left heart failure – since there is no sign of pulmonary edema. This patient has usually the right heart failure common to embolism, pneumonia, COPD, etc. The place of echocardiography can therefore be simplified.

Value of the BLUE-Protocol for Ruling Out Other Diseases

The A-profile, i.e., the normal signal, rules out pneumothorax and pulmonary edema [13–16].

The DVT, when found, is more than a strong argument for pulmonary embolism. However, in the BLUE-protocol, it is advised to begin by the lung (showing an A-profile); this association provides a 99% specificity. If no attention is paid to the lung, the specificity losses *five points*: the positive predictive value of deep venous thrombosis alone was 89 %, but 94 % if associated with the A-profile [12].

The A-profile has a low specificity (50 %): it is seen in quite all cases of COPD, asthma, and posterior pneumonia with no anterior interstitial extension. In all these diseases, there is no reason for finding a DVT. If a DVT has been found in patients with known COPD or asthma, this DVT is likely the cause of the acute exacerbation. The A-profile is seen in all healthy subjects.

Ultrasound Pathophysiology of Pulmonary Embolism

The physiopathology of pulmonary embolism explains the A-profile. There is no factor able to abolish lung sliding. Interstitial signs are not expected. Anterolateral lung rockets are uncommon. The normality of the ultrasound lung examination is the equivalent of the normal chest X-Ray. The PLAPS may be explained by the hemorrhages, infarctions, and atelectatic areas.

Why Not 100 % Accuracy? The Limitations of the BLUE-Protocol

How About Patients With Severe Pulmonary Embolism and No Visible Venous Thrombosis?

The main limitation comes from these 19 % of patients who had no, or no longer, visible DVT. How to manage such cases?

The clue is simple: common sense (a synonym of "Extended BLUE-protocol"). We remind that the BLUE-protocol is only a protocol, and the physician, who has already a diagnosis in mind, must permanently "pilot" this BLUE-protocol. When the clinical setting points on a possible embolism, explorations should go further. A young lady who has no history of asthma, has a recent orthopedic surgery, complains from sudden chest pain and acute respiratory failure, and displays an A-profile, with positive D-dimers and pathologic ECG is a perfect suspect. As a rule, a patient with the nude profile (A-profile, no DVT, no PLAPS, in other words, normal lungs, normal veins) is diagnosed "COPD or asthma" *by the BLUE-protocol*. If the history does not point out such diseases, although we can face a first crisis, pulmonary embolism must be envisaged *by the physician*.

How About Patients with Lung Rockets Instead of the A-Profile?

The B-profile was not seen in the patients of the BLUE-protocol. Its frequency in larger groups stabilizes around 2 % (and the A/B profile in 2 %, study on submission). In these rare cases of lung rockets, they were septal rockets. We still wait our first case of massive pulmonary embolism (not complicating a chronic interstitial syndrome, not complicating an ARDS) with a bilateral ground-glass rocket pattern. In other words, the ground-glass-profile (i.e., bilateral ground-glass rockets) has up to now a 100 % negative predictive value for pulmonary embolism. There is no reason to see a B'-profile. An A'-profile will be seen in all patients with chronic abolition of lung sliding (history of pleural diseases), and there cannot be any lung point there.

Lung Consolidations: Why They Are Not Considered in the BLUE-Protocol

The BLUE-protocol was profiled for proposing a schematic and simple tool. Consolidations are fully considered in the Extended BLUE-protocol (see Chap. 35).

Anterior Consolidations

The C-profile was seen in 5 % of cases in the BLUE-protocol, and 4% in a larger series (under submission). These consolidations are small and centimetric, i.e., these are all C-lines.

C-lines seen in the BLUE-protocol make the C-profile. The C-profile indicated pneumonia in 95% of cases versus embolism in 5 % [12]. This means that severe lung infection was 18 times more likely than pulmonary embolism. In a previous series of 33 cases of patients admitted to our ICU for severe pulmonary embolism, none had anterior small consolidations [17]. Reminder, the A-profile is the rule in massive pulmonary embolism: 95 % in the BLUE-protocol [12].

Reissig and Mathis consider subpleural (read Anecdotal Note 2) alveolar consolidations a major sign of pulmonary embolism [18, 19]. These authors admit that anterior locations are rare: 6 %, i.e., not far from our data [20]. Our rate, slightly lower, may reflect the fact that our patients are severe. The patients in Mathis and Reissig's study are maybe nonsevere (their severity is not specified) and possibly have more consolidations. Pulmonary infarctions are correlated with mild pulmonary embolism: the smaller the embolism, the more distal the disorder (ischemia occurs on distal more than proximal occlusions). In patients with massive pulmonary embolism, C-lines have no time to develop. If they are present at the time of diagnosis, this possibly simply means previous neglected small episodes (read Anecdotal Note 3).

The rarity of the anterior locations explains for half why lung consolidations are not considered in the BLUE-protocol.

Posterior Consolidations

The poor specificity of posterolateral consolidations, roughly 42 %, explains for the other half why lung consolidations are not considered for the diagnosis of embolism in the BLUE-protocol. They are seen in hemodynamic pulmonary edema, pneumonia, pulmonary embolism, and even pneumothorax. We see PLAPS in half of the cases of severe pulmonary embolism and think, since infarctions have no time to develop yet (in theory), that they are mostly due to small atelectasis, secondary to alteration in surfactant and reflex bronchospasm.

Read in the Chap. 35 all clues demonstrating the infectious nature of a lung consolidation.

To summarize, in pulmonary embolism, the BLUE-protocol does not see a lot of anterior consolidations and does not pay major attention to posterior locations. Not sensitive anteriorly, not specific posteriorly, for the sake of simplicity, this item is not required in the diagnosis. Our choice originated however nice exchanges of correspondence [21, 22].

Miscellaneous

The case of the critically ill patient with previous major lung disorders, ARDS usually, is dealt with in the CLOT-protocol (Chap. 28).

The case of nonsevere pulmonary embolism is dealt with in Chap. 36, with interesting perspectives.

How can the BLUE-protocol decrease the rate of medical radiation doses in these diseases (and mostly their suspicion) is dealt with in Chap. 29 on this elegant and realistic potential.

Venography, angio-CT, Doppler, ARM, etc., which is the gold standard for diagnosing DVT? Today, this debate is obsolete. Personal comments can be read in our previous 2010 Edition. Interesting comments on venography were written in our 1992 Edition, when this test was routine. We give a digest in the Anecdotal Note 4.

Anecdotal Notes

1. *Endovenous ultrasound*

   Note that pulmonary embolism is rare (8 % of patients in the BLUE-protocol). Pulmonary embolism without venous thrombosis is five times rarer. We wonder whether such an approach couldn't be developed by ambulatory teams, similarly for bedside caval filter insertion (see in the 2010 Edition, Figure 26.4), showing a filter within the inferior caval vein filter.

2. *Subpleural consolidations*

   It is not useful to qualify these consolidations of "subpleural": if they are seen with ultrasound, they are subpleural. This is the condition for their ultrasound diagnosis.

3. *Small infarctions*

   But visit again the patient, he or she will always tell you about previous episodes of chest pain, which were neglected, not scary enough for calling a doctor.

4. *Venography, CT, MRI*

   Venous ultrasound, a validated field, replaces gradually venography [23]. Venography gives the illusion of an objective document, yet it violates the rules of radiography, by giving only one view instead of two perpendicular views (like bedside chest radiograph by the way). Venography is unable to see the whole venous network (e.g., deep femoral, gastrocnemian veins, etc.). It is operator dependent, with up to 35 % of divergent cases [24], which is scary when one knows that 20–30 % of tests are classified normal in pulmonary embolism [25, 26]. The transportation of critically ill patients, pelvic irradiation, iodine allergy, costs, possible dislodgement of thromboses, and needle insertion at the back of the foot (a nice procedure, especially in the case of iodine extravasation) should be considered too. Doppler is still a highly popular facility. It shows the direction and speed of the flow [25]. Doppler can be advantageous in trauma, since the compression maneuver may be harmful. As the last solutions, angio-CT and angio-MRI are heavy tools for a simple, bedside question. See comments in the section about Doppler in Chap. 37.

References

1. Stein PD, Henry JW (1995) Prevalence of acute pulmonary embolism among patients in a general hospital and at autopsy. Chest 108:978–981
2. Goldhaber SZ (2002) Echocardiography in the management of pulmonary embolism. Ann Intern Med 136:691–700
3. Tapson VF, Davidson CJ, Kisslo KB, Stack RS (1994) Rapid visualization of massive pulmonary emboli utilizing intravascular ultrasound. Chest 105:888–890
4. Haeger K (1969) Problems of acute deep vein thrombosis: the interpretation of signs and symptoms. Angiology 20:219–223

5. Kakkar VV (1975) Deep venous thrombosis: detection and prevention. Circulation 51:8–12
6. Stein PD, Athanasoulis C, Alavi A, Greenspan RH, Hales CA, Saltzman HA, Vreim CE, Terrin ML, Weg JG (1992) Complications and validity of pulmonary angiography in acute pulmonary embolism. Circulation 85:462–468
7. Gibson NS, Sohne M, Gerdes V, Nijkeuter M, Buller HR (2008) The importance of clinical probability assessment in interpreting a normal D-Dimer in patients with suspected pulmonary embolism. Chest 134:789–793
8. Goodman LR, Curtin JJ, Mewissen MW et al (1995) Detection of pulmonary embolism in patients with unresolved clinical and scintigraphic diagnosis: helical CT versus angiography. Am J Rœntgenol 164:1369–1374
9. Levine MN, Hirsh J, Landefeld S, Raskob G (1992) Hemorrhagic complications of anticoagulant therapy. Chest 102(Suppl):352S–363S
10. Mant M, O'Brien B, Thong KL, Hammond GW, Birtwhistle RV, Grace MG (1977) Haemorrhagic complications of heparin therapy. Lancet 1(8022): 1133–1135
11. Hampton AA, Sherertz RJ (1988) Vascular-access infection in hospitalized patients. Surg Clin North Am 68:57–71
12. Lichtenstein D, Mezière G (2008) Relevance of lung ultrasound in the diagnosis of acute respiratory failure. The BLUE-protocol. Chest 134:117–125
13. Lichtenstein D, Menu Y (1995) A bedside ultrasound sign ruling out pneumothorax in the critically ill: lung sliding. Chest 108:1345–1348
14. Lichtenstein D, Mezière G, Biderman P, Gepner A (2000) The "lung point": an ultrasound sign specific to pneumothorax. Intensive Care Med 26: 1434–1440
15. Lichtenstein D, Mezière G, Biderman P, Gepner A, Barré O (1997) The comet-tail artifact, an ultrasound sign of alveolar-interstitial syndrome. Am J Respir Crit Care Med 156:1640–1646
16. Lichtenstein D, Mezière G (1998) A lung ultrasound sign allowing bedside distinction between pulmonary edema and COPD: the comet-tail artifact. Intensive Care Med 24:1331–1334
17. Lichtenstein D, Loubières Y (2003) Lung ultrasonography in pulmonary embolism, Letter to the Editor. Chest 123(6):2154
18. Reissig A, Heynes JP, Kroegel C (2001) Sonography of lung and pleura in pulmonary embolism: sonomorphologic characterization and comparison with spiral CT scanning. Chest 120(6):1977–1983
19. Mathis G, Blank W, Reißig A, Lechleitner P, Reuß J, Schuler A, Beckh S (2001) Thoracic ultrasound for diagnosing pulmonary embolism. Chest 128:1531–1538
20. Mathis G, Blank W, Reißig A, Lechleitner P, Reuß J, Schuler A, Beckh S (2005) Thoracic ultrasound for diagnosing pulmonary embolism. A prospective multicenter study of 352 patients. Chest 128:1531–1538
21. Reissig A, Kroegel C (2009) Relevance of subpleural consolidations in chest ultrasound. Chest 136:1706
22. Lichtenstein D, Mezière G (2009) Response to "relevance of subpleural consolidations in chest ultrasound" (Reissig A & Kroegel C). Chest 136: 1706–1707
23. Lensing AW, Prandoni P, Brandjes D, Huisman PM, Vigo M, Tomasella G, Krekt J, Wouter Ten Cate J, Huisman MV, Büller HR (1989) Detection of deep-vein thrombosis by real-time B-mode ultrasonography. N Engl J Med 320:342–345
24. Couson F, Bounameaux C, Didier D, Geiser D, Meyerovitz MF, Schmitt HE, Schneider PA (1993) Influence of variability of interpretation of contrast venography for screening of postoperative deep venous thrombosis on the results of the thromboprophylactic study. Thromb Haemost 70:573–575
25. Cronan JJ (1993) Venous thromboembolic disease: the role of ultrasound, state of the art. Radiology 186:619–630
26. Hull RD, Hirsh J, Carter CJ, Jay RM, Dodd PE, Ockelford PA, Coates G, Gill GJ, Turpie AG, Doyle DJ, Buller HR, Raskob GE (1983) Pulmonary angiography, ventilation lung scanning and venography for clinically suspected pulmonary embolism with abnormal perfusion lung scan. Ann Intern Med 98:891–899

BLUE-Protocol and Pneumothorax

Why and How the Ultrasound Diagnosis of Pneumothorax, Just This, Can Change Habits in Acute Medicine

The word "pneumothorax" is used several times a day in no less than a dozen of disciplines, not only in ICUs. It is seen in trauma, pre-hospital medicine, emergency rooms, anesthesiology, pulmonology, pediatrics, thoracic surgery, after any procedure, including acupuncture, can be debated in internal medicine, geriatrics, even palliative care, spaceship medicine and world medicine again.

One may consider this diagnosis as the Trojan horse of critical ultrasound. Searching to introduce critical ultrasound for checking gallbladders was the best way to have a noisy *veto* from the radiologists. Considering ultrasound as a machine just for ruling out pneumothorax would have made less noise. Once onsite, other applications would have been easy to develop gradually.

It touches the most vital organ. In trauma, bilateral cases are rapidly deadly. In the ICU, it is a frequent event [1]. The physicians know that severe cases can be radioccult. Traumatized and ventilated patients call for exceptional care, since the risk of a missed pneumothorax is major [2]. Some authors consider that any pneumothorax even occult should benefit from a chest tube before initiating mechanical ventilation [3]. How to make an immediate diagnosis is an issue, since bedside radiographies miss a number of cases. CT makes the diagnosis; this is true, yet two conflicting issues are not envisageable: first, sending all patients to CT, generating irradiation, delays, costs, and lost energy, and, second, losing a patient from such an "illegitimate" trouble. The dilemma is elegantly and perfectly solved by ultrasound. Providentially, the most accessible area is the anterior chest wall, and the A′-profile can be detected in a few seconds. What is difficult on radiography (anterior pneumothorax) is the easiest on ultrasound, which will detect the lung point quite always (when anterior). The most severely injured lungs (ARDS, etc.) are the ones giving the most striking signs ruling out pneumothorax. Ultrasound is a providence for these daily settings.

This is why we really consider that even if it may appear difficult to some (especially those who do not follow the rules), this approach offers so many advantages that a minor investment effort is valuable. The user will benefit from:

- Immediate diagnosis, quicker than the quickest radiograph (and obviously than the quickest CT)
- Immediate ruling out, each time the question is raised (ventilated patients, invasive procedure, respiratory failure, etc.)
- Sensitivity superior to bedside radiography
- Opening to pre-hospital diagnosis
- Major decrease in irradiation
- Major cost-savings, a godsend for most humans on Earth

The interest of lung ultrasound for diagnosing pneumothorax is confirmed by so many works that it becomes impossible to quote all of them [4–13]. The community wakes up, at last, but is well awaken now.

Pathophysiological Reminder of the Disease

The lung is an elastic structure not larger than a hand. It is held under negative pressure in order to be stuck against the pleural cavity. A rupture in this negative pleural pressure results in the physiological need of the elastic forces to come back to a stable status, with massive retraction of healthy lungs.

Idiopathic cases rarely generate acute respiratory failure. Trauma is the most obvious setting. Iatrogenic cases are a classical cause. Cases occurring under mechanical ventilation can lead to major concerns.

The Usual Ways of Diagnosis

If the clinical diagnosis was easy, free from operator dependency, it would raise no problem. Yet in the usual conditions, the need for a confirmation test is quite constant.

Up to 30 % of cases are occulted by the initial radiograph [14–17], many of them evolving to tension pneumothorax [14]. Some tension cases remain even unclear in the bedside radiograph [18]. In dramatic situations, time is lacking for radiological confirmation [19]. CT, the gold standard [20], is a suboptimal option in these critically ill patients.

It is scary to see how often CT was still recently used in the follow-up of a pneumothorax, by doctors aware that the radiograph is not a sensitive tool.

When Does the BLUE-Protocol Proceed? Which Signs? Which Accuracy?

In a dyspneic patient just after a trauma, this is completely part of the physical examination. In these noisy settings, an efficient auscultation is a quandary. This is why lung ultrasound is performed as soon as possible during the physical examination.

The first step is to apply the probe at the anterior BLUE-points. Detecting lung sliding or lung rockets rules out pneumothorax in a few seconds. If lung sliding is absent and no B-line is visible in this area (in one word, an A'-profile), finding a lung point confirms the diagnosis and indicates the volume of the pneumothorax. In the absence of lung point, read below the "Australian variant."

The accuracy using our technique indicates an overall 66 % sensitivity (79 % for occult cases) and a 100 % specificity [21, 22]. This makes sensitivity highly superior to that of radiography for partial pneumothorax, especially anterior cases, regularly radioccult: few millimeters of air thickness are sufficient (read Anecdotal Note 1). The overall sensitivity may appear low, but note that 100 % of patients have the A'-profile (but only 2/3 have the lung point).

Value of the BLUE-Protocol for Ruling Out Other Diseases

The A'-profile is immediately acquired and is highly suggestive. Remember that acute dyspnea can generate the Keyes' sign, i.e., noise above the pleural line, which will not confuse a user following the rules.

Pulmonary edema (B-profile), pneumonia (B'-, C-, A/B-profiles), COPD and asthma (A-profile), and pulmonary embolism (A-profile), these diseases generate profiles distinct from the A'-profile.

Look again at the list of situations able to create an A'-profile in Table 14.1 of Chap. 14 on pneumothorax.

Spending energy to distinguish an A'-profile from pseudo-A'-profiles is a good exercise, allowing to simplify the management of patients who have no pneumothorax.

Ultrasound Pathophysiology of Pneumothorax

Only the parietal pleura is visible at the pleural line. This generates abolished lung sliding. The visceral pleura, even very near (even 1 mm) to the parietal pleura, is hidden by the free gas in the pleural cavity. This generates a homogeneous pattern of the Merlin's space, with regular reverberation of the pleural line, i.e., A-lines. The whole generates the A′-profile. A-lines can be replaced by O-lines without any damage to the concept. "O-lines are A-lines".

The lung point is explained by even a slight increase in parietal contact when the lung inflates, i.e., on inspiration. We reiterate that any lung inflates during inspiration, whether normal or collapsed by a pneumothorax, whether spontaneously breathing, or under mechanical ventilation. This increases the lung volume, even very slightly. If the probe is applied at the boundary area, the very area where the lung increases its contact with the parietal pleura, thanks to real-time, instant response, and zero filter, the user will see sudden lung signs (lung sliding, B-lines) replacing the A′-profile, living air replacing dead air, to make it short.

Why Not 100 % Accuracy? The Limitations of the BLUE-Protocol. How to Circumvent Them

The specificity of ultrasound is 100 %. The sensitivity depends on the existence of a lung point. This raises the following problem: how to do it in a critically ill patient who has an A′-profile, i.e., probably a pneumothorax, but no lung point?

Too much purism would kill patients: mandatorily requiring the lung point would classify cases of pneumothorax as *false-negative*.

Too much laxism would kill other patients. Considering the lung point as a futile sign not really useful would result in correctly managing these patients is true. Yet this simplification would generate *false-positives* of pneumothorax in patients with previous pleural history. To begin with, all these patients who previously received pleural talcage (poudrage) or pleurodesis for iterative pneumothorax are now visited for an acute thoracic pain. These patients would receive a chest tube insertion, not a good idea if they just needed a coronary desobstruction.

The "Australian variant" solves this dilemma. The term, coined in Sydney while we were asked to deal with final details of a consensus conference in full jet lag, trying to understand with the fatigue between accuracy and specificity (two different terms which cannot be compared), indicates one possible solution: just be a doctor. The Australian variant considers a patient with an A′-profile extended to the lateral and posterior chest wall. In such patients seen for acute dyspnea, the slightest clinical sign (lateralized chest pain, lateralized tympanism, lateralized vascular procedure, even *cardiac arrest*) will dramatically increase the possibility of a genuine pneumothorax. Time permitting, traditional tools will be used (X-ray, CT). Time not permitting, in these settings where the blind chest tube insertions were authorized (and sometimes well indicated), the doctor will do the same as he or she did previously, but with a major argument for inserting or not the tube. Remind that abolished lung sliding plus the A-line sign has a 96 % specificity [23]. Tympanism plus A′-profile makes one of hundred examples of Extended BLUE-protocol usage (Chap. 35).

Some Among Frequently Asked Questions

Can ultrasound distinguish a pneumothorax from a giant emphysema bulla?
Absolutely. Using suitable equipment (at best, a simple and old unit), these bullae, even apical, generate all types of pseudo-A′-profile (T-lines, some grains of sand, lung pulse, etc.). In the few cases where they generate a real A′-profile, there will never be any lung point. This prevents to conclude to pneumothorax.

Other questions

What to do if my patient is about to die but has no lung point? (answered just above)
Why do some (prestigious) teams still go on finding this diagnosis difficult? Read Chap. 14 on basic signs of pneumothorax
Why does the literature still speak of "false-positives" of ultrasound? Read Chap. 14
How to deal with an up-to-date sophisticated unit? Read Chap. 14
Can we measure the volume of a pneumothorax? Read Chap. 28

Pneumothorax Integrated in the LUCI-FLR Project

The case of pneumothorax is probably the main target of the LUCIFLR project for decreasing radiographies and CTs.

1. *Spontaneous pneumothorax*

    Ultrasound will be of major help for reducing irradiation while showing the disease better than radiograph, please read Chap. 29, section on Pneumothorax

    During vacuum maneuver, ultrasound has shown us that the lung comes back to the anterior wall very rapidly – less than 1 min sometimes, and we always beware of the sudden changes at the main vital organ. Since ultrasound allows us to control the evolution of the lung point, we prefer to make several short sequences of vacuum.

2. *Pneumothorax in trauma*

    More patients will benefit from hospital CT, because more patients will come alive to the hospital thanks to pre-hospital ultrasound. This will replace the old blind tube insertions, which were long the only alternative.

3. *Pneumothorax under mechanical ventilation*

    Intensivists not fully familiar with ultrasound should ask for a confirmatory radiograph (facing an A′-profile), but meanwhile be prepared for inserting the tube. As soon as the radiograph comes back, the procedure is done, no time is lost. If the patient initiates a bradycardia, the physician will have then little choice but inserting the tube (read again the Australian variant above).

4. *Routine after subclavian cannulation or thoracentesis, or even thoracic pain in the ER*

Ultrasound should definitely replace the traditional check radiograph if the only concern is pneumothorax yes/no.

Asking for confirmatory tools (X-rays, CT) can be valuable in the learning curve of ultrasound, but if they are asked consistently, ultrasound would eventually generate a loss of time.

Anecdotal Note

1. Since the birth of radiography, physicians have feared the delayed pneumothoraces, occurring hours after venous line insertions with normal check radiography. "Delayed" pneumothoraces have probably never existed. The pneumothorax was already present, but just not detected by these supine bedside radiographies, not sensitive enough. This notion highlights a deep insufficiency of the check radiography done on early stage.

References

1. Kollef MH (1991) Risk factors for the misdiagnosis of pneumothorax in the intensive care unit. Crit Care Med 19:906–910
2. Pingleton SK, Hall JB, Schmidt GA (1998) Prevention and early detection of complications of critical care. In: Hall JB, Schmidt GA, Wood LDH (eds) Principles of critical care, 2nd edn. McGraw Hill, New York, pp 180–184
3. Enderson BL, Abdalla R, Frame SB, Casey MT, Gould H, Maull KI (1993) Tube thoracostomy for occult pneumothorax: a prospective randomized study of its use. J Trauma 35(5):726–730
4. Dulchavsky SA, Hamilton DR, Diebel LN, Sargsyan AE, Billica RD, Williams DR (1999) Thoracic ultrasound diagnosis of pneumothorax. J Trauma 47:970–971
5. Sargsyan AE, Hamilton DR, Nicolaou S, Kirkpatrick AW, Campbell MR, Billica RD, Dawson D, Williams DR, Melton SL, Beck G, Forkheim K, Dulchavsky SA (2001) Ultrasound evaluation of the magnitude of pneumothorax: a new concept. Am Surg 67: 232–235
6. Maury E, Guglielminotti J, Alzieu M, Guidet B, Offenstadt G (2001) Ultrasonic examination: an alternative to chest radiography after central venous catheter insertion? Am J Respir Crit Care Med 164:403–405
7. Rowan KR, Kirkpatrick AW, Liu D, Forkheim KE, Mayo JR, Nicolaou S (2002) Traumatic pneumothorax. Detection with thoracic US: Correlation with chest radiography and CT. Radiology 225:210–214

References

8. Kirkpatrick AW, Sirois M, Laupland KB, Liu D, Rowan K, Ball CG, Hameed SM, Brown R, Simons R, Dulchavsky SA, Hamilton DR, Nicolaou S (2004) Hand-held thoracic sonography for detecting post-traumatic pneumothoraces: the Extended Focused Assessment with Sonography for Trauma (EFAST). J Trauma 57(2):288–295
9. Blaivas M, Lyon M, Duggal S (2005) A prospective comparison of supine chest radiography and bedside ultrasound for the diagnosis of traumatic pneumothorax. Acad Emerg Med 12(9):844–849
10. Soldati G, Testa A, Sher S, Pignataro G, La Sala M, Gentiloni Silveri N (2008) Occult traumatic pneumothorax: diagnostic accuracy of lung ultrasonography in the emergency department. Chest 133:204–211
11. Volpicelli G, ElBarbary M, Blaivas M, Lichtenstein D, Mathis G, Kirkpatrick AW, Melniker L, Gargani L, Noble VE, Via G, Dean A, Tsung JW, Soldati G, Copetti R, Bouhemad B, Reissig A, Agricola E, Rouby JJ, Arbelot C, Liteplo A, Sargsyan A, Silva F, Hoppmann R, Breitkreutz R, Seibel A, Neri L, Storti E, Petrovic T (2012) International Evidence-Based Recommendations for Point-of-Care Lung Ultrasound. Intensive Care Med 38:577–591
12. Xirouchaki N, Kondili E, Prinianakis G, Malliotakis P, Georgopoulos D (2014) Impact of lung ultrasound on clinical decision making in critically ill patients. Intensive Care Med 40:57–65
13. Harriott A, Mehta N, Secko M, Romney ML (2014) Sonographic diagnosis of bilatera pneumothorax following an acupuncture session. J Clin Ultrasound 42:27–29
14. Tocino IM, Miller MH, Fairfax WR (1985) Distribution of pneumothorax in the supine and semirecumbent critically ill adult. Am J Roentgenol 144:901–905
15. Kurdziel JC, Dondelinger RF, Hemmer M (1987) Radiological management of blunt polytrauma with CT and angiography: an integrated approach. Ann Radiol 30:121–124
16. Hill SL, Edmisten T, Holtzman G, Wright A (1999) The occult pneumothorax: an increasing diagnostic entity in trauma. Am Surg 65:254–258
17. McGonigal MD, Schwab CW, Kauder DR, Miller WT, Grumbach K (1990) Supplemented emergent chest CT in the management of blunt torso trauma. J Trauma 30:1431–1435
18. Gobien RP, Reines HD, Schabel SI (1982) Localized tension pneumothorax: unrecognized form of barotrauma in ARDS. Radiology 142:15–19
19. Steier M, Ching N, Roberts EB, Nealon TF Jr (1974) Pneumothorax complicating continuous ventilatory support. J Thorac Cardiovasc Surg 67:17–23
20. Holzapfel L, Demingeon G, Benarbia S, Carrere-Debat D, Granier P, Schwing D (1990) Diagnostic du pneumothorax chez le malade présentant une insuffisance respiratoire aiguë. Evaluation de l'incidence en décubitus latéral. Réan Soins Intens Med Urg 1:38–41
21. Lichtenstein D, Mezière G, Biderman P, Gepner A (2000) The lung point: an ultrasound sign specific to pneumothorax. Intensive Care Med 26:1434–1440
22. Lichtenstein D, Mezière G, Lascols N, Biderman P, Courret JP, Gepner A, Goldstein I, Tenoudji-Cohen M (2005) Ultrasound diagnosis of occult pneumothorax. Crit Care Med 33:1231–1238
23. Lichtenstein D, Mezière G, Biderman P, Gepner A (1999) The comet-tail artifact, an ultrasound sign ruling out pneumothorax. Intensive Care Med 25:383–388

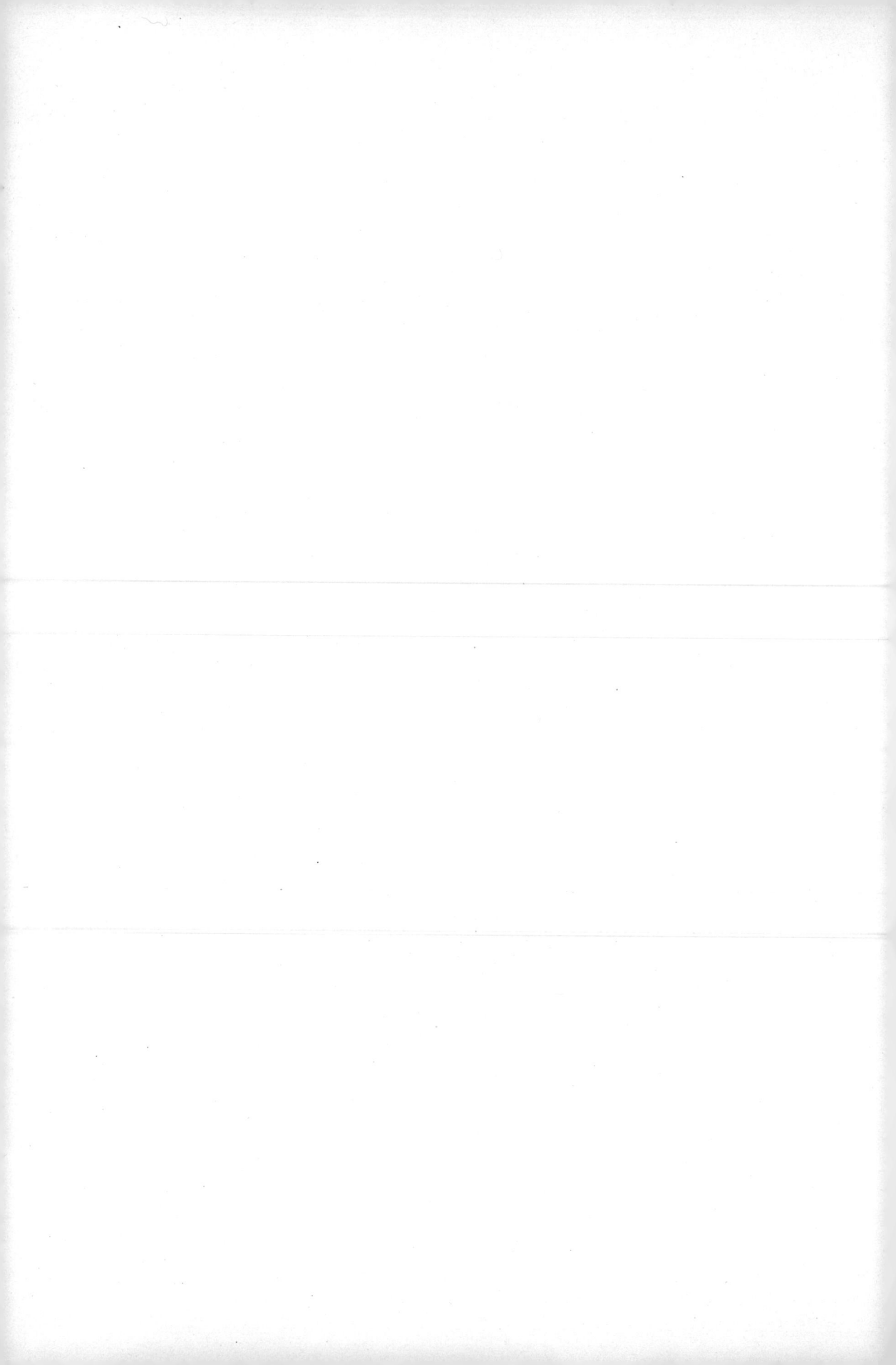

Part III

The Main Products Derived from the BLUE-Protocol

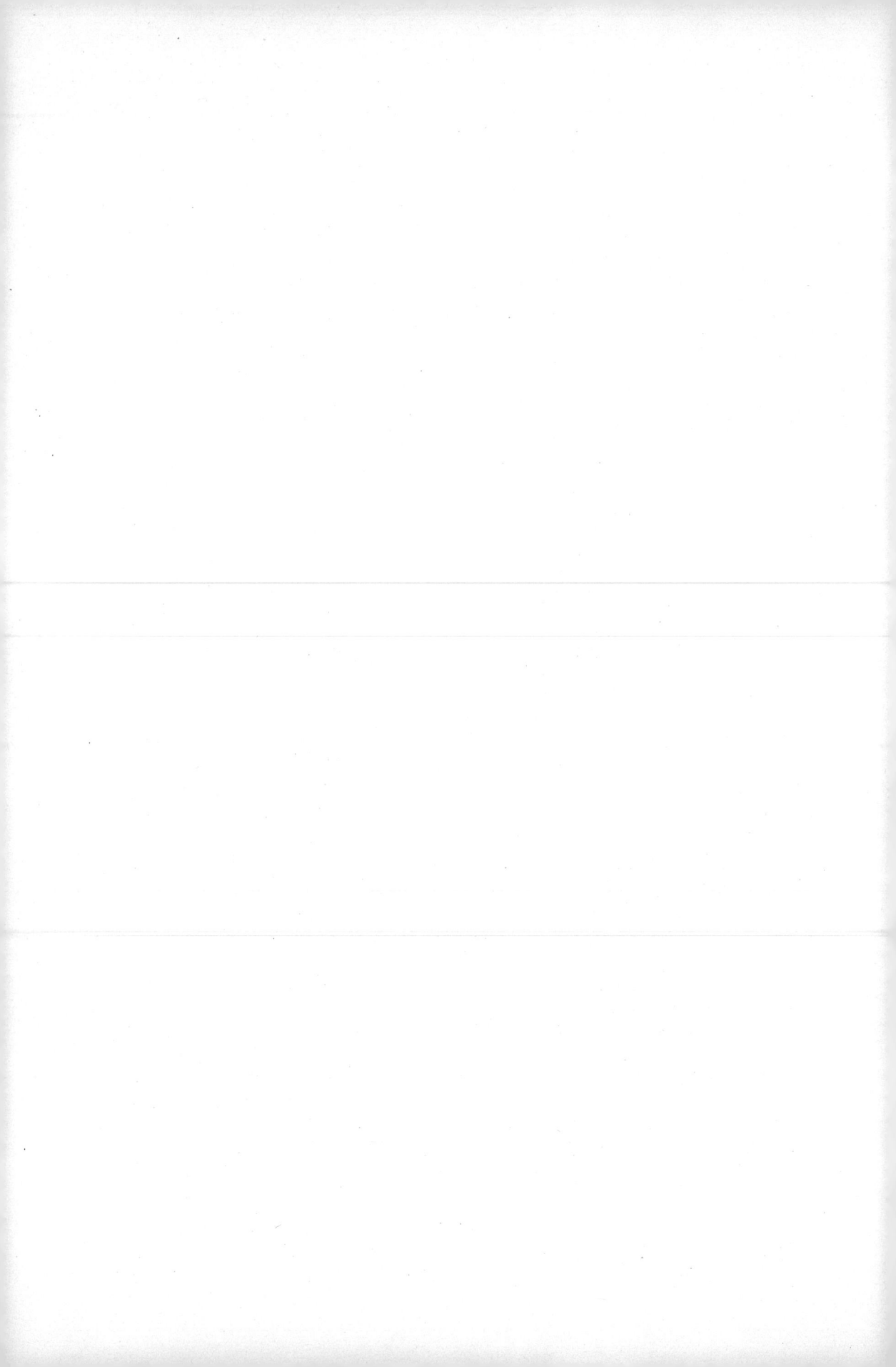

Lung Ultrasound in ARDS: The Pink-Protocol. The Place of Some Other Applications in the Intensive Care Unit (CLOT-Protocol, Fever-Protocol)

Some critically ill patients with massive loss of lung function are not dyspneic, not blue, and have a quiet breathing, just because they are deeply sedated and curarized on occasion and receive pure oxygen. This is mainly the case of ARDS. Lung ultrasound in these patients does not strictly obey to the rules of the BLUE-protocol. This setting was called the Pink-protocol. Not surprisingly in our discipline, the definitions of ARDS changed recently. A homogeneous management is en route, but not fully achieved, with space for discussion [1, 2]. It is peculiar to see that, even if lung ultrasound was of possible use when ARDS was defined [3], in the 2012 definition, this potential was still not fully, deeply integrated (Anecdotal Note 1). Time will correct this. We assume that LUCI will clarify more than confuse, helping in better classifying this multi-faceted disease. The lung is a complex organ, and such an injury (ARDS) can complexify the field even more [4, 5]. Hopingly, an intensive use of ultrasound (lung, veins, diaphragm, heart, etc.) may optimize patient's survival or quicker discharge from the ICU.

Electronic supplementary material The online version of this chapter (doi:10.1007/978-3-319-15371-1_28) contains supplementary material, which is available to authorized users.

This chapter is the opportunity to describe other protocols developed around familiar themes (pulmonary embolism, fever in the ICU, etc.). The reader will find in one chapter elements which made a thick part of our 2010 Edition.

Peculiarities of the Ventilated Patient in the ICU

Because of the quiet breathing with low frequency, the mangrove variant of lung sliding is more marked. Intrications of events will be seen in this battlefield made of victories and defeats, explaining non-frank profiles (that we could maybe call the "Pink profiles"). One finds more b-lines or bb-lines in patients who recover from hemodynamic pulmonary edema, the same with patients initiating ARDS or worsening from nosocomial infections, etc. Apart from ARDS (with B′-profile, C-profile, A/B-profile, etc.), variants of the A-profile will be rather frequent. Venous thromboses are frequent, quite usual once catheters have been inserted. At this step, many patients will have an A-DVT-profile, but it should not be concluded in a pulmonary embolism. The patient is no longer blue; we are not in the BLUE-protocol. PLAPS are quite always present for reasons of gravity; it is true (but we cannot refrain thinking that minor infections and minor infarctions, in addition to gravity atelectases, are possible).

The BLUE-Protocol for *Positive Diagnosis* of ARDS

ARDS can be assimilated to pneumonia, in the terms of the BLUE-protocol. Massive inflammation, lung consolidation, pleural exudate, etc., create the four profiles of pneumonia: the B′-profile, the C-profile, the A/B-profile, and on occasion the A-no-V-PLAPS profile.

The A/B-profile should here be understood as areas, even in the same side, of lung rockets and A-lines ("spared areas" of some Italian literature).

The C-profile can be reduced to minute alveolar syndrome touching the pleural line, resulting in an irregular pleural line ("thickened, irregular pleural line" of some Italian literature). See Fig. 17.4.

In the patients of the BLUE-protocol who initiated ARDS, these four profiles were found in 86 % of cases. The B-profile was seen in 14 % of them [6]. These data indicate that the BLUE-protocol has a substantial role to play for differentiating ARDS from hemodynamic pulmonary edema.

The pathophysiology explains each profile. Lung sliding is frequently abolished (between 33 and 40 % of cases), mainly because of the inflammatory adhesions. The anterior consolidations are due to inflammation (consolidations from hydrodynamic edema reaching the anterior wall in a supine patient would be highly surprising; see again Fig. 24.1).

The Pink-protocol is more subtle than the BLUE-protocol. The patient is visited more quietly. The scanning is more comprehensive. It includes the lateral wall (not used in the BLUE-protocol). The apex is under analysis (we use the ideal probe for this difficult area).

The Extended BLUE-protocol allows bacteriological diagnosis, when a microorganism is isolated from a thoracentesis, among other procedures of interest (read Chap. 35).

Note: the Pink-protocol can be done in any kind of patient on mechanical ventilation, not especially ARDS.

Lung Ultrasound for *Quantitative Assessment* of ARDS

Ultrasound allows to understand and evaluate each component of the disease. The main disorders benefit from a qualitative and quantitative approach – helping for an adapted therapy.

Lung Sliding

It is for sure correlated with lung compliance, provided factors such as tidal volume and abdominal pressure are under control. Currently, there is no available bedside test such as lung sliding. Since there will not be any practical gold standard, we must accept ultrasound as the gold standard. It is possible to define roughly four stages: normal lung sliding, discrete lung sliding, impaired lung sliding with millimetric amplitude, and complete abolition. Discrete lung sliding is normal near the apex and not normal at the base.

We define normal lung sliding when we see that its amplitude comes, on inspiration at the lower BLUE-point, from the lower end of the upper rib to the upper end of the lower rib (this is, anatomically, roughly 2 cm). B-lines help definitely for a finer assessment. If not, some pleural irregularities may be available. If not, the simplest is to give up with the lung and just take a look to the liver or spleen descent. The usual excursion of the (please choose) podal lung sliding, diaphragmatic cupola, liver, and spleen is roughly 2 cm.

We define discrete lung sliding in between (roughly, 5–10 mm).

We define quite abolished lung sliding as a dynamic reduced to a millimetric move.

Abolished lung sliding is an absent dynamic, even one mm.

Pleural Effusion

Volume Assessment

The BLUE-protocol makes a qualitative estimation: PLAPS or no PLAPS. In the Pink-protocol,

Lung Ultrasound for *Quantitative Assessment* of ARDS

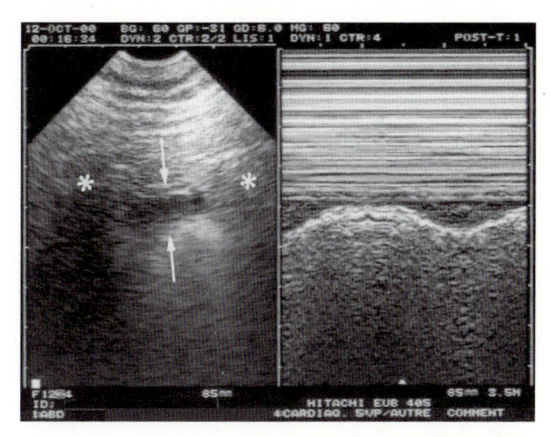

Fig. 28.1 A minute pleural effusion at the PLAPS-point, using the quad and sinusoid sign, between pleural line (*upper arrow*) and lung line (*lower arrow*). We expect a 40–80 ml effusion. Asterix, ribs

intensivists want to know how much fluid is present. We just think that a rough estimation is sufficient: in our practice, the procedure of thoracentesis is so secure that it is quite always done. Withdrawing fluid only when it is >500 cc is not fully satisfactory: patients who have together highly diseased lungs and this restrictive syndrome (even <500 cc) will probably benefit from a procedure. The less the effusion, the more the lung can breathe.

We evaluated several protocols for roughly indicating the volume of the effusion (Accessory Note 1). Different approaches can be consulted [7–11]. We present our most recent approach: the "BLUE-pleural index," which favors simplicity. It requires inserting the probe at the PLAPS-point and simply measuring the distance between the pleural line and lung line. We measure on expiration (on inspiration, the lung line actively moves toward the pleural line). Care must be done for having a probe as tangential as possible to the chest wall. Each centimeter (of probe length, of body habitus) can be a hindrance, resulting in overestimating the dimensions by simple mathematic distortion.

The PLAPS-point shows all volumes of free pleural effusion. A minimal effusion has a millimetric thickness, which anyway generates frank quad sign and sinusoid sign (Fig. 28.1).

Care is done to measure from the pleural line to the lung line. Of no sense would be a measurement from the pleural line to the mediastinum, as seen when made too near to the diaphragm: all cases of effusion able to detach the basis of the lung from the cupola will have a standard 10 ± 1 cm depth. Here is a simple rule for beginners: at the PLAPS-point, the BLUE-pleural index can range from 0 to 4, rarely 5, exceptionally 6, and never 7 cm. A 10-cm value invites to question one's technique. See comment in Fig. 16.5).

One rule must be considered (the principle N°2, of gravity): a quite normal lung should be light like a balloon, allowing pleural effusion to lie dependently. The diagnosis of aerated lung is based, roughly, by the observation of sub-B-lines at the PLAPS-point (see Fig. 16.3). A fully consolidated lung weights and obliges the fluid to spread around. A correction should therefore be made when, below the lung line, the lung is consolidated, not aerated. These rules must be understood as approximate (and, hopingly, sufficient).

And now we can use the BLUE-pleural index. As for consolidations, the BLUE-index is an elementary parameter; the BLUE-volume is an estimated volume, from this index. The following sizes consider adults:

A. When the underlying lung appears aerated:
   Three mm correspond to a *BLUE-pleural volume* of 15–30 ml.
   One centimeter corresponds to 75–150 ml.
   Two centimeters correspond to 300–600 ml.
   Thirty-five millimeters correspond to 1,250–2,500 ml.
   Six cm seem a maximum, and measurements around 10 cm (in our defined conditions) cannot come from a pleural effusion. These numbers are just indicative. This approximation that we use, from simple to double values, is sufficient for clinical practice (has no repercussion on the patient's safety). This also indicates that the accuracy of such measurement is not a major problem in our habits.

B. When the underlying lung is consolidated, these values should be increased. Without yet any confirmatory study, these numbers should be considered as a rough indication:

Lung consolidation	Correction factor
3 cm (roughly 27 cc)	1,1
4 cm (roughly 64 cc)	1,2
5 cm (roughly 125 cc)	1,4
6 cm (roughly 215 cc)	1,7
7 cm (roughly 350 cc)	2

Thoracentesis for Pleural Fluid Withdrawal

For the diagnostic thoracentesis, please refer to Chap. 35 on the Extended BLUE-protocol.

We use this potential of ultrasound to allow safe thoracentesis in ventilated patients, even with PEEP [12]. Fluid withdrawal improves the respiratory parameters [7, 8, 13–15]. The technique for withdrawing fluid is exactly the same than for analyzing some ml. We use the safety criteria explained in Chap. 35. We never use ultrasound during the puncture. Ultrasound just tells us where the needle should be inserted.

Technical Notes

We avoid large tubes, too aggressive, and use a system we have developed with a 16-gauge, 60-mm-long catheter (see Fig. 34.2). Since this multipurpose catheter has no lateral hole, the lung will come into frontal contact with the distal hole, blocking the aspiration in the syringe. The operator should just withdraw the catheter mm by mm and go on aspiration, until this catheter comes out of the pleural cavity.

Using a 60-ml syringe, the fluid is withdrawn with an average output of 1 ml/s, i.e., 20 min for a 1,200 ml effusion. It seems slow but the overall time is decreased: the catheter is withdrawn at the end, a simple family dressing is applied on the skin; this system has the advantages of simplicity, no loss of time, no infectious risk generated by the large tubes (needing dissection of the wall, large wound, the need for making a pouch), no pain, and limited costs. The very limited dressing (1 × 3 cm) allows to make easy post-procedure ultrasound. The procedure can be repeated at will. As

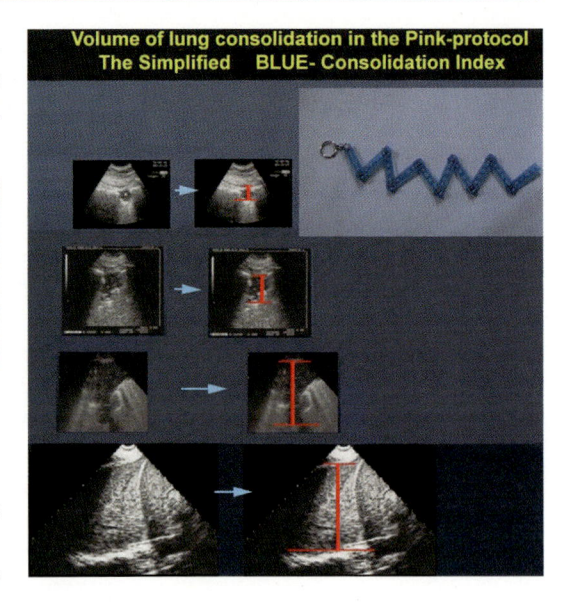

Fig. 28.2 Four different volumes of lung consolidation. It is easy to see that, if occurring in the same patient, it would mean, from *bottom to top*, an improvement or, from *top to bottom*, a worsening. No need of sophisticated approaches for this. Each *red mark* indicates one measurement. The principle of the Pink-protocol, trying to import simplicity in the field of ARDS, is to consider this sole dimension as representative of the consolidation volume. Note that the tool in the cartouche (*upper right*), easy to find in any general shop, was of use twice. Here, it allows to measure lung consolidations in a basic way. Measurements are not emotions. They demonstrated in Chap. 2 that the ultrasound revolution was possible using machines smaller than laptops, far before, more suitable

described, it aims at simplicity more than 100 % fluid withdrawal (some ml can stay on site).

Lung Consolidation: Volume Assessment (During Recruitment)

Many intensivists worry about the volume of the consolidated lung [16]. Some try to make it disappear using PEEP. We will not open the debate on the usefulness of these maneuvers (not in terms of saved respiration but in terms of lost circulation, with potential outcomes on the multiorgan dysfunction) [17]. We just consider, for those who want to monitor this alveolar part, that a simple ruler is sufficient (Fig. 28.2). In other words, we use simplicity as a guide for this assessment (Accessory Note 1).

Lung Ultrasound for *Quantitative Assessment* of ARDS

Sophisticated ways of measurement, as developed by some teams, will give very precise numbers, but is it a true dimension? Critical care teaches us to be cautious if using precise data in a not exact discipline (take the example of the cardiac output measured by the Swan-Ganz catheter). The more precise the measurement, the bigger the risk to be wrong. We have defined a BLUE-consolidation index according to this and two other remarkable points. First, our microconvex probe has the advantage of a sectorial view. Second, observation shows that most lung consolidations behave like compact masses. The three dimensions are roughly the same. Considering two of them – and even one – is sufficient for estimating the other(s), therefore the volume. The BLUE-consolidation index considers the area at the most speaking dimension and assimilates it roughly as one side of a cube. Some would correct this, considering more a sphere than a cube. This may complicate the design, and mostly, the iceberg effect (as we call this) yields underestimations of the volume: massive deep gas collections (air bronchograms usually) can stop the beam, hiding deeper information. The BLUE-consolidation index is expressed in the figures of Chaps. 17 and 35.

Very simply, a BLUE-consolidation index of 1 cm should correspond to a *BLUE-consolidation volume* of 1 ml (2 cm–8 ml, 3 cm–27 ml, etc.).

Note that even if this index is not 100 % exact, its variations should indicate worsening or healing of the disease.

The probe must be as perpendicular as possible to the chest wall for having standardized, consistent measurements. Therefore, just the distance between the pleural line and the end of the consolidation should be measured (if not perpendicular, ultrasound overestimates the consolidation dimension; if you measure a sheet of paper on a table, it can be 0.1 or 300 mm, depending how your tool is oriented). The mediastinal line sign (showing always the same dimension: 10–11 cm) indicates major volume.

A very small consolidation, visible between two ribs, has been called C-line (for Centimetric Cupuliform Consolidation) (see Fig. 17.3).

Teams increasingly use prone positioning. Anticipating many rejections, and years of lost

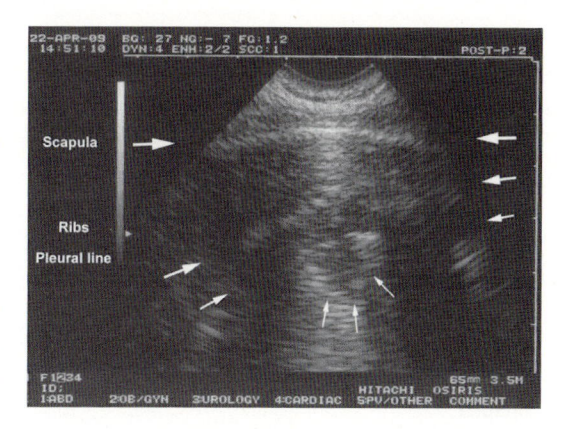

Fig. 28.3 Two dogmas. This single figure invalidates two dogmas, which stipulate that air and bone are insuperable obstacles to ultrasound. On top of the image, the scapula (*large upper arrows*). The intermediate *arrows* indicate the ribs. The *lower, smaller arrows* indicate the pleural line. Arising from the pleural line, a lung consolidation, with a shred sign, is perfectly identified (*vertical arrows*). Even measurements can be done: this piece of consolidation is 12 mm thick (or the BLUE-consolidation volume is roughly 1.4 cc). ARDS in a 35-year-old patient in the prone positioning

time, we confide the principle of our study in progress, for the benefit of the patients. If diffuse interstitial syndrome is not associated with substantial posterior lung consolidation (in a supine patient), this heavy maneuver may not be beneficial. Lobar patients (assuming A-profile plus PLAPS) may benefit from it. In a prone patient, ultrasound remains feasible; the "prone points" can be used (see Fig. 6.7). Even a trans-scapular lung approach is fully possible: see Fig. 28.3, which atomizes two dogmas.

Pneumothorax

In the Pink-protocol, i.e., in ARDS mainly, extensive adhesions, responsible for abolition of lung sliding, may theoretically prevent from pneumothorax, by sticking the lung to the wall. Yet complex pneumothoraces can be seen in these patients. Here, as a rule, lung sliding is abolished everywhere, i.e., in the areas of pneumothorax and in the areas of adherences. Lung rockets and lung pulse help in recognizing the non-detached areas. When there is no B-line nor lung pulse, distinguishing pneumothorax from adhesions is too challenging. This is why the lung point is required for the diagnosis. Knowing the limitations of ultrasound, the physician will not harm the patient. But radiographies can be useful here. If we consider only these cases with large areas of abolished lung sliding with A-lines, associated with radiographies not showing the pneumothorax, CT should answer the question (if clinically relevant). This wise request for CT is fully integrated in the spirit of the LUCIFLR project (next chapter).

How to Evaluate the Volume of a Pneumothorax

This makes no difficulty, yet this raises academical and ethical problems.

Academical: if we use radiography for comparison, poor results will be expected [18–22].

Ethical: if we use CT as a gold standard, whereas radiography has already shown specific signs (even with poor appraisal of the volume), the issue is now ethical: useless irradiation. Any research must bear these heavy limitations in mind. We made a correlation only for radio-occult cases, i.e., cases where CT was the only definite proof [23], showing that 1/3 of patients with radio-occult pneumothorax needed a chest tube, which again shows the poor value of the radiography. Subsequent studies with large use of CT confirmed these results [24].

In our study, the lung point location was correlated with the volume, using one simple criterion: the clinical need of the managing team to insert a chest tube. The chest tube was indicated in 8 % of cases when the lung point was anterior, versus 90 % of cases when it was lateral [23]. The more lateral the lung point, the more substantial the pneumothorax. Major pneumothorax yields very posterior – or even absent – lung point. Anterior lung point is correlated with minimal and generally radio-occult pneumothorax [23].

We must define what a "minute" pneumothorax is. A sheet of A4 paper has a minute thickness (0.1 mm) but an extensive surface (21 × 29 cm). This explains why even "minute" cases are easily detected using the standardized BLUE-points.

Can One Monitor the Volume of a Pneumothorax?

Nothing is more easy. One just has to locate the lung point (if present) and see its evolution. No need for irradiating studies for this.

Interstitial Syndrome

Diffuse ground-glass rockets are correlated with ground-glass areas, a notion of interest for those intensivists who adapt the management according to this pattern (study in progress) [25].

Lung Water

The diagnosis of extravascular lung water (EVLW) is done usually through continuous cardiac output devices. This is a familiar item for many intensivists, not used by others. Combining the measurements of the thoracic fluids, i.e., the pleural free fluid, the fluid within the lung consolidations, and the minute volume of interstitial fluid (paradoxically of high relevance in hemodynamic management of circulatory failure, dealt with in Chap. 30), the intensivist has much more than a lump value of water.

Long-Staying Patients in the ICU: What to Do with These So Frequent PLAPS?

Patients admitted, e.g., for decompensated COPD, difficult to wean, being little by little part of the ICU, often develop PLAPS. What are we speaking of? This can be the fact of a pneumonia (acquired on mechanical ventilation) or postural atelectasis. For distinguishing both, we send to all signs described in Chap. 35. In actual fact, this field is probably not well known. This can come from occult fluid overload (search for even transient B-profiles). Given the frequency of the thromboembolic events in such patients, maybe some of these PLAPS are pulmonary infarctions. In patients full of PLAPS at the onset (e.g.,

ARDS), this is just less visible than in patients with no PLAPS initially. Just read the next section (CLOT-protocol).

Diagnosis of Pulmonary Embolism in ARDS: The CLOT-Protocol

Pulmonary embolism can affect ARDS patients after several days of evolution. The diagnosis, sometimes suggested by sudden clinical worsening after some improvement, is a familiar issue [26]. It seems to appear that in 19 % of ICU patients benefiting from a CT for independent reasons, a pulmonary embolism is found [27]. This notion is of high relevance for the CLOT-protocol.

We don't expect X-rays to make this diagnosis, especially in ARDS. Echocardiography? A right ventricle which has undergone intensive training (e.g., several days of ARDS) has little by little adapted to this increased downstream pressure by getting thicker, i.e., *stronger*, therefore making conditions for not enlarging more (personal opinion). Therefore, a thickened right ventricle, just slightly enlarged, is not of major contribution. D-dimers? They are quite never negative in ARDS. Lung ultrasound is not contributive, quite never showing an A-profile. Daily referrals to CT are not envisageable.

The CLOT-protocol proposes a reasonable approach to this apparent issue.

The CLOT-protocol (Catheter-Linked Occult Thromboses) is defined by daily applying the probe onto areas that show holes from recent or present catheterizations. The dressing of a catheter is a minimal hindrance when using our small footprint/high-resolution microconvex probe. Traditional vascular probes will generate, we guess, ergonomic issues. One or more of the six usual sites (subclavian, jugular, femoral) are checked, making less than 1 min for the six sites (i.e., far less for one site). The CLOT-protocol is routine or goal directed in case of acute impairment. When a DVT is seen, the CLOT-protocol is "activated." This means that the intensivist is free to treat or not such thromboses but is aware of this disorder (our option is to treat; read Accessory Note 2). When the CLOT-protocol is activated, it should be done every day or facing any new event. A positive CLOT-protocol is defined by the sudden disappearing of a thrombosis previously detected. Assuming that the physiological thrombolysis requires much more time for dissolving a thrombosis, the CLOT-protocol just asks the question: "Where is the thrombus now?" For physicians who consider that the only possible answer is "in the pulmonary circulation," a positive CLOT-protocol, associated with suggestive clinical signs (worsening of respiratory parameters), is a possible alternative to spiral CT. Figure 28.4 summarizes the CLOT-protocol.

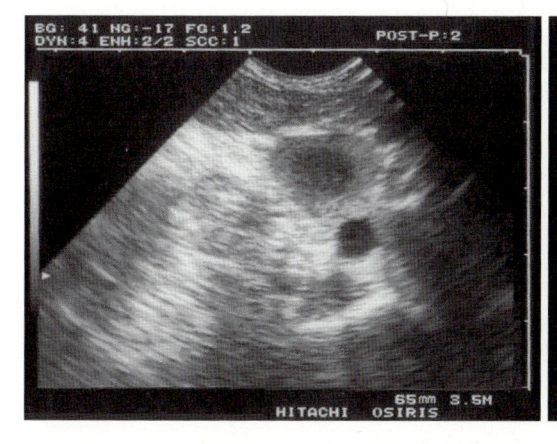

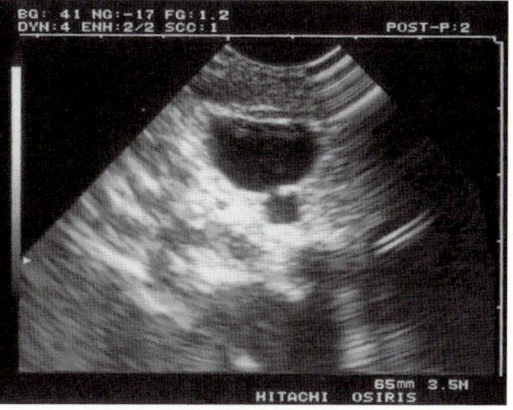

Fig. 28.4 The CLOT-protocol. Transverse scan of a neck, young woman with ARDS. *Left*: a massive internal jugular thrombosis is visible. Real time showed movements inside this thrombosis and any compression was carefully avoided: this scan was diagnostic (i.e., gold standard, to our opinion). *Right*: same patient, same view, 24 h later. The vein is black and compressible. We don't believe a physiological fibrinolysis can dissolve such an occlusive thrombosis in this short time. We can only speculative that the massive clot of the *left image* went somewhere else

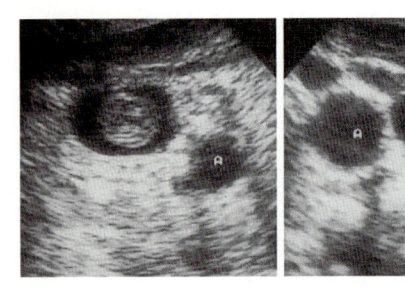

Fig. 28.5 Floating jugular thrombosis. This figure appears in Chap. 18, but its place should be here also. This is the kind of thrombosis often seen at the jugular area in ICU patients with recent catheters. *A* artery

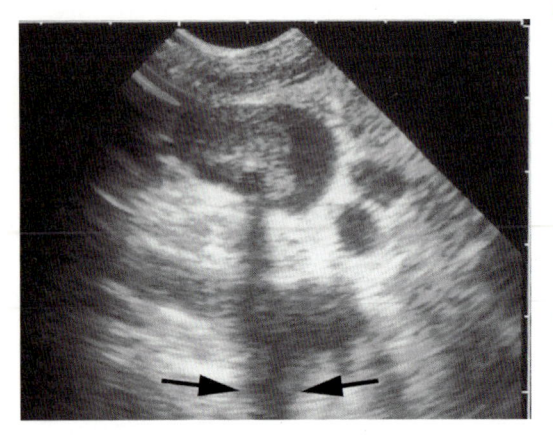

Fig. 28.6 Jugular internal thrombosis on catheter. Typical thrombosis of the jugular internal vein, developing around a venous catheter. The catheter is detected by direct vision or by observing its overt acoustic shadow (*arrows*)

Technique of the CLOT-Protocol

Jugular Internal Vein

Most intensivists and even emergency physicians are familiar with the ultrasound anatomy and approach of this vein; there is nothing to add to the technique rapidly described in Chap. 18 (Fig. 28.5). We just add that our microconvex probe is perfect for this use, especially with the tracheostomy cords. Floating thromboses are frequent (Video 28.1). Jugular internal thromboses appear to be really frequent (Fig. 28.6) [28].

Subclavian Vein

The frequency of subclavian venous thromboses (after catheterization) seems strikingly lower than internal jugular thromboses. The technique

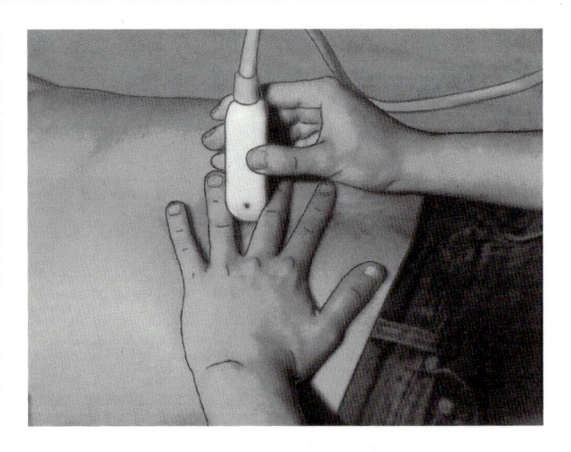

Fig. 28.7 How the CLOT-protocol explores the iliocaval veins. The free hand is spread over the abdomen and the microconvex probe is inserted as shown. The free hand gently controls the pressure and even makes the work of palpation for clinical duties

was briefly recalled in Chap. 18 (for more information, read the comprehensive text of our 2010 Edition).

Common Femoral Vein

There is nothing to add to the technique rapidly described in Chap. 18.

The Iliac Veins

In the ICU, the thromboses are seen after femoral catheterization. The common femoral vein may appear normal if the thrombosis develops downward, at the iliac area, which must therefore be scanned here. Our microconvex probe provides better focused pressure than these cumbersome abdominal probes. Gas is the main hindrance, an issue in more than 1/3 of cases. In most cases, however, iliac veins can be followed and compressed over a more or less long segment (quite always the beginning of the external segment). The primitive iliac vein detection is more chancy.

We routinely use a two-hand technique, applying our free hand with spread fingers on the abdominal wall, inserting the probe between two fingers of the free hand, and applying a more or less important pressure with the free hand in order to gently drive away any gas (Fig. 28.7). A substantial compression by the probe alone would harm the probe, and the patient, and an unstable thrombosis. Most often,

Diagnosis of Pulmonary Embolism in ARDS: The CLOT-Protocol

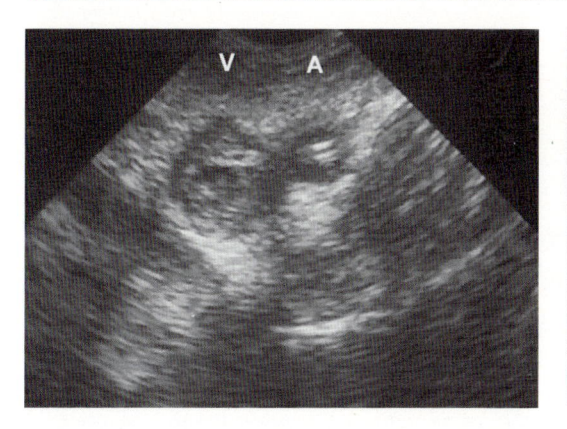

Fig. 28.8 Iliac venous thrombosis. Left external iliac thrombosis. In this cross-sectional pelvic scan, the external iliac vein (below the *V*) is enlarged by an echoic heterogeneous occlusive material. This sole pattern renders the compression technique redundant, hence an inverted risk-benefit ratio of this maneuver. Note at the right of the image an arterial catheter (two parallel hyperechoic lines) inside the iliac artery (below the *A*)

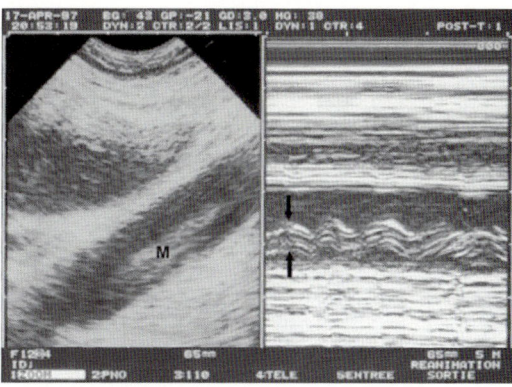

Fig. 28.9 Floating iliac venous thrombosis. Floating iliac thrombosis (*M*). The floating character is demonstrated using the M-mode, at the right: characteristic sinusoid ondulations (*arrows*). If compression of such a structure is attempted, one can calculate a volume of at least 7×7×40 mm of embolus at risk to be dropped toward the lung

the gas barrier is suddenly bypassed, yielding visibility over the target.

The Carmen maneuver is the most efficient way to isolate rapidly the vascular couple from the GI tract. A rectilinear segment of the GI tract locating at the same axis should not mislead. It is single (not a vascular couple) and large and has visible peristalsis, among many signs, making Doppler useless for this task alone. Note that up to now, Doppler does not solve the issue of pelvic gas. When the contrast is suitable, the compression maneuver is less useful, since the DVT is seen within the vein (Fig. 28.8). An echoic flow with dynamic particles can at times be seen, indicating venous patency. Valsalva or sniff-test maneuvers are unrealistic in our tired patients. Floating thrombosis is often detected at these large areas (Fig. 28.9).

Isolated iliac thromboses? Read Accessory Note 3.

Inferior Caval Vein

We use the same two-hand technique at the iliac level (Fig. 28.7). A spontaneous echoic flow, possibly due to agglomerated blood cells, is observed in some cases (see Fig. 13.14 of our 2010 Edition). The flow hesitates on mechanical inspiration or even moves backward – making cheap method of flow analysis without Doppler. The venous caliper is modified by respiratory and cardiac rhythms, with usually inspiratory collapse in spontaneously breathing subjects. Visible flow variations in caliper are signs of venous patency.

A compression maneuver against the rachis, *in the absence of obvious image of thrombosis*, is often able to collapse the IVC, depending on the morphotype. In a segment so near to the heart, one imagines the consequences of an inappropriate compression – if a thrombosis has been seen. Note that a complete venous compression does not affect the real-time blood pressure (immediate derivation through azygos system is a possible explanation).

The signs of caval thrombosis have no peculiarity (Fig. 28.10). The thrombosis is very often floating, a feature obviously favored by the large size of this vein. Detecting hypertrophy of azygos system is a matter for specialists. Extrinsic obstacles, catheters, or caval filters can be observed (see Fig. 13.16 of our 2010 Edition).

Superior Caval Vein

This vein can really not be compressed; Doppler may be useful. Yet before using it, let us point out some clues. Focal, isolated venous thromboses are exceptional (not yet seen in our experience).

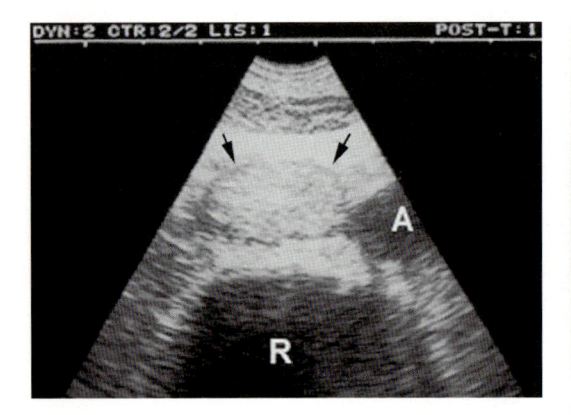

Fig. 28.10 Inferior caval vein thrombosis. Massive thrombosis of the inferior caval vein (*arrows*). Transverse scan of the umbilical area (infrarenal portion). Anterior to the rachis (*R*) and at the right of the aorta (*A*), the venous lumen of the inferior caval vein is filled with echoic material. This recent thrombus is still soft. Hence, a compression maneuver would possibly collapse the venous lumen but may result in dispersing infected miasmas toward the lung. Young patient with multiple traumas

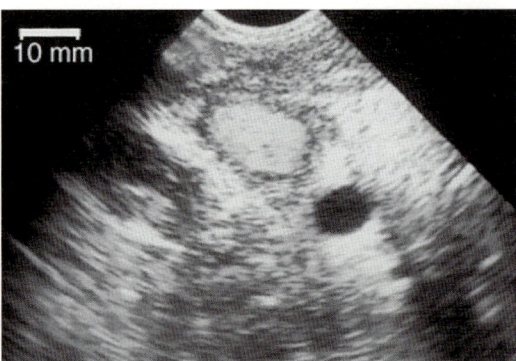

Fig. 28.11 Infected thrombophlebitis. Suppurative thrombophlebitis. Note the markedly echoic pattern and the thickened wall. Complete thrombosis of the right internal jugular vein, transverse scan. Note: we assumed such a fresh, acute thrombosis to be compressible, but we did not try

Indirect signs indicate patency: inspiratory collapse (in a spontaneously breathing patient) of the subclavian or jugular veins indicates absence of an obstacle at the superior caval vein [29]. The sniff test (sudden inspiration by the nose, collapsing normal veins) [29] is not realistic in critically ill patients (and we are not keen on sudden maneuvers in these fragile patients): this would dislodge a thrombosis that was until then stable.

One Particular Extension of the CLOT-Protocol

It is no longer catheter related, but it is a preventing test like the CLOT-protocol. This regards those long-staying patients who can develop spontaneous thromboses because they are simply confined to bed. One can believe in preventive anticoagulation or, alternatively, check (5 s per leg, daily or once/2 days) the lower femoral veins (the V-point, described in Chap. 18). A calf thrombosis extends to the femoral veins in 20 % of cases [30]. This extension always occurs before pulmonary embolism [30]. Taking this notion into account, when the calf analysis is unsatisfactory (or when time really lacks) (or just expertise lacks), we monitor the V-point. If a thrombosis is detected by such monitoring (that we called the V-protocol), it is time for curative treatment. This is a way to minimize the problem of undetected calf thromboses in these patients. The V-protocol is also part of the physical examination that any student will do every day.

Peculiar Patterns Seen on Occasion in the CLOT-Protocol

Infected thromboses, i.e., thrombophlebitis, are seen because CLOT-thromboses have a direct contact with the skin, through the puncture. Instead of the classical gray pattern of those thromboses seen in the ER, the pattern can be hyperechoic (white), due to massive gas within the thrombosis, i.e., severe infection (Fig. 28.11). A thickened wall is often observed (phlebitis). Septic thrombophlebitis is observed preferentially at the internal jugular site, which favors accumulation of all the dirt. An expected sign of infected thrombosis would be the isolation of a microbe within the thrombosis, using minute aspiration of the thrombus under ultrasound guidance, in expert hands. Spontaneous venous thromboses (i.e., without previous catheterization or trauma) have no reason for superinfection.

Fever in the ICU: The Fever-Protocol

We wondered where to insert this section in this textbook and decided that the most logical place was in the present chapter. First, it occurs in critically ill but "pink" patients. Second, the lung, veins, and airways make the main causes of the fever.

FUO (fever of unknown origin) is frequent in the ICU. Once ultrasound is wisely used, "FUSO" (fever of unknown sonographic origin) is rare.

Fever or occult manifestations of sepsis (circulatory, hepatic, or renal failure, fluid retention, muscular shrinking, and multiple signs such as low cardiac output, fall of diuresis, anuria, increase in creatinemia, cholestasis, occlusion, edema of lower or upper extremity, etc.) are some daily situations in the ICU which await the patient. Quite all have a common point: a major place for simple ultrasound [31].

Our 2010 Edition was more comprehensive but the choice was made here to favor lung ultrasound.

There is no acronym in "Fever-protocol," just a daily situation. Those who need acronyms may call it the FICUS-protocol (Fever in the Intensive Care Unit Sonography) or what else would please them.

We won't deal with obvious sources. Some are clinical (cutaneous bedsores, e.g.); a urinary infection is diagnosed far more easily by urine analysis than by a chancy ultrasound kidney analysis (this detail is part of the definition of holistic ultrasound, since such assessments would require sophisticated units, harmonics, CEUS, etc.). Among daily sites of infection in the critically ill in the ICU, the lung is the most familiar [32]. Ultrasound can show a peritoneal collection, rupture of hollow organ with pneumoperitoneum, acute cholecystitis, biliary dilatation, urinary obstruction, deep abscess (liver, spleen, kidney, pancreas), soft tissue abscesses, etc. A severe maxillary sinusitis can be a source of sepsis; a simple sinusitis can create iterative pneumonias (Fig. 28.12) [33]. We look at infected deep venous thromboses, especially from jugular and femoral catheterization, potentially infected by definition (i.e., a use of the CLOT-protocol). The infected thrombosis is sometimes found at the forearm, etc. (Figure 29.6 of our 2010 Edition).

Among rare sites, there is the brain abscess (with optic nerve dilatation), bacterial pericarditis, and endocardial vegetation (seen in many instances using our simple equipment).

Regarding mediastinal collections and mediastinitis, apart from post-cardiac surgical ICU, e.g., we hear two opposed opinions: a frequent cause of fever for some and an exceptional one

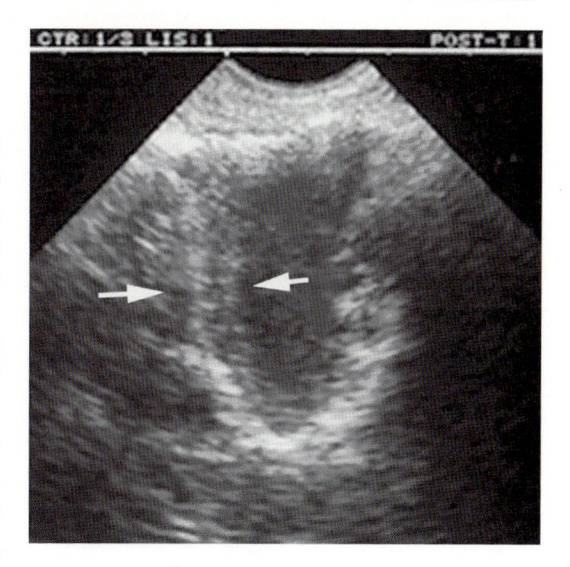

Fig. 28.12 Maxillary sinusitis and the sinusogram. In a few lines (see chapter head of our 2010 Edition for comprehensive details), the thin anterior facial bone allows transmission of the ultrasound flow (like the scapula, iliac aisle). An empty sinus yields an airy (not bony) artifact, looking like an A-line. When the sinus is full, the ultrasound beam crosses the sinus in its totality, displaying its shape, hence the label we suggest: the "sinusogram." Our Japanese 5 MHz probe is suitable for this; its small footprint is an advantage. Ultrasound may overcome the issues of radiographs in supine patients or, worse, transfer to CT. Our study done in the ICU showed a high concordance between complete sinusogram and scanographic complete sinusal opacity: a complete sinusogram (all walls well depicted, like here) is quite specific to sinusitis, whereas an incomplete sinusogram may be due also sometimes to mucosal thickening [33]. Dynamic maneuvers are helpful for diagnosing air-fluid levels. There are other subtleties. Just for the pleasure to demonstrate ultrasound superiority on CT, sometimes, note the mucosal thickening that only ultrasound can see (*arrows*)

for others. In our medical ICU, it is an infrequent cause. Posterior locations but even some anterior locations can be challenging for ultrasound (see Fig. 25.6 of our 2010 Edition).

How is the Fever-protocol in practice done? Well waken up, one can begin by the most likely sites. Tired, one can make the "bulldozer technique," i.e., scan cephalo-podal, i.e., brain first (optic nerves), then maxillary sinus, and so on.

Accessory Notes

1. *Previous assessments*

    "Experience" was our previous way and was rather efficient, but it cannot be easily transmitted, as opposed to the BLUE-index. During some time, for pleural effusion volume assessment, we used the area where the collection stopped to be visible when scanning toward the anterior wall. For lung consolidations, we previously used a rapid, intuitive approach, estimating that a given consolidation occupies something like 1 % (C-line), 5 % (minimal), 20 % (consequent), 50 % (huge), etc., of the lung volume. But it uses experience, which is not a universal tool.

2. *Outcome of these catheter-occult jugular thromboses*

    After cannulations (or worse, multiple attempts), internal jugular thrombosis is common in ICU patients. In rare cases, the thrombosis is not related with a local procedure. Studies in the ICU suggest an occurrence of 70 % [28, 34]. Fewer studies have evaluated the risk of pulmonary embolism as well as septic consequences [32]. Pulmonary embolism from upper extremity veins is estimated as nonexisting for some (corridor talks) and as occurring in 10–12 % of cases, including subclavian source, for others [35, 36]. In both cases, the methodology is unfortunately not optimal. We have evidence that such thromboses can eventually dislodge.

Our (unpublished) observations show an increase of mortality in these patients. Is it an explanation (death from embolism) or just an association (very ill patients may have higher rate of thromboses)? Since death is a daily occurrence in the ICU, all possible factors should be carefully scrutinized.

Unlike the (sterile) lower extremity thromboses, these thromboses come from catheters, therefore in direct communication with the skin, i.e., subject to superinfections. This may explain fever (of "unknown" origin) but also septic pulmonary embolism (so-called pneumonia). This is the hypothesis of the "banderilla": we hypothesize that jugular thrombosis in the long-staying critically ill creates small emboli, likely occult. If they happen repeatedly, they can yield issues, maybe not sudden death but delayed discharge, difficult weaning, dysadaptation episodes, subacute fatigue, or this so-called nosocomial pneumonia. Like a banderilla sunk at the bull's back, maybe these repeated aggressions exhaust the patient, before the deathblow, so to speak.

A catheter surrounded by thrombosis is a frequent finding (Fig. 28.6). We guess that withdrawing the catheter may fragilize the stability of this thrombosis.

Is the "first inspiration" safe? Apart from the first inspiration when we come to life, all ventilated and sedated patients are eventually desedated. At one moment, the positive inspiratory pressure is replaced by a negative inspiratory pressure. When suddenly the pressures are inverted in the bloodstream, what will happen to a floating thrombosis (up to now more or less protected by the relative positive pressure)?

Our solution for these problems is just to avoid the internal jugular route. Please read Chap. 34, section on subclavian vein cannulation, words about our interest for the subclavian route.

3. *Isolated iliac venous thromboses*

Isolated iliac thromboses are reputed to be exceptional, more often visible in the obstetrical or trauma setting [37, 38]. In clinical practice, we assess at least the external iliac vein, quite always accessible. When really the clinical question of a primitive iliac venous thrombosis is raised and no good window is present, there is a space for a referral to CT (far less than one case/year).

Anecdotal Notes

1. ARDS in 1976 and lung ultrasound

By having used pantographic ultrasound machines in 1984 (machines from before the era of real-time ultrasound, developed since 1974), we can tell that precious elements of lung ultrasound could be extracted using this rudimentary but precious tool. It gave (for the youngest) *static* bidimensional images or the same M-mode acquisition that we know today. This would have been of great help in defining even the dynamic patterns of the BLUE-protocol. The real time was a revolution which made ultrasound more easy (Henry and Griffith could even deserve the acknowledgment that ultrasound never had, unlike X-rays, CT, and MRI). Yet experts can use (with some patience for sure) this system for demonstrating quite all signs of LUCI. The physician who, in 2015, activates the button "M-mode" makes suddenly a 40-year travel to the past.

References

1. Ranieri VM, Rubenfeld GD, Thompson BT, Ferguson ND, Caldwell E, Fan E, Camporota L, Slutsky AS (2012) Acute respiratory distress syndrome : the Berlin definition. JAMA 307(23):2526–2533
2. Malbrain M (2014). I don't like the Berlin definitions of ARDS (abstract). 11th Annual critical care symposium. Veerappan Chithambaram, Manchester
3. Ashbaugh DG (1967) Acute respiratory distress in adults. Lancet 2(7511):319–323
4. West BJ. Respiratory physiology. The essentials. 9th Ed. 2012. Philadelphia, Baltimore. Wolters Kluwer, Lippincott Williams & Wilkins
5. Guyton CA, Hall JE (1996) Textbook of medical physiology, 9th edn. W.B. Saunders Company, Philadelphia, pp 212–234
6. Lichtenstein D, Mezière G (2008) Relevance of lung ultrasound in the diagnosis of acute respiratory failure. The BLUE-protocol. Chest 134:117–125
7. Talmor M, Hydo L, Gershenwald JG, Barie PS (1998) Beneficial effects of chest tube drainage of pleural effusion in acute respiratory failure refractory to PEEP ventilation. Surgery 123:137–143
8. Roch A, Bojan M, Michelet P, Romain F, Bregeon F, Papazian L, Auffray JP (2005) Usefulness of ultrasonography in predicting pleural effusion >500 mL in patients receiving mechanical ventilation. Chest 127:224–232
9. Vignon P, Chastagner C, Berkane V, Chardac E, Francois B, Normand S, Bonnivard M, Clavel M, Pichon N, Preux PM, Maubon A, Gastinne H (2005) Quantitative assessment of pleural effusion in critically ill patients by means of ultrasonography. Crit Care Med 33:1757–1763
10. Balik M, Plasil P, Waldauf P, Pazout J, Fric M, Otahal M, Pachl J (2006) Ultrasound estimation of volume of pleural fluid in mechanically ventilated patients. Intensive Care Med 32:318–321
11. Remérand F, Dellamonica J, Mao Z, Ferrari F, Bouhemad B, Jianxin Y, Arbelot C, Lu Q, Ichaï C, Rouby JJ (2010) Multiplane ultrasound approach to quantify pleural effusion at the bedside. Intensive Care Med 36(4):656–664
12. Lichtenstein D, Hulot JS, Rabiller A, Tostivint T, Mezière G (1999) Feasibility and safety of ultrasound-aided thoracentesis in mechanically ventilated patients. Intensive Care Med 25:955–958
13. Depardieu F, Capellier G, Rontes O, Blasco G, Balvay P, Belle E, Barale F (1997) Conséquence du drainage des épanchements liquidiens pleuraux chez les patients de réanimation ventilés. Ann Fr Anesth Reanim 16:785
14. Ahmed SH, Ouzounian SP, Dirusso S, Sullivan T, Savino J, Del Guercio L (2004) Hemodynamic and pulmonary changes after drainage of significant pleural effusions in critically ill, mechanically ventilated surgical patients. J Trauma 57:1184–1188

15. Nishida O, Arenallo R, Cheng DCH, DeMajo W, Kavanagh BP (1999) Gas exchange and hemodynamics in experimental pleural effusion. Crit Care Med 27:583–587
16. Keenan JC, Formenti P, Marini JJ (2014) Lung recruitment in ARDS : what is the best strategy? Curr Opin Crit Care 20(1):63–68
17. Vieillard-Baron A, Charron C, Jardin F (2006) Lung "recruitment" or lung overinflation maneuvers ? Intensive Care Med 32:177–178
18. Tocino IM, Miller MH, Fairfax WR (1985) Distribution of pneumothorax in the supine and semirecumbent critically ill adult. AJR Am J Roentgenol 144:901–905
19. Kurdziel JC, Dondelinger RF, Hemmer M (1987) Radiological management of blunt polytrauma with CT and angiography: an integrated approach. Ann Radiol 30:121–124
20. Hill SL, Edmisten T, Holtzman G, Wright A (1999) The occult pneumothorax: an increasing diagnostic entity in trauma. Am Surg 65:254–258
21. McGonigal MD, Schwab CW, Kauder DR, Miller WT, Grumbach K (1990) Supplemented emergent chest CT in the management of blunt torso trauma. J Trauma 30:1431–1435
22. Gobien RP, Reines HD, Schabel SI (1982) Localized tension pneumothorax: unrecognized form of barotrauma in ARDS. Radiology 142:15–19
23. Lichtenstein D, Mezière G, Lascols N, Biderman P, Courret JP, Gepner A, Goldstein I, Tenoudji-Cohen M (2005) Ultrasound diagnosis of occult pneumothorax. Crit Care Med 33:1231–1238
24. Soldati G, Testa A, Sher S, Pignataro G, La Sala M, Gentiloni Silveri N (2008) Occult traumatic pneumothorax: diagnostic accuracy of lung ultrasonography in the emergency department. Chest 133:204–211
25. Lichtenstein D, Mezière G, Biderman P, Gepner A, Barré O (1997) The comet-tail artifact, an ultrasound sign of alveolar-interstitial syndrome. Am J Respir Crit Care Med 156:1640–1646
26. Schmidt GA (1998) Pulmonary embolic disorders. In: Hall JB, Schmidt GA, Wood LDH (eds) Principles of critical care, 2nd edn. McGraw-Hill, New York, pp 427–449
27. Minet C, Lugosi M, Savoye PY, Menez C, Ruckly S, Bonadona A, Schwebel C, Hamidfar-Roy R, Dumanoir P, Ara-Somohano C, Ferretti GR, Timsit JF (2012) Pulmonary embolism in mechanically ventilated patients requiring computed tomography: prevalence, risk factors and outcome. Crit Care Med 40:3202–3208
28. Chastre J, Cornud F, Bouchama A, Viau F, Benacerraf R, Gibert C (1982) Thrombosis as a complication of pulmonary-artery catheterization via the internal jugular vein. N Engl J Med 306:278–280
29. Gooding GAW, Hightower DR, Moore EH, Dillon WP, Lipton MJ (1986) Obstruction of the superior vena cava or subclavian veins: sonographic diagnosis. Radiology 159:663–665
30. Philbrick JT, Becker DM (1988) Calf deep venous thrombosis: a wolf in sheep's clothing ? Arch Intern Med 148:2131–2138
31. Lichtenstein D (2007) Point of care ultrasound: infection control on the ICU. Crit Care Med 35(Suppl):S262–S267
32. Chastre J, Fagon JY (2002) Ventilator-associated pneumonia. Am J Respir Crit Care Med 165:867–903
33. Lichtenstein D, Biderman P, Mezière G, Gepner A (1998) The sinusogram, a real-time ultrasound sign of maxillary sinusitis. Intensive Care Med 24:1057–1061
34. Yagi K, Kawakami M, Sugimoto T (1988) A clinical study of thrombus formation associated with central venous catheterization. Nippon Geka Gakkai Zasshi 89:1943–1949
35. Horattas MC, Wright DJ, Fenton AH, Evans DM, Oddi MA, Kamienski RW, Shields EF (1988) Changing concepts of deep venous thrombosis of the upper extremity: report of a series and review of the literature. Surgery 104:561–567
36. Monreal M, Lafoz E, Ruiz J, Valls R, Alastrue A (1991) Upper-extremity deep venous thrombosis and pulmonary embolism: a prospective study. Chest 99:280–283
37. Haeger K (1969) Problems of acute deep vein thrombosis: the interpretation of signs and symptoms. Angiology 20:219–223
38. Rose SC, Zwiebel JZ, Miller FJ (1994) Distribution of acute lower extremity deep venous thrombosis in symptomatic and asymptomatic patients: imaging implications. J Ultrasound Med 13:243–250

The LUCI-FLR Project: Lung Ultrasound in the Critically Ill – A Bedside Alternative to Irradiating Techniques, Radiographs and CT

29

> The most severely ill patients are the ones who can benefit less from CT or MRI. Critical ultrasound and lung ultrasound neatly solve this weird paradox while limiting medical radiations.

> The target of the LUCI-FLR project is to decrease in the three next decades bedside radiographies by 1/3 and urgent CT by 2/3.

Some academicians have found that lung ultrasound was a futile idea in light of the technological advances of the modern medicine. The ADR-4000 of 1982, with its 45 cm width, was the basis for an absolute, *disruptive* revolution. At this period, the modern technologies were not mature. CT, D-dimers, and BNP, all these wonderful helps, did not exist. At this remote period, ultrasound mastered countless clinical situations, and those who used this tool first, although working in quite "clandestinity," had a huge advance for night or day management of critically ill patients. Critical ultrasound, more than simple images, allowed to take *immediate* decisions. Today, it is true, the contrast between ultrasound and the rest is less "spectacular" (Fig. 29.1) but remains substantial. In other words, ultrasound currently makes a revolution, but it could have been a historical one. The community just lost three decades of visual medicine (i.e., blood, sweat, and tears for many, many patients).

In this chapter, we will see some occult drawbacks of CT and why ultrasound can avoid most referrals to this giant of imaging through a program which can be perfectly standardized.

Lung Ultrasound and the Traditional Imaging Standards in the Critically Ill: The LUCI-FLR Project

We saw how lung ultrasound performs better than bedside radiography for most indications in the critically ill. It may seem bold to now compare ultrasound with CT. Yet this is what we do daily.

During decades, thoracic ultrasound appeared limited to the sole diagnosis of fluid pleural effusion [1–3], when this application was not forgotten [4]. The alternative for emergency lung assessment was bedside radiography or CT [5]. Ultrasound elegantly solves this quandary.

The LUCI-FLR project (Lung Ultrasound in the Critically Ill Favoring Limitation of Radiation) is in the field of the possible. Its target is to decrease, in the *three* next decades, bedside radiographs by *one-third* and CT by *two-thirds*. One can go far beyond, but we aim at a reasonable, realistic target. The "L" is for limiting. The idea of some aggressive proselytes (who advocate

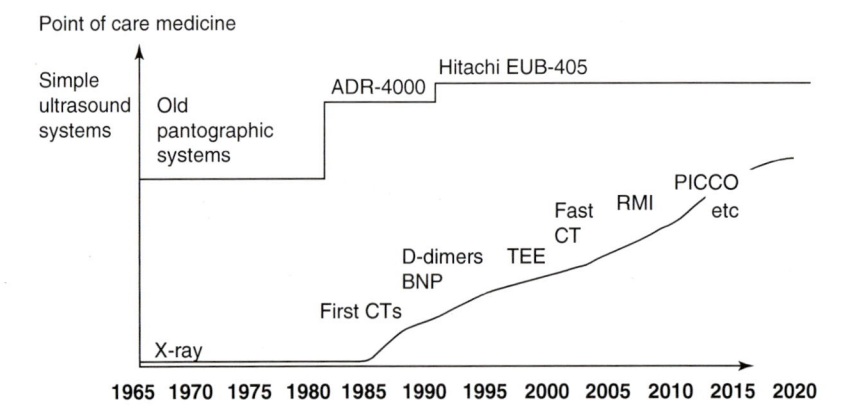

Fig. 29.1 LUCI-FLR and decades. This diagram shows that portable ultrasound, quite perfect since 1982 (the ADR-4000) and even possible before the 1974 revolution of real time, could have made a historical medical revolution, the visual medicine at an era where quite nothing existed (1965, the dark era of kidney tomographies, gas encephalocisternographies, those syringes with glass and metal, etc.). Today, the advances in other fields decrease this gap, which still remains substantial – not to deal with the intrinsic advantages of ultrasound (cost, etc.).

ultrasound for everything) of *eradicating* radiography may appear scary – as well as the resulting acronym. Limiting, not eradicating, is the humble target of LUCI-FLR project.

We must keep radiography, this centenary technique [6, 7], for specific indications (need for overview, exact location of central lines, etc.). On the contrary, all questions clearly answered by ultrasound allow to skip X-rays. Just one example: pneumothorax. Each time the only question is "pneumothorax" and the answer is "no," lung sliding can completely replace any radiograph, *to advantage*. This means, each time there is a chest pain, a thoracic procedure, a desadaptation of a ventilated patient, in an emergency or more quietly.... i.e., a dozen of disciplines and maybe more. Just imagine [8].

We must be aware of the limitations and inadequacies of bedside chest radiography [9–16]. Basic diagnoses are occulted: pneumothorax (even tension cases), pleural effusions (up to 500 ml), lung consolidation (mostly of the lower lobes), and interstitial syndrome (this diagnosis is even not required from a bedside radiograph). The summation of the images makes the disorders difficult to interpret. Some excellent radiologists know how to read some bedside radiographs, but they are not available 24/7/365 in small, nonuniversity-affiliated hospitals. We have evidence that the study of the ten ultrasound signs is much easier to acquire. Either the radiography is normal or highly abnormal (white lung), ultrasound immediately discriminates the alveolar, interstitial, and pleural components, not to speak of subphrenic or mediastinal disorders. Radiography is available only within hospitals (read last §). The irradiating potential of radiography is a concern in each pregnant woman, child, or, by extension, any person.

Tables 29.1 and 29.2 detail why ultrasound usually shows what radiography misses.

Overt and Occult Drawbacks of Thoracic Tomodensitometry

The CT is a giant in imaging. It has the major advantage of providing an easy-to-interpret overview of the chest. We respect this precious tool which has saved many lives. For giving a chance to ultrasound facing this standard, we remind seven of the CT's drawbacks:

1. Cost (machine, maintenance, etc.).
   For us, this is a minor problem. For more than 2/3 of the people on Earth (far more), who will never see a CT, this is a critical, life-threatening issue.
2. Irradiation.
   We who have the privilege of affording CT in each of our wealthy institutions must now face

Table 29.1 Disorders which can be missed or confused with other disorders by bedside radiograph (into brackets, diagnoses that are erroneously done)

	Pleural effusion	Lung consolidation	Interstitial syndrome	Free pneumothorax	Normal subject
False negatives	Retro-diaphragmatic location (*normal*) Extensive but spread posterior location (*normal or alveolar syndrome*)	Too small lesion (*normal*) Consolidation totally hidden by the cupola (*normal*) Consolidation partially hidden by the cupola with blunting of the cul-de-sac (*pleural effusion*) Summation of consolidation without air bronchogram with pleural effusion (*pleural effusion*)	Too small images (*normal*) Too dense patterns (*alveolar syndrome*) Summation with posterior pleural and alveolar images (*alveolar or pleural*)	Pleural line not tangential to the X-rays (*normality*)	Not applicable
False positives	Basal alveolar consolidation blunting the cul-de-sac	Pleural effusion with diffuse posterior location Some interscissural pleural effusions Summation of pleural images with dense interstitial syndrome	None	None	Interstitial syndrome (if poor inspiration) Pneumothorax (skinfolds)

Table 29.2 Disorders which can be missed or confused with other disorders by ultrasound (into brackets, diagnoses that are erroneously done)

	Free pleural effusion	Lung consolidation	Interstitial syndrome	Pneumothorax	Normal subject
False negatives	(1)	Deep lesion (*normal*) Not scanned location (*normal*)	(1)	Absence of lung point (2)	(1)
False positives	(1)	(3)	(4)	(1)	(1)

(1) No condition yet considered
(2) In the case of an A′-profile without a lung point, we remind it is preferable for ultrasound not to conclude
(3) In our previous edition, we featured the thymus and some loculated and echoic pleural collections, but both are distinguished using the thymus line and the lung line, which are not confused with a shred line
(4) The exceptional gooey sign, described in Chap. 12

its high degree of irradiation: 400 times (or more?) that of a chest radiography. Deleterious side effects of CT are now acknowledged [17–21]. Investigation of lung disorders in pregnant women raises concerns [22]. Diagnostic X-rays are the largest source of artificial radiation exposure, the source of 0.6–3.2 % of the cumulative risk of cancer [19, 20]. A CT performed at the chest of a 30-year-old or less woman increases the risk of breast cancer by 35 % [23]. A CT done before the age of 1 year accounts for 3 % of radiation-induced cancers and between 1 and 14 years for 19 % [19]. Authors increasingly point out the drawbacks of chest CT, but without proposing any real alternative [24]. Ultrasound provides an elegant solution.

3. Delay.
   Some experts found lung ultrasound a minor idea, since CT provides all answers in "10 s." Brackets. This vision has resulted in countless rejections, delaying publications, limiting the widespread of a simple approach, with the consequences we can all live now (a whole community equipped with machines which are good, but could have been acquired much sooner, and with *more interesting* performances). But it is far from true. While lung ultrasound was fully implementable, i.e., since 1982 (or less), the CT machines were in their infancy. The image acquisition was long – a deadly issue for some patients. Just for those patients who survived to CT, while bleeding actively, how many blood units were lost. Countless. Rivers of blood. Yet now that CTs are so-called rapid, the real overall time is not "10 seconds." When the managing team comes to the point that a CT is necessary in a given unstable patient, the time for arguing with the radiologist, preparing the patient, moving the patient to the CT department and then on the CT table, waiting the famous 10 s acquisition, understanding the CT results, taking the patient back to the ICU, and being able to manage the disorder according to the CT result, this time is superior to "10 s." Those who can do this incompressible sequence in less than *1 h* can contact us.
4. Need for transportation.
   This is a major drawback in the critically ill. In the intensivist's brain, requiring CT scan is a *decision*.
   - An unstable patient is at permanent risk. Multiple life-support devices (catheters, tubes) can be harmful.
   - Transportation of unstable patients is a strain for the whole medical and paramedical team.
   - The intensivist is condemned to doing nothing during the entire procedure and cannot deal with other emergencies. It should be recalled here that during more than 12 h a day (including the whole night), only one intensivist is present for the hospital's extreme emergencies.
   - Emergency CT scan is not the time to warrant perfect asepsis – the critically ill patient with multiresistant germs behaves as a "bacteriologic bomb" for the whole hospital.
5. Iodine generates vascular overload, anaphylactic shock, and renal injury.
6. Comfort and safety for the patient. The cold temperature of the CT room and the necessary supine positioning can create vasoactive stimulation, with redistribution of fluids, maybe significant.
7. Diagnostic inadequacies.
   - Hindrances for a quality examination
     The signal is impaired by numerous artifacts: intracavitary devices (catheters), arms of the patient when they cannot be shifted, and dynamics of respiration or heartbeats.
   - Low resolution power of CT
     The focal resolution power of CT is inferior to that of ultrasound. Septations within a pleural effusion are not visible [25]. The superior resolution power of ultrasound has been proven for necrotizing pneumonia [26].
   Readers can see Figs. 29.2 and 29.3, and the most skeptical ones can do an in vitro demonstration (Fig. 29.4). The distinction between lung consolidation and pleural effusion usually needs iodine injection. A millimetric effusion can be missed on CT (making by the way one "false positive" for ultrasound). Interstitial syndrome can be hard to detect in ventilated patients. The dynamic features are not detected. The real-time ultrasound is perfectly adapted to this vital, dynamic organ, and all signs using real-time ultrasound will, by definition, be assessed better:
   - Lung sliding allows to know the very function of the lung, unlike no bedside tool.
   - Minimal pneumothorax is minimized since images are acquired at inspiration.
   - The dynamic air bronchogram. When it is seen within a lung consolidation, a nonretractile consolidation can be affirmed.
   - Diaphragmatic static images are much better using longitudinal scans (ultrasound) than transverse CT.
   - Diaphragmatic dynamics can in no way be documented by CT.

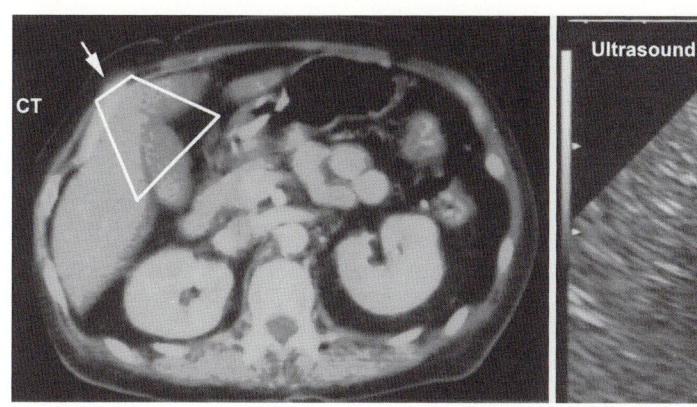

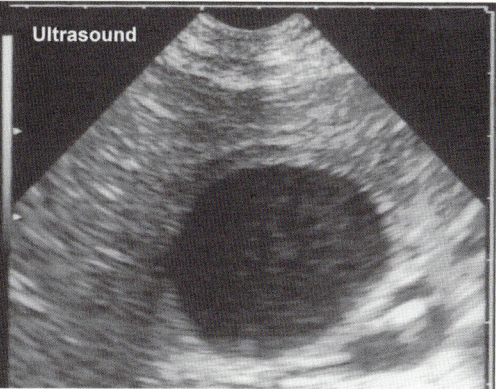

Overt and Occult Drawbacks of Thoracic Tomodensitometry

Fig. 29.2 Ultrasound superior to CT, one example. This couple of figures objectifies strong points of each method. Regarding global overview, CT is superior. Regarding focal spatial resolution, ultrasound's superiority over CT is demonstrated: in the area scanned by ultrasound, (white frame on left figure), the thickness of the gallbladder wall is sharply measured at 3.5 mm, but how could this data be reproduced on the CT image?

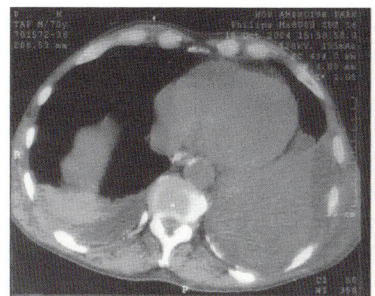

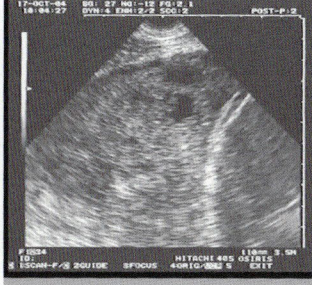

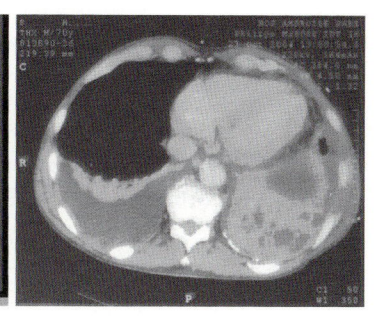

Fig. 29.3 Ultrasound superior to CT, a second example. The *left figure* (CT scan on day 0) indicates an obvious massive left pneumonia, apparently homogeneous. The *middle figure* (ultrasound) shows a pattern typical from necrotizing pneumonia. The *right figure*: CT scan performed on day 5 proves the necrotizing areas. Seen on ultrasound and not on CT: abolished left lung sliding (see Video 35.1)

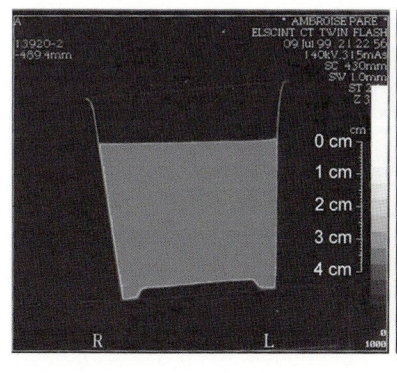

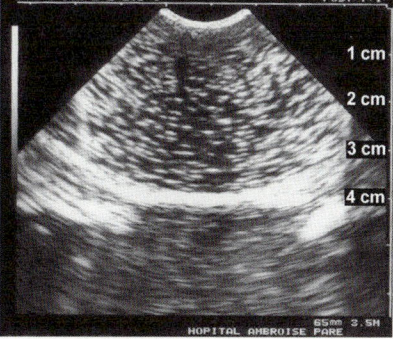

Fig. 29.4 Ultrasound superior to CT, a last example. This simple manipulation uses a transparent container of our Ecolight. The container was shaken before CT and ultrasound acquisitions. From our vision, the fluid seems to be inert. Depth of the bin roughly 4 cm. *Left* (CT): the reader has a nice overview of the bin, but the content is homogeneous, just indicating fluid. *Right* (ultrasound): there is no overview. The bottom of the bin is distorted (the *white stripe* concave to the *top*), but countless particles can be visible. Real time shows random whirling dynamics of these particles. Neither CT nor the eye is able to see these particles or this dynamic whirling. The reader can then chose between a nice overview and a deep vision of the real matter. We thank Marina Perennec who activated the CT scan room for this demonstration

Table 29.3 Published performance of ultrasound compared to CT

	Sensitivity (%)	Specificity (%)
Pleural effusion (*Intensive Care Med* 25:955–958)	94	97
Lung consolidation (*Intensive Care Med* 30:276–281)	90	98
Interstitial syndrome (*Am J Respir Crit Care Med* 156:1640–1646)	93	93
Complete pneumothorax not including lung point (*Intensive Care Med* 25:383–388)	100	96
Occult pneumothorax including lung point (*Crit Care Med* 33:1231–1238)	79	100

All these issues are strong points of ultrasound. Table 29.3 shows that the performance of ultrasound, when compared to high-resolution CT in ARDS patients, is not far from 100 %. Slightly inferior to CT here, clearly superior there, we think that the resultant could make ultrasound a reasonable bedside gold standard in the critically ill. The HICTTUS-exercise allows to reproduce the CT results in function of ultrasound: next section.

Some Legitimate Indications for Traditional Imaging

We fully agree that in a diffuse lung aggression, an initial radiograph would provide an overview. Once in the ICU, probably one radiograph every 2 days would be fine. After a venous line insertion, if it matters to know the exact location of the tip, the radiograph would be indicated. When lung abscesses are suspected, after failure of an ultrasound done in good conditions (good echogenicity, good consolidation windows, etc.), and when complex disorders are suspected (pneumatoceles, multiple adhesions generating complex cases of pneumothorax with bridles, worsening of the clinical and gazometric conditions *with noncontributive Pink-protocol*), the patient can be even referred to CT. The daily practice will specify more clearly, in the decades to come, the real place of radiograph and CT, disease per disease. Overall studies including both the benefits in terms of fast diagnoses, immediate recovery, delayed diseases due to irradiation, and global costs (…) would not be the easiest, we guess. They would raise ethical issues, since control groups where LUCI would not be used at all would have to be defined.

The HICTTUS, a Small Exercise, an Interesting Outcome

We had imagined the RIFLE-exercise (radiography inferred from lung echography), but recently learned that this acronym was taken in the nephrology world before the time to publish ours. Well, the HIBRUU-test, "How Inferring Bedside Radiography Using Ultrasound", was then born. Then, LUCIBIRD (Lung Ultrasound in the Critically Ill at the Blackboard for Inferring Radiographic Disorders) sounded more neutral. Then, for making short, the HIRTUS came, How Inferring Radiography of the Thorax Using Sonography. Quite a game. And in the same time the HICTTUS for… CT, see at the end.

HIRTUS and HICTTUS were not confusing, the exercise was original: the labels were accepted by the SLAM (see the section on "The SLAM" in Chap. 37).

Just take a piece of chalk and a sponge and draw on a blackboard how the bedside chest radiography should look like using LUCI. It begins by a rough lung silhouette. The chalk is gently applied through the lung silhouette for drawing the basic lung parenchyma. The rules of the "game" can be written:

An A-profile will be drawn as no action on the blackboard.
An A'-profile with a lung point: if anterior up to the middle axillary line, no action; if latero-posterior, homogeneous black area (use the sponge) outside a line, the radiological pleural line; if very posterior or absent, fully black area with chalk at the hilum (retracted lung).
The B-profile or B'-profile with septal rockets: no action on the keyboard.

The B- or B'-profile with ground-glass rockets: some haze (put some more chalk).
The A/B-profile: haze images at the B side.
The C-profile: depending on the size, from no change to marked pieces of chalk.
Lung pulse: no action (radioccult phenomenon).
Static air bronchogram: with the small finger, erase linear areas of chalk in creating air bronchograms.
Dynamic air bronchogram: the same (no difference will be seen on radiograph).
PLAPS: using the chalk, blunted sulcus if substantial, direct images of effusion or consolidation if very substantial.
Extensive PLAPS with extensive C-profile: white lung.

Perfectionists can look at the heart and enlarge at will the cardiac silhouette.

One can compete at will. And we let the technicians making the traditional bedside radiograph, wait and compare. HIRTUS just allows to show (to not convinced colleagues) how far lung ultrasound is rich in real information. It will also indicate clearly the limitations of bedside radiography: several ultrasound disorders appear radioccult (mainly anterior pneumothorax, interstitial syndrome, minute PLAPS).

The best experts will use the HICTTUS-exercise, "How Inferring Computerized Tomography of Thorax Using Sonography." Take into account only life-threatening disorders (CT remains a good tool for other lesions). The only risk is to see appear a rictus at the face of some radiologists: they would maybe not like the perspective to have missed (and denied) such a vital potential during so many decades. Please, don't call it the RICTUS-protocol, even if it would be easier to remember.

The LUCI-FLR Project in Action: Example of the Pneumothorax

Patients seen in the ER usually benefit from one anteroposterior radiograph. Let us temporarily accept this tradition, fully foreseen by the LUCI-FLR spirit. On the other hand, we put maximal energy for eradicating useless profile incidences or these dangerous expiratory radiographs. Once admitted, the patient benefits from a chest tube insertion planned according to the lung point location, i.e., far from it. We do not use the traditional clinical landmarks (we forgot them) nor data from radiographs, since usually the patient is not in the same position between radiography (erect) and chest tube insertion (bedside). The tube is fixed, and the nurse makes the vacuum. Ultrasound can check that the return of the lung to the wall is progressive.

Where is the tube? No matter! If an A'-profile is replaced by an A-profile, the tube works. If the tube has been inserted at a distance from the lung point, it cannot be intra-parenchymatous.

Then for every next step (clamping, tube withdrawal), the lung can be monitored on ultrasound alone, especially in a pregnant woman or a child. Lung sliding or equivalents (lung pulse) indicate that there is no need for radiographs. We usually keep an M-mode image of the seashore sign (e.g., with the mention of "upper BLUE-point") as a proof, much more reassuring than a radiograph.

When the tube is clamped, persistence of anterior lung sliding means that the leakage has been sealed, and recurrence of an A'-profile means the opposite.

A last ultrasound view is taken after tube withdrawal, and the patient can go home. With such a management, only the initial radiograph should be found in the patient's file (in the absence of pregnancy). An average number of 8.8 radiographs is taken for an idiopathic pneumothorax [27].

Some colleagues would find pathetical to invest in lung ultrasound for avoiding irradiation, knowing that a CT may be scheduled for documenting this idiopathic pneumothorax, i.e., 200–400 doses of a single radiograph. The main information, i.e., search for contralateral anomalies, is of little relevance: 89 % of patients have such anomalies, and CT cannot predict a recurrence of pneumothorax [28].

The LUCI-FLR Project in Action: Example of the Pulmonary Embolism

The BLUE-protocol is an opportunity to decrease referral to helical CT. Why are all these CTs performed in the ER? Usually because they allow not only to rule out embolism but also to see another cause (pneumonia, edema, etc.). Yet ultrasound also provides these diagnoses. A nude profile (half of the cases of embolism) makes a perfect opportunity to ask not a helical CT but a simple scintigraphy – more elegant and far less irradiating. Usually, the doctors don't ask scintigraphy for the fear of having a noncontributive test. A nude profile allows to foresee that the scintigraphy will be easy to interpret. Just take a look to the uterus for checking the main contraindication: pregnancy (with the same probe: holistic ultrasound, again).

The LUCI-FLR Project in Action: Example of the Pregnancy with Acute Ailments

Once we know that this young lady admitted for lung injury is pregnant, this is the time (now or never) to carefully read the ultrasound user's manual and apply the LUCI-FLR project. The list of complications that can be managed with ultrasound alone is eloquent. In this list, we don't repeat at the end of each application that "irradiating and/or ill-defined radiographies are therefore avoided" and insert "QS" instead:

- This patient can develop pneumonia (aspiration or nosocomial), which is recognized, quantified, and followed up under therapy. QS
- A pleural effusion is directly drained. Some of the complications (e.g., pneumothorax after blind thoracentesis) are also decreased. QS
- Iatrogenic pneumothorax can be drained and followed up. QS
- A subclavian catheter is safely inserted, avoiding pneumothorax, or arterial puncture. QS.
- The correct position of a gastric tube is checked visually. QS
- Abdominal complications such as hollow organ perforation, peritonitis, etc., bring the patient to the operating room directly, QS, including these poorly informative plain abdominal radiographs.
- Venous thromboses and acute dyspnea due to pulmonary embolism directly benefit from heparin. QS
- Maxillary sinusitis is under control. QS

Probably, a whole textbook could be written around this philosophy: using ultrasound as a visual and pacific medicine.

LUCI-FLR Project Can Reduce Irradiation? Fine. But if There Is No Available Irradiation?

Two worlds have a common point: very few spaceships lost in the infinity of the space and disinherited people of countless austere areas of the world. For these few astronauts or these billions of people, there is no alternative. When radiography is not an option, ultrasound's interest does not need long explanations. This is the definite future for these two opposed kinds of patients.

References

1. Mueller NL (1993) Imaging of the pleura, state of the art. Radiology 186:297–309
2. McLoud TC, Flower CDR (1991) Imaging the pleura: sonography, CT and MR imaging. Am J Roentgenol 156:1145–1153
3. Matalon TA, Neiman HL, Mintzer RA (1983) Noncardiac chest sonography, the state of the art. Chest 83:675–678
4. Desai SR, Hansel DM (1997) Lung imaging in the adult respiratory distress syndrome: current practice and new insights. Intensive Care Med 23:7–15
5. Ivatury RR, Sugerman HJ (2000) Chest radiograph or computed tomography in the intensive care unit? Crit Care Med 28:1033–1039
6. Roentgen WC (1895) Ueber eine neue art von Strahlen. Vorlaüfige Mittheilung Sitzungsberichte der Wurzburger Physik-mediz Gesellschaft 28:132–141
7. Williams FH (1901) The Roentgen rays in medicine and surgery. Macmillan, New York
8. van der Werk TS, Zijlstra JG (2004) Ultrasound of the lung: just imagine. Intensive Care Med 30:183–184
9. Greenbaum DM, Marschall KE (1982) The value of routine daily chest X-rays in intubated patients in the medical intensive care unit. Crit Care Med 10:29–30
10. Henschke CI, Pasternack GS, Schroeder S, Hart KK, Herman PG (1983) Bedside chest radiography: diagnostic efficacy. Radiology 149:23–26
11. Janower ML, Jennas-Nocera Z, Mukai J (1984) Utility and efficacy of portable chest radiographs. AJR Am J Roentgenol 142:265–267
12. Peruzzi W, Garner W, Bools J, Rasanen J, Mueller CF, Reilley T (1988) Portable chest roentgenography and CT in critically ill patients. Chest 93:722–726

References

13. Wiener MD, Garay SM, Leitman BS, Wiener DN, Ravin CE (1991) Imaging of the intensive care unit patient. Clin Chest Med 12:169–198
14. Winer-Muram HT, Rubin SA, Ellis JV, Jennings SG, Arheart KL, Wunderink RG, Leeper KV, Meduri GU (1993) Pneumonia and ARDS in patients receiving mechanical ventilation: diagnostic accuracy of chest radiography. Radiology 188:479–485
15. Tocino IM, Miller MH, Fairfax WR (1985) Distribution of pneumothorax in the supine and semi-recumbent critically ill adult. Am J Roentgenol 144:901–905
16. Hendrikse K, Gramata J, ten Hove W, Rommes J, Schultz M, Spronk P (2007) Low value of routine chest radiographs in a mixed medical-surgical ICU. Chest 132:823–828
17. United Nations Scientific Committee on the Effects of Atomic Radiation (2000) Source and effects of ionizing radiation. United Nations, New York
18. Brenner DJ, Elliston CD, Hall EJ, Berdon WE (2001) Estimated risks of radiation-induced fatal cancer from pediatric CT. Am J Roentgenol 176:289–296
19. Berrington de Gonzales A, Darby S (2004) Risk of cancer from diagnostic X-Rays. Lancet 363:345–351
20. Brenner DJ, Hall EJ (2007) Computed tomography – an increasing source of radiation exposure. N Engl J Med 357(22):2277–2284
21. Lauer MS (2009) Elements of danger – the case of medical imaging. N Engl J Med 361:841–843
22. Felten ML, Mercier FJ, Benhamou D (1999) Development of acute and chronic respiratory diseases during pregnancy. Rev Pneumol Clin 55:325–334
23. Hopper KD, King SH, Lobell ME, Tentlave TR, Weaver JS (1997) The breast: in-plane X-ray protection during diagnostic thoracic CT. Radiology 205:853–858
24. Di Marco AF, Briones B (1993) Is chest CT performed too often ? Chest 103:985–986
25. Akhan O, Demirkazik FB, Ozmen MN et al (1992) Tuberculous pleural effusions: ultrasonic diagnosis. J Clin Ultrasound 20:461–65
26. Lichtenstein D, Peyrouset O (2006) Lung ultrasound superior to CT? The example of a CT-occult necrotizing pneumonia. Intensive Care Med 32:334–335
27. Czarnecki F (1998). Diagnostic et surveillance radiologique des patients atteints de pneumothorax. Intérêt potentiel de l'échographie pulmonaire. Thèse (doctorat en médecine), Faculté Necker, Paris
28. Sahn SA, Heffner JE (2000) Spontaneous pneumothorax. N Engl J Med 342(12):868–874

Lung Ultrasound for the Diagnosis and Management of an Acute Circulatory Failure: The FALLS-Protocol (Fluid Administration Limited by Lung Sonography) – One Main Extension of the BLUE-Protocol

30

The potential of lung ultrasound in detecting interstitial syndrome provides an original piece of information which will be used for the sequential diagnosis of a circulatory failure. In the management of shock, it allows to avoid two issues: giving too much fluid, a concern for the modern generation, and keeping a patient in occult hypovolemia, another killer, probably as substantial. The FALLS-protocol may locate the critically ill patient between these two extreme issues, by proposing the appropriate amount of fluid resuscitation.

Using a simple approach considering a focused part of cardiac sonography, some venous sonography, and this simple part of lung ultrasound which visualizes a direct parameter of volemia, an alternative decision tree for hemodynamic assessment can be proposed.

> It is through error that man tries and rises. All the roads of learning begin in darkness and go out into the light.
> Hippocrate de Cos (460 b. JC/370 b. JC), the father of medicine.

Electronic supplementary material The online version of this chapter (doi:10.1007/978-3-319-15371-1_30) contains supplementary material, which is available to authorized users.

A Few Warnings

This chapter is long (those who are happy with their hemodynamic management can skip it). In spite of its length, it considers two simple elements (the A-line and the B-line) which were never yet taken into consideration in the question of hemodynamic assessment. If simplicity is integrated in a complex field, complex explanations must be given. This is why this chapter is the longest of the textbook (we even bet that, like the chapter on the BLUE-protocol of our 2010 edition is now a whole textbook, this chapter will make our next textbook).

The reader is invited to think different. The FALLS-protocol turns around one main idea: in a domain where "everything has been said," but where passion still rules, shouldn't the introduction of a fully new concept (based on logic, on the early detection of a precious data: lung fluid overload) be a help, even partial? We admire the high level and the highly respectable knowledge of most intensivists and world experts in hemodynamics. We are aware that our ambition may appear a bit provocative, and it is with the highest level of humility that we propose a new concept. For achieving this aim, one's current knowledge should temporarily be forgotten, just the time for being able to understand the spirit of the FALLS-protocol. The usual targets (cardiac index changes, etc.) are not used here for instance. After this effort, the readers will take again their usual practice and use a bit, or more, as they feel, of the FALLS-protocol in their daily practice. We know that we ask huge efforts to some.

This chapter is the latest *avatar* of chapter 23 of our 2010 edition. Numerous questions, comments, criticisms heard here and there were answered, resulting in multiple changes. The spirit was unchanged, but many details were adapted for increasing the logic of the FALLS-protocol. We again took great care for making this chapter as moderate as possible and fully open to criticisms. The FALLS-protocol proposes a parameter which can be criticized like all parameters in this field, but whose peculiarity is to provide a *direct* assessment of the clinical volemia.

For performing the FALLS-protocol, which takes mainly simple cardiac sonography and lung ultrasound (both caval veins if needed), our simple unit with its 5 MHz microconvex probe is usually perfect.

Evolution of Concepts Considering Hemodynamic Assessment in the Critically Ill. Which Is the Best One? And for How Long?

The bedside work of the intensivist is to provide adequate oxygen output to the tissues. Our obsessive work is to answer this question: "How to better feed these mitochondria?" All in critical care turns around this.

Before ICUs were created (in the mid-1950s), the patients in circulatory failure died. Then, the physicians in charge of these new units did their best, using the central venous pressure (CVP), until the Swan-Ganz catheter, developed, in the early 1970s, provided more precise data, which gave them the feeling to go in a direction assumed to be the good one [1].

The Swan-Ganz catheter measures the pulmonary artery occlusion pressure (PAOP) [1, 2]. The PAOP informs on left ventricular (LV) end-diastolic pressure [2–5]. This PAOP classically guides fluid therapy [6] and defines risk for hydrostatic pulmonary edema [3, 7].

After decades of use, the Swan-Ganz catheter experiences difficult times. Some considered possible side effects [8], a questionable usefulness [7–23], and others a suboptimal use of a potentially interesting method [24–26]. Alternative techniques were considered such as echocardiography – long accessible by transthoracic approach, and by trans-esophageal approach, a 1976 concept [27], which became so current that we now benefit from disposable TEE probes [28]. These techniques made the Swan-Ganz catheter definitely obsolete [29–39]. Since TEE was not easily accessible (cost, training), other tools were developed, mainly continuous cardiac output devices for assessing lung water (PICCO), esophageal Doppler, pulse pressure variation, pulse contour analysis, pulse analysis of the arterial pressure, sophisticated oxygen transport assessment, or again microcirculation assessment and derived, such as gastric tonometry, sublingual capnometry, laser Doppler flowmetry, near-infrared spectroscopy, gravimetry, and so on [40–51]. Each year, a new tool merges, advocating to definitely solve the problem.

All methods, up to the most recent, are compared to previous ones. The initial reference was the LV catheterization, to which the Swan-Ganz catheter was compared (with accuracy <100 %), and subsequent tools were compared to the Swan-Ganz catheter (with accuracy <100 %). From study to study, the distortion may be substantial with the historical LV catheterization. Even this "floor" is not a direct tool for measuring clinical volemia. Therefore, how about the real value of the most recent tools?

And they provide so many data. If we take a minimal distance, we just may feel disconcerted by the left column of Table 30.1. This impressive list of data extracted from these multiple tools is probably the best proof, ab absurdo, that no gold standard really exists. We know that no isolated, static parameter of preload status is valuable for predicting fluid responsiveness [52, 53]. This assumption indicates that we do not have the direct parameter. The struggle that opposes PAC, TEE, PICCO, etc., gets routine – a godsend for the manufacturers, but some intensivists may feel a little blind in their daily work.

For lack of any perfect gold standard, the point is now to know which patients will increase their

Table 30.1 Usual data and usual therapeutic possibilities in acute circulatory failure

Data derived from various approaches	Therapeutic consequences
Aortic blow velocity	
Arterial pH	Fluids or not
Arterial pulse pressure	
Arterial systolic or pulse pressure variation	Inotropics or not[a]
Capillary wedge pressure	
Cardiac output	Vasopressors or not[b]
Cardiac index	
Central venous pressure	
Central venous oxygen saturation	
Color Doppler regurgitant flow assessment (mitral regurgitation)	
Continuous wave Doppler velocities of tricuspid insufficiency	
Continuous wave Doppler velocities of pulmonary insufficiency	
Cardiac output change following passive leg raising	
Delta PP	
DTE, deceleration time of mitral Doppler Es wave	
E/A waves	
E = maximal Doppler velocity of early diastolic mitral wave	
A = maximal Doppler velocity of late diastolic mitral wave during atrial contraction	
E/E′ – pulsed wave Doppler recorded at the tip of the mitral valve (E)	
E′ = maximal tissue Doppler velocity of early diastolic displacement of the mitral annulus	
End diastolic left ventricular dimension	
End diastolic left ventricular area	
Expired CO_2	
Esophageal Doppler	
Extravascular lung water	
Gastric tonometry	
Global right ventricle size	
Global right ventricle systolic function	
Global left ventricle systolic function	
Heart rate	
Heterogenous left ventricle contraction	
Inferior vena cava collapsibility index	
Intracardiac shunts	
Intrapulmonary shunts	
Laser Doppler flowmetry	
Left ventricle end-diastolic pressure	
Left ventricular diastolic elastance: active relaxation and passive compliance	
Lactic acid	
Mottled skin	
Near-infrared spectroscopy	
Output impedance	
Paradoxical septal motion	
Pulse wave Doppler velocities of right ventricle outflow	
Pulse contour analysis	
Pulse analysis of the arterial pressure	
Pericardial fluid assessment	
Pulmonary artery diastolic pressure	
Pulmonary artery mean pressure	
Pulmonary artery occlusion pressure	
Pulmonary artery systolic pressure	
Pulsed wave Doppler recorded at the tip of the mitral valve	
Pulsed wave Doppler recorded in upper left pulmonary vein	
Pulse pressure variations	
Respiratory systolic variation	
Respiratory variations of maximal Doppler velocity of aortic blood flow	
Right ventricular end-diastolic area	
Right ventricular elastance	
Right ventricle outflow Doppler patterns	
Restrictive flow (E/A ≥2, DTE <120 ms) at the pulmonary vein	
Systemic resistances	
Systolic fraction of the pulmonary vein flow	
Systolic blood pressure	
Systolic pressure variation	
Stressed vascular volume	
Stroke volume variation	
Sublingual capnometry	
Superior vena cava collapsibility index	
Tricuspid annular plane systolic expansion	
Urine output	

[a]Usually decided from two-dimensional left ventricle analysis
[b]Usually deduced from other parameters

cardiac output of more than 15 %. Those who don't would have only the risk of pulmonary edema, for no benefit. This originated elegant concepts. Fluid responsiveness is a concept based on pathophysiology of fluid dynamics [36, 40, 47, 54–56]. It is a current standard, widely used nowadays. Looking at the cardiac Doppler values for knowing the volemic status is an elegant approach, and we take major interest to data extracted from this field: restrictive flows, E/E′ ratio, etc. We just wonder how long is needed for a current investigation, how precise it is (how wide is the gray zone in current practice), how high is the expertise required for a 24/7/365 use in any hospital, and mostly how far these data are direct ways to show the lung damage in case of fluid overload, as elegant can these methods be.

We have the same questions regarding other arising concepts, such as this elegant one of abdominal compartment syndrome [57, 58]. Even if all these techniques would work perfectly, they would just tell that the patient increases (or not) the cardiac output. Do these techniques tell the patient *needed* such an increase is a quandary which we point as central in the spirit of the FALLS-protocol (which as we will see uses a different approach for answering). In late disorders of septic shock comes the far more subtle situation where microcirculation alterations, capillary leak, interstitial and endothelial cell edema, hyperchloremic acidosis, coagulopathy, etc., are mingling, time for multiple organ failure [59, 60]. At this step, it is even not clear whether the tissues really require supplementations in oxygen. The question is probably no longer about the quantity of fluid to administer, whatever the tool used – the usual strategies for hemodynamic optimization become of limited efficiency [61, 62]. Knowing at any price that the cardiac output of a shocked patient increases under fluid therapy is questionable if it is of no benefit to this patient.

Consequently, in the ICU corridors and congresses – a constant phenomenon since the day we began in intensive care (1985) – multiple voices sing dissonant songs. This may confuse those worried by the feeling they may work blindly, whereas the others feel fully reassured using one given approach (PICCO here, ECHO there, etc.). The latter ones argue to the former ones that they did not understand the tool or did not read the user guide, etc. Habits, more than evidence-based medicine, seem to rule. If we are not fully wrong, medicine is not an exact science, and this makes the bed for authoritative behaviors.

In this peak of complexity, where some advocate a return to more simplicity [63], simple maneuvers [32, 64], every point can be debated, even the place of familiar parameters such as cardiac output: not everyone admits its targeting may affect patient's outcome [65], and expert opinions do not recommend its routine measurement [66]. Each current tool has advantages and drawbacks [67]. Table 30.2 shows some of them.

Probably, the modern medicine has progressed with respect to the era of the CVP. Probably, the issues of hemodynamic therapy are partly solved using modern tools. However, we still hear discordant comments in the corridors of the many ICUs we have the privilege to visit trough the world: read Anecdotal Note 1. These comments probably reflect the real life of usual ICUs.

Table 30.2 Comparison between some hemodynamic methods

	Cost	Invasiveness	Technical easiness	Monitoring possibilities	Overall duration[a]	Direct approach to interstitial pulmonary edema	Global rating[b]
PAC	Low – 0	High – 2	Relative – 1	Yes – 0	Long – 2	No – 1	6
TEE	High – 2	Relative – 1	Long training – 2	Limited – 1	Rather long – 1	No – 1	8
PICCO	Relative – 1	High – 2	Easy – 0	Limited – 1	Long – 2	No – 1	7
FALLS-protocol	Low – 0	Nil – 0	Easy – 0	Easy – 0	Fast – 0	Yes – 0	0

[a]Including sterilization, dressings to the patient, etc.
[b]Roughly giving a very approximative notation between 3 and 4 values

To the classical question: Which technique(s) should I introduce in my ICU? Which ones are the good ones? Between progresses and trends, admitting the hypothesis that what is modern is good, may we oppose the notion of the *sinusoidal profile*? A revolutionary novelty of 1 day is forgotten when the next tool is available. Initial enthusiasm for a novelty, full discredit some years later (usually one decade), and more balanced conclusions after prolonged use, this is a familiar tune. Like a single voice, the whole community goes left. Several years after, it makes the opposite turn, and so on. This profile, seen in 100 instances, makes winners and losers of one day. For example, the supranormal value in oxygen delivery in the septic shock was an honorable target [68], before being discredited [69]. Corticoids in sepsis, new immunotherapies in sepsis, etc., up to fluid therapy, typically obey to this sinusoid. During decades, in the hot minutes of shock management, doctors gave fluids cautiously with the fear of the major issue, pulmonary edema [3]. Then they faced this issue of insufficient fluid therapy, keeping the patient in occult hypovolemia (with hemodynamic risk if vasoactive drugs were administered together). Then they were taught to give (early and) massive fluid therapy in septic shock [70]. This has ruled during more than one decade as an evidence. And now, this protocol is thoroughly and completely discredited [61, 71, 72]. This sinusoid music rhythms our life of intensivists. It makes it, it is true, somehow exciting, a "hot" profession definitely, where we can hear prestigious and passionate tenors sharing their point of view on a question which fills the congresses, with complex, thrilling pro/con debates between experts.

So currently, a strong ruling idea, the reality (of today) is a limitation in fluid therapy. Recommendations of yesterday ("early and massive fluid therapy in sepsis") are now erased by modern spectacular teasers: "Dry, the patient survives. Wet, the patient dies." The *must* is the "dry attitude." Without nuance, "fluids kill," etc. These old and new trends arose and arise from prestigious journals (the EGDT as well as its executors). Now, the patient will benefit from the modern trend, built by the Surviving Sepsis Campaign Guidelines, ProCESS, ARISE, and "other" FEAST, FIRST, CRYSTAL, and 6S trial. All in all, the consensus seems to express that the early steps (minutes, hours) should make liberal fluid therapy, whereas the later steps (days, weeks) should be conservative. From all these orders and counterorders which spread from congresses and corridors, we have the confused feeling (possibly completely wrong) that currently the trend is to definitely keep the patient dry to the point that standard physicians feel nearly guilty when they prescribe fluids. There should be no place for emotion, only for facts, yet medicine is still medicine: again, how do we locate our patient within the middle part of this familiar curve indicating the area of optimal volume load [73]?

Some teasers, as far as we understood, seem more balanced than the trend (from Michael Pinsky without mistake): "Dry lungs, happy lungs. Dry liver, dead liver." Would this mean that not all the current voices run in the same direction like one man? Is the problem not completely solved? Other sounds, from respectable key-opinion leaders, seem to point out that the great recent studies which invalidated the EGDT are possibly more of an opportunity to publish than a real advance. They insist on the point that time is of essence. As students, we had the slight idea that in a critically ill patient, it was better to be fast than slow. So none of these guidelines really changed our practice to consider a shock as an emergency.

Fluids kill. Let us admit. Our candid question is: for how long? Should we keep nothing from our previous concepts, without nuance? Physicians now know (or think they know) that too liberal fluid therapy is not good, but do they have the tool which indicates the endpoint with certitude?

We understand that simple ultrasound is introduced in a delicate setting, still open for some [74], less for others who apparently possess the right tool [75].

Can a different approach be considered for the longstanding problem of hemodynamic assessment?

Can our beloved principle of simplicity be used in such a complex field?

Can We Simplify Such a Complex Field? The Starting Point of the FALLS-Protocol

The two basic questions are simple: can this given patient receive fluid therapy? Once initiated, how to determine the endpoint? These questions originated various schools, but did not receive a definite answer admitted by all, *to our knowledge and without mistake*.

An anxious intensivist, willing to give maximal security to this critically ill patient, would insert a Swan-Ganz catheter, plus a PICCO device, make liberal echocardiography, and use all other possible tools. This intensivist would benefit from an impressive list (Table 30.1). Look at a remarkable point: on the left, this huge amount of data (Table 30.1, left column) and on the right, such a limited list of practical options (Table 30.1, right column). Apart from disobstruction of an obstacle (clot, gas, pericardial fluid), apart from specific therapies of given causes of shock (e.g., hemodiafiltration in septic shock, etc.), there are just three options for trying to stabilize a shocked patient: inotropics, vasopressors, and fluids. Just these three limited options – for saving a life – whatever the quality and sophistication of very fine articles [1–76].

Let us study Table 30.1. Shall we say to our nurse that the value of the indexed LV end diastolic volume is 1.23 ml or 109.15 l? What would the nurse understand? She, or he, waits rather precise instructions, to give, or not to give fluids. When we have to give precise instructions, things get suddenly extremely simple in terms of choice (again): inotropics or not, vasopressors or not, fluids or not.

Now, these three options (not a lot) can be reduced to just *one*. Inotropics are usually given from a gray-scale echocardiographic view; the vasopressive option is calculated from the two other parameters. This means that the biggest challenge in the hemodynamic management of a shock is "just" the question of fluid therapy.

The contrast between the left and right columns of Table 30.1 (i.e., the major complexity of usual tests and the so simple alternative "fluids or no fluids") was the starting point of the FALLS-protocol.

How to recognize those lungs which are still dry from those already wet? *Can lung ultrasound be of any help?* While carefully respecting all positions, we felt free to add *one more data* to the impressive left column of Table 30.1: lung ultrasound – A-lines and B-lines precisely. Interstitial edema was one application of ultrasound [77] with clinical uses [78, 79]. Thinking that any new idea in this symphony should be considered – if it can provide any help, even minor, even debatable – our idea is to take, again, our 29-cm wide gray-scale ultrasound unit with its simple microconvex probe, the one which we used already for carrying on 100 life-saving applications.

Would lung rockets help in assessing the lung tolerance to fluid therapy, i.e., fluid administration limited by lung sonography (i.e., FALLS-protocol)? In our 2010 edition, the FALLS-protocol was part of the slightly pompous "limited investigation considering hemodynamic therapy." Now for making short, the FALLS-protocol is this multi-organ approach, including heart and lungs (and veins if needed).

May the FALLS-protocol answer to these two basic questions, purposely recalled:
- Can fluid therapy be initiated in this patient?
- If yes, can the endpoint, where the risk is superior to the benefit, be determined?

Three Critical Pathophysiological Notes for Introducing the FALLS-Protocol

1. *Pathophysiological reminder of pulmonary edema. The relationship between PAOP and ultrasound lung artifacts*

    Pulmonary edema combines hemodynamic and respiratory phenomena, long understood [3, 80–86]. Acute hemodynamic pulmonary edema occurs after the left heart has reached the inflexion point of the Frank-Starling curve, and the end-diastolic LV pressure increases. The capillary pressure and the PAOP are always increased. The transudate invades the interstitial compartment first, with constant interstitial edema. Interstitial edema is an early, *silent step* which precedes alveolar edema. Within this early phenomenon of interstitial edema, the excess fluid first accumulates along the interlobular septa, a non-respiratory part of the interstitial tissue which is not involved in gas exchanges (they occur at the alveolocapillary membrane). The interlobular septa behave like "puisards" (French term, possibly translatable in passive containers), protecting the gas exchanges in the initial step [86]. Then, when lymphatic resorption capacity is exceeded, fluids invade the alveoli. This step initiates alveolar edema, with now clinical signs (dyspnea, rales), radiologic changes, and gas exchange impairment, i.e., the situation that no intensivist wants to reach. At the interstitial step, since the fluids accumulate under pressure, all interlobular septa are filled, including their anterior, nondependent subpleural part – a feature fully accessible to lung ultrasound: lung rockets appear. The B-profile.

Our study in the critically ill showed a correlation between the A-profile and low PAOP values. The A-profile indicates a PAOP ≤18 mmHg with 93 % specificity (Fig. 30.1) (Appendix A.1) [87]. Schematically, A-lines correspond to dry lungs, lung rockets to wet lung, i.e., pulmonary edema, from hemodynamic (with high PAOP) or permeability-induced (with low PAOP) cause [77].

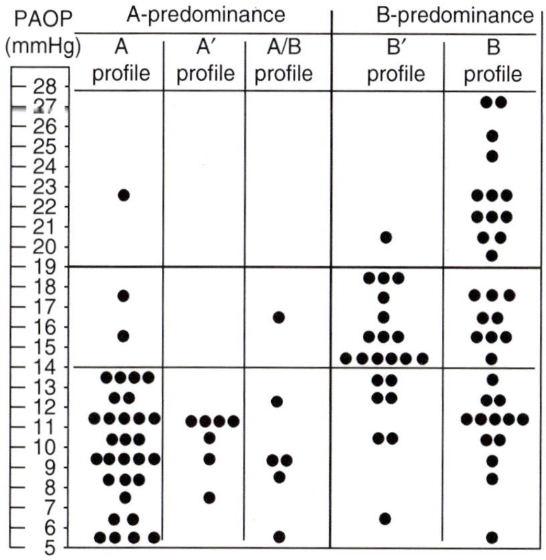

From our study, if an A-profile indicates a PAOP "lower than 18 mmHg," it means that between 0 and 18 mm, the A-profile is the same: healthy subjects and deeply hypovolemic patients display the same A-profile. More relevant, if we see A-lines just transforming into B-lines, the PAOP has just reached the value of 18 mmHg.

2. *A-lines are dichotomous to B-lines: there is no known intermediate artifact*

After 26 years of daily observations, i.e., hours and hours looking at a screen, we were able to describe only two main lung artifacts, one horizontal (the A-line) and one vertical (the B-line). This means that there is no intermediate artifact. This also means that the B-line appears (as well as vanishes) all of a sudden. A-lines are dichotomous to B-lines, without space for other patterns. Lung ultrasound is, definitely, a dichotomous discipline.

The normal subpleural interlobular septa are thin, too thin for being traversed by the ultrasound beam, and this results in A-lines. If we enlarge the septum slightly, by giving fluid therapy while blocking the kidneys, it will first still be too small for generating a change in the artifact. If this fluid therapy is resumed, from a critical amount of fluid, the septum will be enlarged enough for allowing the ultrasound beam to penetrate into the lung. This penetration is minute, less than 1 mm, yet it is sufficient for allowing the B-line to be generated, all of a sudden, like a nuclear chain reaction. We remind the principle N°2 of lung ultrasound: the artifacts come from the mingling between two components with major acoustic impedance gradient: air and water, both present here.

The difference between thin septa and thicker septa, demonstrated by an ON-OFF mechanism generating A-lines then B-lines, is a *volume*. This volume is the fluid capacity of the whole interlobular septal network. Probably the physiologists know this volume, which we guess is small, a few milliliters. However, even small, this volume has a highly strategic relevance for detecting fluid overload. This difference of volume, occurring at the most vital organ, which is normally fluid-free, is accessible to lung ultrasound. This may provide a *direct parameter of volemia*. The way is opened for using the FALLS-protocol (Fig. 30.2).

Fig. 30.1 The correlation between PAOP and lung ultrasound. This graph indicates a quasi-desert area in patients with low PAOP and absence of lung rockets. As expected, lung rockets, indicating either hemodynamic or permeability-induced pulmonary edema, are seen with high and low PAOP, precluding conclusions on the PAOP value. Yet there is an empty space. One empty space? The door opened to scientific rules. Note the other empty space between high PAOP and B′-profile (Permission of CHEST pending)

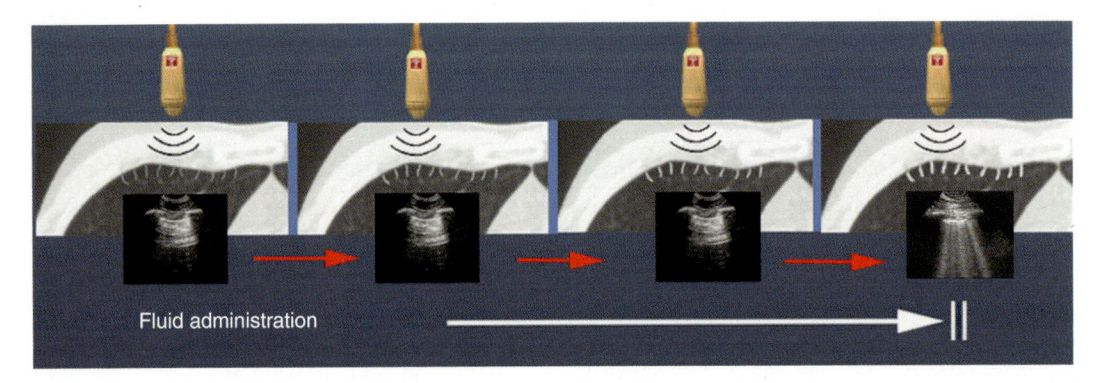

Fig. 30.2 The concept of the swelling septa. Fluid therapy under sonographic control. On the left image (lung CT), subpleural interlobular septa are drawn. Fine, they yield A-lines. Under fluid therapy, on the second and third steps, one can see the septa regularly thickening, without ultrasound change. At the last, right step, from a very level of septal edema, the lung artifacts suddenly become B-lines (here, lung rockets). At this level, we witness a fluid overload at the early, silent step. We see also, of high importance, that whereas the septa gradually enlarge, the artifacts suddenly go up from state A to state B, at a precise threshold. Here, at the fourth step, the PAOP has just reached the value of 18 mmHg: Enough fluid was given. The two vertical lines symbolize the practical action of the FALLS-protocol: discontinuing fluid therapy. This is a dichotomous rule: only A-lines or B-lines have been described, with no intermediate step

3. *Another level of dichotomy*

   Observation in our critically ill patients shows that in terms of fluid overload, in a wide given territory (lateral, anterior), there is little space for intermediate, patchy patterns. Under the influence of hemodynamic changes, all septa of a given area are rapidly invaded by the edema, provided lungs are healthy, spared from scars, focal emphysema, etc. Focusing on this area in a critically ill patient, lung ultrasound offers a qualitative, dichotomous approach: A-predominance versus B-predominance.

Three Critical Tools Just Before Using the FALLS-Protocol

Lung ultrasound was not supposed to exist. It now advocates to provide a direct parameter of volemia. This calls for some precautions, and we will need three critically important tools:

1. *Humility*

   Humility should be the most important: hemodynamic assessment is one of the most complex fields in critical care. The FALLS-protocol does not pretend to suddenly solve all dilemmas met in the daily life of the intensivist. It is completely open to any suggestion, any comment, and any criticism. Up to now, the numerous criticisms made here and there resulted in nice refinements in the concept.

2. *Logic*

   The FALLS-protocol is based upon a pathophysiological approach. Data are available [87].

3. *Pragmatism*

   This is a popular tool in critical care. Each method has limits (Table 30.2). Swan-Ganz catheters are now rarely used. PICCO (apart from its invasiveness) needs some delay to be all set. Echocardiography can be in failure for various reasons: first, most patients on Earth will never see such a technique. Second, the young intensivist needs a long training for this expert discipline. Third, it is never possible to predict that a given patient will have suitable cardiac windows. Fourth, regarding its most advanced development (trans-esophageal echocardiography), apart from the same drawbacks, here exaggerated (access to the planet, etc.), and from the time needed, issues may always appear: non-availability (sterilization on process), failure from breakdown, contra-indication such as recent esophageal surgery. The (good) intensivist (all intensivists are good) is always ready for an alternative tool, the famous "plan B," ready to use.

Practical Progress of a FALLS-Protocol

We visit a shocked patient. The physical examination may be sufficient (typical pulsus paradoxus, etc.) or not. In this case, ultrasound is of major help. We use the Max Harry Weil's classification of shocks [88], slightly adapted for allowing a sequential use of ultrasound (Fig. 30.3). Since the heart is a traditional site for answering this question, we have respected this vital organ by dealing with it first, in a simplified model. The FALLS-protocol suggests to place lung ultrasound immediately after. For a schematic demonstration, we assume the case of a patient victim of an acute circulatory failure with fully unknown origin.

The FALLS-protocol

1) Ruling out obstructive shock

Simple emergency cardiac sonography:
    Pericardial tamponade
    Right ventricle dilatation [1]
BLUE-protocol: Pneumothorax
    (A'-profile)

2) Ruling out (left) cardiogenic shock [2]

BLUE-protocol: Pulmonary edema
    (B-profile)

3) Ruling out hypovolemic shock

    (A-profile)
Correction of clinical signs of shock under fluid administration

4) Detecting distributive shock (septic shock usually)

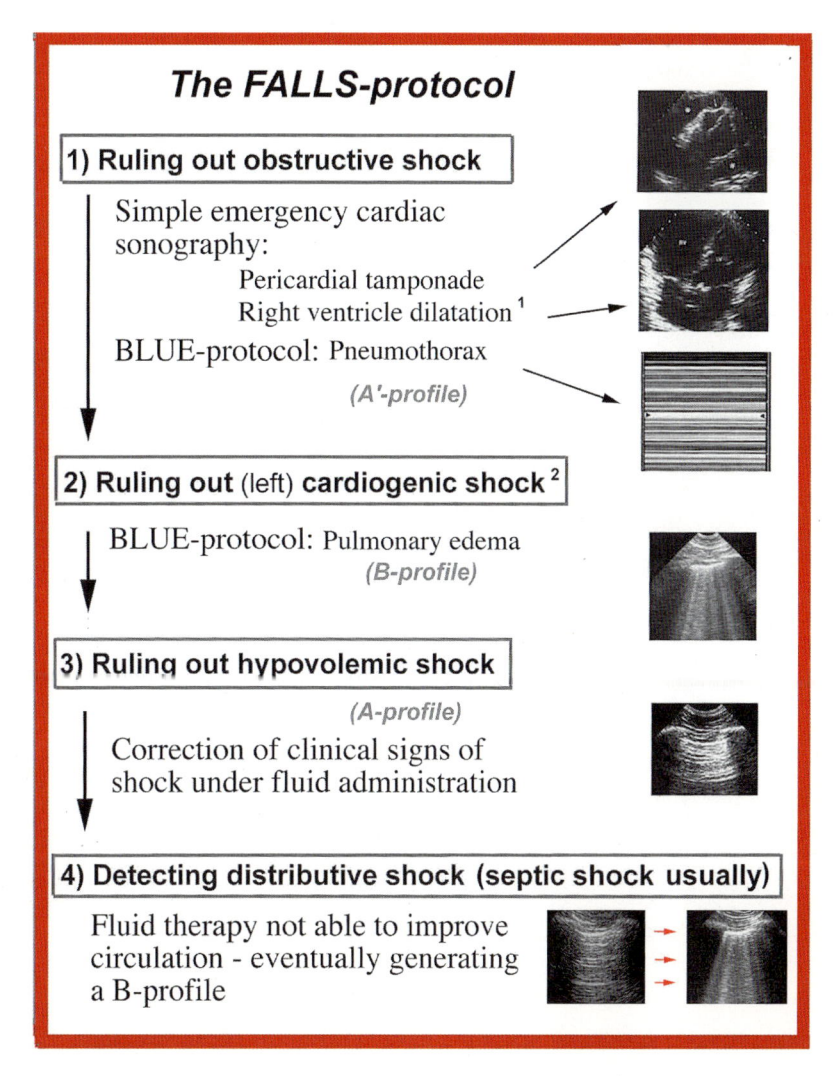

Fluid therapy not able to improve circulation - eventually generating a B-profile

Fig. 30.3 The decision tree of the FALLS-protocol. Using a simple unit, the FALLS-protocol makes a sequential analysis. Obstructive shock is ruled out, and the left cardiogenic shock diagnosed through the constant B-profile. Then fluid therapy is initiated. The hypovolemic shock is diagnosed through an A-profile which remains unchanged while the circulatory failure recovers. The septic shock is diagnosed through the change from an A-profile to a B-profile while the patient remains unstable. Countless subtleties are described in the main text. For sharing a readable, usable decision tree, several branches were cut, such as the withdrawal of fluid once the endpoint has been reached. *1* If there is no cardiac window, the BLUE-protocol can be used instead. The A-profile with a DVT is quite specific to pulmonary embolism. *2* The cardiogenic shock is considered if clinically acceptable. If not, ARDS with shock, or chronic interstitial disease (with shock) should be envisaged. A right cardiogenic shock gives an A-profile (see main text)

Like any traditional shock management, the FALLS-protocol will mingle diagnostic and therapeutic actions. The therapeutic actions will not be "symptomatic" but enlightened.

We use a single probe for expediting the approach of heart, lungs, and veins (and belly): this is holistic ultrasound.

Step 1: Obstructive shock?

The FALLS-protocol begins by the simple emergency cardiac sonography. See in Chap. 19 why and how this approach is different from the numerous protocols developed such as RACE, FATE, FEER, now FOCUS.) (Read Anecdotal Note 2).

(a) *Pericardial tamponade?*

For the novice, Chap. 19 comments on how the diagnosis of pericardial effusion then pericardial tamponade can be simplified. See Video 31.1. Chapter 31 demonstrates how holistic ultrasound allows optimal safe pericardiocentesis (using our microconvex probe better than a cardiac probe).

(b) *Pulmonary embolism?*

In an acute respiratory failure, a RV enlargement is common, seen in COPD, pulmonary embolism, extensive pneumonia, as well as severe asthma. In an acute circulatory failure, such a finding is a major argument favoring pulmonary embolism.

The FALLS-protocol checks the presence of an A-profile, and searches for a DVT. This can also be done without drawback if absent cardiac windows or even routine, since it has a 99 % specificity in the BLUE-protocol [79]: 99 %, just lungs plus veins.

Note: when the FALLS-protocol finds an enlarged RV (or, if no cardiac window, at the next step, an A-profile), an ECG is asked, allowing to detect the exceptional RV infarction. If a B-profile is associated, read below.

(c) *Tension pneumothorax?*

Here, the BLUE-protocol is used without adaptation, same probe, same setting, applied at the anterior BLUE-points (Video 30.1). It will constantly show an A′-profile (Chap. 14).

No substantial pericardial fluid, no cardiac, venous, lung sign of pulmonary embolism, no pneumothorax? The *obstructive shock* is, schematically, ruled out.

At this step, interestingly, note that we did not push on the button "Doppler."

Step 2: Cardiogenic shock?

This is the next step. The B-profile usually indicates hemodynamic pulmonary edema, i.e., here, left (from far) cardiogenic shock. Its origin requires subtle approaches, not dealt with in this textbook (diastolic dysfunction, valvular troubles, etc., diagnosed by expert echocardiography). For the rare cases of cardiogenic shock originating from a right heart failure, please read FAQ N°2.

The B-profile can also come, in a minority of cases, from a lung sepsis. The section on "the case of the B-profile on admission" will show how the caval veins are positioned with respect to the FALLS-protocol.

Chronic interstitial diseases make the last main cause of B-profile on admission. Here, it is bad luck to have a circulatory failure in addition to this respiratory disease, yet in case these two events come by coincidence, Chap. 35 gives the simple clues for distinguishing chronic lung disease from pulmonary edema.

In the absence of a B-profile, a left *cardiogenic shock* can be ruled out.

Note: we still did not push the Doppler button.

Step 3: Hypovolemic shock? The core of the FALLS-protocol. The definition of FALLS-responsiveness

At this step, two major mechanisms of shock have been ruled out. At this step, the remaining causes, i.e., hypovolemic and distributive shock, should practically benefit from one common therapy: fluids.

At this step, how does lung ultrasound look? From the eight profiles of the BLUE-protocol, the B-profile and the A′-profiles have been seen above. Six remain. The three variants of the A-profile make the A-profile. The A/B-profile and the C-profile seen on predominant A-lines around are considered as equivalents of the A-profile. Therefore at this step, the patient has usually the A-profile or equivalents. The B′-profile? Read FAQ 11.

Our study showed that these profiles indicate a low PAOP (Fig. 30.1) [87]. Such patient is decreed FALLS-responder. The state of FALLS-responsiveness implies a clearance for *fluid therapy*. The A-profile, when found at this step, indicates that such patients *can* receive fluid therapy. But it means more. We assume that most physicians will consider that fluids are part of the therapy of distributive shocks. For these physicians, we make our concept explicit: shocked patients, at this step of the FALLS-protocol, *must* receive fluid therapy (Anecdotal Note 4).

A venous line is inserted, fluid therapy is initiated. Which type of fluid (colloid, etc.) is not our debate. One should understand the FALLS-protocol as a therapeutic test – a step expedited at the bedside.

Initiating a fluid therapy with an ultrasound probe applied on the lung, the physician enters into the FALLS-protocol. She/he has determined at this point which patients need fluids, answering to the first of the two main questions.

Fluid therapy begins.

It is administered under the monitoring of clinical parameters (heart frequency, mottling, etc., we let each doctor choose his/her own criteria) and lung ultrasound. Which speed for this fluid therapy and which frequency for the "FALLS-points" (lung ultrasound for analyzing a change in artifacts)? Read FAQ N°4. In the case of an A/B-profile, read Anecdotal Note 3. The physician takes profit of ultrasound for searching a site of hypovolemia, a site of sepsis (an action labelled "round-FALLS-protocol").

Under fluid therapy, two events may occur.
A. The patient improves.
   The improvement of the signs (clinical, biological) of shock under fluid therapy, without change from A-profile to B-profile defines, schematically, the *hypovolemic shock*.
   The origin of this hypovolemia can range from occult bleeding to adrenal failure. This is not in the scope of the FALLS-protocol, which aims at giving a mechanism of shock. Associated signs (not used in the protocol but easy to assess) are a small hypercontractile LV, flattened caval veins.
   For the case of active bleeding, read Anecdotal Note 5.
B. The patient does not improve: time to read the next section.
Still no Doppler used at this step.

Step 4: Septic shock: the climax of the FALLS-protocol. The concept of FALLS-endpoint.

In septic shock, immediate adapted therapy results in a decreased death rate [70, 89, 90]. The last group of the FALLS-protocol is possibly the heaviest.

If the clinical signs of shock resist to fluid therapy, schematically, there is no reason to discontinue it (interrupting at "3,000 ml", e.g., has no scientific basis). Since we obviously reach the conditions of a fluid overload, the more fluid is given, the tighter is the clinical and ultrasound monitoring. Should we introduce norepinephrine at this step? Read FAQ N°13. At one precise moment, a fluid overload will be present and will generate an interstitial syndrome, under the basic rules of pathophysiology (Fig. 30.2). A "new" sign appears, the ultrasound interstitial syndrome. *B-lines replace A-lines*. Lung ultrasound detects the interstitial edema at the earliest step, an infra-clinical and infra-biological step [91]. The lung rockets appear suddenly, although they indicate a soft, continuous change in the septal thickening, with a threshold value, as shown in Fig. 24.1.

The apparition of interstitial changes under fluid therapy indicates that the PAOP is now above (and just above) the value of 18 mmHg [87]. This specific, critical phase has been labelled FALLS-endpoint. At this step, the fluid therapy is discontinued. A hypovolemic shock would have recovered (far before lungs are drowned with fluids). The FALLS-protocol has just answered the second and last main question.

At this step, the protocol orders for several blood tests, including the excellent lactate for assessing the shock, etc., but above all blood cultures. Why several? Why blood cultures?

Why several? A comprehensive answer is made in the FAQ N°5. For hurried readers: this slightly decreases the PAOP.

Why blood cultures? Look carefully at Max Harry Weil's classification. The FALLS-protocol has ruled out, sequentially: obstructive shock, cardiogenic shock, hypovolemic shock. What remains if not distributive shock? And what is distributive shock? In the daily life, anaphylactic shock is usually a clinical diagnosis. The spinal shock is a rarity seen in specific settings. What remains then, if not one of the most familiar challenges in critical care: *septic shock*. Consequently, blood cultures will hopingly find the responsible microbe.

Septic shock is sometimes a simple diagnosis, not requiring the FALLS-protocol (or even ultrasound), and sometimes challenging. The FALLS-protocol just considers the change from horizontal to vertical *artifacts*. Many among the world experts would find this approach a little too simple, not to say bold. This is why we reiterate that, although the FALLS-protocol has been conceived around logic, any comment or criticism is welcome.

For improving the circulation, we can assume that enough fluid was given. It is now time for the vasoactive therapy. The fear of its deleterious side effects if given on still hypovolemic patients has long ruled. At this step, for sure, one can assume these patients are protected – a major potential benefit of the FALLS-protocol. As volemia has been more than optimized, we recommend small initial doses.

All other therapies judged appropriate in this diagnosis of septic shock (renal replacement, etc.) can be given at this step.

Step 4': Other distributive shocks.

The anaphylactic shock requires (among others) fluid therapy [92]. The spinal shock requires (among others) fluid therapy [93]. This means that the FALLS-protocol works here too.

Aside Note of Nice Importance

At this step, we have never used the Doppler button.

The Case of the B-Profile on Admission. Which Management? Are We Still in the FALLS-Protocol? The Place of the Caval Veins

In this latest avatar of the FALLS-protocol, the case of the B-profile is increasingly considered apart.

The B-profile means usually hemodynamic pulmonary edema, and the physician can be satisfied with this diagnosis, if occurring in a suggestive setting. In acute respiratory failure, the B-profile was usually associated with hemodynamic pulmonary edema (in circulatory failure, the word would be cardiogenic shock), rarely pneumonia/ARDS (in circulatory failure, the word would be lung sepsis), exceptionally chronic interstitial lung disease, or CILD (in acute circulatory failure, this would be any coincidental cause of shock); we therefore concentrate only on the first two causes (for CILD, several items, including the simple one of thick free RV wall, usually allow diagnosis, see Chap. 35).

Therefore, when the setting is not simple, cardiogenic shock must be distinguished from lung sepsis with a B-profile. The problem of the FALLS-protocol is simple: a cardiogenic shock does not require fluids (schematically), but a septic shock, yes. The physician has just to gather arguments for lung sepsis. These arguments are numerous, their sum usually allows the diagnosis.

1. First be sure this is a real B-profile (the notion of enlarged B-profile means a liberal scanning for detecting possible C-profiles, or A/B-profiles, or B'-profiles, all fully unusual in hemodynamic pulmonary edema). ARDS, lung sepsis, extensive pneumonia generate a true B-profile in only 14 % of cases. In the other 86 %, we see a B'-profile, C-profile, A/B-profile, or A-no-V-PLAPS-profile [79]. Read Chap. 35 (the section on the diagnosis between pulmonary edema and ARDS).
2. Then make an Extended BLUE-protocol, which is detailed in Chap. 35, and integrates various data:
   - Common sense first.
   - From simple history and simple physical and biological examination: fever, white cells, CRP, BNP, etc.
   - From the simple cardiac sonography:

- *Now* we look at the LV contractility – not at the beginning of the FALLS-protocol (read Anecdotal Note 6). A good contractility slightly favors non-hemodynamic edema (septic shock can generate cardiac hypocontractility). There was no cardiac murmur on auscultation? The possibility of hemodynamic edema with conserved contractility is decreased.
- Now we look at the LV thickness. Absence of hypertrophic LV walls make another small argument against cardiogenic pulmonary edema.
- RV enlargement adds another small element toward lung causes. Note that in the standard sequence, when Step 1 shows a small RV, the protocol goes on to Step 2, which, showing absence of B-line, goes to Steps 3 and 4. Here, we face a RV enlargement with a B-profile. The Extended BLUE-protocol asks a venous analysis (since pulmonary embolism, in 2 % of cases, has the B-profile). No DVT? This association clearly favors the diagnosis of ARDS.

- From the early thoracentesis, which, distinguishing exudate from transudate, quite answers the question.
- From any other tool at the discretion of the clinician, including expert echocardiography-Doppler and any other imaging modality.
- From the caval veins analysis, see below. Only a flattened inferior caval vein (IVC) is a slight more invitation for a fluid therapy. We can see here that the IVC, jammed between major tools, has a rather small place in the FALLS-protocol.

By adding these elements one after another, we eventually benefit from a solid evidence for distinguishing these two basic entities: cardiogenic shock versus ARDS. The BLUE-protocol played a basic role. Now, the question is no longer: what is the diagnosis (the answer is, e.g., lung sepsis); the question is: how to know the needs in fluids of this (septic) shock. Therefore, we are not strictly in the spirit of the FALLS-protocol. The caval veins assessment is rather a tool allowing us to manage a patient with a known diagnosis.

In this perspective, we will take a look at the caval veins, since it may be able to drive our fluid management. Caval vein or any other method, at the present state of knowledge, the needs for fluid therapy in this septic shock answer to more traditional rules, and invite to more traditional tools. One should understand that the lung can no longer be used as a guide for fluid therapy (since diffuse sliding rockets are present).

Caval Veins: (1) Inferior Caval Vein (IVC)

The venous compartment contains 65 % of the systemic blood. Draining half of the venous return, the crossroad of lower extremity thromboses, the IVC has a strategic situation. A whole chapter in our 1992 edition [94], long considered by CEURF of interest [95], it is now located in the position N°5 in the sequence of the FALLS-protocol, used for lack of anything better. It is unable to provide an ON-OFF answer to the question: when should I give the last tolerable drop of my fluid therapy? However, it shows a volume, i.e., a part of volemia (Video 30.2). When nothing else is available, this tube becomes precious (read Anecdotal Note 7). Here (for the first time), we make measurements (never done during the whole FALLS-protocol). Our study used the CVP as gold standard. The CVP is a "dynamic" concept, only its evolution is of interest (meaning that an isolated data has limited value). The inspiratory (insp.) IVC caliper decreases in spontaneous breathing, increases in ventilated patients. The expiratory (exp.) caliper is quite not modified after intubation and sedation, as opposed to insp. caliper. We showed that an exp. caliper <10 mm was correlated with a CVP <10 cm H_2O with a 95 % specificity, 84 % sensitivity [95]. More interestingly, the changes of IVC caliper under fluid therapy were parallel to the CVP changes (Fig. 30.4).

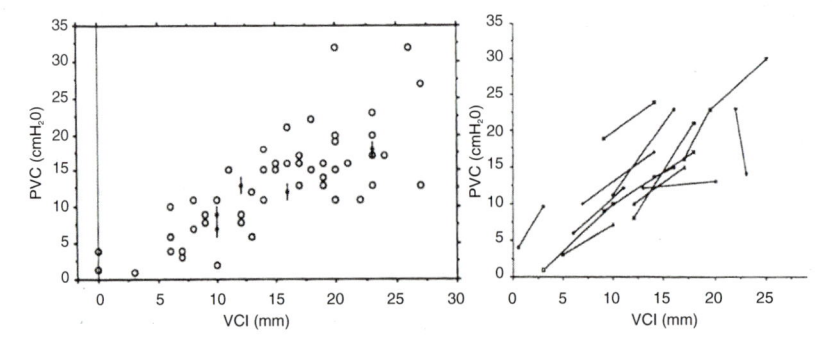

Fig. 30.4 Inferior caval vein and central venous pressure. *Left*: correlation between expiratory caliper of the IVC (*VCI*) at the left renal vein and CVP (*PVC*) in 59 ventilated patients. *Right*: caliper of the IVC when the CVP is modified. Note that the relative dispersion seen at the *left panel* is quite absent at the *right panel* (From Lichtenstein and Jardin [95])

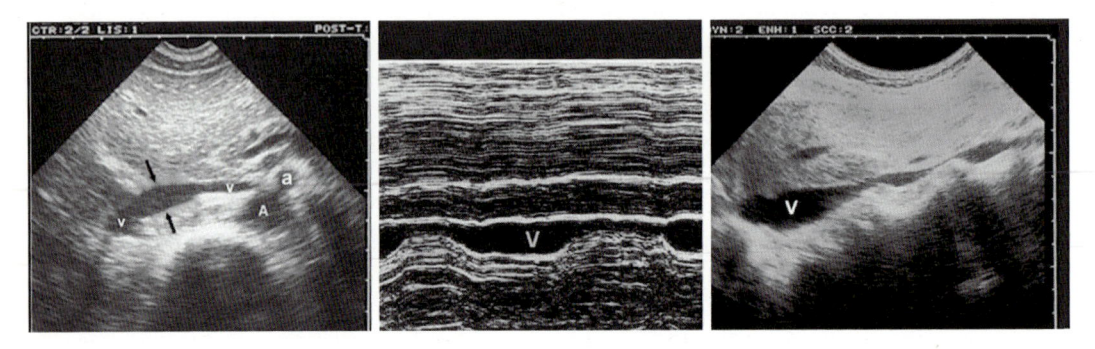

Fig. 30.5 Inferior caval vein. *Left*. IVC and left renal vein. This transverse epigastric view shows the point of arrival of the left renal vein (*v*). This vein is seen between the aorta (*A*) and the superior mesenteric artery (*a*), a really accessible landmark, the point where we measure the IVC caliper. Measurement should be from face to face (not from border to border), on expiration. See how the *arrows* follow the slight obliquity (20°) of the vein, in order to have meaningful measurement. Here, an expiratory caliper of 8 mm (*arrows*) indicates a low CVP. See the renal veins in frontal view in Fig. 18.1. *Middle*. IVC in M-mode. Inspiratory collapse, showing a 12-mm diastolic caliper (*V*) which collapses to 4 mm at inspiration in a spontaneously breathing patient with bleeding. *Right*. Moniliform IVC. Irregular pattern, mostly collapsed. Hypovolemic patient with the A-profile. Note the bulge (sabre profile) near the heart (where the letter V is located): the area where precisely we do not measure IVC caliper

How We Measure (and Why)

A transversal abdominal scan in a supine patient immediately detects the IVC. We measure it far from the heart, using a reproducible, easy-to-find landmark: the left renal vein arrival (read Anecdotal Note 7). This level produces our correlation with the CVP [96]. An indexation to surface body (i.e., weighting unstable patients) is risky, and useless: IVC dimensions don't correlate with the patient's size (Sykes study in *JUM* 1995:14:665). The collapsibility index – in spontaneous ventilation – is now a popular data [97, 98] (Fig. 30.5). An insp. collapse can be explained by hypovolemia, or dyspnea with use of accessory respiratory muscles, since the insp. collapse of thoracic pressure creates aspiration of the systemic blood, with Venturi effect. A flattened IVC in a shocked patient indicates low CVP (Fig. 30.5). An enlarged exp. IVC (Fig. 7.5 of our 2010 edition) is seen in RV failure, fluid overload, or can again be normal, with low CVP (Fig. 30.4). Figure 30.4 shows that the correlation was narrow with small caliper values.

Usual Errors Daily Seen

In the present edition, we still need to warn on frequent mistakes: (1) A noncontrolled compression of the abdomen for hiding gas decreases the IVC caliper. See our technique in Fig. 28.7. (2)

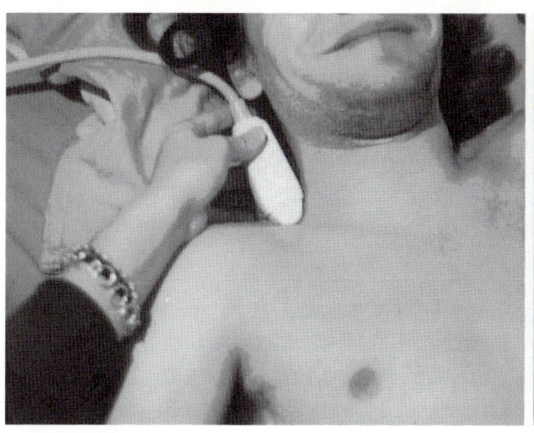

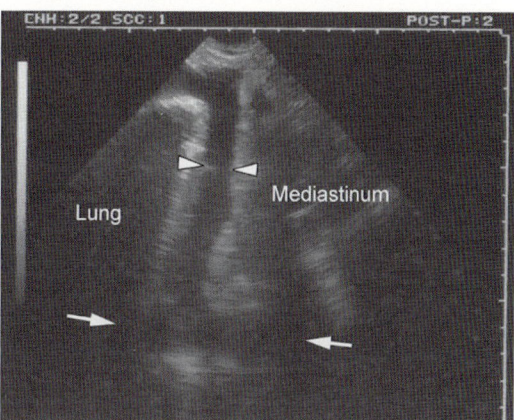

Fig. 30.6 A simple, noninvasive access to the superior caval vein (SVC). *Left*: this figure shows how we search for the SVC. We take the IJV in transversal approach, descend to the SVC, then progressively position the probe parallel to the neck long-axis. The rear part of the probe is slightly oriented backward for exposing the SVC. *Right*: the SVC (*arrowheads*) is seen through its entire length (8–9 cm) in this view. The right pulmonary artery is discretely seen, posterior to the vein (*arrows*). The ascending aorta, pulsatile and turning to the left, was previously seen just inside the SVC, making any confusion impossible. The arrowheads indicate a 10-mm laterolateral caliper. Respiratory collapse can be detected in the best cases. No probe but a microconvex one can be applied on such a narrow area and provide this image quality. This approach is an alternative for all those who cannot afford the TEE approach, or those who are hurried to manage the patient

The hepatic vein syndrome: doctors often measure a hepatic vein instead of the IVC (see Fig. 4.5 of our 2010 edition). (3) The palsy syndrome. They measure just near the heart. Their hand seems stuck to the heart, unable to displace caudally. Usually seen in doctors trained only in echocardiography, the palsy syndrome results in measuring the IVC where there is a bulge (where the IVC receives the hepatic veins) (Fig. 30.5) (see Fig. 4.2 of our 2010 edition). In addition, the IVC is an embryologic puzzle, with venous tissue near the cardiac tissue in this area, i.e., possibly, not a good idea for measuring there. Measuring at this bulge does not give our correlations, done at the left renal vein. (4) Considering a flattened IVC as a sign of hypovolemia. CVP values range normally from 12 to 0 mmHg.

Some Limitations of the IVC Assessment, of the CVP Value

Poor acoustic window is an absolute concern for those who believe in the IVC. Intra-abdominal hyperpressure squashes the IVC. All constraints relative to the CVP: definition and control of hydrostatic zero, supposed location of right auricle depending on habits, need for interrupting drugs flow for each measurement.

Caval Veins: (2) The Superior Caval Vein (SVC)

The IVC became a popular tool, then the SVC arrived. It was nearer to the heart, a zone maybe more prestigious than this IVC lost among stinking guts. In this respect, maybe the SVC is superior. Its analysis shows hypovolemia [34]. It needs however the TEE. Keeping our usual distance since the gold standard is still not defined, holistic ultrasound opens anyway fully to this elegant potential. Therefore, we take once again our basic 5 MHz microconvex probe and just insert it at the neck (Fig. 30.6). Only a microconvex probe has the ergonomy and the suitable resolution. We obtain a noninvasive, bedside, immediate measurement that can be done successfully in roughly 78 % of the patients (probably more, on study). We benefit from a medio-lateral dimension and assess a possible insp. collapse. Correlations with the semi-invasive method (TEE) are ongoing. Right atelectasis, not a rare situation in the ICU,

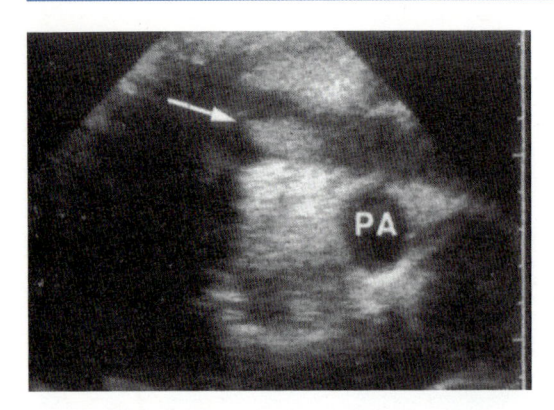

Fig. 30.7 Superior caval vein (SVC) floating thrombosis. This patient had a right lung atelectasis, yielding a nice right longitudinal parasternal window to the SVC. The thrombus (*arrow*) appeared highly floating within the venous lumen. The only immediate thing one could do (apart from immediate fibrinolytic therapy, if possible) was to position this patient on the right lateral decubitus, hoping that the thrombus, when dislodged, would choose the dependent right lung. An idle observer, searching for spectacular movie, could take prolonged observation for eventually seeing the thrombus dislodgement, followed by a few fractions of seconds later by the embolus fleetingly visible through PA, the right pulmonary artery (hopingly). The issue of an SVC thrombosis? Read about the CLOT-protocol in Chap. 28

attracts the SVC and makes it accessible using a parasternal approach (Fig. 30.7).

Case of the Patient in Extreme Hemodynamic Instability with Imminence of Cardiac Arrest

Between severe shock and cardiac arrest, the gap is sometimes weak. The critical need for a fast diagnosis creates an inversion of the priorities, with lung coming first. Imminent cardiac arrest and cardiac arrest, put together for simplifying, are dealt with in the SESAME-protocol, a concept mingling mechanism and cause for immediate diagnosis (Chap. 31).

By the Way: Whole Body Ultrasound of a Septic Shock? A Treasure Hunt

From Step 3 of the FALLS-protocol, the sepsis sites are under investigation. For relieving this long chapter and keeping hemodynamics on focus, please refer to the Fever-protocol of Chap. 28. Most of these findings can benefit from an ultrasound-guided tap (empyema, peritonitis, and bile; see our 2010 edition) with maximal safety using this visual control [99]. The sample is promptly sent to the laboratory. This authorizes immediate and adapted (*not probabilist*) therapy [100]. The use of simple ultrasound should change the usual management of septic shock.

FALLS-Protocol: Again a Fast Protocol. Its Positioning with Respect to the Early Goal-Directed Therapy and Its Recent Troubles

The traditional recommendation has taught us to provide early and massive fluid in septic shock [70]. It is now highly questioned, at the light of recent breaking studies [61, 71, 72]. Yet, we are not sure whether 100 % of the concept must be rejected. Just simply note that an "early" and "massive" fluid therapy is exactly what the FALLS-protocol does, with two slight peculiarities.

Early fluid therapy? The FALLS-protocol did not wait to know that this given circulatory failure was due to a sepsis. How long does it take to recognize a sepsis? Hours. Many hours. Probably time is lost at this step; read the relatively important Anecdotal Note 8. The FALLS-protocol has administered fluids just after steps 1 (obstructive shock) and 2 (cardiogenic shock), i.e., 1 min for recognizing a state of FALLS-responsiveness and initiate fluid therapy.

Massive fluid therapy? Now that this attitude has been completely discredited (but for how long?), we simply remind that the FALLS-protocol has discontinued the fluid therapy at the last tolerable drop, from a pathophysiological basis at an infra-clinical and infra-biological step of fluid overload, at the value of roughly 18 mmHg of PAOP, likely providing an *appropriate* volume of fluid.

Strong Points of the FALLS-Protocol: The Basic Advantages

Table 30.2, comparing various tools, shows that in terms of cost, invasiveness, technical easiness, monitoring possibilities, time spent, and direct approach to interstitial lung water, the FALLS-protocol is positioned first. Let us detail.

Rapidity (a few minutes)

In critical settings, *speed* is an advantage.

Simplicity: a steep learning curve

Look at the decision tree. This is visual medicine. No measurement is made at any step. The youngest doctors take the highest responsibilities, in the night (maybe on us, tomorrow). The mastery of lung artifacts and the simple emergency cardiac sonography is rapid using appropriate training.

Sensitivity

Lung ultrasound shows interstitial edema, i.e., the initial signature of fluid overload, the clinically occult, radio-occult step.

Accuracy

The concept of a dichotomous approach may allow to decrease the gray zone of other methods. The fact is that the FALLS-protocol detects the very beginning of tissular edema in the most sensitive and fragile organ. The earliness is a major advantage.

Monitoring fluid therapy

The possibility of detecting at a glance a change between A-profile and B-profile (a few seconds) makes the FALLS-protocol different from other tools, in particular complex Doppler-echocardiography.

An independent parameter of volemia

The FALLS-protocol provides a parameter *independent* from many limitations of the other methods (needing subtle calculations, ponderations, consideration of transmural pressures, cardiac rhythm, type of ventilation, esophageal or arterial contra-indications, etc.)

A direct parameter of volemia

The FALLS-protocol introduces for once a direct parameter of clinical volemia (used for allowing clearance for fluid therapy).

A tool able to measure more than lung water: interstitial lung water

Lung water can be measured using invasive methods. The FALLS-protocol not only detects lung water (and noninvasively), but also makes more: it assesses the interstitial component. The access to *interstitial lung water*, i.e., the step occurring before the alveolar step, gives to the intensivist one step ahead for limiting fluid therapy: a notion similar to Guyton's concept of a safety margin factor [83].

Figure 23.2 of our 2010 edition showed three containers: one quasi-empty, one quite full, one overflowing. This figure showed that deep hypovolemia and normal volemia yield the same A-profile. The FALLS-endpoint shows the upper limit of normovolemia. Lung ultrasound is nicely positioned to protect against both deep hypovolemia and fluid overload.

The direct assessment of the capillary pressure?

Maybe lung ultrasound allows to better approach the value of the *capillary pressure*, a basic data that PAOP only tries to reflect.

Maybe the main advantage of the FALLS-protocol: a new tool for diagnosing hypovolemia

In a few seconds and schematically, the recognition of A-lines provides a major piece of information: this given patient *can* receive fluids. In the sequence of the FALLS-protocol, we can add that this patient *must* receive fluids.

The detection of an A-profile will be of interest in these many difficult settings: the perioperative patient, the bariatric patient, these occult and prolonged states of hypovolemia. Patients receiving too high levels of drugs (epinephrine, norepinephrine) would be interested too in receiving more fluids and less drugs.

In complex and hemorrhagic abdominal surgery, the upper BLUE-points can be made easily accessible by the anesthesiologist, hence a simplified management.

Maybe a role for preventing late, torpid complications of prolonged underdiagnosed hypovolemia

Could these prolonged states of occult hypovolemia make the bed for the microcirculation disorders, the multiple organ failure, and the scary irreversible hypoxemia of septic shock? Let us hypothesize that the "golden hours," these decisive steps of management, belong to the early ones. Would an efficient

early fluid therapy, in the first minutes, create optimal conditions for decreasing these late disorders? To be sharply confirmed of course.
One more reason to choose a simple, cost-effective unit

We have a direct parameter of clinical volemia. This contribution (not every day, a tool for direct measurement of volemia is found) is likely able to counterbalance the absence of Doppler – not to say more. If confirmed, the last major interest of Doppler in critical ultrasound would vanish. This would allow to democratize a little more critical ultrasound. We like to remind that this application was achievable using the portable 42-cm wide ADR-4000 of 1982. Pantographic systems of the years 1960s were technically suitable for the lung part of the FALLS-protocol.

Weak Points of the FALLS-Protocol: The Limitations and Pseudo-limitations

The use of too sophisticated machines, which do not respect the artifacts, is the main pseudo-limitation.

The B-profile on admission (read p. 238).

The FALLS-protocol has not been validated. If it is, the reference must be perfect, and we know the issues, at the present time, to provide a gold standard admitted by all. We work on this.

The FALLS-protocol is probably not suitable for all patients. A fulminans sepsis will generate a quandary: all the fluids pour outside all organs, lung included. Hemodynamic and permeability-induced edema coexist, in addition with a potential massive hypovolemia (if the lung is suddenly wet, the patient is suddenly hypovolemic – these patients are too wet and too dry). The mastery of these acute changes is a challenge. Traditional approaches should be used (if they succeed in changing the dramatic prognosis of these patients). Some cases of fulminans pulmonary edema (with massive lung rockets) benefit from fluid therapy, which will worsen the hemodynamic pulmonary edema. Of note, if an A-profile is initially seen, and becomes B-profile during or even before fluid therapy (in a fulminans pneumonia), even if it is difficult to say where the edema (hemodynamic or not) comes from, consider that the initial diagnosis provided by the FALLS-protocol is a sepsis. Pulmonary edema (hemodynamic or not) appears as a complication, not a cause (of shock).

The FALLS-protocol focuses rather on the left heart. For those who wish to avoid the right heart failure, for the case of a fully asymmetrical right heart failure, read FAQ 6 and 8.

There are probably other limitations not yet seen. Let us keep it open.

FAQ on the FALLS-Protocol

We anticipate many questions, here are a dozen.
1. *How about the PAOP as a reference value?*

   Like everything in medicine, this choice can be debated. We know PAOP values do not reflect LV performances such as stroke volume index, etc. [6, 23, 101–105] but, obsolete or not for reflecting downstream pressures, the PAOP still indicates the risk of pulmonary edema. For some, it remains a precious tool, valuable when restrictions are applied [106, 107]. The PAOP value is unknown from numerous physicians who are now deprived of the Swan-Ganz catheter but have no access to TEE, or just miss this precise value. The FALLS-protocol will be appreciated by those intensivists who envision fluid therapy based on low PAOP values and consider that our concept of a safety factor is logical.
2. *How about cardiogenic shock with low PAOP?*

   In practice, this deals with the RV infarction *with shock* – not a frequent event. For simplifying, we would say: "The FALLS-protocol requires an ECG, in these cases:
   1. enlarged RV
   2. if there is no cardiac window, in the case of an A-profile without DVT

   It is not necessary (for the diagnosis) if pericardial tamponade, pulmonary embolism, pneumothorax, hypovolemia are detected."

But we guess normal doctors will not wait for any advice, restriction, or protocol for making an ECG in a shocked patient. This concept is just an academic exercise.

Now, and apart from unavoidable controversies, the usual therapy of the RV infarction includes precisely fluid therapy. Precisely, these patients will display the A-profile, which calls for fluid therapy. The right cardiogenic shock is fully in the scope of the FALLS-protocol. We just aim at keeping its decision tree simple, not hampered by rarities. Integrating this diagnosis would add a branch which will quite never be used.

We remind that in the RV infarction, the traditional ultrasound patterns (dilated RV and dilated IVC) invite not to give fluids.

3. *Why not search for lateral or even posterior lung rockets during fluid therapy?*

    Why not, indeed? The anterior area of the FALLS-protocol was our first step for sharing a simple message (we aimed at increasing the chance of acceptation of the manuscript). Lateral approaches may inform on even lower values of PAOP. As to posterior B-lines, we remind that they may indicate gravitational changes [86]. Yet if they are initially absent, this makes a target for a prompter detection. We just think that the difference will not be major: a posterior approach should theoretically save a few points of mmHg of PAOP, not more; then the B-lines should rapidly invade the whole lung surface (study in process).

4. *Which speed for fluid therapy, which frequency of checking?*

    If we deal with a young patient, if the IVC is very flattened, we can administer quantities of fluid and make quiet regular "FALLS-points," up to the FALLS-endpoint. A FALLS-point is a flash ultrasound test including at least the two anterior BLUE-points (and - if indicated - the PLAPS-point and a lateral point) of a chosen lung, sufficient since fluid overload yields bilateral patterns of edema: 15 s or less! This makes the FALLS-protocol a reasonable monitoring tool.

    In an old patient with cardiac history and already dilated IVC, we will be slower in the fluid administration and check with higher frequency. Please come back to the concept of the PUMA (see Fig. 2.2). We remind that a (theoretical) coffee machine is located at the top, for the main reason that this possibility quietly invalids the interest of the laptop philosophy (there is space for such a device, the important dimension is lateral, not the ceilings). Here, the coffee machine – a symbolic image – indicates that the physician should remain beside the patient. Once fluid therapy has been initiated, once the round-FALLS-protocol has been done, he or she has nothing else to do but wait for one of the two events (clinical recovery or lung rockets), making from time to time, then more and more frequently a FALLS-point (in parallel to the cardiac frequency, mottlings, etc.). This is not wasted time. From the moment where B-lines appear (if the patient did not improve meanwhile from a hypovolemic shock), the action comes back suddenly: stopping fluid therapy, blood cultures, initiating vasopressors, etc. And here, the "lost" time is transformed into saved time regarding the patient's management, therefore the shock prognosis. Users can take tea instead of coffee if they prefer.

    In other words, the IVC analysis gives us, initially, a rough indicator on the frequency of our FALLS-point monitoring.

5. *When a B-profile appears, isn't the heart already on the flat slope of the Frank-Starling curve?*

    We assume such a question may concern some readers. Even asymptomatic, the generation of an interstitial syndrome under fluid therapy means that the physician has intentionally initiated a slight but genuine fluid overload, i.e., he/she has positioned the patient's heart after the inflexion point of the curve (Fig. 30.8).

    Let us consider critical points.

    1. The FALLS-endpoint, a pure interstitial fluid overload, is an early step, locating the heart at the beginning of the flat portion of the curve.

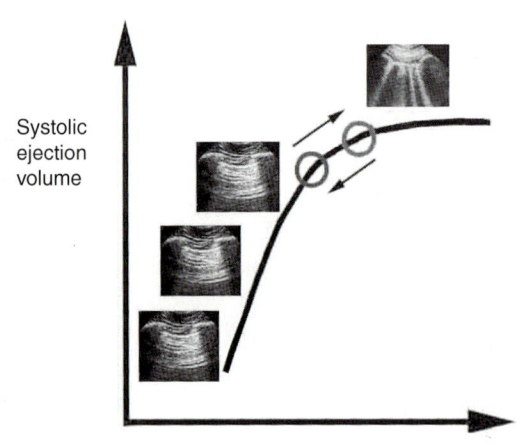

Fig. 30.8 Positioning of the heart on the function curve. FALLS-protocol and cardiac function curve. The fluid therapy is controlled by the physician. When lung rockets appear, we can consider we are at an early phenomenon on the inflexion point of the curve of the ventricular function (*upper circle*). A minimal fluid withdrawal will move the patient near to the lower target (*lower circle*), with the aim of positioning the heart at the ideal point of the curve

2. How to assess the danger of such a cardiac positioning? Is it real or hypothetical, would well-profiled studies answer? Please note that physicians who make a fluid responsiveness maneuver usually don't use LUCI, and possibly make such positioning blindly, maybe without too much harm. We ask the question. But see the fourth point.
3. Septic shock is a setting of high mortality. We consider that a very acutely ill patient needs an energic management. This is nearly a philosophic positioning, yet we saw that this energy is controlled. We remind that the tool "pragmatism" is part of the FALLS-protocol. Any shocked patient will die promptly if not treated, and many of those admitted to the best ICUs will also die. We are in a logic of death. Solutions are urgently needed. The aim of the FALLS-protocol is to decrease the death rate.
4. Mainly, once the physician has discontinued the fluid therapy, the slight fluid excess is immediately withdrawn. We use one of these solutions:

A. Usually we ask to the nurse, simply, for *seven blood tests*.

Why seven? Not only is this a biblical number (even if rational behaviors are preferred in such settings), but this maneuver allows to withdraw blood: nothing less than a genuine *blood-letting*. Advocating a blood-letting may initiate some smiles, at the modern era of recombinant human activated protein-C therapies, ultrafast multi-bar CT, etc., and we apologize for this, not searching for any provocation. But let us come three centuries (and more) back. In the 1600s, at the era of Molière, this was the recommended therapy – sometimes efficient – of fluid overload (the French term was "fluxion de poitrine"). Completely useless in 1000 other applications, here it worked! It worked because after all it was based on pathophysiology: even at these obscure, old times, these patients had a cardiac function curve, a pulmonary artery occlusion pressure, and the blood-letting resulted in decreasing this pressure. It worked.

This maneuver is done in the spirit of positioning the heart at the ideal point of the function curve: standard blood tests on admission withdraw roughly 50 ml (making however 1 % of the total blood). Yet remember we asked the question, at the end of page 233, which volume can the interstitial compartment accept before saturation? The answer will be subtle, require fine studies, distinguishing the blood in the pulmonary capillary from the plasma from the interstitial tissue. Would the value of saturated interstitial lung water be similar to the blood-letting, nice perspectives would follow the implementation of the FALLS-protocol.

Some would find it questionable to withdraw blood in a shocked patient. Probably they have in mind that this

may be a hemorrhagic shock. This diagnosis is déjà vu, step 3 of the FALLS-protocol. It is a non-problem.
B. A traditional hemodiafiltration (HDF), if already on-site, would be an elegant solution. No doctor will initiate HDF just for withdrawing a few milliliters of excessive fluid, but do not forget that at this step, the diagnosis is septic shock: many teams use early HDF for various targets.
C. Third solution, for those who would be reluctant to withdraw any blood volume, we share here the FALLS-PLR-protocol: simply rise passively the legs of your patient with the A-predominance, check that this maneuver does not generate B-lines, then fill the patient, until B-lines appear, and then lay the legs down again. Using simplicity, the FALLS-PLR-protocol allows noninvasive optimization of volume therapy.
D. Diuretics? Some colleagues spoke of this option, but we are not sure it would work in a septic shock when the hemodynamic is, by definition, not optimized.

6. *But we have been taught that too much fluid (liberal management) was more deleterious than conservative management.*

The FALLS-protocol is neither liberal nor conservative. In between, it aims at providing the appropriate fluid therapy without excess. Let us take the problem at the source.

Several studies have shown that a liberal fluid therapy is not good. But did they use the potential of the lung artifacts for measuring the threshold between liberal and conservative? Apparently not. The FALLS-protocol gives fluid, stops at the limit between normo- and hypervolemia (in the lungs), and withdraws some. This would position the volemia below the risk of fluid overload. But let us go further anyway. The real risk of fluid overload should be perfectly known and controlled. This risk seems different according to sources.

For most, the absolute risk is the pulmonary edema, and it should be considered before the issues of abdominal organs' edema, at least in the extreme emergency.

For some, the edema of the abdominal organs is worse than their hypoperfusion.

For others, the septal interference will add a cardiogenic shock to the initial problem.

For others again, the increase of the right pressures is a hindrance to the coronary circulation at the RV, especially in the cases where a pulmonary hypertension is present. We remind that pulmonary embolism has been detected at the first step of the FALLS-protocol.

Other sources fear issues with idiopathic pulmonary hypertension – a rare event (where simple signs of simple cardiac sonography will alert).

Once again, so many envisaged complications may indicate a certain confusion. We remain on maximal attention on this point, but wait for scientific proof, in this fragile field. The fear of creating an abdominal edema is legitimate, but we must not forget the essential: it is minimal, it is transient since immediately compensated. Again, well-designed studies should assess the real danger of this fleeting fluid overload, compared with the usual mortality of septic shock. We repeat this basic truth, written earlier regarding the LV.

7. *How will the FALLS-protocol work in massive pulmonary embolism?*

Fluid therapy is often considered as double-edged, and many recommend modest volumes – in order to avoid septal interference. But why give fluids? This is the behavior of a physician facing a circulatory failure and wanting to do something before having the diagnosis. No therapy here but disobstruction is fully efficient. The question of the fluid therapy is not really appropriate. The diagnosis is given in the first step of the FALLS-protocol (read below and in the Chap. 26).

8. *How to use the FALLS-protocol if a predominant RV failure is feared?*

Shelton Magder noticed at a recent conference that the FALLS-protocol should have more respect for the RV function.

For fully answering this concern, we may first ask how frequent a fully asymmetrical right heart failure in the real life of an ICU is. Aren't there simple ways to detect such cases with simple tools taken from simple emergency cardiac sonography? Obviously, in such settings, a simple look to variations of volume at the RV during fluid therapy is not a big deal. But let us see further.

The FALLS-protocol does not assume specifically that the weakest pump is the LV. It just considers that, in the case of slight asymmetry, the interstitial pulmonary edema will be the first change promptly and easily detected (maybe ultrasound markers of abdominal organs edema have been described – if existing, they should be rather subtle). What about patients with a very asymmetrical heart? A charicatural example is the post-cardiac surgery with open pericardium: under fluid therapy, the right heart enlarges, enlarges, without any septal interference. The septal interference is a concept fully used in the FALLS-protocol, precisely because it may protect both circulations from fluid overload, read below.

When is an asymmetrical RV failure expected? We remind that pulmonary embolism has been ruled out at the first step of the FALLS-protocol (or confirmed in roughly 80 % of cases using the BLUE-protocol – not to deal with the cardiac approach, showing enlarged RV). We remind that an ECG is done in the FALLS-protocol, for detecting the rare cardiogenic shock due to RV infarction.

Patients with a history (known or revealed by the current episode) of chronic right heart failure, including rare causes (pulmonary hypertension) will raise the problem of a dilated RV on admission. Apart from the epidemiological factor (idiopathic pulmonary hypertension is not exactly the daily life), the detection of a thickened RV free wall should immediately alert on a chronic history [108]. These patients will obviously be treated apart, with high care to the RV status.

Once this exceptional setting is put apart, we search for the frequent causes of acute right heart failure without free wall thickening, and we have difficulties in finding many. Pulmonary embolism or RV infarction is déjà vu. The septic cardiomyopathy: why should it attack the RV more than the LV? But let us admit, just for a demonstration considering the worst hypothesis.

Take a fully asymmetrical right heart failure, with a closed pericardium. Give fluid to this patient (Fig. 30.9). One main event will be the occurrence of a septal interference [109]. This interference creates an increase of the left pressures, possibly sufficient for generating a mild interstitial edema, precisely the one detected at an early step by the FALLS-protocol. This would be the signal for the FALLS-endpoint. In other words, it is difficult to imagine a severe RV failure, with deleterious edema of abdominal organs, without a slight increase of the LV pressures. The principle of the FALLS-protocol should therefore preserve both ventricles. If the RV "explodes," the LV should be (a bit or more) "splashed." They are such close neighbors. In real life, if the disease comes from the right heart, the asymmetry should maybe not be charicatural, i.e., the fluid therapy may increase the pressures of both ventricles (more at the right, but enough at the left for generating B-lines). We therefore speculate that the FALLS-protocol should work, even in the case of asymmetrical right heart dysfunction. We wait of course for a confirmation or an infirmation on the way.

The case of a hypovolemic shock in a patient with a chronic lung disease. Let us place the concepts in their right place, and consider a patient with a history (known or not) of right heart disease, here in your ER/ICU for what will be eventually a hypovolemic shock (with initially and supposedly, absence of marked RV enlargement). This patient will likely receive fluids, suggested by the FALLS-protocol. But under fluid therapy, which event will appear *first*? A huge RV dilatation (sufficient for creating a septal interference)? Rather a clinical improvement,

FAQ on the FALLS-Protocol

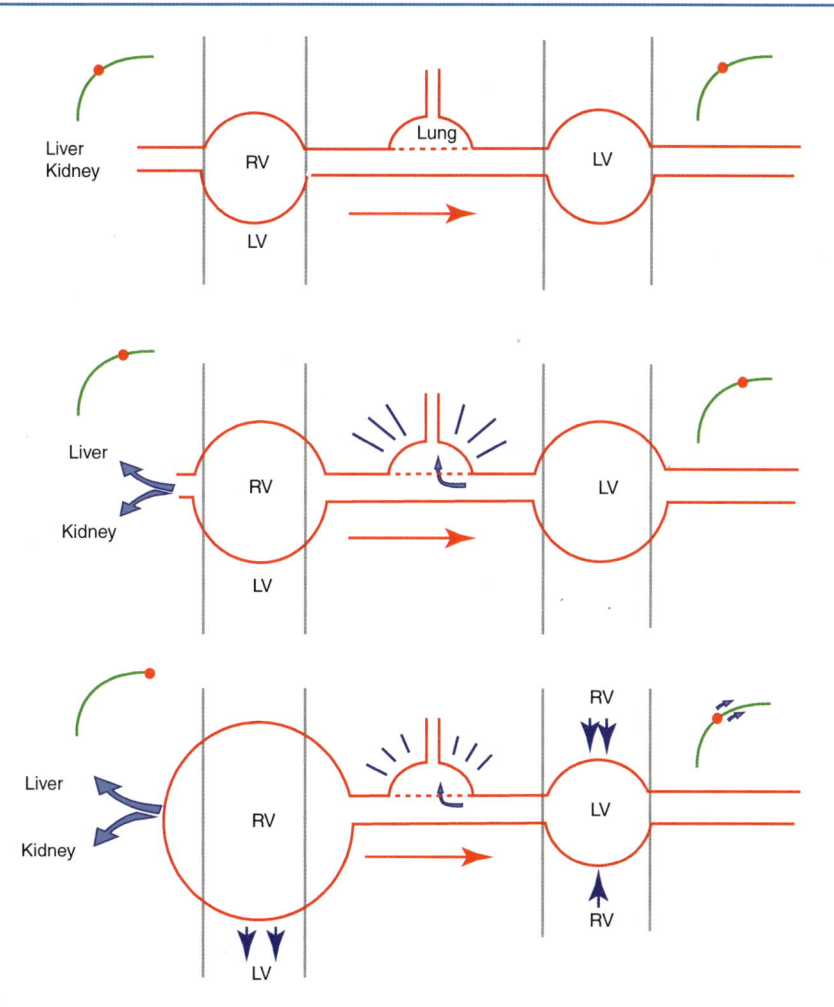

Fig. 30.9 FALLS-protocol in the case of asymmetrical heart. *Top*: two (cardiac) pumps assumed to work in parallel, lung in between (*green*: cardiac function curve). *Middle*: an increase of both ventricles work under fluid therapy, resulting in upstream phenomena: possible edema of the abdominal organs, but also lung interstitial edema, immediately detected: lung rockets. *Bottom*: charicatural asymmetry, where only the RV dilates under fluid therapy. This generates increase of upstream pressure (abdominal edema), but also a septal interference, which will create a decreased LV volume with elevated left heart pressures, enough in our hypothesis for generating this mild lung interstitial edema recognized by the FALLS-protocol. Note: these are schematic representations, not taking into account (for simplicity) the anatomic realities (septal interferences) nor pressure/volume instant phenomena (the *middle image* would suppose a very compliant pericardium, etc.)

likely. Again, nothing forbids the physician to take a frequent look to the RV volume (a data that is, as opposed to the FALLS-protocol, not dichotomic. What is the endpoint value?). We just aim at not complicating the daily FALLS-protocol for such causes, but are ready to revisit our concept if necessary.

To conclude the long development of this FAQ, patients should be protected by successive shelters from deleterious right heart events:
- Embolism and infarction were usually detected straightaway (*déjà vu*).
- Exceptional settings (open pericardium) are known by simple history.
- Most cases of chronic right heart failure are known through the history.
- A simple look at the RV volume and free wall is not a big deal.

- The septal interference should protect both ventricles from fluid overload using LUCI.
- Last, how really deleterious are the consequences of a minimal, *transient* right fluid overload?

9. *But how about the cardiac output (CO)? Can one really manage a critically ill patient without such a basic parameter?*

    Without problem. We have just to think different and forget (for a few moments) the usual tools we have always used. The community has the mind fixed at tools which measure the CO because they are at advanced steps of management: they know the initial diagnosis. They possibly occult the fact that a CO assessment does not provide a diagnosis, as opposed to the FALLS-protocol. See Table 30.1 and consider first that the nurse will take advantage of knowing not the CO, but which one of the three therapeutic actions to prepare (fluid, inotropic, vasopressor). The FALLS-protocol does not tell whether the CO is low, or high, or high but not high enough, or not increasing under fluid therapy. It tells which patients must receive fluids, it tells when to discontinue the fluid therapy.

    Knowing the CO can be of interest, once the diagnosis is done, for following any therapy. But do not forget that its instant value in a given septic patient can be meaningless: for instance high, but not high enough for the tissular needs of oxygen.

    We imagine that patients with a B-predominance are at risk of being those very patients who will no longer increase their CO (and will be non-*fluid* responders, for using traditional words, study in progress, trying to find a gold standard maybe better than the increase of CO >15 %).

10. *But where is the LV contractility in the FALLS-decision tree?*

    In our 2010 edition, the assessment of the inotropic function was placed early. Change by change, the place of this item was relegated, exactly like in the BLUE-protocol, same logic. The FALLS-protocol allows different perspectives. The A-profile, regardless the LV contractility, indicates that the left filling pressures are low. Facing the B-profile, the priority diagnosis is (left) cardiogenic shock.

    Since the LV function can be impaired in septic shock – always, even occult, according to some studies [110] – to see the LV contractility first would generate the risk of considering the cardiac failure as the origin of the shock (cardiogenic shock) whereas it can be the consequence (septic shock).

11. *In Fig. 30.1, the B'-profile seems associated with a low PAOP. Can this be exploited?*

    As shown in Chap. 13, standstill lung rockets indicate ARDS, not hemodynamic pulmonary edema. For simplifying (and favoring the acceptance of our manuscript), we did not bring this item on the first line, but further studies will assess the potential of this finding.

    A shocked patient with the B'-profile is a septic patient with a lung sepsis. Should fluid therapy be beneficial? The FALLS-protocol cannot be used. Use the IVC here, or any traditional tool.

12. *Can I use the FALLS-protocol in a given patient with ARDS and septic shock, in the ICU, for the daily needs of fluid? I often have the feeling that fluid therapy in these patients full of lung rockets, of peripheral edemas, with a high lactate rate, etc., is sometimes of benefit to their circulation, so what to conclude?*

    One detail must be pointed out: we are no longer at the time where there is a need for a diagnosis of shock (obstructive, etc.). Here, the patient is in the ICU, with a known diagnosis (here, septic shock). The rules of the FALLS-protocol should not apply at this step, unless the tool would definitely appear too provocative. Let us wait a few decades, time for the community to get accustomed to its basic principle.

    After some days, the lung may suffer from various insults: sepsis, nosocomial infections, and mechanical complications. ARDS patients are the most likely to exhibit lung rockets. They can experience occult hypovolemia as well as occult hypervolemia with high PAOP [111]. All this can deeply affect the nature and distribution of lung artifacts.

How much fluid today for this ARDS patient? The FALLS-protocol does not give the answer, temporarily. *The FALLS-protocol has not the pretention to define the needs of fluids in long-staying, septic patients.* This period is no longer part of the FALLS-protocol and we send readers to more traditional tools.

Regarding the future, just imagine: since the FALLS-protocol takes into account a direct parameter (interstitial fluid saturation), nothing prevents the intensivist to, little by little, extend the patient management of the first hours for a few later hours. Hour per hour, fine studies may assess the place of LUCI, of the FALLS-protocol. Let us assume that a given patient has a roughly symmetrical heart, with two cardiac pumps working roughly the same. In this hypothesis, the lung interstitial edema would be an indicator of other organs edema, and may be of help for determining whether fluid therapy begins to be toxic for the whole organism. Maybe lung rockets could be this early sign predicting brain edema, or abdominal organs edema. As always, we wait a solid study with a solid gold standard, but if the theory of the roughly symmetrical heart would happen to work, there would be a nice future for LUCI in the late hemodynamic management of septic shock.

13. *In Step 3, can't we introduce some early norepinephrine, in addition to the fluid therapy?*

This is a current comment. We should keep in mind that we are in a search of a diagnosis. Those who mix some fluids and some vasopressors have already in mind the *septic* shock. But consider that we are discovering a shocked patient. We have ruled out obstructive and cardiogenic shock, and we have given a lot of fluids. Giving a vasopressor now may spread confusion: just imagine a patient with a (still unknown) hypovolemic shock. You have already given huge volumes, say 3 l. The patient did not improve (but is just on the point to improving – but you can't foresee this). The temptation is high to now introduce the vasopressor. Likely at this precise step, this would improve a *moderate* hypovolemia, and we may consider instead the diagnosis of vasoplegia. The real diagnosis (hypovolemia) remains occulted by this action. Time is lost.

Now imagine you strictly follow the FALLS-protocol: additional fluid therapy begins to be efficient (with A-profile unchanged): you have just diagnosed a deep hypovolemic shock. Maybe the patient needed 3,001 cc (not 3,000) for beginning to initiate signs of recovery.

The FALLS-protocol tries to be consistent: one action at a time.

14. *Can't we see a continuation between FALLS-protocol and BLUE-protocol?*

Critical states can more or less mingle circulatory and respiratory phenomena. Any shock even septic creates respiratory troubles (e.g., metabolic dyspnea). Even the SESAME-protocol (next chapter) is not far from the FALLS-protocol. Making a SESAME-protocol in a shocked patient will not provide confusing elements. Just the order is adapted for respecting logic, brain function, time, and academic standardization. If a FALLS-protocol is done in a real acute dyspnea, finding a pericardial effusion would be incidental (acute pericarditis does not generate real respiratory failure).

15. *Can the FALLS-protocol be associated with traditional tools of hemodynamic investigation?*

Without any problem.

A Schematical Synthesis of the FALLS-Protocol

How do we proceed in practice? We are called, e.g., at the emergency room for visiting a shocked patient. We make the normal doctor's work (physical examination, etc.). Our machine switches on in 7 s. The look at a normal pericardium needs usually a few seconds. The look at a non-dilated RV takes a few seconds. In the absence of cardiac window, the sequential search of the BLUE-protocol finds the A-profile (20 s) then a DVT in most cases of pulmonary embolism (<2 min). The absence of an A′-profile takes less than 5 s per lung. *Obstructive shock* is ruled out. The absence of the B-profile, checked in 20 s, indicates that there is no pulmonary edema, i.e., no left *cardiogenic shock*. At this step, the order of giving fluids is given. Two events can occur.

A. Under fluid therapy, the shock decreases (mottling vanishes, etc.). The fluid therapy can be discontinued. Patient's improvement under fluid therapy (with unchanged A-profile) defines *hypovolemic shock*.
B. Under fluid therapy, the shock resists. Eventually, B-lines replace A-lines. This interstitial syndrome likely indicates hydrostatic interstitial edema: the endpoint has been reached. This is time for stopping fluid therapy – and introducing another agent for improving the circulation (norepinephrine here). The transformation from A-lines to B-lines indicates, schematically, distributive shock, i.e., in daily practice, *septic shock*.

An Attempt of (Very) Humble Conclusion

In the field of hemodynamic assessment, it is always a bit bold to use the word "Conclusion." Only the doubt and the wish to improve the patient's prognosis drive our efforts. It is not really a conclusion, just the wish to stimulate a field in the search of a gold standard, which seems a longstanding issue up to now [112].

The FALLS-protocol must again be highly open to any criticism. It would like to be compared to other tools (provided the gold standard is solid). It aims, between these two inappropriate options (those which drown the cells and those which keep them too dry) at finding the equilibrium.

In light of recent studies, we should make conservative fluid policies. Today, critically ill patients die less but still die. This means there is a place for new approaches, the FALLS-protocol humbly desires to be a new indicator of clinical volemia, and we consequently suggest to redesign and do again these multicentric studies which concluded that the fluid therapy had to be conservative. Including lung ultrasound, a critical piece of information, would help redefine hypervolemia, and more precisely, the threshold between normovolemia and hypervolemia.

We would like to remind the essence of holistic ultrasound. If the FALLS-protocol works, this would mean that our simple equipment, without Doppler, with one probe, our "antique" 1992 machine, may become a stethoscope of tomorrow (read Appendix A.2). This would justify the theme of CEURF ("tomorrow's medicine using the tools of ever"). This would definitely be the recognition of a research life: helping to provide a gold standard in this field.

Some Small Story of the FALLS-Protocol

No later than 1996, we were able to see some threshold values where the lung rockets appeared: it was first 13 mmHg, then 16 mmHg, then stabilized at the value of 18 mmHg, with a 97 % specificity. In 1996, B-lines, lung rockets, were still not published in the international peer-review literature [77]. The BLUE-protocol was even far to be submitted [79]. Therefore, from the first conclusions to the last publications, 13 years passed.

In 1996, we had the aim to favor the respiratory failure and made it an absolute priority, because dyspneic patients suffer so much, likely more than shocked patients. The acceptance in 2008 of the BLUE-protocol by CHEST simply allowed us to submit the FALLS-protocol (Manuscript N° CHEST-09-0001).

Are rejections a good thing? Yes! Our choice to favor human priorities (BLUE before FALLS), combined with the watchful work of our reviewers, was a great opportunity for numerous smart research teams. Precisely, some among them, not far from us (roughly 888 km), just opened our 2002 edition at the right page (p. 130), and just changed the label "lung rockets" for "lung comets" for making elegant articles in the cardiologic literature. Anyone can replace a word by another (e.g., "Stalingrad" can suddenly become "Volgograd"). The point is that lung comets *are not* lung rockets. The term "lung rockets" is equivalent to interstitial syndrome, the term "lung comet" is not. We hope this term will not add too much confusion in such a field.

If the words may confuse, the technique also must be adapted to time-dependent patients. Our studies focus in critically ill patients, and use a dichotomous protocol allowing to define in a few seconds a characteristic profile, considering a limited, anterior, chest area. The comprehensive counting of B-lines (up to more than 500 in some studies) can be interesting for subtle publications in non-time-dependent patients. We aim at avoiding to our readers this boring task in critically ill patients: the FALLS-protocol *is* a fast protocol!

Anecdotal Notes

1. *Some comments frequently heard from the corridors*[1]

    "This patient has received already 3,000 cc. I consider this is enough fluid!"

    "What is the good hemodynamic tool? It depends. Probably all of them. If you have just a PICCO in your institution, you will use the PICCO. If you have two tools, you can choose, case per case. This given patient will be better assessed using a TEE, e.g."

    "I don't believe too much in PICCO. What are my arguments? No precise argument, I just don't believe."

    "I love PICCO."

    "I succeeded to maintain this patient only at the price of massive doses of epinephrine and norepinephrine, he was definitely extremely severe."

    ---
    [1] All these comments have been heard, here or there (and even said by the young author). They are inserted here, not in order to highlight our ignorance, but rather to show, by the text, that the traditional tools are all indirect ones.

    "I lost this patient in spite of massive doses of epinephrine and norepinephrine, he was definitely too severe."

    "Before sending the patient to CT (for a diagnosis), I stabilized him."[2]

    "I don't care the first value of this measurement (CVP, etc.). What I care is the evolution under my therapy."

2. *Simple emergency cardiac sonography*

    The choice of the word "sonography" was deliberate, for avoiding confusions between the traditional territories of "ECHO" (prestigious cardiac approach of the cardiologist – valvular regurgitations, etc.) and "ultrasound" (abdominal approach of the radiologist – rather some gallstones, etc.).

3. *The A/B profile*

    Finding an A/B profile, the user can make the FALLS-points only on side A, and save time.

4. *The reed*

    Like the reed of the fable, we should always consider the FALLS-protocol, as just a "protocol," i.e., a tool to be used wisely. Too much rigidity would break it. Each decision in critical care can be debated again and again, we keep each physician free of his/her management.

5. *Active bleeding*

    The only deleterious fluid therapy in a hypovolemic shock is the particular case of the active bleeding. The round-FALLS-protocol (i.e., a standard ultrasound to the peritoneum, aorta, etc.) usually solves this "non-quandary." Blindly giving fluids ad nauseam to a bleeding patient would result in replacing the blood by pure saline, but which doctor would not diagnose an active bleeding? FALLS is just a protocol, there is a pilot behind.

    ---
    [2] Supposedly, blindly.

6. *LV contractility*

    The non-inclusion of the LV contractility in the decision tree of the FALLS-protocol is reasoned. On the other hand, not looking at the LV while applying a probe at the heart would be really excessive. In practice, we always take a look at it with one eye, while ruling out obstructive causes (tamponade, embolism) with the other, at the same step for saving time. LV contractility data are not used for immediate therapeutic change, especially when there is no B-profile.

7. *IVC and left renal vein*

    Of all manuscripts we proposed to François Jardin for a signature, the IVC was the privilege of the unique one he agreed to cosign (apart from the letter to the editor on the IJV thrombosis in *Intensive Care Med* 23:1188–1189). Honest, having no frank opinion on lung ultrasound for lack of time but trusting us, he let us publish our research. Then he wanted the French article to be enriched by new data, for a submission in English-speaking literature. We were then asked to measure the IVC at the bulging area, just near the heart, for the fear that getting far from the heart for measuring at the left renal vein would be an impossible task for intensivists trained in echocardiography. In spite of François Jardin's warning, we did not think this was a fully scientific thought process. Now, by observing the quite lethargic dynamic of the intensivists during decades (2.6 currently), who still position the probe just against the heart for studying the IVC, we could realize a posteriori how insightful he was.

8. *Sepsis, a daylight diagnosis*

    Septic shock is a *daylight* diagnosis. Look at the time of admission in your institutions: usually at open hours, the initial team talks with the ICU team, the patient is transferred and taken in charge by the ICU. This means that the initial team has taken some time for envisaging the diagnosis. This means that maybe little was done in the night, while the inflammatory cascade was debuting its deadly coil. Possibly, the golden hours of septic shock are the earliest ones. By a prompt bedside diagnosis, the FALLS-protocol would like to decrease the huge mortality rate of septic shock – a major healthcare challenge.

Glossary

Clinical volemia This part of volemia which determines the beginning of fluid overload at the main vital organ, normally fluid-free.

FALLS-endpoint The instant where B-lines replace A-lines under fluid therapy.

FALLS-PLR-protocol Passive leg raising initiating a fluid therapy.

FALLS-point Applying the probe at anterior lung watching for a change from A-lines to B-lines during fluid therapy.

FALLS-protocol Protocol analyzing the cause of a shock using simple cardiac sonography and lung ultrasound.

FALLS-responsiveness Defined by an A-profile (or equivalents) in a patient without ultrasound signs of obstructive or left cardiogenic shock. Clearance for fluid therapy.

Round-FALLS-protocol Ultrasound search for a site of sepsis or hypovolemia done during the FALLS-protocol.

Appendix A

A.1 Short Reminder of Our Study

A prospective 5-year study evaluated 102 critically ill ventilated and sedated patients, receiving a PAC for complex hemodynamic situations in medicosurgical ICUs (62 men, mean age 57, PEEP between 0 and 7 mmHg, mean tidal volume 7 ± 1 ml/kg, plateau pressure <32 cm H_2O), hemodynamic measurements done at the discretion of the managing team. The ultrasound operators, blinded to hemodynamic measurements, checked for pressure head at the correct location, catheter line flushed, zero level, radiography, appropriate pressure curves surrounding balloon inflation. The PAOP curve displaying characteristic and logic curves (respiratory variations of PAOP remaining under respiratory variations of pulmonary artery diastolic pressure) was considered. The patients remained connected with the ventilators. The probe was applied on the BLUE-points. We slightly adapted the nomenclature of the BLUE-protocol [79], defining the A-predominance as predominant areas of anterior A-lines, including the A/B profile, and the C-profile surrounded by A-lines. The B-predominance was defined as predominant anterior areas of lung rockets. For a PAOP value ≤18 mmHg, the A-predominance had a 93 % specificity and a 97 % positive predictive value (PPV) (sensitivity 50 %, negative predictive value (NPV) 24 %). If the value of 13 mmHg was considered, the specificity of a PAOP ≤13 mmHg was 90 % and the PPV 91 % (sensitivity 67 %, NPV 65 %) [87] (Fig. 30.1).

A.2 Application of the Grotowski Law to the FALLS-Protocol

A shocked patient has little chance to survive, spontaneously. Admitted in a hospital of any quality, and taken in charge by an intensivist of any quality, the chances of survival dramatically increase, from zero to maybe 60 % in what we will call "average ICUs," and 75 % in the best institutions of our world, using TEE, etc. (called "top ICUs"). These numbers are author's very rough estimations. Accepting them, the difference between the average and the top ICU would be roughly 15 points.

If we introduce holistic ultrasound (i.e., the BLUE-protocol, the FALLS-protocol, the Fever-protocol, the SESAME-protocol, venous line insertion, etc.) in the "average ICUs," with our simple gray scale unit, we just bet that this gap of 15 % will be reduced. If we make the free hypothesis that holistic ultrasound will provide just a small 14 % improvement, it would mean that the whole investment of top ICUs (intellectual investment plus financial investment for PICCO, sophisticated echocardiography, etc.) would allow a 1 % improvement of care quality. If LUCI would provide a 16 % improvement, the average ICUs would increase up to 76 %, which would here, in this hypothetical case, raise solid questions. We advocate the launching of multicentric studies for giving scientific answers (not assumptions) of how LUCI can impact the daily life of an ICU.

References

1. Swan HJ, Ganz W, Forrester J, Marcus H, Diamond G, Chonette D (1970) Catheterization of the heart in man with use of a flow-directed balloon-tipped catheter. N Engl J Med 283:447–451
2. Cholley BP, Payen D (2003) Pulmonary artery catheters in high-risk surgical patients. N Engl J Med 348:2035–2037
3. Braunwald E (1984) Heart disease. W.B. Saunders Company, Philadelphia, p 173
4. Braunwald E, Rahimtoola SH, Loeb HS (1961) Left atrial and left ventricular pressure in subjects without cardiovascular disease. Circulation 24:267–274
5. Flores ED, Lange RA, Hillis LD (1990) Relation of mean pulmonary arterial wedge pressure and left ventricular end-diastolic pressure. Am J Cardiol 66:1532–1533
6. Pinsky MR (2003) Clinical significance of pulmonary artery occlusion pressure. Intensive Care Med 29:175–178

7. Boldt J (2000) Volume therapy in the intensive care patient – we are still confused, but.... Intensive Care Med 26:1181–1192
8. Connors AF Jr, Speroff T, Dawson NV, Thomas C, Harrell FE Jr, Wagner D, Desbiens N, Goldman L, Wu AW, Califf RM, Fulkerson WJ Jr, Vidaillet H, Broste S, Bellamy P, Lynn J, Knaus WA (1996) The effectiveness of right heart catheterization in the initial care of critically ill patients. SUPPORT investigators. J Am Med Assoc 276:889–897
9. Krausz MM, Perel A, Eimerl D, Cotev S (1977) Cardiopulmonary effects of volume loading in patients in septic shock. Ann Surg 185:429–434
10. Packman RI, Rackow EC (1983) Optimum left heart filling pressure during fluid resuscitation of patients with hypovolemic and septic shock. Crit Care Med 11:165–169
11. Zion MM, Balkin MM, Rosenmann D, Goldbourt U, Reicher-Reiss H, Kaplinsky E, Behar S (1990) Use of the pulmonary artery catheter in patients with acute myocardial infarction. Chest 98:1331–1335
12. Mimoz O, Rauss A, Rekik N, Brun-Buisson C, Lemaire F, Brochard L (1994) Pulmonary artery catheterization in critically ill patients: a prospective analysis of outcome changes associated with catheter prompted changes in therapy. Crit Care Med 22:573–579
13. Wagner JG, Leatherman JW (1998) Right ventricular end diastolic volume as a predictor of the hemodynamic response to a fluid challenge. Chest 113:1048–1054
14. Wilson J, Woods I, Fawcett J, Whall R, Dibb W, Morris C, McManus E (1999) Reducing the risk of major elective surgery: randomized controlled trial of preoperative optimisation of oxygen delivery. Br Med J 318:1099–1103
15. Rhodes A, Cusack RJ, Newman PJ, Grounds RM, Bennett ED (2002) A randomised, controlled trial of the pulmonary artery catheter in critically ill patients. Intensive Care Med 28:256–264
16. Richard C, Warszawski J, Anguel N, Deye N, Combes A, Barnoud D, Boulain T, Lefort Y, Fartoukh M, Baud F, Boyer A, Brochard L, Teboul JL (2003) French Pulmonary Artery Catheter Study Group – Early use of the pulmonary artery catheter and outcomes in patients with shock and acute respiratory distress syndrome: a randomized controlled trial. J Am Med Assoc 290:2713–2720
17. Sandham JD, Hull RD, Brant RF, Knox L, Pineo GF, Doig CJ, Laporta DP, Viner S, Passerini L, Devitt H, Kirby A, Jacka M (2003) A randomized, controlled trial of the use of pulmonary artery catheters in high-risk surgical patients. N Engl J Med 348:5–14
18. Monnet X, Richard C, Teboul JL (2004) The pulmonary artery catheter in critically ill patients. Does it change outcome? Minerva Anestesiol 70:219–224
19. Shah MR, Hasselblad V, Stevenson LW, Binanay C, O'Connor CM, Sopko G, Califf RM (2005) Impact of the pulmonary artery catheter in critically ill patients: meta-analysis of randomized clinical trials. JAMA 294:1664–1670
20. Sakr Y, Vincent JL, Reinhart K, Payen D, Wiedermann CJ, Zandstra DF, Sprung CL (2005) Use of the pulmonary artery catheter is not associated with worse outcome in the ICU. Chest 128:2722–2731
21. Simini B (2005) Pulmonary artery catheters in intensive care. Lancet 366:435–437
22. Harvey S, Harrison DA, Singer M, Ashcroft J, Jones CM, Elbourne D, Brampton W, Williams D, Young D, Rowan K (2005) PAC-Man study collaboration. Assessment of the clinical effectiveness of pulmonary artery catheters in management of patients in intensive care (PAC-Man): a randomised controlled trial. Lancet 366(9484):472–477
23. Osman D, Ridel C, Rey P, Monnet X, Anguel N, Richard C, Teboul JL (2007) Cardiac filling pressures are not appropriate to predict hemodynamic response to volume challenge. Crit Care Med 35:64–68
24. Gnaegi A, Feihl F, Perret C (1997) Intensive care physicians insufficient knowledge of right-heart catheterization at the bedside: time to act? Crit Care Med 25:213–220
25. Squara P, Bennett D, Perret C (2002) Pulmonary artery catheter: does the problem lie in the users? Chest 121:2009–2015
26. Pinsky MR, Vincent JL (2005) Let us use the pulmonary artery catheter correctly and only when we need it. Crit Care Med 33:1119–1122
27. Stoddard MF, Liddell NE, Vogel RL, Longaker RA, Dawkins PR (1992) Comparison of cardiac dimensions by transesophageal and transthoracic echocardiography. Am Heart J 124(3):675–678
28. Vieillard-Baron A, Slama M, Mayo P, Charron C, Amiel JB, Esterez C, Leleu F, Repesse X, Vignon P (2013) A pilot study on safety and clinical utility of a single-use 72-hour indwelling transesophageal echocardiography probe. Intensive Care Med 39(4):629–635
29. Jardin F, Valtier B, Beauchet A, Dubourg O, Bourdarias JP (1994) Invasive monitoring combined with two-dimensional echocardiographic study in septic shock. Intensive Care Med 20:550–554
30. Benjamin E, Oropello JM, Stein JS (1996) Transesophageal echocardiography in the management of the critically ill patient. Curr Surg 53:137–141
31. Costachescu T, Denault A, Guimond JG, Couture P et al (2002) The hemodynamically unstable patient in the ICU: hemodynamic vs. transesophageal echocardiographic monitoring. Crit Care Med 30:1214–1223
32. Boulain T, Achard JM, Teboul JL, Richard C, Perrotin D, Ginies G (2002) Changes in BP induced by passive leg raising predict response to fluid loading in critically ill patients. Chest 121:1245–1252
33. Axler O, Megarbane B, Lentschener C, Fernandez H (2003) Comparison of cardiac output measured with echocardiographic volumes and aortic Doppler methods during mechanical ventilation. Intensive Care Med 29:208–217
34. Vieillard-Baron A, Chergui K, Rabiller A, Peyrouset O, Page B, Beauchet A, Jardin F (2004) Superior vena

caval collapsibility as a gauge of volume status in ventilated septic patients. Intensive Care Med 30:1734–1739
35. Slama M, Masson H, Teboul JL et al (2004) Monitoring of respiratory variations of aortic blood flow velocity using esophageal Doppler. Intensive Care Med 30:1182–1187
36. Monnet X, Rienzo M, Osman D, Anguel N, Richard C, Pinsky MR, Teboul JL (2005) Esophageal Doppler monitoring predicts fluid responsiveness in critically ill ventilated patients. Intensive Care Med 31:1195–1201
37. Poelaert JI, Schupfer G (2005) Hemodynamic monitoring utilizing transesophageal echocardiography: the relationships among pressure, flow, and function. Chest 127:379–390
38. Via G, Braschi A (2006) Echocardiographic assessment of cardiovascular failure. Minerva Anesthesiol 72:495–501
39. Price S, Nicol E, Gibson DG, Evans TW (2006) Echocardiography in the critically ill: current and potential roles. Intensive Care Med 32:48–59
40. Perel A (1998) Assessing fluid responsiveness by the systolic pressure variation in mechanically ventilated patients. Systolic pressure variation as a guide to fluid therapy in patients with sepsis-induced hypotension. Anesthesiology 89:1309–1310
41. Shoemaker WC (1996) Oxygen transport and oxygen metabolism in shock and critical illness. Invasive and noninvasive monitoring of circulatory dysfunction and shock. Crit Care Clin 12:939–969
42. Taylor DE, Simonson SG (1996) Use of near-infrared spectroscopy to monitor tissue oxygenation. New Horiz 4:420–425
43. Tavernier B, Makhotine O, Lebuffe G, Dupont J, Scherpereel P (1998) Systolic pressure variation as a guide to fluid therapy in patients with sepsis-induced hypotension. Anesthesiology 89:1313–1321
44. Michard F, Boussat S, Chemla D, Anguel N, Mercat A, Lecarpentier Y, Richard C, Pinsky MF, Teboul JL (2000) Relation between respiratory changes in arterial pulse pressure and fluid responsiveness in septic patients with acute circulatory failure. Am J Respir Crit Care Med 162:134–138
45. Michard F, Teboul JL (2002) Predicting fluid responsiveness in ICU patients: a critical analysis of the evidence. Chest 121:2000–2008
46. Reuter DA, Felbinger TW, Schmidt C, Kilger E, Goedje O, Lamm P, Goetz AE (2002) Stroke volume variation for assessment of cardiac responsiveness to volume loading in mechanically ventilated patients after cardiac surgery. Intensive Care Med 28:392–398
47. Pinsky MR (2004) Using ventilation-induced aortic pressure and flow variation to diagnose preload responsiveness. Intensive Care Med 30:1008–1010
48. Perel A, Minkovich L, Preisman S, Abiad M, Segal E, Coriat P (2005) Assessing fluid responsiveness by a standardized ventilatory maneuver: the respiratory systolic variation test. Anesth Analg 100:942–945
49. Combes A, Arnoult F, Trouillet JL (2004) Tissue Doppler imaging estimation of pulmonary artery occlusion pressure in ICU patients. Intensive Care Med 30:75–81
50. Pavlinic I, Tvrtkovic N, Holcer D (2008) Morphological identification of the soprano pipistrelle in Croatia. Hystrix It J Mamm 19:47–53
51. Magder S (2005) How to use central venous pressure measurements. Curr Opin Crit Care 11:264–270
52. Pinsky MR (2003) Hemodynamic monitoring in the intensive care unit. Clin Chest Med 24:549–560
53. Pinsky MR, Payen D (2005) Functional hemodynamic monitoring. Crit Care 9:566–572
54. Vincent JL, Weil MH (2006) Fluid challenge revisited. Crit Care Med 34:1333–1337
55. Michard F, Teboul JL (2000) Using heart-lung interactions to assess fluid responsiveness during mechanical ventilation. Crit Care 4:282–289
56. Rex S, Brose S, Metzelder S, Huneke R, Schalte G, Autschbach R, Rossaint R, Buhre W (2004) Prediction of fluid responsiveness in patients during cardiac surgery. Br J Anaesth 93:782–788
57. Fietsam RJ, Villalba M, Glover JL, Clark K (1989) Intra-abdominal compartment syndrome as a complication of ruptured abdominal aortic aneurysm repair. Am Surg 55:396–402
58. Malbrain ML, Cheatham ML, Kirkpatrick A et al (2006) Results from the international conference of experts on intra-abdominal hypertension and abdominal compartment syndrome. Intensive Care Med 32:1722–1732
59. de Backer D, Creteur J, Preiser JC et al (2002) Microvascular blood flow is altered in patients with sepsis. Am J Respir Crit Care Med 166:98–104
60. Sakr Y, Dubois MJ, De Backer D et al (2004) Persistent microcirculatory alterations are associated with organ failure and death in patients with septic shock. Crit Care Med 32:1825–1831
61. Dellinger RP, Levy MM, Carlet JM, Dion J, Parker MM et al (2008) Surviving Sepsis Campaign. International guidelines for management of severe sepsis and septic shock. Intensive Care Med 341:17–60
62. Abid O, Akca S, Haji-Michael P, Vincent JL (2000) Strong vasopressor support may be futile in the intensive care unit patient with multiple organ failure. Crit Care Med 28:947–949
63. Magder S (1998) More respect for the CVP (editorial). Intensive Care Med 24:651–653
64. Walley KR (2005) Shock. In: Hall JB, Schmidt GA, Wood DH (eds) Principles of critical care, 3rd edn. McGraw Hill, New York, pp 249–265
65. Jardin F (1997) PEEP, tricuspid regurgitation and cardiac output. Intensive Care Med 23:806–807
66. Antonelli M, Levy M, Andrews P, Chastre J, Hudson LD, Manthous C, Meduri GU, Moreno RP, Putensen C, Stewart T, Torres A (2007) Hemodynamic monitoring in shock and implications for management. International Consensus Conference, Paris, April 27–28, 2006. Intensive Care Med 33:575–590
67. Teboul JL (1991) Pression capillaire pulmonaire. In: Dhainaut JF, Payen D (eds) Hémodynamique, concepts et pratique en réanimation. Masson, Paris, pp 107–121

68. Schumaker PT, Cain SM (1987) The concept of a critical oxygen delivery. Intensive Care Med 13:223–229
69. Hayes MA, Timmins AC, Yau EH et al (1994) Elevation of systemic oxygen delivery in the treatment of critically ill patients. N Engl J Med 330(24):1717–1722
70. Rivers E, Nguyen B, Havstad S, Ressler J, Muzzin A, Knoblich B, Peterson E, Tomlanovich M (2001) Early goal-directed therapy in the treatment of severe sepsis and septic shock. N Engl J Med 345:1368–1377
71. ProCESS Investigators, Yealy DM, Kellum JA, Huang DT, Barnato AE, Weissfeld LA, Pike F, Terndrup T, Wang HE, Hou PC, LoVecchio F, Filbin MR, Shapiro NI, Angus DC (2014) A randomized trial of protocol-based care for early septic shock. N Engl J Med 370(18):1683–1693. doi:10.1056/NEJMoa1401602
72. Peake SL, Delaney A, Bailey M, Bellomo R, Cameron PA et al, ARISE Investigators (2014) Goal-directed resuscitation for patients with early septic shock. N Engl J Med 371(16):1496–1506
73. Bellamy MC (2006) Wet, dry or something else? Br J Anaesth 97(6):755–757
74. Hollenberg SM, Ahrens TS, Annane D, Astiz ME, Chalfin DB, Dasta JF, Heard SO, Martin C, Napolitano LM, Susla GM, Totaro R, Vincent JL, Zanotti-Cavazzoni S (2004) Practice parameters for hemodynamic support of sepsis in adult patients: 2004 update. Crit Care Med 32:1928–1948
75. Vieillard-Baron A, Slama M, Cholley B, Janvier G, Vignon P (2008) Echocardiography in the intensive care unit: from evolution to revolution? Intensive Care Med 34:243–249
76. Vieillard-Baron A, Slama M (2008) Prise en charge hémodynamique du sepsis sévère et du choc septique à l'aide de l'échocardiographie. In: Vignon P (ed) Echocardiographie Doppler chez le patient en état critique. Elsevier SRLF, Paris, pp 97–114
77. Lichtenstein D, Mezière G, Biderman P, Gepner A, Barré O (1997) The comet-tail artifact : an ultrasound sign of alveolar-interstitial syndrome. Am J Respir Crit Care Med 156:1640–1646
78. Lichtenstein D, Mezière G (1998) A lung ultrasound sign allowing bedside distinction between pulmonary edema and COPD: the comet-tail artifact. Intensive Care Med 24:1331–1334
79. Lichtenstein D, Mezière G (2008) Relevance of lung ultrasound in the diagnosis of acute respiratory failure – the BLUE-protocol. Chest 134:117–125
80. Lemaire F, Brochard L (2001) ARDS. In: Réanimation Médicale. Masson, Paris, pp 807–810
81. Walley KR, Wood LDH (1998) Ventricular dysfunction in critical illness. In: Hall JB, Schmidt GA, Wood LDH (eds) Principles of critical care, 2nd edn. McGraw Hill, New York, pp 303–312
82. Staub NC (1974) Pulmonary edema. Physiol Rev 54:678–811
83. Guyton CA, Hall JE (1996) Textbook of medical physiology, 9th edn. W.B. Saunders Company, Philadelphia, pp 496–497
84. Chait A, Cohen HE, Meltzer LE, VanDurme JP (1972) The bedside chest radiograph in the evaluation of incipient heart failure. Radiology 105:563–566
85. Safran D, Journois D (1995) Circulation pulmonaire. In: Samii K (ed) Anesthésie Réanimation Chirurgicale, 2nd edn. Flammarion, Paris, pp 31–38
86. Rémy-Jardin M, Rémy J (1995) Œdème interstitiel. In: Imagerie nouvelle de la pathologie thoracique quotidienne. Springer, Paris, pp 137–143
87. Lichtenstein D, Mezière G, Lagoueyte JF, Biderman P, Goldstein I, Gepner A (2009) A-lines and B-lines: lung ultrasound as a bedside tool for predicting pulmonary artery occlusion pressure in the critically ill. Chest 136:1014–1020
88. Weil MH, Shubin H (1971) Proposed reclassification of shock states with special reference to distributive defects. Adv Exp Med Biol 23:13
89. Natanson C, Danner RL, Reilly JM, Doerfler ML, Hoffman WD, Akin GL, Hosseini JM, Banks SM, Elin RJ, MacVittie TJ et al (1990) Antibiotics versus cardiovascular support in a canine model of human septic shock. Am J Physiol 259:H1440–H1447
90. Cariou A, Marchal F, Dhainaut JF (2000) Traitement du choc septique: objectifs thérapeutiques. In: Actualités en réanimation et urgences 2000. Elsevier, Paris, pp 213–223
91. Gargani L, Lionetti V, Di Cristofano C et al (2007) Early detection of acute lung injury uncoupled to hypoxemia in pigs using ultrasound lung comets. Crit Care Med 35:2769–2774
92. Quilici-Ancel N, Laxenaire MC (2001) Choc anaphyllactique. In: "Etats de choc", Réanimation Médicale. Masson, Paris, pp 719–745
93. Brooks A et al (2007) Major trauma. Elsevier, Edinburgh, p 841
94. Lichtenstein D (1992) [Inferior caval vein and central venous pressure]. In: L'Echographie Générale en Réanimation. Springer, Paris/Berlin/Heidelberg, pp 84–88
95. Lichtenstein D, Jardin F (1994) Noninvasive assessment of CVP using inferior vena cava ultrasound measurement of the inferior vena cava in the critically ill. Réanim Urgences 3:79–82
96. Lichtenstein D, Jardin F (1996) Calibre de la veine cave inférieure et pression veineuse centrale (Lettre à la Rédaction). Réanim Urgences 5(4):431–434
97. Barbier C, Loubières Y, Schmitt JM, Hayon J, Ricôme JL, Jardin F, Vieillard-Baron A (2004) Respiratory changes in IVC diameter are helpful in predicting fluid responsiveness in ventilated, septic patients. Intensive Care Med 30:1740–1746
98. Feissel M, Michard F, Faller JP, Teboul JL (2004) The respiratory variation in inferior vena cava diameter as a guide to fluid therapy. Intensive Care Med 32:1832–1838
99. Dénier A (1946) Les ultrasons, leur application au diagnostic. Presse Med 22:307–308
100. Lichtenstein D (2007) Point of care ultrasound: infection control on the ICU. Crit Care Med 35(Suppl):S262–S267

References   259

101. Thys DM (1984) Pulmonary artery catheterization: past, present and future. Mt Sinai J Med 51:578–584
102. Raper P, Sibbald WJ (1986) Misled by the wedge? The Swan-Ganz catheter and left ventricular preload. Chest 89:427–434
103. Tousignant CP, Walsh F, Mazer CD (2000) The use of transesophageal echocardiography for preload assessment in critically ill patients. Anesth Analg 90:351–355
104. Pinsky MR (2003) Pulmonary artery occlusion pressure. Intensive Care Med 29:19–22
105. Kumar A, Anel R, Bunnell E, Habet K, Zanotti S, Marshall S, Neumann A, Ali A, Cheang M, Kavinsky C, Parrillo JE (2004) Pulmonary artery occlusion pressure and central venous pressure fail to predict ventricular filling volume, cardiac performance, or the response to volume infusion in normal subjects. Crit Care Med 32:691–699
106. Boldt J, Lenz M, Kumle B, Papsdorf M (1998) Volume replacement strategies on intensive care units: results from a postal survey. Intensive Care Med 24:147–151
107. Teboul JL et le groupe d'experts de la SRLF (2004) Recommandations d'experts de la SRLF. Indicateurs du remplissage vasculaire au cours de l'insuffisance circulatoire. Réanimation 13:255–263
108. Jardin F (1986) Cœur pulmonaire chronique. In: Jardin F, Dubourg O (eds) L'exploration échocardiographique en médecine d'urgence. Masson, Paris/New York/Barcelone, pp 125–133
109. Jardin F, Farcot JC, Boisante L, Curien N, Margairaz A, Bourdarias JP (1981) Influence of positive end-expiratory pressure on left ventricle performance. N Engl J Med 304(7):387–392
110. Vieillard-Baron A (2011) Septic cardiomyopathy. Ann Intensive Care 1(1):6. doi:10.1186/2110-5820-1-6
111. Ferguson ND, Meade MO, Hallett DC, Stewart TE (2002) High values of the pulmonary artery wedge pressure in patients with acute lung injury and acute respiratory distress syndrome. Intensive Care Med 28:1073–1077
112. de Backer D (2012) Predicting fluid responsiveness: what to do with all these indices? Réanimation 21:123–127

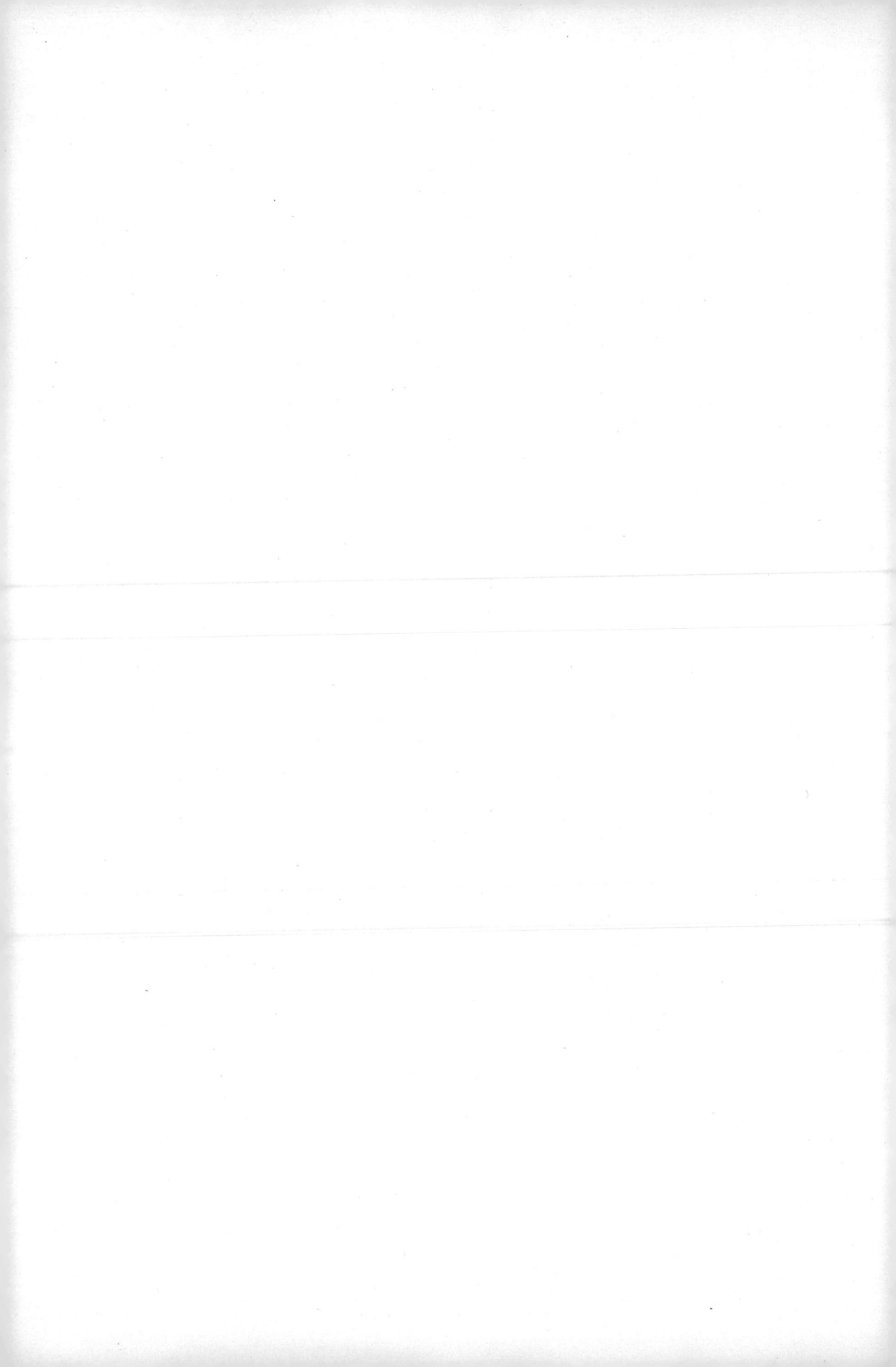

Lung Ultrasound as the First Step of Management of a Cardiac Arrest: The SESAME-Protocol

31

In cardiac arrest, the SESAME-protocol proposes to scan first the lung for two major targets: pneumothorax and clearance for fluid therapy. This information can be obtained in less than 5 s, i.e., a minimal hindrance in the course of resuscitation.

The SESAME-protocol then scans the lower femoral veins and the belly (first if trauma), for detecting pulmonary embolism or massive bleeding.

Then a pericardial tamponade is sought for.

Cardiac causes then follow, in position 5.

Our small, compact ultrasound unit (with the 5 MHz microconvex probe) allows for whole body exploration. How does it work in practice, considering the ultimate emergency: cardiac arrest?

Electronic supplementary material The online version of this chapter (doi:10.1007/978-3-319-15371-1_31) contains supplementary material, which is available to authorized users.

The Concept of Ultrasound in Cardiac Arrest or Imminent Cardiac Arrest, Preliminary Notes

No need to write that we deal here with the highest degree of skill, responsibilities, and emotion (Fig. 31.1). Slight warning: the diagnosis of a cardiac arrest is usually easy and does not require ultrasound. The SESAME-protocol should not be used by doctors knowing the cause of this given cardiac arrest. It is mainly devoted to the arrest of unknown origin, assuming that we have no clinical clue for orientation. It is also devoted to the young intensivist not sure to give his or her best. The author is not young but uses this protocol in almost all cases. The word "usually," written 8 lines above, becomes obsolete with the use of ultrasound.

Cardiac arrest and imminence of cardiac arrest have many common causes. The SESAME-protocol was initially built for extremely severe shocks with imminence of cardiac arrest, but rapidly extended to cardiac arrest. To consider both together allows making the thinnest possible textbook. Few subtleties are not significant enough for changing the spirit.

The best medicine is to anticipate cardiac arrest, by detecting the reversible causes. In the dark ages, these were usual errors in diagnosis, yielding so many avoidable deaths in the night of admission – before the era of visual medicine. The concept of the SESAME-protocol was

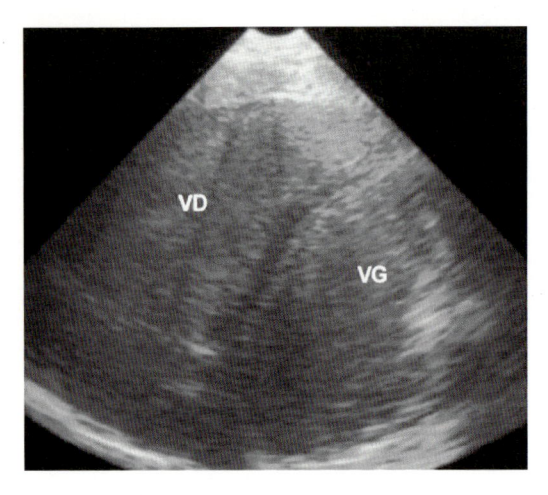

Fig. 31.1 Cardiac sludge. In this subcostal view, all chambers have echoic homogeneous content. This sludge pattern is the result of cardiac arrest (hypoxic asystole in a chronic lung disease). The chambers will become normally anechoic after the recovery of a spontaneous cardiac activity (*VD* right ventricle, *VG* left ventricle)

to find the compromise combining the most frequent situations, the most easy to diagnose using ultrasound, and the most accessible to immediate management – apart from shockable causes. Obstructive causes (pneumothorax, pericardial tamponade, pulmonary embolism) and hypovolemic causes (hemorrhage, etc.) are the most easy to manage. Pneumothorax is probably the best example. In other causes, ultrasound plays a modest role: myocardial infarction, hypoxia (no need for ultrasound for administrating oxygen in a cardiac arrest), hypothermia, toxins, etc.

All settings are considered together (home, trauma, ward, ICU, rich or poor institutions, war settings, etc., resulting in a thin textbook, etc.). In critical situations, the signs are usually blatant (apart from massive pulmonary embolism with no low femoral DVT nor cardiac window, since only subtle signs must be sought for).

Holistic ultrasound will be exploited here to its best, resulting in a really fast protocol where each second is devoted to a specific task. Our daily 26-year work aimed at optimizing each step. We invite to follow a sequential order.

SESAME-Protocol: Another Fast Protocol

Our sequential echographic screening assesses the mechanism *or* origin of a shock of indistinct cause. SESAMOOSIC was a long abbreviation that we shortened in the convenient SESAME-Protocol. Our personal examination regarding shock using adapted sonography indicating origin *or* nature (yes, PERSUASIO*O*N) is rather for those who would prefer tortuous acronyms.

From its own words (see the italic O of the native label), one of the main peculiarities of the SESAME-protocol is to take into account the mechanism *or* the cause of the drama. The user permanently travels from cause to mechanism, according to what comes first to the screen. Finding blood in the abdomen (suggesting hypovolemic cause), or hypercontractile heart (suggesting mechanism of hypovolemia), or again the A-profile, all go to the same action: immediate fluid therapy. There is no time for academic considerations.

Time for scanning both lungs is usually 10 s. Then detecting leg venous thrombosis, abdominal fluid, or pericardial fluid can be done during cardiac compressions (24 more seconds). Then 12 s are devoted to the heart, with the necessity to stop the compressions.

Cardiac Arrest: Time for Technical Considerations

The SESAME-protocol assesses the lung (far) before the heart, because in 5 s pneumothorax can be discounted and clearance is given for fluid therapy. This apparently futile property upsets the choice of equipment. This textbook will reflect our direct positioning without compromise (Anecdotal Note 1).

Nowadays machines are often laptops with three probes, each one having devoted applications (vascular, cardiac, and abdominal). Multiple filters, harmonic modes, and various facilities allow image refinements. Is it an advantage or a hindrance in critical ultrasound, especially cardiac arrest?

This chapter is an opportunity to remind that the unit that allowed us to define critical ultrasound was the perfectly suitable ADR-4000 from 1982, then the Hitachi-405 since 1992 (updated 2008), which was slightly superior. Since this is so important, we repeat it here briefly, with critical adaptations, the best of Chaps. 2 and 3, on the seven points that make the difference.

1. *Size.* Each saved centimeter is critical. Our machine is 32 cm wide on the cart, i.e., narrower than laptops. This size plus the wheels allow to bring the unit quicker at the bedside of busy settings (ICU, OR, ER, etc.). Imagine we organize a race, each one would take his preferred machine (always fixed on carts of course), all in the same line. At the start, we may see a beautiful mess, with all these large machines running for avoiding the hospital obstacles. A steeple-chase. Who will be the winner? The slimmest machine, regardless laptop or not. Pocket machines? Read the last FAQ, below.
2. *Start up time.* Each second is critical. Our unit starts up in 7 s. In machines with longer start up time (from 30″ to 3′), there is nothing to do but wait. We don't care to have informatic programs – we need an immediate access.
3. *The probe.* Which probe first if pneumothorax, bleeding, and tamponade are all possible (trauma)? Respectively (in this order if the user wishes to follow the SESAME-protocol), the linear then the abdominal and then the cardiac? This probe swapping is time-consuming (not to forget probe/cable disinfection, here theoretical, usually a critical point). The SESAME-protocol skips this chancy guessing game by using a universal microconvex probe. It is a high-level compromise allowing in a few seconds, a lung-vessel-abdomen-pericardium-heart assessment exploiting its 0.6–17-cm range (see Chap. 3). Its shape allows insertion at any site, narrow or large, linear or not.
4. *Simple technology, plus a life-saving detail.* It is permanently configured with the setting of cardiac arrest, which is the same used for everyday applications (venous line insertion, check for bladder distension, etc.). We have *no* setting "LUNG." Our setting is "critical ultrasound," or "SESAME," or "zero filter," or again, "CEURF." There is no change to do for being immediately operational. No destructive filter, no confusing time lag, no harmonics that alter the artifact detection. Complex keyboards, a hindrance for novices, are a hindrance for all in critical, stressing settings. Remember we advocated three buttons for practicing critical ultrasound. Not a lot, yet this is too much in cardiac arrest. Gain? When the unit starts up, it is at the optimal setting. B/M mode? It will not be touched, this is why we advise to get accustomed to recognizing immediate, real-time lung sliding. Depth? A special paragraph for this critical detail.

    The depth: we have fixed a default value, at start-up, of 85 mm. This range is the compromise that allows us to see with maximal relative accuracy those targets: the pleural line, the Merlin's space, the lower femoral vein, the peritoneum, most GI tract, and the pericardium in most cases. If we have to arrive to the heart (Step 5), time may be devoted to push the button up to 140 mm. This setting has been worked out for saving an optimal number of neurons. Everyone can define a different setting (child setting, etc.), just think that depth is time.

    We insert in this section our contact product, Ecolight®, since its use (apart from resulting in a clean discipline) warrants a fast protocol. It saves precious time – with Ecolight®, time for changing a region of interest (lung, veins, belly, pericardium, etc.) is less than 1 s. Read also at the cardiac step, another unexpected advantage.
5. *Compact design.* It is flat, cleanable.
6. *Image quality.* Just see the figures of this textbook. No time to play guesses here, with suboptimal equipment.
7. *Cost.* Its low cost was an opportunity for most patients on Earth since 1992 and even before: the year 1982 was the time for the revolution.

Each detail interacts with others. Our single probe lies on top, not laterally, a detail that saves lateral width: one example among dozens of holistic ultrasound. Some manufacturers begin to build machines inspired by this 1992 technology.

- Unexpected limitations can suddenly appear at any step, potentialized by the extreme stress. An issue is the permanent risk to face unsuitable cardiac windows. Several probes make cables inextricably mixed. Nervously pulling the cable results in drawing the knots tighter, etc. Among apparently futile causes, cables lying on the floor favor the risk of a machine tip over when suddenly mobilized. When each of these small (or bigger) difficulties is added to each other, it is maybe wiser, sadly, not to use ultrasound, and do like doctors always did, i.e., working clinically. Ultrasound must save time, not the opposite.

  This section was an opportunity to insist again on the interest of our universal probe among others. Repeating and repeating is sometimes worth it.

Practical Progress of a SESAME-Protocol

For simplifying the concept, we consider a cardiac arrest occurring in a hospital. It allows the physician to intubate the patient, and then pilot the resuscitation. One solid help makes the cardiac compressions. One delicate help makes the ventilation. One nurse prepares the drugs, etc. (Technical Note 1). For less than four actors, see Technical Note 2.

It is assumed that the intubation was wisely done, i.e., not inserting a demesurate number of meters of endotracheal tube within the thorax. This is important first because ventilating both lungs allows correct oxygenation. If there is no cardiac pulsation, there is *no lung pulse*, and the one-lung intubation would simulate a pneumothorax, etc. A reasonable length is inserted (3 cm after the vocal cords is highly sufficient). Common sense is more useful than ultrasound here. Ultrasound-assisted ABCDE? Read Anecdotal Note 2.

We assume all details not pertaining to ultrasound (sternal punch, check for airway patency, etc.) are covered as usual.

Now, we can manage this cardiac arrest. Figure 31.2 indicates the optimal timing, done with quite no interruption of cardiac massage.

The Lung: First Step of the SESAME-Protocol

Here is no time for politeness (read Anecdotal Note 3). In spite of what was written since ever in the stone regarding lung ultrasound [1], the SESAME-protocol not only includes the lung, but also, and without any complex, begins with the lung. We have all reasons, diagnostic, therapeutic, technical. To begin with the lung allows to benefit from a series of seven providential features:

1. A highly reversible cause of cardiac arrest is detected: pneumothorax.
2. Finding an A-profile makes half of the diagnosis of pulmonary embolism, following the rules of the BLUE-protocol [2]. The diagnosis will be confirmed just after by the venous step (or 24 s later at the cardiac step – window permitting).
3. The detection of an A-profile is a signal of immediate clearance for fluid therapy, following the rules of the FALLS-protocol [3, 4].

Fig. 31.2 The SESAME-protocol. A logical order suggested for assessing cardiac arrest or extreme circulatory failure. SESAME-protocol in a kind of explicit decision tree. Note the quasi-absence of dichotomy: the causes are sought for sequentially, mingling frequency, easiness of ultrasound detection, and possibility of active therapy. *Steps 1, 2, 3, 4* are devoted to highly reversible causes: pneumothorax, pulmonary embolism, hypovolemia, and pericardial tamponade. *Step 5*, more expert, more chancy (depending on favorable windows), asks for the interruption of cardiac compressions. This figure indicates the optimal timing in the best conditions (patient in bed, readily accessible regions of interest), the type of probe used for each step (i.e., here, for all steps), and the depth chosen. The timing includes any change of region of interest, expedited using Ecolight®

Practical Progress of a SESAME-Protocol

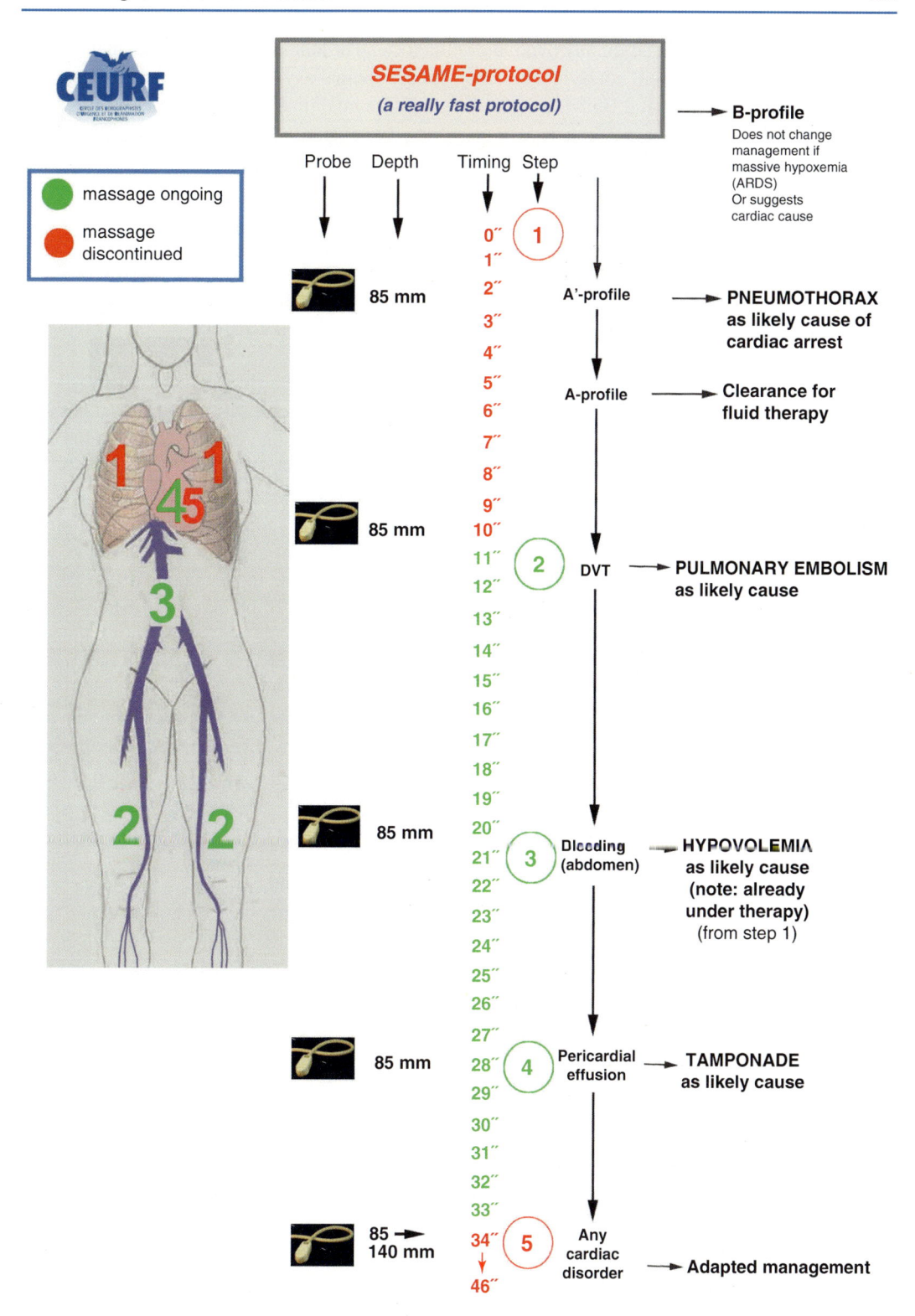

SESAME-protocol
(a really fast protocol)

→ **B-profile**
Does not change management if massive hypoxemia (ARDS)
Or suggests cardiac cause

Probe | Depth | Timing | Step

- 🟢 massage ongoing
- 🔴 massage discontinued

Probe	Depth	Timing	Step		
	85 mm	0″–1″	1		
		2″		A'-profile	→ **PNEUMOTHORAX** as likely cause of cardiac arrest
		3″–4″			
		5″–6″		A-profile	→ Clearance for fluid therapy
		7″–9″			
	85 mm	10″			
		11″–12″	2	DVT	→ **PULMONARY EMBOLISM** as likely cause
		13″–19″			
	85 mm	20″			
		21″	3	Bleeding (abdomen)	→ **HYPOVOLEMIA** as likely cause (note: already under therapy) (from step 1)
		22″–26″			
	85 mm	27″–28″	4	Pericardial effusion	→ **TAMPONADE** as likely cause
		29″–33″			
	85 → 140 mm	34″ ↓ 46″	5	Any cardiac disorder	→ Adapted management

This fluid will be beneficial for any hypovolemic cause (step 3), and will not be lost for any obstructive cause (steps 1, 2, and 4).

4. Lung windows are always `"generous": no need for chancy search, like in echocardiography. The correct window is obtained in 1 s.
5. A pneumothorax able to generate a cardiac arrest is substantial: one point is sufficient.
6. In cardiac arrest, the patient breathes very quietly. This makes the perfect conditions for an optimized detection. No dyspnea, no Keye's sign, no pseudo-A′-profile here: ultrasound is a providence.
7. All this information is obtained in less than 5 s, i.e., a minimal hindrance in the course of resuscitation.

We check at the lower BLUE-point, roughly, while the compressor's hands are positioned on site, ready to work (Technical Note 3). If a pneumothorax is suspected, the CEURF has described some fast solutions. Searching for a lung point may cost time. If decided, it should be done first very posteriorly. Finding (especially in bilateral cases) an extended (anterolateral) A′-profile, detecting just lung sliding posteriorly is a nonacademic makeshift, a common sense maneuver instead of the pathognomonic lung point. The Australian variant can be perfectly used here (see Chap. 27 on pneumothorax): we can consider an A′-profile as a pneumothorax in the case there is a strong clinical argument. The patient is here in cardiac arrest: do we need a stronger clinical argument? Read Anecdotal Note 4. We strengthen this suspicion by here just sounding the thorax by percussion. At this step (cardiac arrest with A′-profile), the slightest tympanism at the suspected side makes the decision. Manually sounding the thorax before ultrasound would be a loss of time each time there is no pneumothorax (and is not a 100 % easy sign in routine medicine). When the Australian variant is positive, the hands of the cardiac compression begin or resume their work, time for finding any large needle, and saving a life.

If the first scanning shows disseminated lung rockets, fluid therapy will not be the immediate option. It means likely that the problem is not related to a low preload. Cardiac causes are usually on focus. The lungs are wet and a fluid therapy may hinder optimal oxygenation (Technical Note 4).

In trauma (mainly frontal mechanism with lung contusion), anterior lung rockets are expected (in the absence of pneumothorax).

No pneumothorax? The probe comes to the femoral veins.

The Veins: Second Step of the SESAME-Protocol

Compressions Begin (or Are Resumed)

A deep venous thrombosis found in a patient with cardiac arrest is quite diagnostic for pulmonary embolism, following the rules of the BLUE-protocol, where the specificity is 99 %.

In the mind of radiologists or vascular physicians, venous scanning is a comprehensive, long work. Here, we use the technique of the BLUE-protocol adapted to the extreme emergency. By applying the probe at the V-point (lower femoral vein), the operator has the best compromise between the following:

- Sensitivity: almost half cases with massive embolism had a lower femoral venous thrombosis, twice as many as the common femoral vein (still under submission). Likewise, scanning the inferior caval vein would be a loss of time: here, the likeliness to still see floating iliocaval thrombosis is near zero. In our series of massive pulmonary embolism under submission, there is no inferior caval location, and we don't devote energy (in the BLUE-protocol) or time (in the SESAME-protocol).
- Speed: in this setting, it is much faster to scan the V-point than the popliteal vein.
- Good sense: the calf area would be even more sensitive, but more difficult. Expert users should begin by the calf veins.

Which side first? Our data slightly favor the right side, paradoxically, but large numbers must be studied.

The venous step limited to the lower femoral vein takes 10 s for both legs and does not interrupt the cardiac compressions. The diagnosis of pulmonary embolism is therefore done with less damage to the brain than if using cardiac echo.

Particular settings. In medical patients with high suspicion of pulmonary embolism, our simple V-point analysis can be extended. In trauma patients, in children, the search for a DVT makes little sense and should really be limited to the V-point (or even skipped). In ICU patients, a CLOT-protocol (i.e., jugular or iliofemoral axes, see the CLOT-protocol in Chap. 28) should be preferred. A slight problem is that DVTs are frequent after catheterization. Yet why should'nt they be responsible for severe disorders, including cardiac arrest?

The BLUE-Protocol as Providing a Direct Proof of Pulmonary Embolism?

If no DVT is found at this area, this does not rule out embolism, far from it. But if the cardiac step, done 14 s later, is unable to show the familiar dilated RV for lack of window, we can enrich the protocol with a kind of sixth step. We know that the only proof of embolism is a direct visualization of clots within pulmonary arteries. CT cannot be performed during cardiac arrest. Transesophageal echo appears, apparently, as the sole tool able to confirm pulmonary embolism at the bedside [5]. Everything seems to have been said regarding this disease [5, 6]. Yet here is our solution: searching for a clot in the right pulmonary artery. We have in hands the perfect tool: our microconvex probe, whose ideal shape and resolution allow an insertion at the suprasternal notch, the best combination for favoring the inconstant exposition of the right pulmonary artery: holistic ultrasound (Fig. 31.3). The CEURF approach can be done much faster than the fastest TEE. Finding a clot within the right pulmonary artery, a rare event it is true, allows a definite diagnosis.

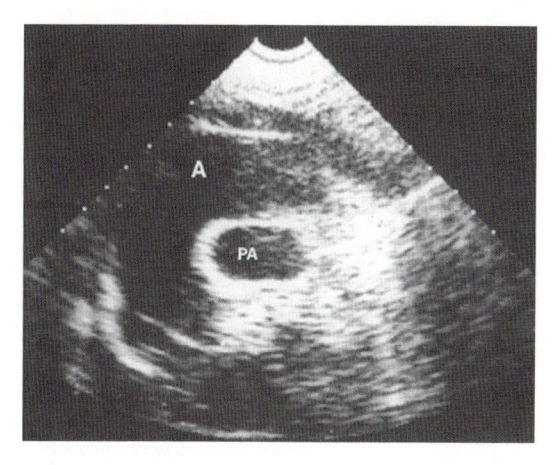

Fig. 31.3 A bedside proof of pulmonary embolism. In cardiac arrest, likeliness to see a clot in the pulmonary artery is much higher than in any other situation. Our small microconvex probe is easily inserted at the suprasternal notch, its resolution allows most often, not always, to expose the aortic arch (*A*), and in its concavity, the right pulmonary artery (*PA*). Clots should be sought for there. They can be seen floating even without circulatory activity

Finding abdominal blood, the fluid therapy is just massive, there is nothing more to do (apart from calling a surgeon, finding fresh blood units, compress the belly).

This is why, outside trauma, the SESAME-protocol considered the veins before the abdomen (detecting a DVT leads to an immediate specific therapy).

We here proceed to a fast scanning for any source of fluid, i.e., peritoneal and intra-digestive. Don't be obsessed only by the Morrison's pouch, etc.: substantial amounts of digestive fluid is likened to an hypovolemic cause of cardiac arrest. See what GI tract hemorrhage looks like in Chap. 34, Video 34.3. This section remains short (See Anecdotal Note 5).

The Belly: Third Step of the SESAME-Protocol

No Need for Discontinuing Compressions

A bleeding can explain the cardiac arrest, and its detection concludes the SESAME-protocol. Note that it will not provide immediate changes: the A-profile already ordered massive fluid therapy.

The Pericardium: Fourth Step of the SESAME-Protocol

No Need for Discontinuing Compressions (Usually)

Usually, the abdominal hypotony favors a subcostal window. We therefore first try this approach. In the unlikely event there is no

window, the probe is applied at the thorax, meaning the necessity of withdrawing the hands of the cardiac compression. The SESAME-protocol splits pericardium from heart since five solid reasons have decided so:
1. The pericardium is quite immediate to learn, does not require anatomical efforts: we see two heart circles instead of one.
2. It is a reversible cause of cardiac arrest.
3. It is easy to treat, usually.
4. It enlarges the "cardiac" windows, which makes it particularly suitable for ultrasound diagnosis.
5. No need to enlarge the 85 mm depth usually: saved time, the pericardium is a superficial organ (unlike the heart, a deeper organ).

A substantial effusion in cardiac arrest *means* pericardial tamponade (Video 31.1). If the right chambers are collapsed, this speculation becomes even more of a reality. We don't need Doppler.

Our adapted technique of visually assisted pericardiocentesis will be described here (more than in Chaps. 19 or 30), in a devoted appendix for not breaking the rhythm of this paragraph (Appendix 1).

How to drain the pericardium fully pertains to holistic ultrasound. We have in hands the universal probe, allowing both to diagnose the tamponade, and to drive our needle with maximal ease. With cardiac probes in hands, physicians do not have the perfect tool for detecting a needle. They developed sophisticated protocols for avoiding a cardiac wound, e.g., microbubble injections, etc. This is time-consuming (see special note on pericardiocentesis in Chap. 3).

The Basic Heart: Last Step of the SESAME-Protocol

Need Here for Discontinuing Compressions

When pneumothorax, pulmonary embolism, hypovolemia, and pericardial tamponade have been ruled out (four highly reversible causes), the very heart is then scanned.

At this step, mystical colleagues should devote 1 s for a short prayer, for the blessing of a cardiac window. As opposed to the lung, the absence of correct cardiac window is a constant possibility. Insisting eats precious time. One profits of this short prayer for enlarging the depth from 85 to 140 mm. Now, recognizing at first glance all cardiac structures is obvious for skilled users, but beginners must devote substantial time for being really operational. We first try a subcostal view (cardiac compressions are discontinued, hands on-site). If there is no window, the operator takes the responsibility of withdrawing the compression hands.

When the heart is not rapidly visible (10–12 s is probably a maximum), it is given up (temporarily if necessary) for resuming massage and privilegiating (shockable causes aside) hypovolemic or embolic causes (e.g., see other sites of DVT, bleeding, aortic aneurysm, massive pleural effusion). This "sixth step" can also include the optic nerves (brain hemorrhage).

Our contact product, Ecolight, has one more major relevance: at the cardiac step, time for withdrawing the amounts of gel for resuming cardiac compressions (unless the area would be *slippery*) is skipped.

Some are free to use – at this step – a transesophageal approach.

Hundreds of subtleties arc available for favoring a cardiac window. We always ask the ventilator help to stop ventilation at end of expiration. We can ask the strong compressor help to turn the thorax to the left. These details pertain to ultrasound too.

If a window is acquired, we will see various dynamics, from *simple* to *subtle:*
- To see a dynamics means that the patient is not fully dead. One can complicate (read Anecdotal Note 6).
- A LV hypercontractility with virtual systolic volume (kissing walls): *déjà vu*. This invites to consider huge hypovolemia as a cause (detected in Steps 1 and 3, usually redundant).
- The swinging heart: *déjà vu*. It was seen at Step 4 (pericardial tamponade).
- A RV enlargement with sometimes some contractility: *déjà vu*. This suggests massive pulmonary embolism (a diagnosis done in half the cases at Steps 1 and 2). Devote 2 s for detecting a clot within the heart. The cardiac

compressions are resumed (very energetically for some, in the hope of fragmenting a voluminous clot), a fibrinolytic therapy is injected.
- Ventricular tachycardia and ventricular fibrillation make a continuum. In ventricular tachycardia, contractions are still visible. Here, in principle, the place of ultrasound is limited when the semi-automatic device (EAD), now more widely available, gives the suggestion to defibrillate. When the tachycardia degrades into ventricular fibrillation, one may detect in favorable cases a shivering myocardium. This sometimes mimics asystole on ECG. Ultrasound may possibly show more sensitive (and much faster, a nice advantage) than ECG, skipping the limitations of those EADs, which may in a few instances suggest not to push the red button. In these disorders, the cardiac arrest is rather sudden, and the usual steps of the SESAME-protocol (if done, in the absence of any EAD), can be adapted. It is true also that with the current progresses in cardiology, these causes get less frequent nowadays – a nice beginning. One day maybe, it will be forbidden to die from the heart.
- Torsade de pointe gives more marked contractions (in our observations, it does not completely stop the circulation). We had not yet time to see if the torsade itself can be detected.
- In high degree atrioventricular block, the auricle systole is independent from ventricle systole, a characteristic asynchronism.
- Clearly, many other dynamic signs exist, complementary to the ECG or quicker. Slightly apart from cardiac arrest, in the left bundle branch block, a delay in septal contraction is typically a subtle sign.
- Asystole, i.e., a standstill heart. This is a rather easy diagnosis (Video 31.2), with however a poor prognosis [7]. This is another reason why CEURF teaches lungs before heart.

When cardiac output is interrupted, the blood becomes visible in the heart chambers (Fig. 31.1, Video 31.2). The SESAME-protocol inserts some 4T4P causes here: toxic drug, hyperkalemia, hypothermia. Here, other tools are used for the diagnosis. The usual therapy is given (epinephrine or any drug *à la mode*), cardiac compressions are resumed, time for drugs to come on site. Devices for automatic massage, ECMO, all possible tools are welcome at this step.

Interventional Ultrasound in the SESAME-Protocol

The drainage of a tamponade is detailed in Appendix 1.

Fast central venous access, by simple checking for a favorable venous caliper, or ultrasound-guided procedure, can be useful. Here, this is no time for traditional catheterism: we take our ELSISCEC system, with the multipurpose 60-mm long catheter, described in the section on urgent procedures of Chap. 34, and Fig. 34.2. This catheter is on site on the ultrasound cart (one more reason for having a cart, one more reason among many for not finding major interest in the laptop philosophy). For young users, the femoral route is the best since the massage can be maintained (have in mind that the arterial pulse is difficult to detect). For experienced users, less than 20 s are sufficient for the internal jugular or subclavian access.

If an electrosystolic probe must be inserted, ultrasound has a double advantage: immediate venous access and guiding the probe within cardiac cavities.

Inserting a radial artery for distinguishing shock without pulse from PEA [8]? With therefore the necessity of purchasing in a haste the sempiternel vascular probe? Read Technical Note 5.

Limitations of the SESAME-Protocol

Pseudo-limitations are all ultrasound configurations that may generate loss of time, loss of suitable vision.

Pneumothorax: mainly, massive subcutaneous emphysema.

Pulmonary embolism: obviously, those cases with no visible DVT, no fine cardiac window, no supra-aortic window for the pulmonary artery.

Table 31.1 Correlation between 4T/4P and SESAME-protocol

Traditional 4T/4P (slightly adapted and modified)	SESAME-protocol
Tension pneumothorax	Step 1
Thrombosis (pulmonary artery)	Step 2 (sometimes 5)
Tamponade	Step 4
Thrombosis (coronary artery)	Step 5 or AED
Toxics	Step 5
Hypovolemia	Steps 1 and 3
Hyperkalemia and other metabolic causes	Step 5
Hypothermia	Step 5
Hypoxia	One may envisage a Step 6, PLAPS-point investigation (with no added therapy)

Abdominal bleeding: cases with poor echogenicity.

Pericardial tamponade: these cases we heard about of loculated effusions that can create hemodynamic dramas, but are impossible to drain from percutaneous approaches (if posterior), a therapeutic issue common to traditional CPR.

Any cardiac cause: no cardiac window.

Everywhere (lungs apart): poor windows, unsuitable body habitus.

Frequently Asked Questions on the SESAME-Protocol

We guess many questions will arise. Here are some.

Q: *The "4 H and 4 T": not considered by the SESAME-protocol?*

A: Yes, fully, but dispatched in another logic (and with a probe in hands). See Table 31.1.

Q: *Does it work as well in adults and children?*

A: Adults are more likely to make cardiac arrest. In the neonate, the DVT is unlikely. Bleeding from a difficult delivery is a cause. It can be abdominal, intra-cerebral, intra-ventricular, immediately diagnosed using the microconvex probe, whose raison d'être was initially, as far as we understood... the transfontanellar use...

Q: *Mahmoud ElBarbary, a name in critical ultrasound, also a smart mind, asked us whether it was legitimate to search for a venous compressibility in a state where the blood was not circulating.*

A: One may answer that, if a cardiac arrest is managed at a step where the blood has already massively clotted, a bolus of fibrinolytic agent would be an idea as valuable as any other idea. We will nevertheless pay high attention to this remark. At the time given, we make profit of it for giving one more suggestion for researchers eager for publications: would ultrasound be able to *date* a cardiac arrest?

Q: *But has the SESAME-protocol been validated?*

A: The SESAME-protocol does not require validation: It uses applications already validated. Pneumothorax, fluid detection, pericardial tamponade, etc., belong to the domain of ultrasound. The SESAME-protocol just asks to make these steps faster, using a sequence just adapted to the likely origin of cardiac arrest, using a concept (unit, probe, contact product, etc.) where every step has been worked out for being expedited.

Q: *SESAME-protocol apart, are there solid validations in the use of ECHO in cardiac arrest?*

A: Each of us has spectacular stories where ultrasound saved lives. Strong signals are perceptible on the usefulness of the concept [9]. Our friends have developed nice studies for cardiac arrest [7, 10]. Papers begin to merge. Yet cardiac arrest is not the most favorable setting for academic studies with accurate gold standards. We expect countless fresh, enthusiastic studies to be published – bewaring all sudden studies that sometimes, time passing, lose their flashy colors – but we should take care of every detail, trying to catch any information with both a critical and open mind in this sensitive field. Up to now, comparing the SESAME-protocol with other studies has not yet been achieved.

Q: Pocket machines?

A: We must identify two kinds. One of them, cardio-centered with Doppler, may not be suitable. We did not study it in depth, given a really insufficient resolution (point 2 in our seven requirements). Permanently wearing this cumbersome device (which does not take one pocket but two) (plus one pocket for the gel, do not forget) (plus the disinfectant) (and the needles) is a bit constraining. Keeping the unit round the neck is, at the time being (apart from a flashy image), not fully pleasant, and it is rather harming and noisy, since the two parts repeatedly knock against each other – a detail which may rapidly become boring for an event which does not occur every day. Another kind, from Australia, has the suitable resolution according to our criteria. This is a simple grayscale concept that respects the artifacts, works in instant response, has a long range microconvex probe, and a simple setting (two buttons). It was built in the spirit of the Hitachi-405 technology. The small screen and the long probe are defaults we can accept here. A major advantage: a possible use when the patient is lying on the ground, in the street, or again a use in a crowded room, where even a small cart may be difficult to insert very rapidly (see Fig. 2.5).

The SESAME-Protocol: Psychological Considerations

Academic readers will wonder how far will this use decrease mortality and neurologic sequela of such a drama. While keeping the question open, and apart from huge satisfactions of saving lives and brains in our carrier, we highlight one point that is not insignificant: our profession is based on a lot of (prestigious) technique and knowledge, but also some emotion. Managing a cardiac arrest using *visual* assistance allows to see that everything is done for this patient. This enables to endure our profession, year after year. This is good for the doctor and is consequently good for the many patients he or she will manage. Several of our colleagues (or sometimes, their wives, a real achievement for us) tell us how they feel serene, using this visual medicine here. "Be fast, not nervous" may be the discrete theme of the SESAME-protocol. Critical ultrasound is an *anti-aging* drug.

Critical Notes for Concluding

Like a certain kind of computer compared with others, we have tried to do the whole work for avoiding any time-consuming work to the users. They have just to push the button, everything is ready for scanning and saving a life (one unique probe, one setting, one default depth, etc., every technical detail behind has been optimized, worked out for expediting each step).

However, we should keep in mind that ultrasound is only a tool. Sometimes, it is of great contribution, such as immediately detecting the tension pneumothorax and giving clearance for fluid therapy, not too bad for an application (lung) not supposed to exist [11]. Yet, even if it usually provides a luminous way, its contribution can like any tool unexpectedly, for infrequent but countless reasons, be a failure. Be a doctor, always, more than ever. Not a magic wand, ultrasound should be used with major humility and seriousness.

> **Technical Notes**
> 1. *How to practically initiate the SESAME-protocol*
>
>   We are called for a cardiac arrest (ward, ER). We leave our ICU, run on site with the red bag of Fig. 2.6, at best followed by our student who takes the ultrasound machine. The saved time allows a prompt intubation, while the unit is switched on. We (before or during intubation) hear the available clinical information, always very limited – and we decide, either to follow the five steps of the SESAME-protocol or to adapt them to the specific setting. The SESAME-protocol aims at being

flexible. In some cases, ultrasound is useless (if an EAD is already on site, ready to defibrillate, or any other reason).

2. *How many actors*

EAD, etc., aside, assuming the patient in a hospital bed, and no orientation, here is a possible guideline.

One single doctor (with ventilation equipment)

If the cardiac arrest has just happened, this physician benefits from many seconds before the fated three minutes (i.e., 180 s, a lot). Considering any possibility, we first intubate, inflate balloon, fix the tube at best, then ventilate with one hand and scan the lung with the probe in the other hand. This is technically possible (in less than one minute after short training), and probably better than compressing the thorax blindly during hours in the case of a pneumothorax (this should have happened more than once in the old times). Then we make Steps 2, 3, 4, and 5 with no ventilation, no compression. Then we do as any doctor. If the physician has just the ultrasound unit and nothing for ventilating the patient, then Step 1 (pneumothorax) should be assessed using clinical tools.

With one help

We find better to ventilate the patient, make Steps 1, 2, 3, 4, and 5 (without compression), then do traditional CPR as long as necessary.

With two helps

One for the ventilation, one for the circulation, the physician makes a "quiet" SESAME-protocol.

3. *Compression first, or lung ultrasound first?*

If cardiac compressions are done but interrupted, the coronary perfusion pressure drops immediately, and it is longer to find the previous values. This is why, if it is only a matter of 10 s, our habit is to begin by lung ultrasound scanning, then initiate compressions. As a concept, this can be debated.

4. *Fluid therapy if wet lungs?*

Once a ROSC obtained (easy in the case of hypoxic arrest), one can scan the PLAPS-point, find huge bilateral PLAPS, which confirm the diagnosis of hypoxic arrest. Knowing that liters of fluid have invaded the lungs, i.e., have left the vascular compartment, some will consider these patients as suddenly and deeply hypovolemic, and will give fluids, anyway, favoring circulation over oxygenation.

5. *Radial artery*

Willing to insert a radial artery under sonography would mean a new change of probe, from the last used (cardiac) to a vascular one. For them, we give again our simple solution (shown in Fig. 3.4), allowing to keep the same microconvex probe: keep ready somewhere in the cart some *tofu*. The tofu gives 1 cm of superficial view, which allows to see the very first millimeter (Fig. 31.4).

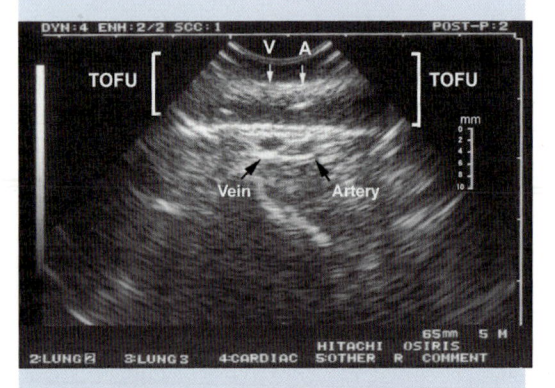

Fig. 31.4 The radial artery using our microconvex probe. Located 3 mm deep to the skin, it is perfectly visualized, small, and pulsatile, if we interpose a piece of *tofu* in order to get the skin 1 cm far from the probe head. We kept the *arrows* at a distance for not spoiling the image. This (not futile) figure means that one probe for the whole body in critical ultrasound is fully realistic, whatever the application

Anecdotal Notes

1. *Why wise water in wine?*

    Each time we were invited to write (solicited) review articles, our manuscripts compared our equipment with the usual laptops. Each time, this was argued by the respected reviewing committees, and we were highly advised to add water in our wine (French expression, roughly meaning, tone down our talks). Here is a space for expressing our experience *as it is*.

2. *ABCDE*

    Some ultrasound courses highlight the A (for airways in life support protocols). Once again, colleagues are free to insert ultrasound everywhere, but we think it is wiser just to learn to intubate correctly. Don't make very exceptional cases the rule. Make the airways free using your vision, aim at the right hole, resist to the longing to penetrate the whole tracheal tree, etc.

3. *Lung first in CPR?*

    When managing cardiac arrest using ultrasound, we did not first begin by the lungs. In 1985, the idea of just using ultrasound appeared "crazy." In these underground years, such a management in such a dramatic setting would have scared our colleagues and chairs (and definitely threatened the rest of our carrier). Even using cardiac ECHO was not in the thought processes. Colleagues were so much interested in other topics (oxygen transport, nitrite oxide in ARDS, etc.), or just had no time for "this." An intensivist using ultrasound? And scanning the *lungs?* This doctor was clearly on an ejection seat. Maybe also, some among these colleagues had in mind these cumbersome machines that needed to be carried out, or even "modern" laptops (not less cumbersome) with endless minutes of start-up, these multiple probes, choosing the setting, etc.., and they found the idea futile. With such a tool, the patient would have it is true no chance of surviving. "Imagination" was *not* "at work" there. In these remote years, we tried to work as far as possible in accordance with the guidelines. Since 1989, the period of lights at François Jardin's ICU, far before the advent of the laptop machines, an embryo of the SESAME-protocol was used, focusing on the heart. Scanning the lung was progressively prepared, time for building scientific evidence, and making it come little by little at the first place, before becoming an irreversible step: all reluctance was then lost for this use, for sharing this image – in 1985 nearly a blaspheme, three decades later the image of a normal modern physician.

4. *Grotowski law*

    Here is one more illustration of Grotowski's law. If we scan thousands of pedestrians in the street, we will probably see some A'-profiles (history of pleural disease, poudrage, pleurodesis, etc.). Immediately piercing the thorax of these poor people right on the street would make more harm than good. If an A'-profile is found during a cardiac arrest, the insertion of any tube/needle would make much more sense, most of the time.

5. *GI tract bleeding plus DVT*

    This note is more sophisticated than anecdotal and could be summarized so: "always, be a doctor" (as Bowra would say). Bleeding plus DVT can coexist. Just consider a bleeding under too generous heparin therapy of a known pulmonary embolism: only the bleeding needs to be fixed. Note that these patients have here two reasons for showing an A-profile: pulmonary embolism, hypovolemia.

6. *PEA*

    A persistent activity recorded on ECG defines pulseless electric activity (PEA), previously called electromechanical dissociation, but still a severe accident. If necessary, respectable works are available [7, 9, 10]. If an echocardiographic dynamics is seen, this is a pseudo-PEA. Half of these cases can benefit from ROSC.

Appendix 1: Our Adapted Technique for Pericardiocentesis

Technically, the cardiac compressions are discontinued, the subxiphoid area is disinfected, and the needle and the microconvex probe make a rather sharp angle (like 30°). Our special 60-mm 16 G catheter is used (ELSISCEC protocol, described in Chap. 34). Thick fluid requires larger catheters. The section on venous cannulation in Chap. 34 describes our extremely simple way of ultrasound-assisted procedures. No need for a 65-statement ICC, just check that the four points are aligned two by two, and go.

Now the needle is inserted, through some liver parenchyma (large vessels, clearly seen, are avoided). If the tip is lost, slight (millimetric) Carmen maneuvers find it back. When a metallic structure penetrates a large fluid rounded cavity, plenty of arciform artifacts can be generated (a "firework sign" should be a self-speaking term). The physician must concentrate only on the needle tip.

Our habit is to keep the end of the needle open, at atmospheric pressure, without syringe: the pericardial fluid under tension will spontaneously spout out (try to collect some fluid for analysis, and volume assessment). This allows to keep the needle in the pericardial sac *and* far from the heart. These good sense maneuvers simplify the technique.

Once fluid pours out, two options are possible: keep the entire catheter as it is, and withdraw it when a reasonable amount of fluid has been evacuated, in order to avoid harm to the heart (initially protected by the pericardial fluid). Or withdraw the metal part for making no risk of cardiac harm, but consider the obliquity of the needle tip (usually 4 mm) and secure this procedure by inserting at least 5 mm of needle within the pericardial sac. A syringe can be mounted, vacuum can be made (two operators may be wise, one firmly maintaining the catheter). According to the volume-pressure curve of the pericardium, a minimal amount is sufficient for fixing the adiastole, allowing a return of spontaneous circulation. If the pericardial effusion is 25 mm large, the first few milliliters of withdrawn fluid will decrease the pressure far more than the volume, and this is the target. If inserting 5 mm of the whole needle, there are still 20 mm (or slightly less) of safety distance from the heart. In the ultrasound domain, this is a comfortable margin.

Several other protocols may be imagined after – we let the user free of his/her own technique.

References

1. Fuhlbrigge A, Choi A (2012) Diagnostic procedures in respiratory diseases. In: Harrison's principles of internal medicine, 18th edn. McGraw-Hill, New York, p 2098
2. Lichtenstein D, Mezière G (2008) Relevance of lung ultrasound in the diagnosis of acute respiratory failure. The BLUE-protocol. Chest 134:117–125
3. Lichtenstein D, Mezière G, Lagoueyte JF, Biderman P, Goldstein I, Gepner A (2009) A-lines and B-lines: lung ultrasound as a bedside tool for predicting pulmonary artery occlusion pressure in the critically ill. Chest 136:1014–1020
4. Lichtenstein D (2015) BLUE-protocol and FALLS-protocol, two applications of lung ultrasound in the critically ill. Chest 147:1659–1670
5. Goldhaber SZ (2002) Echocardiography in the management of pulmonary embolism. Ann Intern Med 136:691–700
6. Schmidt GA (1998) Pulmonary embolic disorders. In: Hall JB, Schmidt GA, Wood LDH (eds) Principles of critical care, 2nd edn. McGraw Hill, New York, pp 427–449
7. Blaivas M, Fox JC (2001) Outcome in cardiac arrest patients found to have cardiac standstill on the bedside E.R. department echocardiogram. Acad Emerg Med 8:616–621
8. Soleil C, Plaisance P (2003) Management of cardiac arrest. Réanimation 12:153–159
9. Salen P, O'Connor R, Sierzenski P et al (2001) Can cardiac sonography and capnography be used independently and in combination to predict resuscitation outcomes? Acad Emerg Med 8:610–615
10. Breitkreutz R, Walcher F, Seeger FH (2007) Focused echocardiographic evaluation in resuscitation management: concept of an advanced life support-conformed algorithm. Crit Care Med 35:S150–S161
11. van der Werf TS, Zijlstra JG (2004) Ultrasound of the lung: just imagine. Intensive Care Med 30:183–184

Part IV

Extension of Lung Ultrasound to Specific Disciplines, Wider Settings, Various Considerations

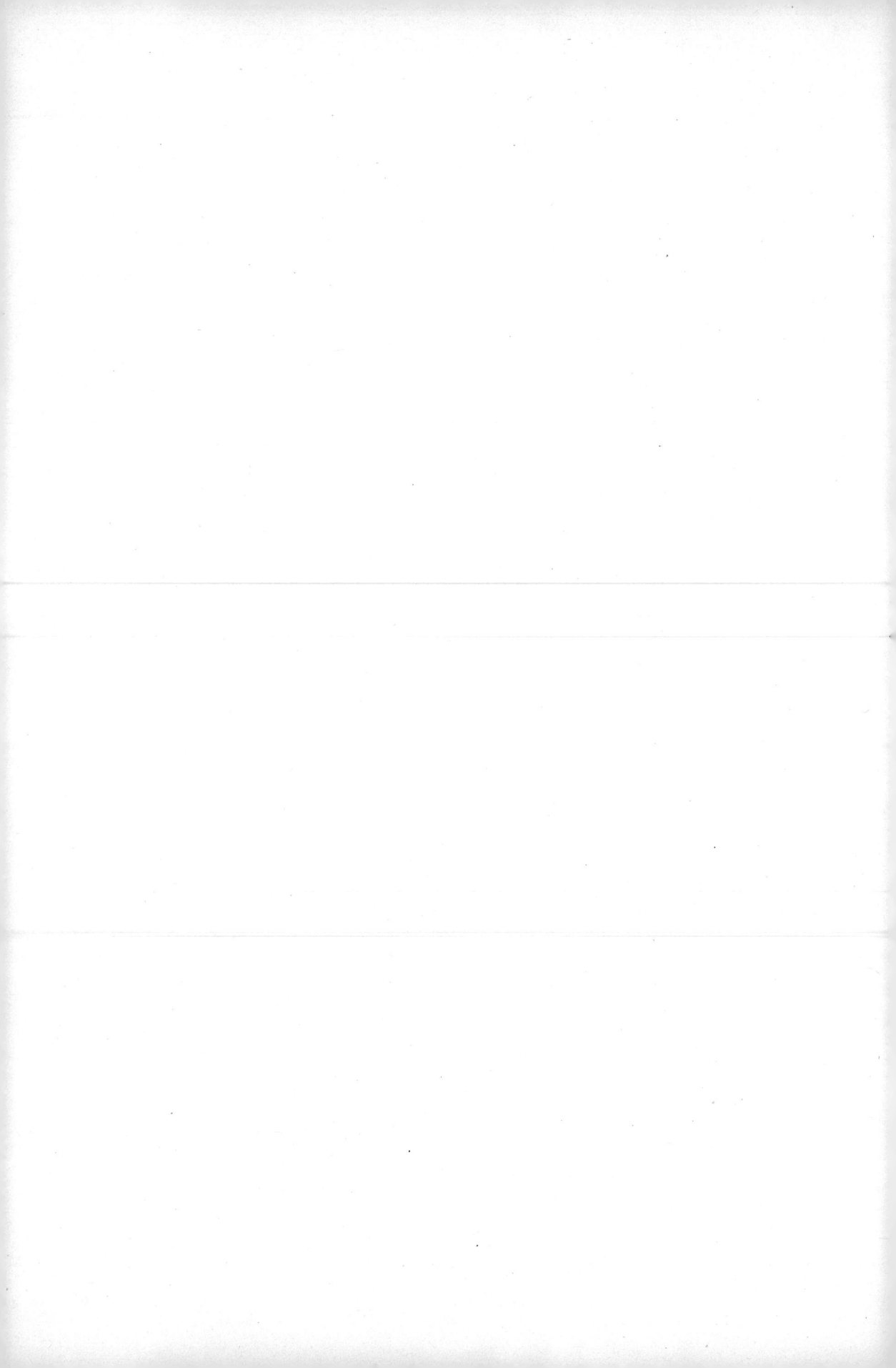

Lung Ultrasound in the Critically Ill Neonate

32

The lung is the main vital organ, and the child is our most precious priority. Any concept which could link the lung and the child is therefore of interest. Up to now, the usual tool is the radiograph. CT should be more accurate one guesses, yet its radiation hazards are difficult to accept here [1–4].

How about using ultrasound, lung ultrasound, a non-irradiating technique, repeatable at will, in the neonate? Born for the privilege of having completed an experience in the critically ill neonate, this chapter will see how LUCI can be introduced in this precious setting. We will demonstrate, without gold standard, why it is possible and urgent to implement lung ultrasound in the neonate.

A 5 MHz microconvex probe will maybe not be sufficient in very small children. Frequencies such as 8–12 MHz should probably be preferred. The use of a high frequency offers the finest resolution.

Lung Ultrasound in the Newborn: A Major Opportunity

The bedside chest radiography is the usual tool used for assessing the neonate's lung. This is striking to see that (without deep mistake) this tool was never assessed. All conclusions can therefore be drawn. In the adult, the bedside radiograph has a rough sensitivity of two-thirds for life-threatening disorders [5].

It is classical (and correct) to say that the child is not a miniature adult. But is it true as regards lung ultrasound? In particular, would pneumothorax generate the same signs? Would the edematous interlobular septa of a neonate (10 or 20 times smaller than the adult) generate the same B-lines? Interstitial changes are hardly visible in adult radiographies, this is worst in neonates.

Rare works had the opportunity to overcome the obstacle of the reviewing processes in this sensible setting [6–10], while we were stuck with the task of submitting just the *signs* of lung ultrasound before being able to reach the following step: showing their relevance [11–13]. We congratulate these authors, hoping our underground work has helped a little.

We analyzed newborns (35± days) admitted in a PICU after cardiac surgery, for 3 years. We used the technique and semiotics described, assessed, and standardized in the adult.

We took maximal care avoiding crossed infections. This is quite impossible with most machines, since the profusion of buttons and probes makes futile any attempt of cleaning.

We avoided the use of Doppler, since we are still not confident on the absence of side effects [14–16].

We had no choice but using a Philips Sonos 5500 (Philips, Andover, Netherlands) unit with a phased array 12 MHz probe. This was not ideal for many reasons. By fully exploiting our previous experience, it was possible to draw conclusions, but we guess young users would have found more difficulties.

An acronym for such an application? Read our comments in Chap. 37.

The Design of Our Study

We assessed whether the ten signs that make lung ultrasound in the adult were found again in the newborn:
1. The pleural line (with the bat sign)
2. The A-lines
3. Lung sliding (with the seashore sign)
4. The quad sign (with the lung line)
5. The sinusoid sign
6. The tissue-like sign
7. The shred sign
8. The B-lines
9. Lung sliding abolished (with the stratosphere sign)
10. The lung point

Basic Technique

The BLUE-points, described in Chap. 6, are used with no adaptation (Fig. 32.1). They replace previous landmarks (Accessory Note 1). Lung ultrasound in the neonate is more easy than in the adult. The 8-cm length of the probe is relatively long here, for the PLAPS-point investigation, but the light weight of the baby makes easier the rotation of the thorax (keeping in mind the fragile endotracheal tube).

The Signs of Lung Ultrasound (Seen and Assessed in Adults) and Rough Results

Basic normal signs: Signs N° 1–3
The pleural line (with the bat sign) was found in all examinations (Fig. 32.2). Lung sliding was either present (with the seashore sign) or abolished. The A-lines were visible in enough cases to note that a newborn lung surface was able to generate A-lines.

Pleural effusion: Signs N° 4 and 5
The quad sign and the sinusoid sign were found in some cases (Fig. 32.3). It was possible to make precise measurements. Further studies should convert these measurements into volumes, using standardized points.

Lung consolidation: Signs N° 6 and 7
All signs described in the adult were present, i.e., the tissue-like sign, the shred sign, the air bronchograms, the dynamic air bronchograms, etc. (fluid tubulograms and others) (Fig. 32.3). They were seen in more than half the cases. A BLUE-consolidation index was available for each. Regarding the mediastinal line, the distance with the pleural line, 9–11 cm in adults, should be here (as well as in adults) four times the length of the pleural line.

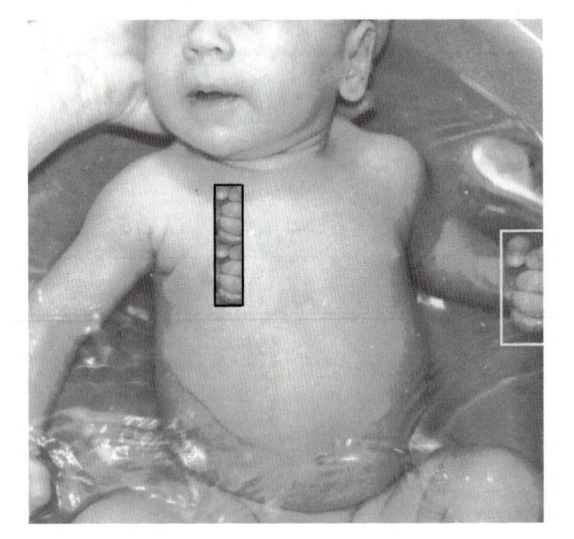

Fig. 32.1 The BLUE-points in the neonate. This figure shows a simple way to determine the anterior chest wall. One takes the size of two hands of the baby, side by side, without thumbs, from the lower border of the clavicula. The lower finger indicates the lower end of the lung (note that the left hand (*white frame*) is in a nearer plane, and we corrected the projection of the hand for the need of the picture)

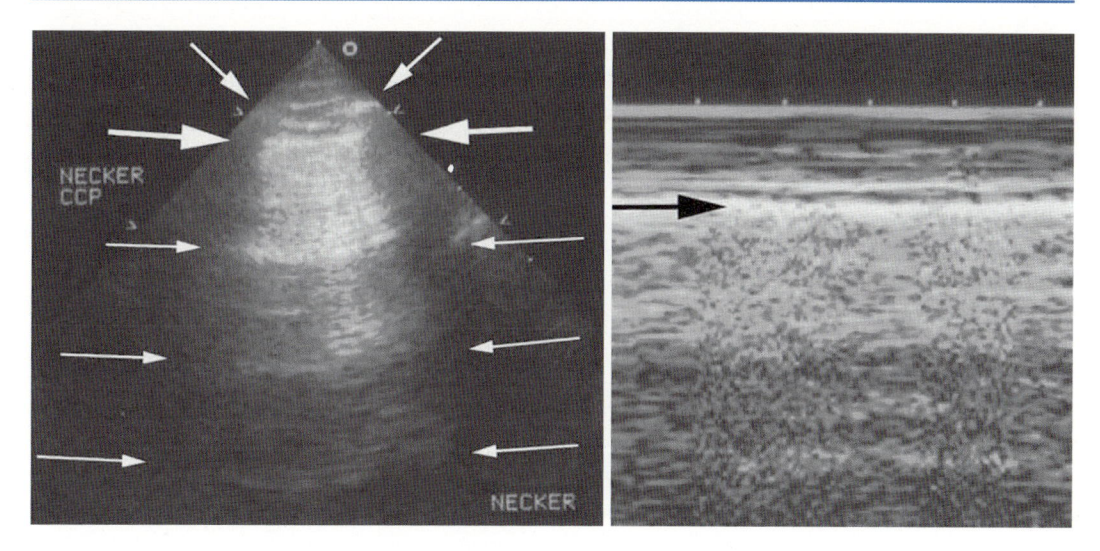

Fig. 32.2 Normal lung surface (A-profile) in the neonate. *Left*: as in the adult, the ribs of the mature neonate give acoustic shadows, and a bat sign can be depicted, with proportions identical to the adult. In this child, the pleural line between two ribs is visible through 9 mm, and the rib line/pleural line distance is 2.5 mm. The fine *horizontal arrows* indicate A-lines. *Right*: a seashore sign, exactly similar to an adult's one. Note the Keye's sign (also similar to the adult's one), above the pleural line (*arrow*). All these data indicate that this child has a (quarter of) A-profile, meaning that the BLUE-protocol may be applied to children (Image acquired with a Hewlett-Packard Sonos 5500)

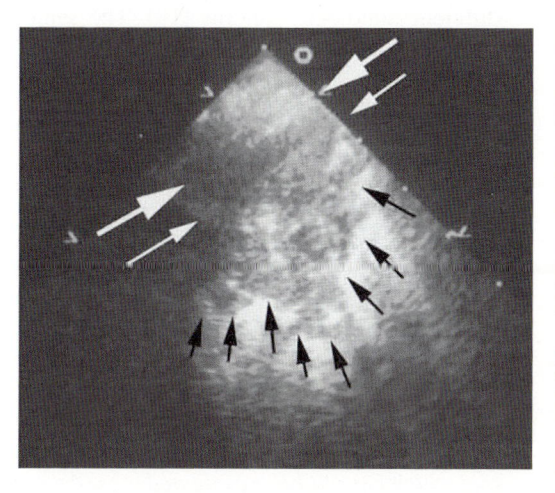

Fig. 32.3 PLAPS in the neonate. From *top to bottom*: the large *arrows* indicate the pleural line. The *small white arrows* indicate a lung line, demonstrating a (small) pleural effusion. Surrounded by the black arrows, a tissular pattern with a shred sign, i.e., a lung consolidation. Example of PLAPS (detected at the PLAPS-point). Once again note the poor resolution quality (Image acquired with a Hewlett-Packard Sonos 5500)

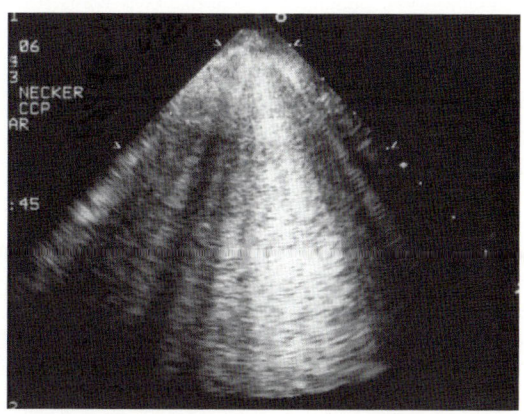

Fig. 32.4 Lung rockets in the neonate. Massive lung rockets at a neonate's lung surface, as in the adult, indicating an interstitial disorder (inflammatory lung syndrome after cardiac by-pass) (Image acquired with a Hewlett-Packard Sonos 5500)

Interstitial syndrome: Sign N° 8

The characteristic sign of interstitial syndrome, i.e., the disseminated lung rockets, were recorded in many cases (Fig. 32.4).

Pneumothorax: Signs N° 9 and 10

The A′-profile and the lung point were observed in a few cases.

The profiles of the BLUE-protocol

It is too early to affirm that the BLUE-protocol works in the neonate. Just note that *all* its profiles were seen again in critically ill neonates: we saw all BLUE-profiles dispatched among these babies, by order of increasing frequency: the B, A/B, C, A then B′ profiles. We let the physicians either imagine what they can infer from these data or drive any necessary studies using any appropriate gold standard.

Demonstration of the Potential of Ultrasound to Replace the Bedside Radiography as a Gold Standard

We found in this series roughly the same discrepancy than the one long highlighted in the adult (where CT clearly demonstrated ultrasound's superiority). Our experience has no solid gold standard such as CT, and we expect many rejections of our work (warning on the value of bedside chest radiography in the light of ultrasound data).

When two tests disagree, one is right, one is wrong, without space for intermediate possibilities in one given patient. We propose two ways (one logical, one scientific) for demonstrating the superiority of ultrasound, even without a gold standard.

For the Hurried Reader, the Logical, and Intuitive Proof

Our 3-year experience driven in a neonate ICU showed that the 10 basic, standardized signs that were assessed in the adult (who benefited from CT correlations) were all found again in critically ill newborns. During all this observation, we did not see any "new" sign particular to the neonate that had not been observed previously in the adult. What else to add? When finding a fractal sign, which disease to expect (but a non-translobar lung consolidation)?

For Non-hurried Readers, a Scientific Proof

Here is a ten-step demonstration. In spite of the absence of CT correlation, the discrepancy found between radiography and ultrasound should favor ultrasound.

Step 1: The ultrasound signs assessed in the adult are exactly the same in the neonate

See our comments just above ("for the hurried readers").

Step 2: A discrepancy between ultrasound and radiography is highlighted in the critically ill neonate

Our experience in neonates showed that the correlation with the radiography, read by skilled blinded radiologists, made appear a discrepancy in roughly the same proportions as the one long observed in adults – where CT clearly showed ultrasound's superiority.

Step 3: The anatomic features of each syndrome (pneumothorax, etc.) are the same in both adults and neonates

Regarding the assessed disorders, no radiologic distinction was made to our knowledge between adults and children [17]. There is no physiopathological argument for assuming that these two populations should generate different radiologic patterns [18]. The same reasoning is valuable as regards ultrasound. This is the only speculation of our demonstration.

Step 4: Adult bedside chest radiography is imperfect

The limitations of radiography have been clearly demonstrated in the adult [19–27] (Table 32.1).

Step 5: Ultrasound has accuracy near to CT in the adult

As opposed, ultrasound proved in the adult a sensitivity and a specificity near to CT [5, 26–32] (see Table 29.3), on occasion superior [33].

Step 6: Bedside radiography in the neonate is a tool which has not been evaluated

No work to our knowledge has assessed chest radiography's value in neonates. Some works comment the interest of daily routine radiographs in the PICU when showing unexpected

Table 32.1 Accuracy of radiography compared to CT in the adult ARDS

	Sensitivity (%)	Specificity (%)
Pleural effusion	39	85
Lung consolidation	68	95
Interstitial syndrome	60	100

From Lichtenstein et al. [5]

findings [34–36], but none investigated the interpretation of negative findings (as well as critical appraisal of positive results).

Step 7: In the adult, bedside radiography is more specific than sensitive

Assessment of bedside radiography in the critically ill adults highlighted a low sensitivity. The specificity was far better. False-negatives were six times more frequent than false-positives, i.e., a false-negative/false-positive ratio of 6 (Table 32.1) [5]. Keep in mind this proportion for the next step.

Step 8: If compared to radiography, ultrasound in the neonate seems more sensitive than specific.

In our experience, if taking radiography as a gold standard, ultrasound showed much more false-positive cases than false-negatives. The overall false-positive/false-negative ratio was precisely 5.3. This rate is strikingly similar to the adult false-negative/false-positive ratio. This similarity will now be exploited.

Step 9: In the present study, ultrasound had the worst results in the areas where radiography is known for having precisely the worst results

We now use the Step 3 speculation. Demonstrating that a method (lung ultrasound in the neonate) has apparently low specificity precisely in the areas where radiography showed poor sensitivity (in the adult) amounts to saying that ultrasound false-positives would have been in fact true-positives, if compared with a solid gold standard. Our experience showed that ultrasound had the *worst* specificity precisely in the areas where radiography had the *worst* sensitivity.

Radiography's specificity is good as regards pneumothorax [31] and interstitial syndrome [5]. In these fields precisely, ultrasound showed high sensitivity.

Step 10: Our few CT correlations

They have no statistic power, but, precisely, they show what had to be demonstrated. Of this very beginning of definitive proof, cases of lung consolidation which were frank on ultrasound and absent or uncertain on radiograph were clearly proven – as expected – on CT.

Finding again the 10 assessed standardized ultrasound signs is not due to hazard. Conceptually, it is not possible to imagine which disease can mimic a sinusoid sign if not a pleural effusion (or a lung point, if not a pneumothorax, etc.).

Some Comments

An explanation is available for each of our results (see Tables 29.1 and 29.2).

Bedside radiography lacks sensitivity. Mainly, bedside radiography in supine neonates misses small and retrodiaphragmatic consolidations. When they are visible, but slightly (cul-de-sac blunting), they are easily interpreted as pleural effusions. Bedside radiography misses small pleural effusions (that are easily seen on ultrasound), subtle interstitial changes, small pneumothoraces when the pleural line is not tangential to the X-ray beam. Precisely, the children in our series had postoperative chest tubes. This generated a small size of pleural effusions (if any), well detected on ultrasound, missed on X-ray.

Bedside radiography lacks specificity in precise cases: it proceeds by summation. The summations images can confuse alveolar and pleural disorders, not a problem with ultrasound, which does not make any summation.

As opposed to radiography, ultrasound has both a high sensitivity (principle N°7, nearly all the disorders abut the surface and have usually extensive contact) and a high specificity (since there is no summation effect, mainly). Minute pleural effusions are identified at the PLAPS-point. Minute pneumothoraces are identified at the BLUE-points. For lung consolidations, the problem is slightly different, since their location is not standardized (an incomplete scanning can miss some), and some (1.5 % in the adult) do not abut the wall. Not surprisingly, here we found most "false-negative" ultrasound results when compared to radiography.

The case of interstitial syndrome is the most interesting. We first saw that the B-line, as rigorously defined in adults, was present at the neonate's chest wall. Neonates were able to display lung rockets. Our experience being done in a neonate post-cardiac surgery ICU, a high prevalence of interstitial syndrome was expected, since most of them received cardiopulmonary by-pass, a condition known for generating diffuse inflammatory changes [37]. Note that just a few cases among these numerous ones was detected using bedside radiography. We conclude that ultrasound detects a pattern that is most of the time radio-occult. The anterior Kerley lines, those which are quite never detected on anteroposterior bedside radiographies, are immediately accessible using ultrasound. Septal rockets as well as ground-glass rockets were observed, suggesting that ultrasound can distinguish simple septal edema from ground-glass lesions also in the neonate. This will maybe have a future impact for urgent therapeutic decisions.

Limitations and Pseudo-limitations of Lung Ultrasound in the Newborn

An hypertrophic thymus is a tissular image which will not confuse with a consolidation: first it is located in a standardized parasternal area, second its deep limit is smooth and regular (not shredded). Third, lung sliding is visible in the depth. Note that the thymus can make a challenge in some front radiographies.

The limitations found in adults will be the same in the neonate (parietal emphysema, dressings).

Among theoretical limitations, if someone can demonstrate that lung consolidations in the neonate do not reach the wall in the same proportion than adults, i.e., 98.5 % of cases, this would decrease ultrasound sensitivity. Our few CT correlations indicate the opposed conclusions: consolidations have the same look as in adults, with large parietal contact (Fig. 32.5). We are ready for this rendezvous with science.

Various Diseases Seen in the Neonate and the Baby

Here is what we saw from our travel in the pediatric world.

The lung of a *fetus* is full of fluid and would show in theory a massive C-profile with massive PLAPS (massive consolidation without effusion), both translobar of course. At birth, the alveolar fluid is rejected outside from the pressure created by the mother's vagina. It is normal to see B-lines on the first hours (should disappear after some hours).

Some neonates have still some water in the lungs at birth. After Caesarean birth, the lungs are not expressed as efficiently as by natural birth. These babies can show *transient tachypnea*. It is transient since it improves after 1–2 days. The

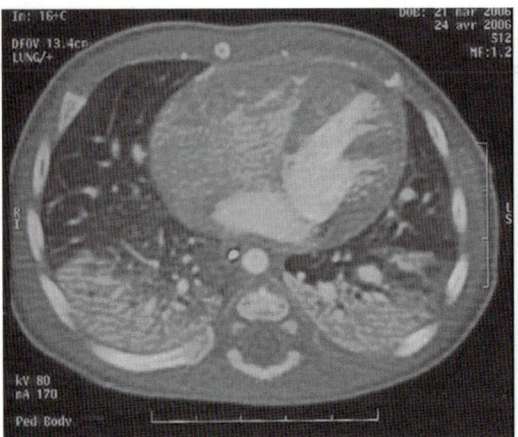

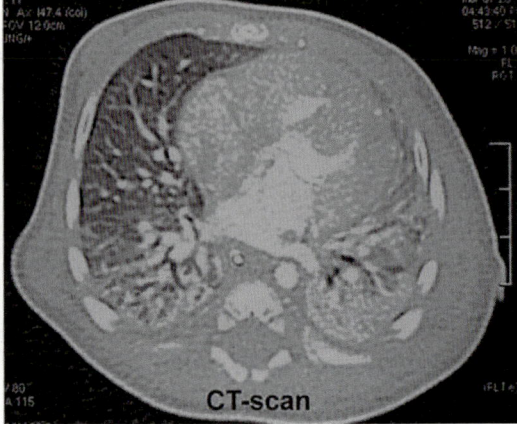

Fig. 32.5 CT in the neonate. Two babies (see centimetric scale) CTs required by the managing team of this pediatric and neonate post-cardiac surgery ICU. As a main piece of information we can exploit, the disorders (lung consolidations here) have the same morphology as in adults

pattern is the upper half A-profile, lower B-profile, for being schematical [6].

Some premature babies develop the *hyaline membrane disease*, a genuine ARDS where B-profiles, B′-profiles, and ground-glass rockets are frequently seen. Eventually, some of these babies will develop bronchopulmonary dysplasia from all traumas of the disease, plus oxygen plus barotraumas. We could see a conserved or impaired lung sliding, and equivalents of A/B-profile (sometimes at the same lung area), of C-profile (many C-lines, sometimes just a thickened, irregular pleural line).

The *acute bronchiolitis* generates patchworks of A/B-profile (we call it micro-A/B-profiles), ground-glass and septal rockets, C-lines, substantial lung consolidations, not including complications (pleural effusions, pneumothorax). This can be described using different terms [9]. The Downes score should be probably connected with these lung ultrasound profiles.

In specific settings such as *post-cardiac surgery*, there is a mingling between "natural" inflammatory response and various aggressions such as ventilator-acquired pneumonia. The result is a mixing of B, B′, C, A/B, A-no-V-PLAPS profiles.

The *pneumothorax* can be seen in various events (traumatic, iatrogenic, lung diseases).

Safety of Lung Ultrasound in the Newborn

We are cautious to any issue that may hamper the use of critical ultrasound. As regards asepsis, we have described our policy in Chap. 4, and will repeat our reluctance for usual laptop keyboards in Chap. 37. As regards the issues of a bad training, we do our best for an efficient training in Chap. 38. As regards Doppler [14–16], we answered by not using this sophistication. As regards the possible side effects of simple ultrasound, we have no knowledge of a particular disease generated by ultrasound since 1951. Which kind of disease has been generated by the way?

For anticipating any issue from fussy users, we give two practical pieces of advice.

1. Lung ultrasound can be done without any decrease of quality with the control button of emission power settled at the *minimal* position.
2. The BLUE-protocol is a fast protocol which can be used with no adaptation in these neonates, meaning that just three points per lung are assessed, each one needing a few seconds. The examination can in addition be recorded, allowing quiet subsequent analysis. All signatures, from lung sliding, lung rockets, etc., to PLAPS, can be detected immediately.

One FAQ: How About the Intermediate Steps Between Neonates and Adults?

Analyzing first with the neonates was time-saving: if neonates have the same signs as adults, it can be safely extrapolated that the sucklings, toddlers, young children, teenagers, etc., will benefit from the same approach. Instead of submitting several manuscripts with endless rejections, we will have enough troubles by just sending one.

Lung Ultrasound in the Neonate, Conclusions

Our observations showed that the ultrasound signs described and standardized in the adult were found again in the newborn. This invites to consider that as regards ultrasound, the newborn's lungs are small adult's lungs [12].

The high degree of standardization of the signs made lung ultrasound a reasonable bedside noninvasive reference test for the critically ill adult (Table 32.1). Its implementation in the child or the neonate must be considered as an absolute priority target [38].

In addition to providing immediate and accurate data, lung ultrasound will be fully integrated in the LUCIFLR project for successfully decreasing radiation doses.

We wait for proofs that only CT will provide. We expect that some cases, gathered here and there, will give the necessary statistic power for convincing the skeptical ones. Meanwhile, we invite pediatric physicians to read the chest radiographies twice, when ultrasound shows discordant items.

Critical ultrasound accustomed us to surprises. Why was it not used sooner? Why was the lung so rigidly prohibited? Why do they sell us this wacky gel? Why this craze for Doppler? Why laptop machines in hospitals? When the problem regards a new life, in a pediatric or neonate ICU, all these questions must be answered seriously. Academic, or opportunist opinions must be balanced only for the benefit of science.

> **Accessory Note**
> 1. Previous landmarks: The mamillary line was a practical landmark in the adult, but is high located in the neonate. We used also the mid-distance between the lung apex and lower costal border as a basic landmark.

References

1. Brenner DJ, Elliston CD, Hall EJ, Berdon WE (2001) Estimated risks of radiation-induced fatal cancer from pediatric CT. AJR Am J Roentgenol 176:289–296
2. Berrington de Gonzales A, Darby S (2004) Risk of cancer from diagnostic X-rays. Lancet 363:345–351
3. United Nations Scientific Committee on the Effects of Atomic Radiation (2000) Source and effects of ionizing radiation. United Nations, New York
4. Brenner DJ, Hall EJ (2007) Computed tomography – an increasing source of radiation exposure. N Engl J Med 357(22):2277–2284
5. Lichtenstein D, Goldstein I, Mourgeon E, Cluzel P, Grenier P, Rouby JJ (2004) Comparative diagnostic performances of auscultation, chest radiography and lung ultrasonography in acute respiratory distress syndrome. Anesthesiology 100:9–15
6. Copetti R, Cattarossi L (2007) The "double lung point": an ultrasound sign diagnostic of transient tachypnea of the newborn. Neonatalogy 91(3):203–209
7. Copetti R, Cattarossi L (2008) Ultrasound diagnosis of pneumonia in children. Radiol Med (Torino) 113(2):190–198
8. Tsung JW, Kessler DP, Shah VP (2012) Prospective application of clinician-performed lung ultrasonography during the 2009 H1N1 influenza A pandemic: distinguishing viral from bacterial pneumonia. Crit Ultrasound J 4:16
9. Caiulo VA, Gargani L, Caiulo S, Fisicaro A, Moramarco F, Latini G, Picano E (2011) Lung ultrasound in bronchiolitis: comparison with chest X-ray. Eur J Pediatr 170:1427–1433
10. Shah VP, Tunik MG, Tsung JW (2013) Prospective evaluation of point-of-care ultrasonography for the diagnosis of pneumonia in children and young adults. JAMA Pediatr 167:119–125
11. Lichtenstein D, Mezière G (2008) Relevance of lung ultrasound in the diagnosis of acute respiratory failure. The BLUE-protocol. Chest 134:117–125
12. Lichtenstein D (2009) Ultrasound examination of the lungs in the intensive care unit. Pediatr Crit Care Med 10:693–698
13. Lichtenstein D, Mezière G, Lagoueyte JF, Biderman P, Goldstein I, Gepner A (2009) A-lines and B-lines: lung ultrasound as a bedside tool for predicting pulmonary artery occlusion pressure in the critically ill. Chest 136:1014–1020
14. Taylor KJW (1987) A prudent approach to Doppler ultrasonography. Radiology 165:283–284
15. Miller DL (1991) Update on safety of diagnostic ultrasonography. J Clin Ultrasound 19:531–540
16. Barnett SB, Ter Haar GR, Ziskin MC, Rott HD, Duck FA, Maeda K (2000) International recommendations and guidelines for the safe use of diagnostic ultrasound in medicine. Ultrasound Med Biol 26:355–366
17. Tuddenham WJ (1984) Glossary of terms for thoracic radiology: recommendations of the Nomenclature Committee of the Fleischner Society. Am J Roentgenol 143:509–517
18. Guyton CA, Hall JE (1996) Textbook of medical physiology, 9th edn. W.B. Saunders Company, Philadelphia, pp 496–497
19. Greenbaum DM, Marschall KE (1982) The value of routine daily chest X-rays in intubated patients in the medical intensive care unit. Crit Care Med 10:29–30
20. Janower ML, Jennas-Nocera Z, Mukai J (1984) Utility and efficacy of portable chest radiographs. AJR Am J Roentgenol 142:265–267
21. Peruzzi W, Garner W, Bools J, Rasanen J, Mueller CF, Reilley T (1998) Portable chest roentgenography and CT in critically ill patients. Chest 93:722–726
22. Wiener MD, Garay SM, Leitman BS, Wiener DN, Ravin CE (1991) Imaging of the intensive care unit patient. Clin Chest Med 12:169–198
23. Tocino IM, Miller MH, Fairfax WR (1985) Distribution of pneumothorax in the supine and semi-recumbent critically ill adult. AJR Am J Roentgenol 144:901–905
24. Hendrikse K, Gramata J, ten Hove W, Rommes J, Schultz M, Spronk P (2007) Low value of routine chest radiographs in a mixed medical-surgical ICU. Chest 132:823–828
25. Henschke CI, Pasternack GS, Schroeder S, Hart KK, Herman PG (1983) Bedside chest radiography: diagnostic efficacy. Radiology 149:23–26

References

26. Lichtenstein D, Mezière G, Lascols N, Biderman P, Courret JP, Gepner A, Goldstein I, Tenoudji-Cohen M (2005) Ultrasound diagnosis of occult pneumothorax. Crit Care Med 33:1231–1238
27. Lichtenstein D, Hulot JS, Rabiller A, Tostivint I, Mezière G (1999) Feasibility and safety of ultrasound-aided thoracentesis in mechanically ventilated patients. Intensive Care Med 25:955–958
28. Lichtenstein D, Lascols N, Mezière G, Gepner A (2004) Ultrasound diagnosis of alveolar consolidation in the critically ill. Intensive Care Med 30:276–281
29. Lichtenstein D, Mezière G, Biderman P, Gepner A, Barré O (1997) The comet-tail artifact, an ultrasound sign of alveolar-interstitial syndrome. Am J Respir Crit Care Med 156:1640–1646
30. Lichtenstein D, Menu Y (1995) A bedside ultrasound sign ruling out pneumothorax in the critically ill: lung sliding. Chest 108:1345–1348
31. Lichtenstein D, Mezière G, Biderman P, Gepner A (1999) The comet-tail artifact, an ultrasound sign ruling out pneumothorax. Intensive Care Med 25:383–388
32. Lichtenstein D, Mezière G, Biderman P, Gepner A (2000) The lung point: an ultrasound sign specific to pneumothorax. Intensive Care Med 26:1434–1440
33. Lichtenstein D, Peyrouset O (2006) Lung ultrasound superior to CT? The example of a CT-occult necrotizing pneumonia. Intensive Care Med 32:334–335
34. Spitzer AR, Greer JG, Antunes M, Szema KF, Gross GW (1993) The clinical value of screening chest radiography in the neonate with lung disease. Clin Pediatr 32:514–519
35. Hauser GJ, Pollack MM, Sivit CJ, Taylor GA, Bulas DI, Guion CJ (1989) Routine chest radiographs in pediatric intensive care: a prospective study. Pediatrics 83:465–470
36. Greenough A, Dimitriou G, Alvares BR, Karani J (2001) Routine daily chest radiographs in ventilated, very low birth weight infants. Eur J Pediatr 160:147–149
37. Day JR, Taylor KM (2005) The systemic inflammatory response syndrome and cardiopulmonary bypass. Int J Surg 3:129–140
38. van der Werf TS, Zijlstra JG (2004) Ultrasound of the lung: just imagine. Intensive Care Med 30:183–184

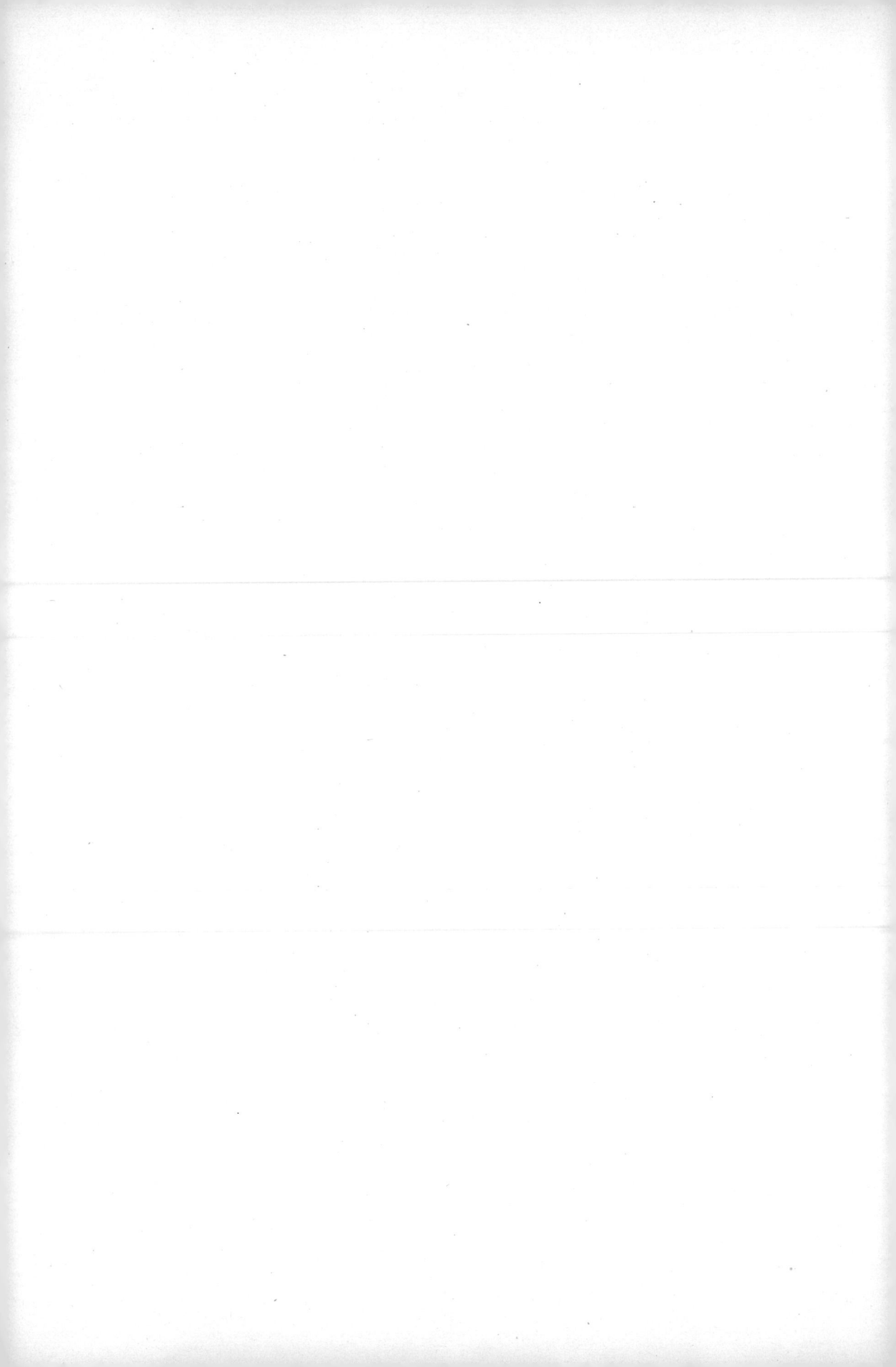

Lung Ultrasound Outside the Intensive Care Unit

33

The intensive care unit is the priority step for developing the BLUE-protocol, but ultrasound is welcome everywhere: the intensivist's experience can be extrapolated to several disciplines and countless settings. We estimated that a dozen of clinical disciplines would be interested. The best for making it a reality would be to implement lung ultrasound in the medical studies: the shortest way. Not whole body ultrasound, because this would result in making longer medical studies. Just lung ultrasound, because it is the simplest, and because all future doctors dealing with the lung would benefit from it. Another aspect of the paradox of LUCI. Therefore, please expect some decades (hopingly less) for seeing ultrasound a natural component of each of these specialties.

Specialties Dealing with Critical Care

The Intensivist

The book is quite fully dedicated for the frontline critical care physician, from medical intensive care or anesthesiology.

Pediatrics and Critical Care, the Neonatologist, the Neonate Intensive Care Unit

This is our priority target. Although our findings were assessed in adults, our experience showed that the signatures were exactly the same with critically ill neonates, with no adaptation.

Given the potential hazards of radiations, each time a child in less critical settings will have ultrasound *instead of* CT, his or her long-term health will be preserved. Cough and fever should expedite an ultrasound test, indicating here no need for antibiotics, or there adapted antibiotics, and there again, admission for tight control (if ultrasound shows disseminated lung disorders).

The Trauma Physician

When we wrote our 1992 edition, the road accidents created severe lesions, and CT was an adventure in these patients. Facing countless minutes for image acquisition, many patients never came back from the CT department. The year 1982 (ADR-4000®) was a golden opportunity for critical ultrasound to develop – a revolution for a complete autonomy. Countless stars in the sky are souls that were not saved since these times.

Now, not only road accidents are much less frequent, but also each small hospital counts several ultra-rapid CT units, the doctors have just to push the button and have a whole body analysis in 10 s, which provides a complete study of the deep organs, the skeleton, a functional study by iodine injection that shows vascular ruptures or parenchymal lesions at the liver, spleen, kidneys, etc. Highlighting CT scan as the first tool in trauma is therefore natural – now [1].

We will not underline again CT's drawbacks. CT is still reserved to the most stable patients, and to be fair, we know some remote villages in the far world that are not yet equipped with hypermodern CTs. We hope that the development of pre-hospital ultrasound will allow more patients to come alive to the hospital. Let us also consider that CT access may become restrained in the future for limiting irradiation – making ultrasound of major interest in focal trauma [2].

We saw about hemothorax, pneumothorax, one lung intubation, etc. Lung contusion [3] yields lung rockets and lung consolidation, better than radiography, only 63 % sensitive [4].

The second principle of lung ultrasound (the sky-Earth axis) will be used if the patient is not strictly supine, but for example a prisoner in an upside down crashed automobile.

We assess the diaphragm using longitudinal scans, an indisputable advantage of ultrasound when compared to the transversal views of CT (see some slides of cupolas in Chaps. 16 and 17 and video in Chap. 36). As usual, radiography lacks specificity. Ultrasound here again plays a role [5]. We put emphasis on indirect signs of rupture: ectopic locations of subphrenic organs – spleen (liver more rarely), GI tract, and abolished lung sliding in spontaneous ventilation.

Pre-hospital Medicine: Lung Ultrasound for Flying Doctors

In an airplane, room is a true concern. Handheld units are *here* a providence. We had the privilege to drive in 1996 the first medical experience of pre-hospital ultrasound [6]. It was made from a medical helicopter in a mission over Morocco, Mauritania, Mali, and Senegal – we are glad to see that this princeps paper initiated a wide use in pre-hospital ultrasound. In our pilot study, the physicians answered to vital clinical questions on site. A focus on life-saving traumatic problems (pneumothorax, hemothorax, hemopericardium, abdominal bleeding) provided the answer to 90.6 % of the questions. The local conditions (sun of the desert, sand, vibrations, interferences from rotor in the helicopter) affected in no way the ultrasound examination.

So, without mistake, the first pre-hospital ultrasound diagnosis of pneumothorax was made in the Mauritanian desert (January 8, 1996), using a 3.5 kg perfectly portable machine

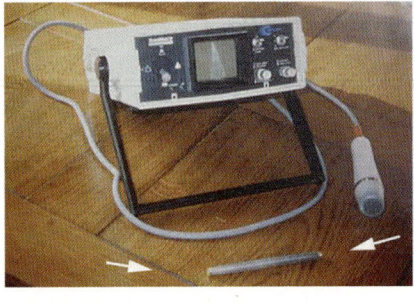

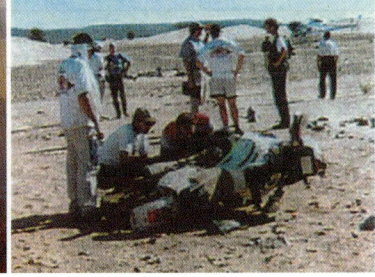

Fig. 33.1 Portable ultrasound in the desert in 1996. A lot to describe in these coupled figures. At the *left*, the antique Dymax TM-18, the unit we took in the Sahara desert and the helicopter of the Paris-Dakar rally, i.e., probably the first extra-hospital experience. This unit had five buttons, no lost space for storing any image, only one probe and a battery. This was a fully autonomous "stethoscope," since December 1995. The pen (*arrow*) indicates the size of the machine. At the *right*, we can witness a first: January 8, 1996, in the Saharan desert of Mauritania. A pneumothorax is diagnosed in a crashed biker of the Dakar rally. Maybe the first pre-hospital diagnosis of a life-threatening disorder. The concept we defined in our 1992 textbook is fully illustrated in this image: the exercise of critical ultrasound, the setting of point-of-care ultrasound, and lung (LUCI) as the main target in the critically ill

(Fig. 33.1). We then used for our flying missions the 1.9 kg compact machine for more than one decade (Fig. 33.2) then the 0.4 kg machine described in Chap. 2. We would feel really naked without it. Read if needed words about the light units in Chap. 2. We have designed the ULTIMAT-protocol, an ultrasound report dedicated to medical transportation (Table 33.1). The SLAM made some difficulties with the "L" (lump), found it a bit artificial, but eventually accepted the lump acronym.

In some countries with low-density population (Australia), physicians willingly use the air route, and may feel reinforced by this clinical tool.

Few adaptations should be done. Turbulences (air, road, sea, space, battlefield, etc.) can be a source of difficulties. One relevant issue is the monitoring of a pneumothorax. We describe the van-Dravik protocol (with his authorization): before the transportation, we search for an anterior b-line. This is a frequent event at the minor fissure. We carefully mark its location. During the transportation, in case of vibrations, detecting this b-line is easier than subtle lung sliding. We regularly take the blood pressure, saturation, cardiac frequency, van-Dravik sign, and the trip goes on safely.

Physician-Attended Ambulances

What was possible in a small helicopter is even easier in an ambulance. Should one be destitute in the full arid desert of Mauritania or medicalized in an Alma tunnel in the heart of Paris, one may feel the need for a lifesaving diagnosis. The traditional quandary "scoop and run" versus "play and stay" can be elegantly smashed when visual medicine is used on site.

Our experience of pre-hospital medicine has been followed in the ambulances by exciting papers [7]. All the content of this book can be achieved without any adaptation in such a setting. We are concerned to see attempts of developing sophisticated Doppler echocardiography (without care for LUCI) in ambulances. This begins to be the past, fortunately.

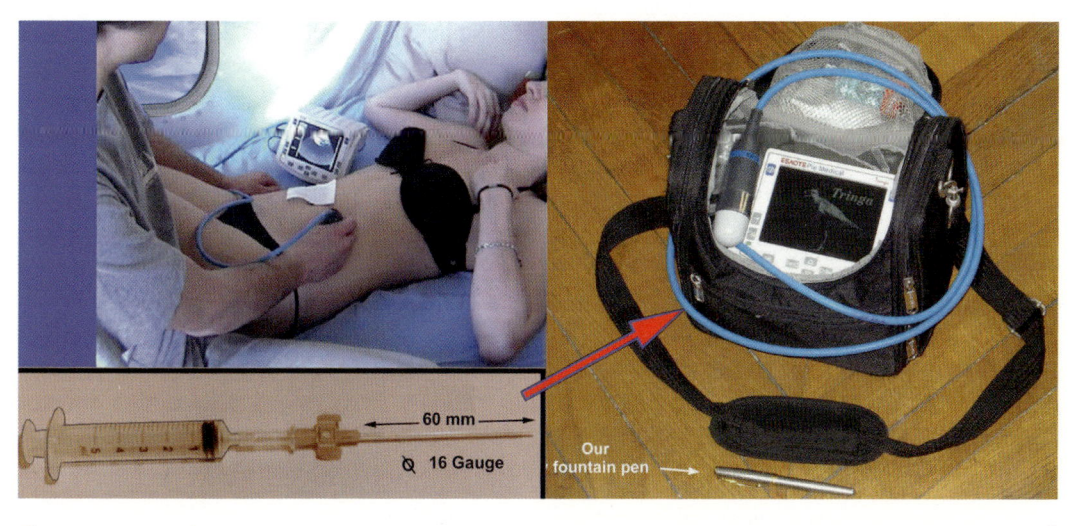

Fig. 33.2 Air medicine since the year 2000. This machine, which allowed us to conduct countless medical retrievals of critically ill patients through the sky from 2000 to 2012, was devoted to *veterinarians*, with a smart system for fixing the unit on the forearm, for checking using the other hand whether lady pigs were pregnant. In critical ultrasound, we need our two hands, and we quickly fitted this system into a suitable bag. Using our one-probe philosophy and a light screen, this Tringa unit from Netherlands was clearly one (large) step ahead. Note how small it is (look at the pen). It is perfect for jet medicine. Note on the front pocket of the bag (*arrow*), material such as this universal 16 G 60 mm catheter, for life-saving procedures (pneumothorax, pericardial tamponade, deep venous line insertion, etc.), making a diagnosis and therapeutic unit. We are approaching the concept of the PUMA (see Fig. 2.2)

Table 33.1 The ULTIMAT-protocol: ultrasound lump test initiating medical airway transportation protocol

Name:	Date:	
Setting:		
Indication: checking for the absence of occult disorders which may influence safety of the air medical transportation		
Operator:	Ultrasound unit: Signos RT, 5 MHz probe	
Technique: two-dimensional technique only	Various parameters (ventilated patient, etc.)	
Lungs		
Screening for pneumothorax (2″ × 2)	ABSENT	PRESENT[a]
Screening for hemothorax (10″ × 2)	ABSENT	PRESENT[a]
Screening for one lung intubation (5″)	ABSENT	PRESENT[a]
Screening for interstitial disorder (6″ × 2)	ABSENT	PRESENT[a]
Heart		
Screening for pericardial effusion (10″)	ABSENT	PRESENT[a]
2D impairment of LV contractility (10″)	ABSENT	PRESENT[a]
Abdomen		
Screening for pneumoperitoneum (5″)	ABSENT	PRESENT[a]
Screening for hemoperitoneum (30″)	ABSENT	PRESENT[a]
Screening for mesenteric ischemia (30″)	ABSENT	PRESENT[a]
Screening for distended bladder (5″)	ABSENT	PRESENT[a]
Central veins		
Screening for a venous thrombosis involving a strategic area or with instable pattern:		
Internal jugular axes (6″ × 2)	ABSENT	PRESENT[a]
Ilio-femoral axes (15″ × 2)	ABSENT	PRESENT[a]
Head		
Screening for optic nerve changes indicating intracranial hypertension (7″ × 2)	ABSENT	PRESENT[a]
Miscellaneous data seen during this examination which will not affect the safety of the transportation, but may be of clinical relevance		

Note: average timing if all items are checked, using 15 changes of site: possible in 4 min by trained users
[a]If the answer is "PRESENT" in one or some of these items, the safety of the transportation should be questioned

The Emergency Physician

Developing ultrasound in the emergency room is of interest. We don't deal here with the critically ill patient, promptly managed in a private circuit and rapidly sent in the ICU. We deal with all patients, who make the main problem of the emergency room: a recurrent accumulation. They write that ultrasound is a good *triage* tool. We are not keen in this word: ultrasound provides a diagnosis, not a triage indication. An impressive number of situations (renal colic, rib fracture, withdrawal of foreign body, even spinal tap, and 100 others) can be quickly managed. Excellent and numerous textbooks are now available.

Just this word: in the ER, the laptop units were a commercial solution to a scientific problem, which was to just think different. We invite the readers to use the instrument featuring in Fig. 28.2 for measuring the width of the units currently invading their ERs, and above all to consult Fig. 2.2 about the image resolution, which shows how the community lost 33 years of progress. See more details in Chap. 37.

Gyneco-obstetrics

Pregnant ladies can suddenly fall in the scope of the BLUE-protocol or the FALLS-protocol. Massive bleedings and gravidic hypertension generate situations where the optimal fluid therapy can be really challenging, and the risk of pulmonary edema an obsession. The FALLS-protocol will easily see the early, infra-clinical stage of interstitial edema – A-lines, lung rockets, same music.

Other Medical Specialties

The Anesthesiologist Outside the ICU

This important part of any hospital would have been able since 1982 to immediately insert central venous catheters with nearly zero fault and control the fluid losses of some abdominal interventions, among examples. TEE is useful where there is really no access to the thorax. Lung ultrasound may be a nice alternative, provided a small space is devoted at the upper lungs (or, even used by the surgeon, or any person able to apply a probe on a chest). Enough for performing a FALLS-protocol – including settings where the thorax has been opened (one limitation of TEE, since the pleural variations are unavailable).
- Before any surgery
- Recognizing high-risk patients is a sharp task. The cardiac function, the BNP are useful, but how about a fast protocol just scanning the lung for identifying these patients with uncertain cardiac function?
- During general surgery
- Assessing the necessary volume for replacing the losses uses indirect tools and is operator-dependent. New habits in the OR should include, during abdominal surgery, some place for the anesthesiologist to scan the lungs (reminder).
- We wrote in our last editions: "If it succeeds penetrating in the prestigious operating room, ultrasound can initiate a small revolution." Now this step is behind us, fortunately. One can regret that they waited so long. Waiting for the laptop era was useless (ceilings are high enough in operating rooms). The 1992 technology was perfect.

The Cardiologist

There is no need for long explanations. They have the probe in hand. They have just to push it slightly outside the heart windows for having a new vision of the patient (not as optimal as with our probe, but some "cardiac" probes are better than others for imaging the lung more or less). They will see not only cardiac functions, but simultaneously their consequences on the lung. Fortunately, our friends attempt to show them the way [8]. Just a question of decades, maybe less.

The Pulmonologist

There is no need for long explanation here. They have an extremely wide field for daily use, and this is a positive point to see that since very recently, they get interested in lung ultrasound. Let us just cite:
- The control of irradiation: read the LUCI-FLR project.
- The diagnosis of any chronic interstitial syndrome, from idiopathic pulmonary fibrosis to any rarity, can be detected during ambulatory duties: diffuse lung rockets.
- Diagnosis and management of any pleural syndrome.
- Location and biopsy of superficial masses.

We have no space for detailing all diseases – each one should have its own profile. Just for citing some, cystic fibrosis should yield a normal profile, so far as the cystic elements are usually central, not extended to the periphery. Just one word: regarding cancer. Here, given the risk of misuse, we need scientific proof more than uncontrolled enthusiasm. If the enthusiasm is supported by scientific data, we promise the best future to ultrasound, and the word "revolution" will not be spoilt here.

The Thoracic Surgeon

Many concerns can be controlled.

During surgery, a lung exclusion should be checked using ultrasound.

After pulmonectomy, the initial pattern is the A′-profile, without any lung point. A swirl sign can be visible when the cavity is little by little filled with fluid. After a pulmonectomy, the intra-thoracic pressures must be balanced, between the residual air and the contralateral lung. The gold standard (mediastinal location on bedside radiography) may be replaced by ultrasound.

The Nephrologist

One obsession here is the assessment of volemia, and how to schedule a hemodialysis. Same song, lung rockets indicate wet lungs, A-lines dry lungs [9].

In Internal Medicine

Each time the word "lung" is pronounced, i.e., 50 times a day here, ultrasound can inform, easily, at the bedside. This means gaining time and cost savings. A suspicion of diffuse systemic disease involving the interstitial tissues? Just take a look at the lungs.

The Physiologist

They will better understand lung physiology by using ultrasound. The lung sliding is one of the main interests, since no test (even fluoroscopy) can figure out the subtleties of this physiological entity.

Any Specialty Dealing with:

Bariatric Patients

We deal here with a major advantage of lung ultrasound. Fat people are usually disadvantaged when they fall ill, whatever the level of courage of the managing team. The physical examination is disappointing, as is the bedside chest radiography. CT would be of interest, but, in addition to its known drawbacks, not only is the transportation a big issue, but above all these referrals have broken many tables (plus vertebras of the teams).

For this patient, apparently isolated by this excessive fat thickness, lung ultrasound will be one more time providential. Let us follow the seven principles of lung ultrasound.

1. Will a simple machine, without Doppler suit? Figure 33.3 answers the question (Fig. 33.3).
2. Air and fluid are mixed together. When the beam crosses the chest wall, even very fat, and suddenly meets the air tissue of the lung, the reverberation can be detected. The high impedance gradient between gas and fluids makes this distinction rather easy.
3. Lung is the most voluminous organ. Whereas a novice user would be confused by where to apply the probe, the BLUE-points provide an immediate and standardized answer for locating the lung.
4. The pleural line: using our probe (of substantial depth), it can be visualized, as well as the shadow of the ribs (Fig. 33.3).
5. Lung sliding: see Fig. 33.3 that speaks for itself (Fig. 33.3).

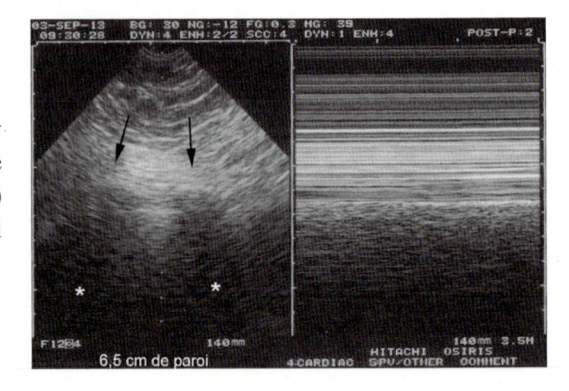

Fig. 33.3 LUCI in bariatric patients. *Left*: the ultrasound flow crosses nearly 7 cm of good old fat before reaching the pleural line. The rib shadows, more than the ribs, are recognized (*stars and arrows*). The Merlin's space seems free – at last there are O-lines but no B-line. *Right*: the seashore sign clearly appears, with a quiet Keye's space in this well-ventilated patient. Although the radiograph showed white "lungs," the BLUE-protocol infirmed easily the clinico-radiological diagnosis of cardiogenic pulmonary edema. This mixture between BLUE-protocol and FAT-protocol suggested pulmonary embolism among others, a diagnosis confirmed using some tests including venous ultrasound

6. Lung artifacts: with a probe such as ours, A-lines as well as B-lines easily appear on the screen.
7. Most critical acute disorders are superficial. This principle is of prime importance since most of them will be detected.

The PLAPS-point is certainly difficult in bariatric patients. We have aimed at optimizing this step. The standardized location of the PLAPS-point helps. Distinguishing abdominal fat from lung consolidation is possible, but requires expertise. Using the PLAPS-point, this issue is skipped. The detection of posterolateral A-lines or B-lines is possible in extreme depth. It indicates that the Merlin's space is artifactual, and this means "no PLAPS," of major relevance. Venous ultrasound, usually more difficult at iliocaval areas, is sometimes quite impossible at the calf areas, sometimes, paradoxically, very easy.

In other words, the FAT-protocol (which is not an acronym, and any resemblance with the FAST-protocol would be pure coincidence) has the peculiarity to have no peculiarity.

Skinny Patients

Just a word to highlight, for those who advocate one unique probe (but a cardiac one), that in the extreme emergency, the analysis of a too near pleural line can raise issues. Again, vascular probes on very skinny patients will not always fit.

Burned Patients

The change of dressings is the opportunity for routine lung ultrasound. One can use sterile gel, just apply the probe on the thorax and see the same signs as when the skin is not damaged. One understands here that the less probes are used, the less buttons are prominent, and the best the asepsis is warranted.

Doctors of Scarce-Resource Areas: *Ultrasound of the World*

No major loss of ink is necessary here. The *same approach*, valuable for sophisticated ICUs of wealthy countries, using this cost-effective system, will perfectly fit all these regions of the world, where a simple radiographic unit is a luxury. Ultrasound here more than ever acts as a terminal for therapeutic decisions.

All doctors implied in austere medicine, mass casualties, and other areas will discover an impressive potential. The others, in wealthy countries, who see CT, MRI, etc., with admiration, should think in terms of global health (not to forget the drawbacks of these giants, too heavy for critical care).

We congratulate the WINFOCUS and its founders, Luca Neri, Enrico Storti, and Mike Blaivas as prominent members, and so many names that this book would suddenly become too heavy. Many of them are, in fact, imbedded through the text. In the field of critical medicine, WINFOCUS has hoisted our 1985 spirit of considering ultrasound as a tool for visual medicine through difficult parts of the world. We are glad to have been part of its pioneering debuts and are certain they will adopt the spirit of holistic ultrasound. Special thanks to Larry, Mahmoud, Rocky, and so many – may all those who are not featuring here consider our closeness and not feel frustrated.

Doctors of Remote Areas

We come back to "wealthy" settings. Ocean ships, remote islands, airplanes, rural areas – there are many areas where an urgent need for a diagnosis is present (read Anecdotal Note 1).

Family Doctors

They may immediately detect whether this child has a pneumonia or not, a sinusitis – not to speak to all extra-lung applications.

Acupunctures

In this popular discipline, pneumothorax is pointed out as a potentially life-threatening complication. A simple ultrasound unit in the office would allow immediate post-procedure diagnosis.

Physiotherapists

This discipline should deserve a whole chapter, especially those working in the ICUs. Ultrasound should change many aspects of the protocols, since the result can be seen on site.

"Last But Not Least": LUCIA – Lung Ultrasound for the Critically Ill Animals, Lung Ultrasound for Vets

Our 26-year research, which was initiated, improved, and refined with success on human beings without side effect, can now be fully applied on animals safely. We extrapolate exactly the same signs, provided they have lungs (whales, bats, etc.). Like in human critical care, animals can express themselves with difficulty. Usually, some morphine and many tears are used when a critical disorder occurs in our beloved pets, without space for sophisticated diagnosis. Imagine the benefit. Note that veterinarians were not the last to have understood the (commercial) interest for ultrasound (for knowing pregnancy states). Ironically, from 2000 to 2013, we have been using for our aeronautic missions a hand-held machine from the vet world, which contributed in saving human lives from time to time (Fig. 33.2).

Anecdotal Note

1. While many Terrians have to face the difficult life on Earth, some others devote their life to make long interplanetary travels (initiating other difficulties). Here, and maybe only here, a hand-held ultrasound unit is really welcome. It makes a unique opportunity to diagnose acute disorders that can be managed on site, typically pneumothorax [10]. Although we bet such a possibility will *never* happen (during our life at least), why not be prepared for this, especially by choosing the method with the fastest learning curve? And the NASA can purchase a cheap hand-held unit without Doppler – not a question of cost here! Just a question of quality.

References

1. Van Gansbeke D, Matos C, Askenasi R, Braude P, Tack D, Lalmand B, Avni EF (1989) Echographie abdominale en urgence, apports et limites. In: Réanimation et médecine d'urgence. Société de Réanimation de Langue Française. Expansion Scientifique Française, Paris, pp 36–53
2. Brenner DJ, Elliston CD, Hall EJ, Berdon WE (2001) Estimated risks of radiation-induced fatal cancer from pediatric CT. Am J Roentgenol 176:289–296
3. Soldati G, Testa A, Silva FR, Carbone L, Portale G, Silveri NG (2006) Chest ultrasonography in lung contusion. Chest 130(2):533–538
4. Schild HH, Strunk H, Weber W, Stoerkel S, Doll G, Hein K, Weitz M (1989) Pulmonary contusion: CT vs plain radiograms. J Computed Assist Tomogr 13:417–420
5. Blaivas M, Brannam L, Hawkins M, Lyon M, Spiram K (2004) Bedside emergency ultrasonographic diagnosis of diaphragmatic rupture in blunt abdominal trauma. Am J Emerg Med 22(7):601–604
6. Lichtenstein D, Courret JP (1998) Feasibility of ultrasound in the helicopter. Intensive Care Med 24:1119
7. Lapostolle F, Petrovic T, Lenoir G, Catineau J, Galinski M, Metzger J, Chanzy E, Adnet F (2006) Usefulness of hand-held ultrasound devices in out-of-hospital diagnosis performed by emergency physicians. Am J Emerg Med 24:237–242
8. Gargani L, Volpicelli G (2014) How I do it. Lung ultrasound. Cardiovasc Ultrasound 12:25
9. Noble VE, Murray AF, Capp R, Sylvia-Reardon MH, Steele DJR, Liteplo A (2009) Ultrasound assessment for extravascular lung water in patients undergoing hemodialysis: time course for resolution. Chest 135:1433–1439
10. Dulchavsky SA, Hamilton DR, Diebel LN, Sargsyan AE, Billica RD, Williams DR (1999) Thoracic ultrasound diagnosis of pneumothorax. J Trauma 47:970–971

Whole Body Ultrasound in the Critically Ill (Lung, Heart, and Venous Thrombosis Excluded)

34

The present textbook is labelled *Lung Ultrasound in the Critically Ill*. This respects the trust that the community shows to our few publications. This also limits us to lecture quite only on this restricted topic. We have the feeling that the whole body can benefit from the same approach, mainly by using a single probe with equivalent results.

We will be brief: the 2010 edition contains all details, there is not much to add.

Some figures shown here have all been taken using our Japanese 5 MHz microconvex probe.

Basics of Critical Abdomen

Most acute abdominal disorders can be detected using ultrasound, usually superior to plain abdomen radiographies. It is often able to replace CT for indicating prompt surgery. In a few lines (see 2010 edition for details), we expose the main problem. Twenty organs, 20 diseases per organ: This is ultrasound, i.e., this traditional, expert, operator-dependent world. We know that many emergency physicians have used a lot of energy for investing in this hard field, and, today, we assume each reader is at ease with some diagnoses, such as fluid in the abdomen, kidney dilatation, bladder distension, aortic aneurism, etc.

How to make a logical presentation of abdominal ultrasound? Using frequency? Severity of the diseases? Anatomic classification (from outside to inside for instance)? Why not alphabetic order (aorta, bladder, colon, duodenum, etc.)? We will just, in this small paragraph within a small chapter, show some of the diseases which are the most severe and the less known by the radiologists, in an order less than academic.

Pneumoperitoneum

We aimed at describing signs more standardized than just "gas barriers at the abdomen." In a very few words, it shows the same logic as pneumothorax. The physiological peritoneal sliding is abolished (with a stratospheric pattern on M-mode) (Video 34.1). Our study showed a 100 % sensitivity and a 92 % specificity [1]. Below the peritoneal line are only artifacts, like A-lines (and Z-lines too), called GA-lines (and GZ-lines) since they do not arise from the pleural line. GA-lines are observed with a 100 % sensitivity. At the periphery, a "gut point," equivalent to the lung point, is found in 50 % of the cases. Gut sliding, splanchnogram (vision of abdominal viscera), and GB-lines (equivalent of lung B-lines) rule out pneumoperitoneum. See more details in the caption for Fig. 34.1.

Electronic supplementary material The online version of this chapter (doi:10.1007/978-3-319-15371-1_34) contains supplementary material, which is available to authorized users.

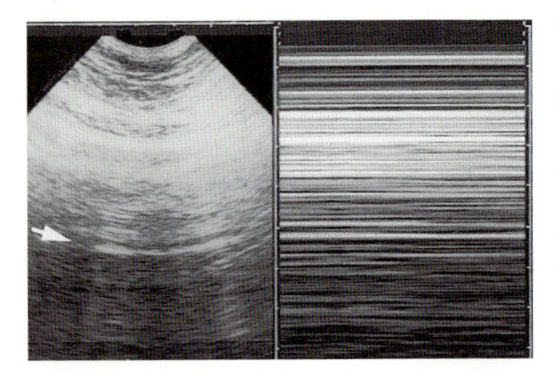

Fig. 34.1 Pneumoperitoneum. The free gas collects at nondependent areas, making the diagnosis accessible. Gut sliding is the label we give to the respiratory dynamic of the visceral layer against the parietal layer: an equivalent of the seashore sign (see Fig. 5.12 of 2010 edition). The splanchnogram is how we called the detection of real, not artifactual structures (liver, bowel loops, etc.), showing that there is no free gas interposition between these structures and the probe. The aerogram is how we called all these gas in the GI tract. The artifacts generated were called G-lines, with the same features as A, B, and Z-lines, hence the labels GA, GB, and GZ-lines for making zero confusion with lung artifacts. GB-lines are like B-lines, apart from the fact that they do not arise from the pleural line. No rib at the abdomen, there is no bat sign here. *Left*: GA-lines (and GZ-lines) of a pneumoperitoneum (*arrow*). *Right*: M-mode shows the abolition of gut sliding, with a stratosphere sign (gut sliding is also abolished in surgical adherences, absence of diaphragmatic motion, peritonitis with antalgic hypopnea). GA-lines plus abolished gut sliding is labelled the Gut-A'-profile. The gut point is an equivalent of the lung point. Countless other signs can be added, such as postural changes (but we don't like to mobilize these fragile patients). *Previsible pitfall*: A distended stomach will come against the anterior wall, making gut sliding hard to detect and able to generate GA lines. Consequently, analysis of gut sliding contributes more if the stomach was previously localized in one way or another

Mesenteric Ischemia/Infarction

For summarizing a very long text (read our 2010 edition), the GI tract is a vital organ, therefore in permanent dynamic. To see loops of GI tract without any motion should be a major sign alerting of something wrong in the abdomen of a patient with unusual abdominal pain or shock (Video 34.2). The data show a correlation which should be enhanced using simple, clinical elements: 87 % sensitivity, 88 % specificity when compared with patients having suspicion of ischemia [2]. Portal gas is dealt with below.

Various GI Tract Disorders

Either no part of the GI tract can be analyzed or the whole of the GI tract appears with fine details. In this unforeseeable case, the physician can see all these items: gut sliding, wall thickness (pseudomembranous colitis), wall content (bullous pneumatosis of infarction), content caliper (occlusion), echogenicity of lumen (blood, stools, etc.), massive fluid content (sequestration), gastric repletion (acute gastric dilatation), and so on.

Various Parenchymal Disorders

One can see liver or splenic abscesses (round hypoechoic heterogeneous areas), pancreatic enlargement (pancreatitis), areas of infection or infarction in various parenchymas (kidney, spleen, etc). Hepatic gas from mesenteric infarction (portal gas) yields small disseminated hyperechoic images – this was in our previous editions the only major indication of assessing the liver in critically ill patients.

Various Hollow Structure Disorders

Cholecystitis is a wide field, but in the ICU, an enlarged wall is more often a sign of acute right heart failure. We wrote a whole development in our 2010 textbook with this statement: "in a medical ICU patient, a gallbladder wall enlarged of more than 7 mm should invite to find a cause (of the trouble, pain, fever…) different from an acute acalculous cholecystitis." Numerous data that we will never have time to submit for publication indicate that probably too many gallbladders are removed. The main issue is that the real cause (e.g., pneumonia) of the trouble (e.g., RUQ pain) is not cured.

An obstacle from urinary cavities is a basic diagnosis, especially the bladder, maybe an invitation to initiate one's training in critical ultrasound. Anuria was extensively dealt with in our previous edition. Now, it is simply one sign of acute circulatory failure, read Chap. 30. Anuria is simply confirmed when the bladder is empty.

Vascular Disorders

An aortic aneurism enlarges the aortic lumen (what more to write?).

GI Tract Hemorrhage

Ultrasound is not mandatory for the management, but it can allow immediate diagnosis of acute deglobulization in extreme settings. We remind that the SESAME-protocol (cardiac arrest) has placed the abdomen in the third position (after lungs and veins, before pericardium and heart). We describe it here: substantial amounts of fluid are detected within the belly. They are not concave outside such as peritoneal effusions, they are convex outside, meaning the fluid is within the GI tract compartment. The fluid can be black or gray, once again it does not matter (Video 34.3).

Ultrasound can see the massive fluid before it is accessible to rectal examination or gastric tube. Anecdotal but interesting applications are the detection of esophageal varices, signs of cirrhosis – a help for inserting a Blakemore tube, the detection of complications of the Blakemore tube insertion, mainly esophageal rupture (pleural effusion, pneumothorax, subcutaneous emphysema, etc.). An anecdotal cause of GI tract bleeding, the aortic aneurism leaking inside the GI tract can be detected. Ultrasound can again see cardiac anomalies, enolic disease associated. All figures of these diseases feature in our 2010 edition, in the chapters on abdomen mainly.

Free Peritoneal Blood

This is dealt with below, in the section on trauma.

Miscellaneous

Some are familiar to any ultrasound user, such as wall disorders (hematoma, abscess), retroperitoneal hematoma, mesenteric venous thrombosis (visible without Doppler in good conditions). Some thoracic disorders simulate abdominal emergencies: pneumonia, pleural effusion, pneumothorax, sometimes myocardial infarction.

Basics in Any Urgent Procedure in the Critically Ill

The possibility of visual insertion of any needle within any area was already a small revolution: vein, pleural cavity, peritoneal cavity, pericardium, mainly. We emphasize our message around a catheter devoted to all these life-threatening emergencies. The Emergency Life-Saving Insertion of a Short Central Endovenous Catheter, or ELSISSCEC-protocol, never mind, uses a remarkable device: a multipurpose 60-mm, 16 gauge catheter (Fig. 34.2). It can be inserted with little training under sterile conditions. Inserting a short (60 mm, not so short, but not 45 cm) catheter in a central vein may appear unusual; this is what we do when time is of essence. The problem of the central venous access is solved in a few seconds, avoiding spectacular alternatives such as the transosseous access (useful it is true if there is no ultrasound).

In all cases, the rules of any needle insertion should be respected.

The impaired hemostasis, frequent in critically ill patients, should be a contra-indication, but ultrasound helps to avoid the main obstacles, usually vessels in the route of the needle. On the road, arteries such as the epigastric or internal mammary arteries should be avoided. Our nonvascular microconvex probe is able to see them (see if needed Fig. 5.16 of our 2010 edition)

At the end of the road, vascular masses (aneurisms), hydatid cyst, pheochromocytoma, and other nice subtleties must be suspected before any attempt. We should beware of any round, extraparenchymatous mass, a golden rule in our approach. Aneurisms can be highly suspected even without Doppler, using some history, the notion of a thrill, the location, etc. An echoic flow, regular, pulsatile, with whirling dynamic is rare but specific to vascular masses (see Fig. 25.5 and the text in our 2010 edition). Conversely, the detection of a slow, hectic flow within the mass indicates the absence of pressurized blood (plankton sign, see Fig. 35.10). When really the physi-

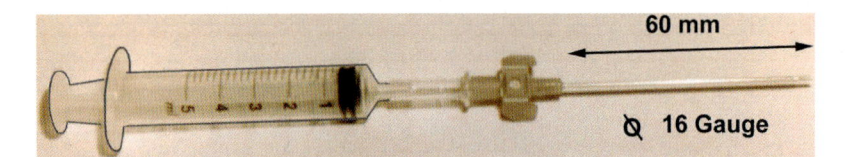

Fig. 34.2 ELSISSCEC-protocol. A universal interventional device. In the same way we use one probe for the whole body, this simple catheter has the length and the cross-section relevant for, at will, inserting central (or less central) venous lines, withdrawing pleural, pericardial, or peritoneal fluid, withdrawing pleural gas of gas tamponade in tension pneumothorax, i.e., a simple but really universal tool

cian is embarrassed, he or she can always ask for the DIAFORA approach, described in Chap. 2.

All technical details for safe pleural puncture are in Chap. 35. For the gallbladder, a transhepatic approach limits the risk of biliary leakage in the peritoneum (we don't overburden this textbook, see if needed our 2010 edition). There are many details at any area. In the thorax, the lung line of the pleural effusion avoids confusion with an ectopic, intra-thoracic stomach. At the groin, an abscess will not be confused with an inguinal hernia.

Basics of Subclavian Venous Line Insertion

This section will be useful only for the physicians who think that the blind approaches do not work all the time, or want to take no risk for their patients. The others can do as they will. To our opinion, the ability to find any vein in a few seconds is a reason per se to have a unit in each ICU. In our 1992 edition, this section was a whole chapter: we had to explain the interest of the concept. Now, this kind of propaganda is obsolete. We all know that blind insertions of catheters are difficult in the extreme emergency [3, 4]. The image of the physician so near to the patient and so "useless" is even ironic.

The interest of the venous cannulation under ultrasound is a revolution in the habits (read Anecdotal Note 1). This new trend, still not shared by all, will nonetheless help in making the present textbook thinner. Countless articles have been published yet with some distance, we see the same points repeated and repeated: they use the same target (jugular internal vein), the same approach (short axis), the same probe (vascular). Therefore, the reader will find here the CEURF philosophy, once again point-by-point opposed to the usual habits (apart from the main point: using ultrasound). We could have shared our experience since 1990 in peer-review literature, but our submissions on lung ultrasound prevented this, apart from just one abstract [5].

We summarize our previous editions since 1992, keeping only technical points.

Which Patients?

If one wants to take zero risk, or zero discomfort for the patient, check all the patients. Some authors keep it after failure of blind attempt, when there is contraindication of a blind attempt, or for controlling costs [6].

How to Train Before On-Site Use

One can acquire the skill first on inert material. Our method for simulating parenchymas for cheap is described in the caption of Fig. 34.3. There is no difficulty. Any person able to write, for instance, the simple letter "O" recruits without thinking agonists and antagonist muscles in an admirable synchronism.

Which Machine?

We tried recently with a modern laptop machine, failed in locating the needle and were a bit intrigued before realizing that the lag created by

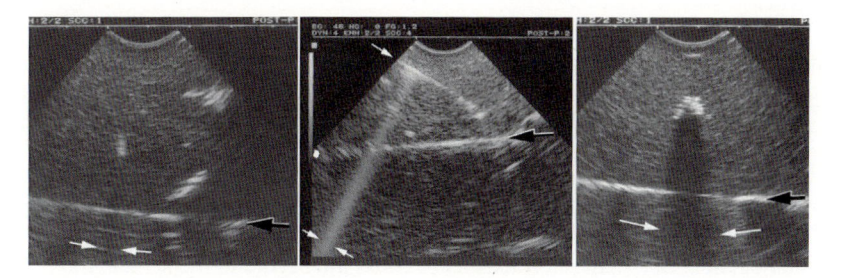

Fig. 34.3 A phantom for cheap. Using a simple piece of tofu, for 1 $, one can observe: *Left*, the appearance of a metallic wire (note the acoustic shadow between *arrows*). *Middle*, a needle (*arrow*) aiming at a target created by a simple match; note a beautiful V-line (*arrows*), read p. 363. *Right*, the outlook of a nasogastric or chest tube (it easily penetrates the tofu parenchyma), with its large acoustic shadow (*arrows*). Note: these images, easy to produce in vitro, are reproduced the same in clinical conditions. The *black arrows* indicate the bottom of the tofu piece, roughly 4 cm thick. Tofu can be conserved far more than 1 month for such use

the non-instant response filters is not suitable for an instant control of our movements. We use our 1992 unit.

How to Do on Site

Our approach was self-taught: in 1989, there was no teaching center to tell us what and how to do. Based on simplicity, the CEURF approach is summarized in Fig. 34.4. We fail to understand why linear probes (called vascular), why the short-axis and why the jugular vein, not to speak of *human cadaver* workshops are used so often. Our approach makes the field much simpler. Since 1989 with the ADR-4000, since 1992 with the Hitachi-405, we are accustomed to cannulate the subclavian vein (below the clavicula) this simple way [5]. Our published results are featured in Technical Note 1.

From the 10 points which CEURF highlighted in the Chap. 18, we briefly remind those pertaining to venous cannulation: one probe for the whole body. Not a vascular probe. A 5 MHz microconvex probe, perfect for this use. No Doppler. A long-axis approach. A particular emphasis for the (infraclavicular) subclavian vein. This venous area is the best choice in terms of infectious issues [7]. We will therefore deal only with this vein, neglecting the femoral and jugular internal ones, supposed mastered by the community.

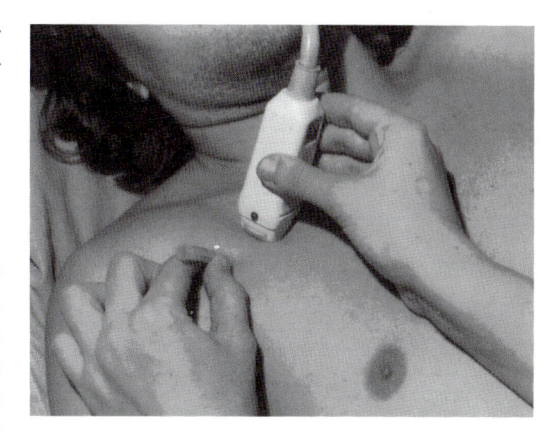

Fig. 34.4 Subclavian venous cannulation. This simple figure provides *nine* pieces of information. The right hand holds a microconvex probe, ideal for this nonlinear area (subclavian vein). Note the available space due to the probe's small footprint. The probe is applied quietly, with minimal pressure, by a hand lying on the thorax. The probe is applied tangential to the thorax (90°): just above the region of interest. The probe exposes the vein on a long-axis view. The left hand holds the needle, quietly, with no crispation since the vacuum of the syringe is not required here. The needle is applied 45° on the thorax. Roughly 2 cm separate the needle from the probe head extremity. The needle quietly aims at the landmark of the probe (note this intelligent landmark, easy to locate). There is no sophisticated device attaching the needle to the probe. For simplifying the image in this fictitious procedure, no syringe, no sterile equipment

First point, the patient, needle, probe, and screen must be roughly in a same visual site for minimizing basic difficulties, such as moving one's head all the time. We take our single microconvex probe, insert it in a sterile sheath we use since 1992 (see the whole procedure if needed in Fig. 26.1 of our 2010 edition). Note that the microconvex probe has a size making it glide into a sheat more easily than a large vascular one. We search for the vein in a longitudinal scan below the clavicle, immediately detect its short axis and the satellite artery. We check for its patency by gently compressing it, using if needed our free hand above the clavicle, the "Doppler hand" described in Chap. 18 (Fig. 34.5).

Other signs can show the venous patency (apart from Doppler, which we don't use): spontaneously floating valvulae within the vein (the free valvula sign), spontaneously visible echoic flow, and spontaneous respiratory changes in dimensions. The subclavian vein had the reputation of being always open and large, suitable for cannulations. Our experience using ultrasound shows it is untrue, at last at the external two-thirds of the vein. An inspiratory collapsus can be seen: a scary image since we guess the risk of gas embolism is maximal. The vein can be permanently collapsed, i.e., obviously not ready for cannulation. Here, we search for alternatives (other vein, or fluid therapy, or Trendelenburg).

Once the vein is seen – and safe, the probe gently rotates like unscrewing with a screwdriver, permanently using the Carmen maneuver. A microconvex probe is not only perfect but also

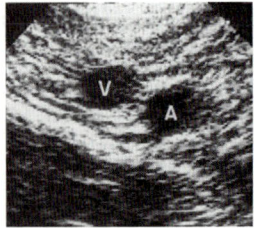

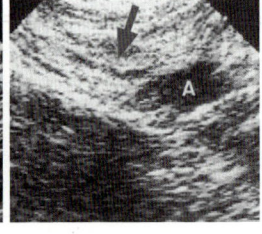

Fig. 34.5 Subclavian compression maneuver. The *left image* shows how the subclavian couple immediately appears on a longitudinal scan of the thorax below the clavicula. The *right image* shows the complete collapsus of this vein when pressure is exerted by a probe (*arrowhead*). Cross-sectional scan of the subclavian vein (*V*), with the satellite artery (*A*). Image taken in 1989 using 1982's ADR-4000 at the bedside

mandatory, since we face here one of the less linear areas of the human being. Then the whole of the long axis of the vein appears. The probe is then held firmly, tangential (90°) to the skin like quite always in critical ultrasound. Then the needle is applied at 45°, aiming a point located 1–2 cm far from the probe (too far, you risk to miss the needle in the screen, too near you risk to pierce the precious probe).

Servocontrol or any of these countless helps, Doppler, multidimensional devices, etc., special needles developed by sly manufacturers? Useless. It complicates a very simple procedure.

How many operators? Just one. In the blind techniques, the users had to make the vacuum and needed their two hands. This allowed to withdraw low-pressure blood and diagnose (a little too late) pneumothorax or arterial puncture. With ultrasound, one hand holds the probe, the other hand takes the needle like a pen: no need for vacuum. Just one operator.

It is even possible to insert just a needle, at atmospheric pressure, without syringe: in sedated patients, the increase of inspiratory venous caliper is always correlated with a centrifuge flow of venous blood during disconnection of the syringe.

Then FOUR POINTS are aligned: *tip of needle facing landmark of the probe, end of the needle facing end of the probe*. That's all. That's not more difficult. No need to be a ballistic expert. Once these two axes are aligned, the needle is inserted. It is directly seen, through its entire length (unlike the simple spot in the short-axis technique), penetrating the parietal tissues, arriving at the vein, pushing then piercing the proximal wall, and penetrating the vein. The deed is done. The needle traverses only the plane that is visible on the screen. If the pleural line is not visible in the screen, it cannot be pierced by the needle. If the artery is not visible in the screen, it cannot be pierced by the needle. We guess the vascular probes make this long axis approach difficult (they make every step more difficult in fact).

By the way, we have heard of an international consensus conference reporting 65 statements. *Sixty-five statements for this basic application? We fail to understand and suspect the "vascular"* probes to generate complicated procedures, and in addition to be unsuitable for all nonlinear areas, mainly the subclavian vein (read Anecdotal Note 2). If the needle is not well seen (it occurs in 15/20 % of the cases), provided the four points are aligned, the needle is in the axis of the probe, driving to the vein, there is therefore no risk of accident, and eventually the tip of the needle is seen touching the vein, etc. No need for sophisticated and costly devices.

In our training center (CEURF), we don't use *cadavers*, but for one dollar we get a piece of *tofu* with some materials inside, which the attendees usually succeed to cannulate at the *first* attempt (Fig. 34.3).

There are many tricks, and minor details can be added at this step (read our 2010 edition).

Some may prefer just to look at the vein using ultrasound, then switch off the machine and puncture a vein once they know it is large, free and here, making a landmark before puncturing (semi-visual approach so to speak). This can work for large jugular internal veins, meaning also that they would be easy to puncture without ultrasound, meaning also that the relevance of the pre-procedure ultrasound was just to predict a fast success using blind puncture. It was long proven that large veins were easier to cannulate than small ones [8] (read Anecdotal Note 3). The subclavian vein is too deep (and usually smaller) and is not an application for this procedure. A minor change in angulation drives to the failure. Nonetheless, some teams, closing their eyes on this very basic rule, published in respectable literature that ultrasound was of no benefit there [9].

For those who would use the semi-visual approach, we remind that the internal jugular veins are asymmetrical in 62 % of the cases, to the benefit of the right side in only 68 % of the cases [10]. We remind that on admission in the ICU, 23 % of these veins had a cross-sectional area less than 0.4 cm^2 [10]. The Trendelenburg maneuver changes theses dimensions only slightly. The "semi-visual technique" prevents to cannulate a too small caliper or a fully thrombosed vein, and to be confused by aberrant anatomy [11].

What to Do After the Procedure

Ultrasound checks for the absence of a pneumothorax (just because it takes 1 s – not because there is a serious risk), with much higher sensitivity than bedside radiograph done too early. Ultrasound checks also the absence of an ectopic positioning toward the jugular vein. If a jugular malpositioning is the only question, ultrasound can really be done instead of the radiography (LUCIFLR project).

Why the Subclavian Vein

Why did we choose the subclavian vein? Mainly because it is, from far, the cleanest area for venous cannulation [7]. The jugular choice condemns to do with these hair falls, nasal drops, eye tears, mouth droppings, ear miasmas, leaking substances from tracheostomy, not to forget the sweat which detaches the dressing. There is no such thing at the infraclavicular subclavian vein, remote from this mess. It is more comfortable for the patient and the nursing team. Remote infectious complications may also decrease [12]. Using ultrasound, the patient benefits from all advantages of this route with no drawback (no risk of pneumothorax or arterial puncture, even in patients with impaired hemostasis, obesity, and other classical contraindications). Among other advantages, the visual guidance usually allows a unique puncture, minimizing the damage to the vein (some nephrologists are scared when they have the perspective of future hemodialysis – not such a frequent event in addition). The rate of catheter-linked thrombosis seems strikingly lower in our experience when compared to the jugular internal vein, with a possible explanation linked to the difference of output between the territories (in submission). Cannulating dirty sites (jugular vein) whereas we have the visual guidance comes possibly from the ergonomy of the vascular probes, which makes this procedure too difficult. Briefly, the subclavian vein appears as the most elegant choice. When we hear that physicians are reluctant to use this vein for the fear of pneumothorax, whereas they have ultrasound, we fail to understand, apart from the explanation that they have the wrong tool: The ergonomy of these large vascular probes is simply unsuitable.

Philosophic Considerations

The practice of ultrasound-guided puncture does not help to progress in the blind technique, since the landmarks are different. We cannot answer to a critical question: should these blind approaches be forgotten? This should make the operator dependent from the ultrasound machine. Yet how to select the patients who will benefit from this "refresher" technique will be an ethical issue without solution.

For Concluding This Section

Vascular probes are, in our use, not fully suitable for all vascular accesses. The label "vascular" makes doctors believe that they are adapted to the vessels. They are adapted to some vessels, in some orientations. Our microconvex probe can be applied on any vein of the body.

Basics of Optic Nerve (and Elevated Intracranial Pressure)

Optic nerve is part of holistic ultrasound, i.e., our microconvex probe shows not only sufficient but above all more suitable than these vascular probes which generate *artifacts* below the retina, making all publications more or less wrong. Only lack of time prevented us to share our approach, apart from a remote abstract [13]. The whole chapter on head of our 2010 edition dealt with it (with the maxillary sinus), and we don't reiterate many details. In very few lines, we remind that intracranial pressure (ICP) is usually assessed using transcranial Doppler, and we propose an alternative written in our 1992 edition, the consideration of the *optic nerve* as part of the brain (Fig. 34.6). Since the optic nerve is part of the very brain, therefore surrounded by meninges, it is expected that the cerebrospinal fluid, under pressure, will fill these spaces, resulting in an apparent enlargement of the caliper.

Our first observations showed a difference of optic nerve caliper in patients with or without elevated ICP. Based on a cut-off value ≥ 4.5 mm, our observations showed that the caliper of the optic nerve on normal subjects was 3.4 mm (range, 2.1–7.0 mm). An enlarged optic nerve was observed in the study group, with a caliper of 5.1 mm (range, 2.8–7.0 mm). These results pointed out a lack of absolute concordance with the gold standard (edema on CT), with 80 % sensitivity and 83 % specificity [13]. This potential went to interest for many teams, we apologize for quoting just less than a few [14]. Some of these studies show quite perfect results, *not* ours. This makes a problem regarding such a fragile organ. We would have preferred a 100 % accuracy. Read many details for how to improve ultrasound accuracy on our 2010 edition. We optimized the method by using a microconvex probe, which does not generate any acoustic shadow. Linear probes used by the community in all subsequent studies required a measurement 3 mm behind the eyeball because they measured in actual fact an acoustic shadow, unlike our probe – showing one more time how universal it is. See in Fig. 11.3 how the artifacts enlarge with depth. An artifact is easy to distinguish from an optic nerve: the former is straight, linear, unlike the sinuous latter one.

Transcranial Doppler? The development we made in our 2010 edition is too long for being inserted in a textbook mostly devoted to the BLUE-protocol, and we apologize for this.

Safety of spinal tap in meningitis? Read 2010 edition.

Basics of Soft Tissues

"Soft tissues" includes a lot. Fat, fluids, nerves, lymph nodes, cysts, spine... Abscesses are usually well-defined, hypoechoic, with possible bacterial gas. A posterior enhancement (never used by CEURF in lung and venous ultrasound) can here demonstrate the fluid nature (without painful and risky pressure) but a needle insertion is the simplest way for expediting the diagnosis. This also allows the distinction with the hematoma, also well-limited, first anechoic but rapidly heterogeneous. In both cases, just beware vascular masses (pseudo-aneurism e.g.) when the collection is rounded: use clinical data, the absence

Basics of Airway Management (and a Bit of ABCDE)   303

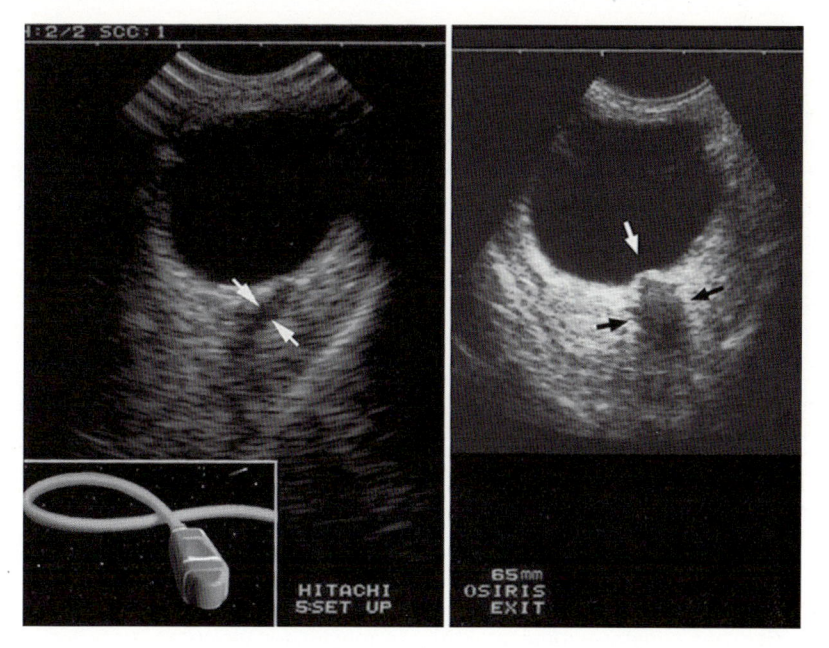

Fig. 34.6 Optic nerve and elevated intracranial pressure (IP). One practical use of optic nerve. In any comatose patient, the question of elevated IP should be raised. Sending any alcoholic coma or drug abuse to CT would not be realistic, but missing a neurosurgical emergency in the same alcoholic patient would be a dramatic mistake. The gold standard (the measurement of the IP, using direct transcranial device) has several issues (invasive, time-consuming, not of proven efficiency). In the absence of strong clinical evidence or either extreme surgical emergency, or ordinary drug/alcohol abuse, patients having values <4.5 mm are monitored at the bedside, those with higher values referred for CT. *Left*: normal optic nerve. The microconvex probe is gently applied on the eyelid, like a fountain pen, the operator's hand lying on the patient's face. No pressure should be exerted on the eye so that any vagal reaction is avoided. The eye must be in the axis (for not scanning ocular muscles instead of optic nerve). This application requires some skill. Posterior to the eyeball, a sinuous hypoechoic tubular structure usually well outlined by hyperechoic fat is detected by slight scanning. This optic nerve (*arrows*) has a normal caliper (2.6 mm). Note its sinuous route. *Right*: brain edema. In this scan, the apparent caliper of the optic nerve is markedly enlarged: 5.3 mm (*black arrows*). In addition, the papilla (*white arrow*) bulges in the lumen of the eyeball. There was diffuse brain edema on CT. Note in the cartouche that a microconvex probe has been used in our studies, generating a real, sinuous optic nerve, i.e., not an artifact (generated by a refractory conflict between papilla and acoustic properties of the vascular probes)

of auscultatory thrill, the absence of systolic dynamic on real-time ultrasound. In necrotizing cellulitis, the pattern is diffusely ill-defined with hypoechoic areas. Subtleties distinguish myonecrosis from simple gangrenous cellulitis. In malignant hyperthermia, the muscle would show a heterogeneous and grainy pattern. Rhabdomyolysis shows hypoechoic muscular pattern with increased volume. The analysis of muscular trophicity in long-staying patients can generate nice studies (see our 2010 Edition). Not soft tissues really but superficial structures, we find strategical parietal vessels (epigastric, internal mammary). If needed, take our tofu solution (see our Fig. 31.4). We have withdrawn from this edition, devoted to the lung mainly, one of the two sole picturesque images of our 2010 Edition, the Fig. 25.9, which showed an intervertebral disk, with the sign of the gorilla in the mist, and mainly the vision of the CSF.

Basics of Airway Management (and a Bit of ABCDE)

We try to give to ultrasound its real place. A difficult airway management is rare, and now so many tools make the procedure safer (Eschman device, visual laryngoscopy, etc.). As to the one-lung intubation, we ask doctors not to insert kilometers of tube once the vocal cords are crossed. Of course, ultrasound will show a pseudo A′-profile with a lung pulse, usually [15], a stand-still left cupola whereas the right cupola has exaggerated amplitude, but first let's intubate wisely. These images are, indeed, spectacular, but this should be learned far after the vital points. Don't let ultrasound be a mental disease.

Esophageal intubation is a clinical diagnosis, which it is true can be confirmed in a few seconds (see if needed Fig. 24.11 of our 2010 edition). We try not to confuse "critical" ultrasound with "spectacular" ultrasound. In the famous "ABCDE" management (which we call "ABCBE," read the reason why in Chap. 37, Sect. SLAM, the "A" is done clinically, then ultrasound is used for breathing (B) and circulation (C), four first-line applications, two major targets. For the brain (B again, not D?), ultrasound can wait a few minutes.

Basics on Sepsis at Admission

An impressive list of targets can be detected at the bedside using our simple equipment [16]. Read again on sepsis and ultrasound in Chap. 30.

Basics on Fever in the Long-Staying Ventilated Patient

This setting made a didactic problem, because it deals also with the lung (excluded from the present chapter), and is rather seen after several days of stay in the ICU. It has been located in Chap. 28 – read the section on Fever-protocol.

Basics of Basics on Trauma

We do not intend to write an atlas. Excellent textbooks exist already. Take these lines as free talks.

At the thorax, an aortic rupture can be suspected, or again detected, in patients with favorable morphotype. In a tracheal rupture, ultrasound will show parietal emphysema, pneumothorax, abolished or pseudo-abolished lung sliding or lung pulse. The main bronchus rupture can yield atelectasis. The pneumomediastinum is to our knowledge a subtle diagnosis. A hemopericardium should be sought routinely in a traumatized patient. There is no need for an acronym for this.

At the abdomen, the detection of peritoneal fluid is a basic step familiar for many [17]. Fluid in the peritoneal cavity can be urine, bile, or digestive fluids (easy to diagnose, although mingled with blood, using the principles of interventional ultrasound). It can also be pure blood. This finding made 12 lines in our 1992 textbook [18] and 1 line in our 1993 article [19]. Not for lack of major relevance, just because there were hundred other relevant targets. How to label this, and is it important? We did not use any specific word in our 1992 edition because acronyms were not on fashion in our debuts (1985). We just wrote "ultrasound search for free blood." We could have created the not flashy at all OCCARBOST-protocol (one can create a revolution by opening sonographer's textbooks) (One Can, etc.). One word about this protocol: For many young physicians, finding free blood is the symbol of the revolution of critical ultrasound, its very begin. Is it serious to imagine that the absence of a flashy acronym would have cost *lives*? That a life can be saved because you are on fashion? Normal doctors do not need flashy acronyms for understanding what is important or not in their profession. This is not, on purpose, inserted as an anecdotal note. Read instead the section on SLAM in Chap. 37.

Ultrasound signs of pneumoperitoneum mean rupture of hollow organ. The parenchymal analysis (liver, spleen) should not delay management – but yields characteristic signs: heterogeneous (usually hypoechoic) images of contusion (Fig. 28.4 of 2010 edition), hyperechoic lines of fracture (Fig. 28.5 of 2010 edition), and biconvex external images of subcapsular hematoma. A pancreatic trauma mimics acute pancreatitis. The diagnosis of vascular rupture (renal artery) is better approached by Doppler, CT, or angiography.

At the head and neck, the eyeball integrity can be checked, signs of frank cervical vertebra rupture are accessible to ultrasound from C1 to C7. Carotid artery dissection makes us penetrate into a complex field, as opposed to most applications seen previously. The diagnosis usually refers to Doppler. Enlarged caliper, segmentary ectasis, offset stenosis, radish-tail tapered occlusion, double lumen, intimal flap, anomalies of velocities, and pulsatility index with flow inversions when compared to contralateral artery are sought for [20], yet heavy concerns are present. The skill required is high. Fine analysis is compromised by the cervical collar, or worse, if carefully withdrawn, by the usual agitation of the patient. Heparin therapy can be double-edged in these traumatized patients. Eventually, when experts write that a Doppler study of the carotid artery has no sense if not integrated to the clinical context, they make the tacit acknowledgement of insufficiencies of arterial Doppler. In lung ultrasound, the signs can be interpreted independently from the clinical setting (an effusion is an effusion, etc.), indicating its high degree of standardization. We would like to see, in this delicate context, the same conclusions that were made in the areas of the veins, the hemodynamic and many others as regards the real utility of Doppler.

Basics on Acute Deglobulization

In trauma, a hemothorax, a hemoperitoneum, a hemopericardium, a capsular hematoma (liver, spleen, kidneys), a retroperitoneal hematoma, a soft tissue collection (femoral fracture), and in other settings, a GI tract hemorrhage are quickly recognized. In any doubt, a puncture will show that the fluid is blood. Multiple small collections can explain a hemorrhagic shock.

Basics on Non-pulmonary Critical Ultrasound in Neonates and Children

This paragraph has no pretention to replace comprehensive textbooks written by experts. Our experience was deeply hampered by the equipment we had, a traditional echocardiographic machine. In these times, we were like all these teams who today discover critical ultrasound using unsuitable units.

Head

The transfontanellar approach is a standardized field. A profuse literature is available. This window is used in cardiac arrest in the neonate for searching brain, ventricular hemorrhage. The sequence of the SESAME-protocol (designed for adults) should be adapted for searching earlier at the brain the origin of a cardiac arrest.

Neck

Correct placement of endotracheal tubes is a basic application.

Veins

Central venous line insertion will be greatly facilitated. Their correct placement can be checked with the same limitations as in the adult. Ultrasound will detect the catheter-linked thromboses [21].

Heart

The heart as a target is a matter of specialists (congenital malformations). The heart as an indirect marker of hemodynamic disorders is accessible to a simple protocol (see Chap. 30).

Circulation and Volemia

The volemia control is a sensitive issue in these babies. We see around us various options, from the clinical assessment to PICCO devices, not easy to implement in small weight babies. Why wouldn't the FALLS-protocol be used here? We currently work on this theme, assuming that the parameter offered by lung ultrasound, i.e., the B-line as a direct marker of increase of pulmonary artery occlusion pressure, should be extrapolated in the neonate [22].

Lung

See devoted Chap. 32.

Diaphragm

Its anatomy and function can be precisely analyzed.

Abdomen

The organs of the adult are present: aorta, inferior vena cava, GI tract, liver, spleen, kidneys, pancreas, adrenals, gallbladder, bladder, all in order. Some fields are more characteristic of the child, but here we get too far from the subject, which could include various digestive disorders such as pyloric stenosis, esophageal atresia, intussusception: a whole discipline [23].

Basics on Futuristic Trends

A therapeutic use of ultrasound has been evoked in the years 1960 [24]. Studies point out the potential role of therapeutic ultrasound in strokes [25]. High intensity focused ultrasound may be used at the kidney, liver, pancreas, breast, bones, lung, etc.

Basic Conclusion

This chapter, reduced to the minimal vital (13 chapters in our 2010 edition), shows that ultrasound, a multifaceted tool, should change medical habits in countless settings. Just note this point: one simple grayscale machine and one simple probe were used. The spirit of simplicity may rule not only at the main vital organs (heart, lungs, veins) but with the same results for the whole body.

Technical Note

1. *Summary of our abstract*

    In a study of 50 consecutive procedures carried out in subclavian veins in ventilated patients, with no selection (which will probably never be submitted for lack of time and high risk of multiple rejections), we had a success rate of 100 % [5]. In 72 % of the cases, success (frank flow within the syringe) was obtained in less than 20 s, in 16 % of cases in less than 1 min. Twelve percent of the cases were considered long, but success was nonetheless obtained in less than 5 min. In other words, ultrasound has accustomed us to immediate success (5 min seems a long time). Basically, all patients were *consecutive*, meaning that the usual factors of reluctance – or exclusion – were not considered. Twenty-five percent of the patients were plethoric (with distance from the skin to the subclavian vein >30 mm). The procedure was immediate in 84 % of these challenging patients.

Anecdotal Notes

1. *Venous ultrasound for who*

    We use ultrasound in each patient for avoiding any risk, but also any discomfort to the patient. It is seen in the literature that ultrasound guidance is suggested after the failure of a blind attempt, or when there are official contraindications, or again when costs have to be controlled: ultrasound should use 40 % less material than blind techniques [6].

2. *65 statements?*

    So many statements for such a simple application? Probably because the choice of vascular probes makes everything more complicated. The probe has to be held by the whole hand, crispated whereas our microconvex probe is held like a pen, quietly. The cumbersome vascular probe is so long that long-axis approaches are made difficult, and users prefer these short-axis procedures, at the neck. The vascular probe cannot be rotated in the natural anatomical axes of the veins, and the operator must adapt to the probe, while we do the opposite. As self-taught sono-intensivist, we suspect that the tradition which created venous ultrasound (vascular probes, etc.) and the one which wrote in the stone the unfeasibility of lung ultrasound were created by the same users.

3. *The spirit of the ATACCS poster*

    When we presented these data in the international ATACCS congress (in our beloved fifth Parisian district: no costs for flight or hotel) in 1994, some had a smile, so obvious was the conclusion. They should have read the real message: one application among 100 that justified the purchase of simple ultrasound units in each ICU – for a visual medicine since 1994 or before [7].

References

1. Lichtenstein D, Mezière G, Courret JP (2002) Le glissement péritonéal, un signe échographique de pneumopéritoine. Réanimation 11(Suppl 3):165
2. Lichtenstein D, Mirolo C, Mezière G (2001) Abolition of GI tract peristalsis, an ultrasound sign of mesenteric infarction. Réanimation 10(Suppl 1):203
3. Sznajder JI, Zveibil FR, Bitterman H, Weiner P, Bursztein S (1986) Central vein catheterization, failure and complication rates by three percutaneous approaches. Arch Intern Med 146:259–261
4. Skolnick ML (1994) The role of sonography in the placement and management of jugular and subclavian central venous catheters. AJR Am J Roentgenol 163:291–295
5. Lichtenstein D, Saïfi R, Mezière G, Pipien I (2000) Cathétérisme écho-guidé de la veine sous-clavière en réanimation. Réan Urg 2(Suppl 9):184
6. Thompson DR, Gualtieri E, Deppe S, Sipperly ME (1994) Greater success in subclavian vein cannulation using ultrasound for inexperienced operators. Crit Care Med 22:A189
7. Merrer J, De Jonghe B, Golliot F, Lefrant JY, Raffy B, Barré JP, Rigaud JP, Casciani D, Misset B, Bosquet C, Outin H, Brun-Buisson C, Nitenberg G (2001) Complications of femoral and subclavian venous catheterization in critically ill patients. A randomized controlled trial. JAMA 286:700–707
8. Lichtenstein D (1994) Relevance of ultrasound in predicting the ease of central venous line insertions. Eur J Emerg 7:46
9. Mansfield PF, Hohn DC, Fornage BD, Gregurich MA, Ota DM (1994) Complications and failures of subclavian vein catheterization. N Engl J Med 331:1735–1738
10. Lichtenstein D, Saïfi R, Augarde R, Prin S, Schmitt JM, Page B, Pipien I, Jardin F (2001) The internal jugular veins are asymmetric. Usefulness of ultrasound before catheterization. Intensive Care Med 27:301–305
11. Denys BG, Uretsky BF (1991) Anatomical variations of internal jugular vein location: impact on central venous access. Crit Care Med 19:1516–1519
12. Karakitsos D, Labropoulos N, De Groot E, Patrianakos AP, Kouraklis G, Poularas J, Samonis G, Tsoutsos DA, Konstadoulakis MM, Karabinis A (2006) Real-time ultrasound-guided catheterisation of the internal jugular vein: a prospective comparison with the landmark technique in critical care patients. Crit Care 10(6):R162
13. Lichtenstein D, Bendersky N, Mezière G, Goldstein I (2002) Diagnostic de l'hypertension intra-crânienne par la mesure échographique du nerf optique. Réanimation 11(Suppl 3):170s
14. Blaivas M, Theodoro D, Sierzenski PR (2003) Elevated intracranial pressure detected by bedside emergency ultrasonography of the optic nerve sheat. Acad Emerg Med 10:376–381
15. Lichtenstein D, Lascols N, Prin S, Mezière G (2003) The lung pulse: an early ultrasound sign of complete atelectasis. Intensive Care Med 29:2187–2192
16. Lichtenstein D (2007) Point of care ultrasound: infection control on the ICU. Crit Care Med 35(Suppl):S262–S267
17. Rozycki GS, Ochsner MG, Feliciano DV, Thomas B, Boulanger BR, Davis FE, Falcone RE, Schmidt JA (1998) Early detection of hemoperitoneum by ultrasound examination of the right upper quadrant: a multicenter study. J Trauma 45(5):878–883
18. Lichtenstein D (1992) L'échographie générale en réanimation, 1st edn. Springer, France, p 27
19. Lichtenstein D, Axler O (1993) Intensive use of general ultrasound in the intensive care unit, a prospective study of 150 consecutive patients. Intensive Care Med 19:353–355
20. Ter Minassian A, Bonnet F, Guerrini P, Ricolfi F, Delaunay F, Beydon L, Catoire P (1992) Carotid artery injury: value of Doppler screening in head injury patients. Ann Fr Anesth Reanim 11:598–600
21. Hanslik A et al (2008) Incidence and diagnosis of thrombosis in children with short-term central venous lines of the upper venous system. Pediatrics 122:1284–1291
22. Lichtenstein D, Mezière G, Lagoueyte JF, Biderman P, Goldstein I, Gepner A (2009) A-lines and B-lines: lung ultrasound as a bedside tool for predicting pulmonary artery occlusion pressure in the critically ill. Chest 136.1014–1020
23. Kairam N, Kaiafis C et al (2009) Diagnosis of pediatric intussusception by an emergency physician-performed bedside ultrasound: a case report. Pediatr Emerg Care 25(3):177–180
24. Dénier A (1961) Les ultra-sons appliqués à la médecine. L'Expansion Scientifique Française, la Tour du Pin, pp 70–133
25. Alexandrov AV, Mikulik R, Ribo M, Sharma VK, Lao AY, Tsivgoulis G, Sugg RM, Barreto A, Sierzenski P, Malkoff MD, Grotta JC (2008) A pilot randomized clinical safety study of sonothrombolysis augmentation with ultrasound-activated perflutren-lipid microspheres for acute ischemic stroke. Stroke 39:1464–1469

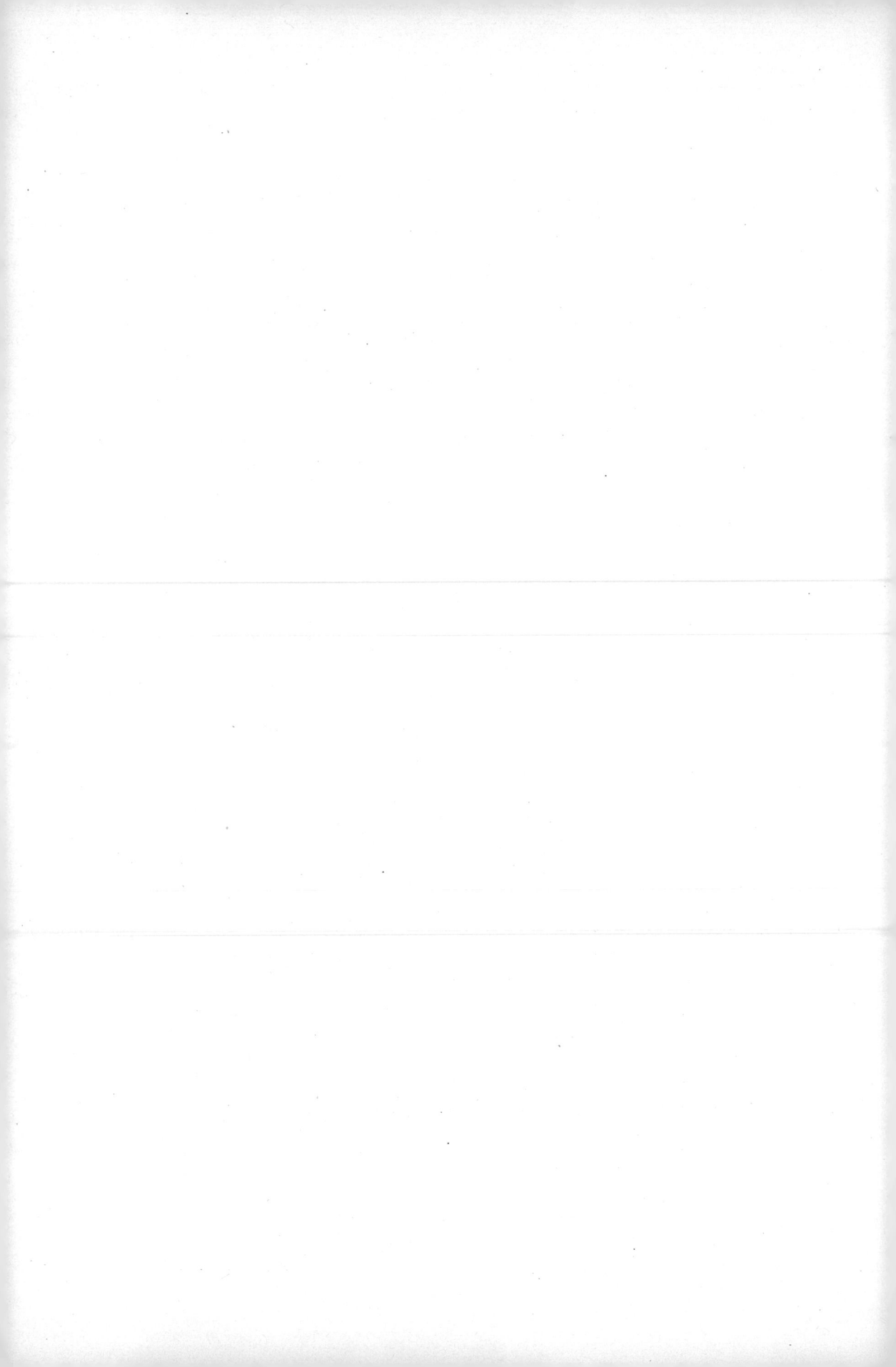

The Extended-BLUE-Protocol

35

Warren Zapol wrote us one day: ".... As for rejections, they continue, even with age and celebrity. Persistence and resubmitting is what counts. *Illegitimus non caborundum est.*" We now know with years how right he was (regarding age). Regarding celebrity (and not losing time waiting its hypothetical arrival), we anticipate difficulties and delays and prefer to have less publications and give instead our non-peer-reviewed experience through this textbook. We share here the main aspects of the Extended BLUE-protocol. This is a concept considering the multiple interactions between diseases for increasing the accuracy of the BLUE-protocol (which was a preliminary work), from the initial 90.5 % to a value as near as possible to 100 % (Fig. 35.1). The value of 90.5 % is not bad for a discipline which was not supposed to exist, but we have now to answer more scientifically to issues heard here and there (why didn't they include the heart? etc.).

The Extended BLUE-protocol refines diagnoses of frequent diseases. It includes rare diagnoses, double diagnoses. It gives diagnoses to patients without official diagnoses.

The Extended BLUE-protocol: a giant work we should normally submit in 20 years (reasonable foreseen delay, because of priority submissions and endless rejections). This delay considers full

---

Electronic supplementary material The online version of this chapter (doi:10.1007/978-3-319-15371-1_35) contains supplementary material, which is available to authorized users.

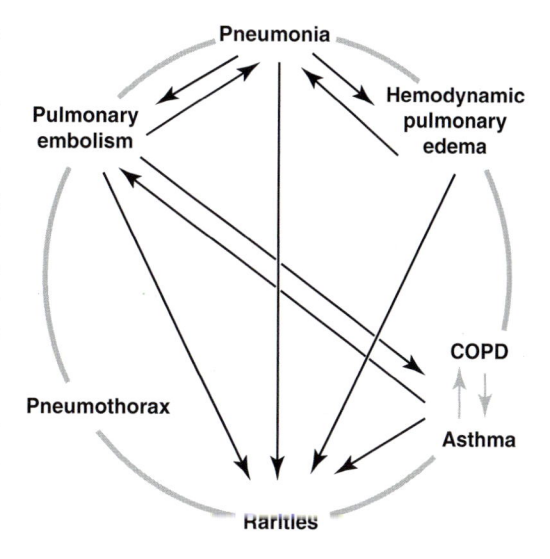

Fig. 35.1 The circle of the Extended BLUE-protocol. This figure, as simple as possible, shows that, in real life, intrications are possible. Frequent causes of acute dyspnea can interfere with each other, and with rare diseases

mastery of pathophysiology pertaining to critical ultrasound by physicians, of any available data from modern lung physiology and imaging [1–6].

It will include the following:

1. Simple but selected clinical data (history, auscultation), simple biological data for refining diagnoses (D-dimers). One may add here epidemiologic data (frequency of given diseases).
2. Refined ultrasound LUCI data: splitting the simple concept of PLAPS into pleural effusion and lung consolidation, assessing

consolidation volume, bronchogram dynamics, lung pulse, etc.
3. Simple emergency cardiac sonography (ventricle behavior, free wall thickness, etc.)
4. Interventional weapons, such as ultrasound-assisted thoracentesis
5. Time (i.e., assessing the ultrasound evolution under therapy of the supposed disease)

And, if necessary, other tools such as Doppler or even CT (although the aim of the Extended BLUE-protocol is to by-pass this heavy test). The place of the simple radiography can be considered either here in step 5, or more realistically, in step 1; this can be debated.

We use this protocol every day in actual fact. We use a bit, or the whole of it depending in the setting. Before being experts in Extended BLUE-protocol, doctors must first master the basic BLUE-protocol. We aim at making it widespread using appropriate teaching methods (please refer to Chap. 38). Once accustomed, they will sophisticate its decision tree by adding basic branches.

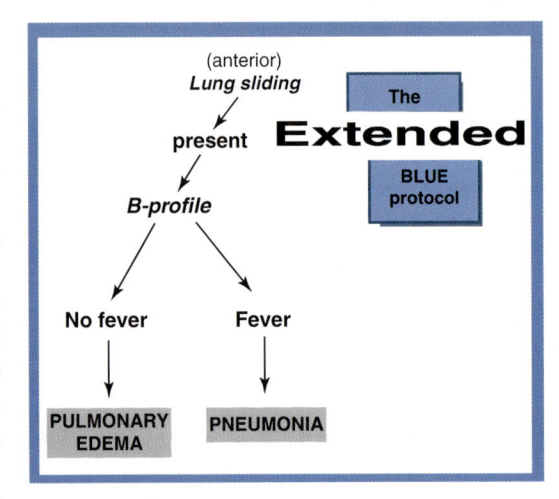

Fig. 35.2 Extended BLUE-protocol integrating one clinical sign. One comprehensive tree showing the potential of the Extended BLUE-protocol may be probably too complicated to draw, too bushy, just because it integrates the BLUE-protocol to many other data, from current knowledge, fine lung ultrasound signs, simple cardiac sonography, etc. Here is featuring one basic example: for refining the left branch that drives to hemodynamic pulmonary edema, but includes some cases of interstitial pneumonia. One has just to consider, at this step, the temperature, usually normal in hemodynamic pulmonary edema, usually present in pneumonia. This is the most schematical, basic example

What Is the Extended BLUE-Protocol, Three Basic Examples

We can enrich the BLUE-protocol to various extents. By just adding *one* data, it will already be improved.

One Basic Example: Hemodynamic Pulmonary Edema Versus Pneumonia with the B-Profile, Integrating Just One Clinical Data

The most basic example, charicaturally simple but significant, is the consideration of fever. Fever is an important and not important data. Let us take the example in the title. The small branch, at the left of the BLUE-protocol decision tree, drives to the B-profile and concludes to hemodynamic pulmonary edema. With scientific reserves: "only" 95 % specificity. The few cases of B-profile that do not come from a hemodynamic cause are some pneumonia, and chronic interstitial diseases, mainly. The Extended BLUE-protocol just aims at improving this rate of 95 % by diagnosing these few cases. We remind that in the absence of a B-profile, there is no hemodynamic pulmonary edema, and the need for a sophisticated "ECHO" should not generate exaggerate energy.

This part of the B-profile can be refined, precisely by adding fever, at this step. If fever was really discriminative, things would be simple: dyspnea with fever is pneumonia. Yet medicine is medicine. Because of previous antibiotherapy, or comorbidities, of limit value of temperature, because some say that fever is "often" seen in hemodynamic pulmonary edema, or any other confusing factor, things are less simple. Here, the BLUE-protocol becomes interesting. The inclusion of the item "fever" *there*, once a B-profile detected, may add points. It should not be done at every step: for instance, the A-profile plus DVT with, or without, fever remains a pulmonary embolism. Yet the B-profile with fever is not the most typical from pulmonary edema. Here, a fever makes a simple and efficient alert. The consideration of this basic piece of information, of never yet debated interest, can refine this small branch of the B-profile that drives, *usually*, to hemodynamic pulmonary edema (Fig. 35.2).

Fig. 35.3 Extended BLUE-protocol integrating one sign of LUCI. A substantial volume of lung consolidation favors the diagnosis of pneumonia more than pulmonary embolism. This is based on observation. The volume should be defined according to strict rules (see ours in Chap. 28). The threshold volume should be defined using sharply designed studies, taking into account the severe cases, for making homogeneous groups of patients

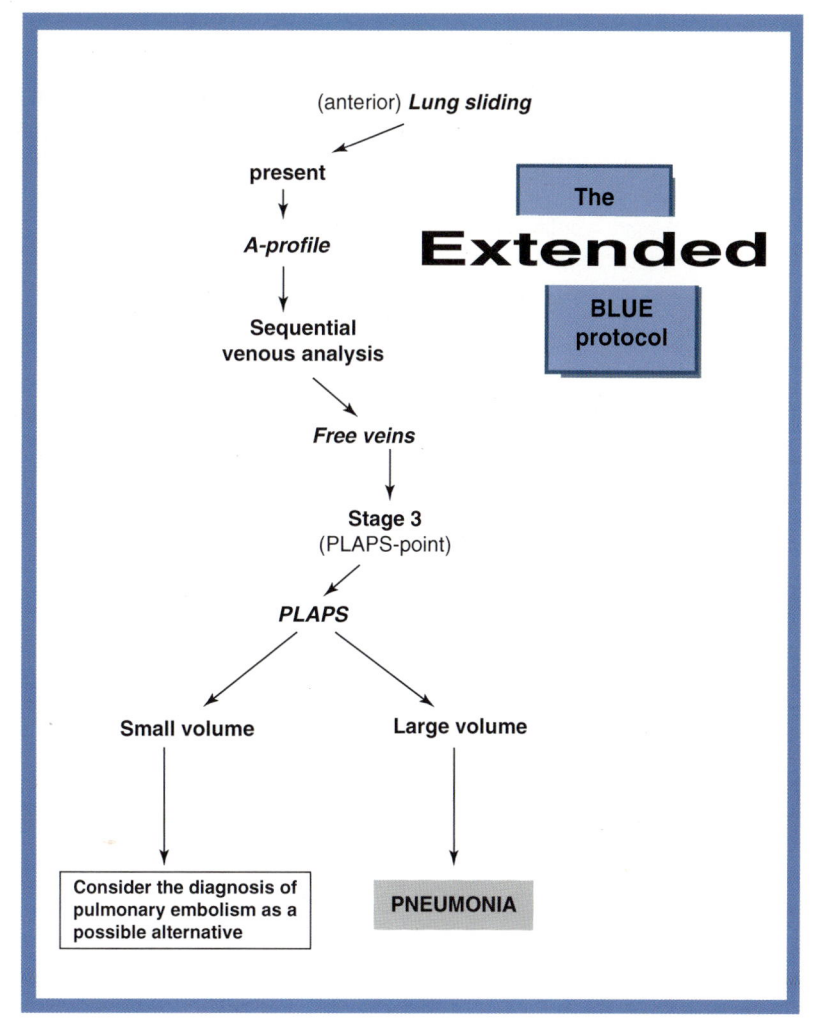

This is the simplest example of what is, basically, the Extended BLUE-protocol. Works should of course specify the discriminative value of the temperature (37°8? 38°2?). Hundreds of examples can be added here for the relevance of the physical examination, we let the book as thin as possible.

Another Example for Better Diagnosing Pneumonia from Pulmonary Embolism, Integrating Just One Data from Lung Ultrasound

The consideration of the volume of lung consolidation should matter. A respiratory failure due to pneumonia on healthy lungs (i.e., not including patients with previous chronic respiratory insufficiency), generates a rather substantial volume of excluded lung tissue. The volume of consolidation is usually limited in pulmonary embolism. This can make another small branch in the E-BLUE-protocol (Fig. 35.3).

A Last Example for Diagnosing Pulmonary Edema from Chronic Interstitial Disease, Integrating Just One Data from Simple Emergency Cardiac Sonography

Once again, we consider the branch driving to the B-profile. In exceptional cases, a chronic interstitial disease can be the diagnosis. By inserting the item "right ventricle enlargement with thickened free wall and well contractile left ventricule" (RVETFWWCLV), the few patients having a B-profile coming from a chronic interstitial disease would be immediately detected – and the therapy would be adapted. Note that colleagues not making lung ultrasound but making echocardiography instead would see a "right" disease, but they would not be able to discriminate a bronchial disease (COPD, etc.) from a chronic interstitial disease (especially when radioccult), which requires other therapies.

The Extended BLUE-Protocol: An Opportunity to Use the Best of the Clinical Examination

We are confident that the physical examination and the history are probably the most important tools. Yet the consideration of the BLUE-protocol allows to hierarchize them. Instead of a use without discrimination, we will pay high attention to such sign, less to another.

The stethoscope (the one you apply at your ears) plays a major role in one setting: searching for an acute bronchial stenosis, i.e., usually, asthma. The bronchial tree is the only element not really assessed using lung ultrasound, because it does not reach the lung surface (principle N°7 of LUCI). Bronchial diseases have to be *heard*. This is a main interest of the stethoscope, at the era of lung ultrasound.

The auscultatory data, especially wheezings (and mitral, aortic valve murmurs), are fully included in the Extended BLUE-protocol.

Pulmonary Embolism: How the Extended BLUE-Protocol Integrates Lung Consolidations? When Should Anterior Consolidations Be Connected to This Diagnosis?

The principle of the Extended BLUE-protocol is simple. The detection of a C-profile (usually small consolidations, i.e., C-lines) (see Fig. 17.3) concludes a BLUE-protocol: the BLUE-diagnosis is "pneumonia." Anterior lung consolidation indicated pneumonia in 95 % of cases (versus 5 % for embolism), meaning that pneumonia was 18 times more likely than embolism. If the physician decides to make an Extended-BLUE-protocol, the venous analysis will be done systematically. In the 5 % of patients with a C-profile but a (final) diagnosis of pulmonary embolism, the same proportion of DVT should be found, i.e., 4/5th of the patients [7].

One can go deeper in details, considering sliding and non-sliding C-profiles (read Anecdotal Note 1).

Note. Let us remember that when there is no anterior lung consolidation, the A-DVT profile in a severe dyspnea has an 81 % sensitivity and a 99 % specificity. Associated with chest pain, the specificity quite reaches 100 %. The BLUE-protocol should result in a decrease of helical CT of roughly 4/5th, which is more than the aim wished by the LUCI-FLR project (2/3 would be enough for the three next decades).

Distinction Between Acute Hemodynamic Pulmonary Edema and ARDS

We compared patients in the BLUE-protocol who had acute hemodynamic pulmonary edema ("AHPE") and pneumonia initiating ARDS. These last patients were included as "pneumonia" for keeping the decision tree simple, the therapy being roughly similar. Patients with AHPE had the B-profile (97 % of cases). In 86 % of cases, patients with ARDS had either the B', A/B, C, or A-no-V-PLAPS-profile, and the 14 % remaining had a B-profile. The B', A/B, and C-profile have a high specificity for pneumonia.

These results are explained by pathophysiology.

The B'-Profile

The exudative process invades the subpleural interlobular septa and sticks the lung (like countless small nails) to the chest wall. This explains the frequent B'-profile of ARDS [4]. Facing diffuse interstitial edema, the BLUE-protocol distinguishes patients with lung sliding (suggesting transudative process) from those with abolished lung sliding (indicating exudative process).

The C-Profile

Infectious processes, including ARDS, can widespread through airway routes, according to non-hemodynamic rules, and the gravity law is less expressed here. This is why lung consolidations can develop anteriorly (the C-profile). The C-profile cannot be seen in AHPE (see pathophysiologic discussion, and Fig. 24.1). The term of "enlarged" B-profile indicates that the user went beyond the four anterior BLUE-points and made a liberal scanning, searching for C-lines, even minute, not finding any. If a C-line is found, the classification changes, from the B-profile to the C-profile. And the diagnosis is shifted from AHPE to pneumonia.

The A/B-Profile

Asymmetry can be seen if the disorder comes from one lung infection, which explains A/B profiles. An extended definition of the A/B profile includes, at the same lung, areas of predominant lung rockets with areas of predominant A-lines. Unilateral hemodynamic pulmonary edema? These famous cases are very rare, and this is a radiological definition – our very few observations showed more PLAPS at the edematous side, but a symmetrical (anterior) B-profile. To be confirmed on large series.

The A-No-V-PLAPS Profile

Most of these patients have lateral lung rockets. This may be considered as an extreme variant of an A/B-profile, i.e., anterior areas without and lateral areas with interstitial patterns. Fluids in AHPE, submitted to hydrostatic pressure, move up actively to the anterior areas through the interlobular septa – toward the sky. Fluids in permeability-induced edema passively descend to the dependent areas (principle N°2 of LUCI). White X-rays with absence of anterior lung rockets are therefore suggestive of ARDS.

The B-Profile? How to Manage Then?

Some cases of pneumonia are expressed by a diffuse interstitial injury with no, or not yet, impairment of lung sliding (B'-profile) or anterior consolidation (C-profile). Because of a low accuracy, this profile is not considered as indicating pneumonia in the design of the BLUE-protocol (which, reminder, provides profiles with a high likeliness of diseases, rarely a 100 % certitude, read cartouche of the native decision tree, Fig. 20.1). Other tools can be added, in the order of the E-BLUE-protocol: from clinical, LUCI, simple emergency cardiac sonography, and interventional ultrasound data, up to classical tests if needed.

1. *All clinical and paraclinical elements*

    Some drops of clinical information are priceless. We refer here to the usual tools, from fever to CRP, that any doctor masters. Many diagnoses are done clinically, we just find it more elegant, however, to aim at the zero fault and make ultrasound for all cases. Remember that a systematic use of ultrasound in all patients admitted to the ICU found 1/4th of unexpected data [8].

2. *LUCI*

    Volume of consolidation

    It is fully considered in the Extended BLUE-protocol. PLAPS seem more substantial in pneumonia than in hemodynamic pulmonary edema (under sharp analysis).

    Advanced ultrasound features of pneumonia (search for abscess or necrosis)

    Read next section.

    Analysis of lateral chest wall

    In 3 % of cases of AHPE, lung rockets are not anterior but lateral. This is found three to five times more often in cases of pneumonia. This makes schematically the A-no-V-PLAPS-profile (the lateral wall is not considered in the BLUE-protocol).

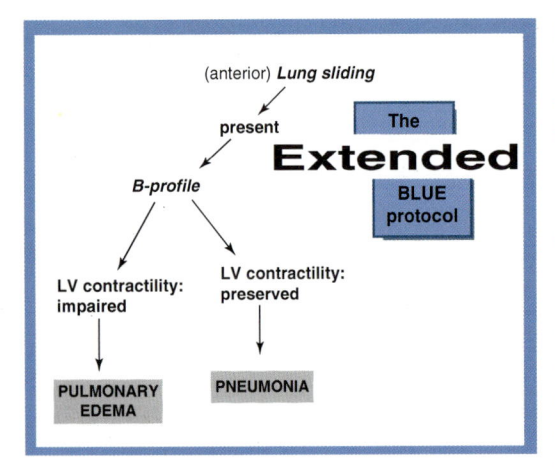

Fig. 35.4 Extended BLUE-protocol integrating one sign from the simple emergency cardiac sonography. Some intensivists may find that the correspondence between the B-profile and the diagnosis of hemodynamic pulmonary edema is too basic. First, the specificity is 95 %, not so bad. Rare cases of pneumonia with the B-profile were detected using Fig. 35.2. Now, exceptional cases of chronic interstitial diseases will be detected by just including the item of the LV contractility, which should be, schematically, impaired in hemodynamic pulmonary edema, conserved in chronic lung diseases. One could have instead used the thickening of the free RV wall (choosing the best item results in the most simple tree)

3. *Echocardiography*
   When a B-profile is seen, the Extended BLUE-protocol considers the LV contractility. If decreased, this is a banal, quite redundant, sign of hemodynamic pulmonary edema. It can also be a sign of septic cardiomyopathy, sometimes. If conserved (with no sign, clinical or even echocardiographic, of valvular regurgitation, it should increase the probability of a pneumonia or ARDS (Fig. 35.4)). Read Anecdotal Note 2.
4. *Direct analysis of the pleural fluid: thoracentesis*
   Read below. The lung puncture should also be envisaged, if studies confirm the safety shown by our initial data.
5. *Time*. Septic lung rockets do not vanish rapidly.
6. *Other tests*
   If the diagnosis resists to these successive tools.

Distinction Between Pulmonary Edema and the Few Cases of Pulmonary Embolism with Lung Rockets

The B-profile, seen in 2 % of our cases of severe pulmonary embolism apart from ICU-acquired cases (under submission) may be explained by the septal interference, which generates elevated pressures from the left ventricle [9]. There is a paradox: this profile would be more often seen, given that all these patients had a severe failure. This raises interesting potential of research, for knowing how far the left heart pressures are increased (relatively, with exact measure of transmural pressures) in the case of a paradoxical septum.

The clue in the E-BLUE protocol is simple – instead of concluding "pulmonary edema," the test includes the following:
1. Clinical signs (pain).
2. The simple cardiac sonography, which detects an enlarged right ventricle: the suspicion of embolism is immediately raised.
3. Search for DVT. Keep in mind that among these few cases of pulmonary embolism with lung rockets, 4/5th of them should have visible DVTs. This is the Extended BLUE-protocol.
4. In the few (among the few) cases with no clear answer, more expert signs should be added: paradoxical septum, sophisticated ECHO signs, up to CT if needed.

Distinction Between Bronchial Diseases and Pulmonary Embolism with No DVT

Both yield the nude profile. Here, we can just rebuild all familiar pre-probabilities tests, and insert some of them in the Extended BLUE-protocol. We pay special attention to:
1. *Clinical step*
   - History. A dyspnea in a patient without any history of asthma or COPD favors the embolic cause.
   - Epidemiology. A bronchial disease is four times more frequent in the BLUE-protocol

- Simple clinical signs such as wheezings. Wheezings are not part of pulmonary embolism. Young patients with wheezings usually do not require any BLUE-protocol: the diagnosis of asthma is done. The BLUE-protocol is used here, not for making the diagnosis, already done clinically, not especially for confirming it (nude profile), but mostly for rapidly searching for any complication. One can also easily detect the *cardiac asthma* in a patient with wheezing plus B-profile. Some cases of asthma don't display any wheezing. Here, if pulmonary embolism is suspected, the Extended BLUE-protocol selects only patients without wheezing. Only this group, which includes patients with pulmonary embolism, and the few asthmatic patients without wheezings, may have a more invasive confirmatory test.
- Chest pain has nothing to do with bronchial diseases.
- Classical tests such as D-dimers and ECG.

2. *LUCI*

Nothing to be expected: nude profile in both cases. We intentionally do not insert signs of lung distension (subtle, and we don't need them critically).

3. *Simple cardiac sonography*
- One can add the RV free wall thickness (fine: embolism or asthma – thickened: rather COPD).

All these simple data build evidence; the aim is to decrease the number of CTs, following the LUCIFLR project. Typically, a young woman who has no history of asthma, had a recent orthopedic surgery, complains from sudden chest pain and acute respiratory failure, and displays an A-profile, with positive D-dimers and pathologic ECG (Stein signs), is a perfect suspect (and should benefit from scintigraphy first).

Just a note: wheezings can be heard in cardiac asthma, as we understood of an edematous decreasing of bronchial caliper. Here, ultrasound makes an immediate distinction: A-profile of true asthma versus B-profile of cardiac asthma. Nothing more to say.

Distinction Between Hemodynamic Pulmonary Edema and Exacerbation of Chronic Lung Interstitial Disease

Both display the B-profile.

1. *Clinical, epidemiological data*

Edema was seen 16 times more frequently than exacerbated chronic interstitial lung disease, first. Yet rarity should not be a punishment for these unhappy few. The notion of known chronic lung disease is present in most cases.

2. *LUCI*

PLAPS have nothing to do with a "simple" exacerbation of chronic lung disease. PLAPS would favor hemodynamic edema. PLAPS seen in a genuine chronic lung disease means any complication, such as pneumonia, embolism, or pulmonary edema, as the factor of decompensation.

3. *Simple cardiac sonography*

If the patient makes the first episode (of chronic lung disease), this simple test shows subtle right heart anomalies, no left heart anomalies, schematically.

4. *Time*

The B-profile should vanish if the episode of pulmonary edema is under control. If it does not, in a stabilized patient, this makes a major argument for a non-hemodynamic interstitial syndrome.

The "Excluded Patients" of the BLUE-Protocol Revisited by the Extended BLUE-Protocol

The Extended BLUE-protocol allows to include patients excluded from the native BLUE-protocol (detailed in Chap. 21).

1. *Rare diagnoses* (per order of frequency)
- Exacerbation of chronic interstitial disease: read the devoted section.
- Massive pleural effusion. A BLUE-pleural index of 5 cm indicates that the volume of the effusion is certainly responsible for the dyspnea.

- Atelectasis: read the devoted section in the following text.
- Tracheal stenosis: an anterior approach may find tracheal granulomas (see Figure 24.10 of our 2010 edition).
- Sterile aspiration pneumonia. This disease is seen more often in settings such as neurosurgical ICUs. Since the insult comes from inside, an alveolar injury is expected, with alveolar signs visible before interstitial signs.
- Fat embolism. This may generate a patchy B-profile. This disorder is under deeper investigation.

Among diagnoses not seen in the BLUE-protocol:
- Acute gastric dilatation: critical ultrasound includes the scanning of the stomach (using our microconvex probe).
- Phrenic palsy, Guillain-Barré syndrome: a standstill cupola is one of the easiest diagnoses.
- Metabolic dyspnea: it is more a hyperpnea than a dyspnea. A nude profile is expected if there is no lung origin nor complication.
- Pneumonia linked to amiodarone or other drugs: under investigation.

For the countless very rare diseases, years of large-scale multicentric studies will be necessary for gathering enough patients. The BLUE-protocol favors the daily life, the E-BLUE-protocol is an expert approach, for again decreasing the need for traditional tools, urgent CT first.

2. *Double diagnoses*

Do not forget the limitation evoked in Chap. 21. One never knows if the two diagnoses participate in a 50/50 % ratio – it can be 51/49 % or 99/1 %: a real methodological issue.

Here are some examples:
- Pulmonary edema plus pneumonia: in a patient with cardiac history, the B-profile with impaired left ventricle contractility and large posterior consolidation (plus an exudative pleural effusion) (plus the item of Fig. 35.2, fever) (etc.) invites to a double therapy.
- Pulmonary edema plus COPD: if the B-profile disappears after specific therapy of edema, but not the dyspnea, the diagnosis of associated COPD is suggested.
- Pulmonary edema plus chronic fibrosis: the fibrosis is often known on admission by the history. PLAPS have nothing to do in a simple exacerbation of fibrosis. PLAPS plus apyrexia suggest an associated hemodynamic pulmonary edema, PLAPS plus fever suggest a pneumonia, and PLAPS plus DVT a pulmonary embolism. If the diagnostic is still obscure, a thoracentesis may prove beneficial.

3. *No diagnosis*

We remind a critical point: all these patients had anyway one among the eight BLUE-profiles. The future will hopefully give credit to the BLUE-protocol, with maybe no need for an Extended-BLUE-protocol in these patients. Don't search for rarities in this group of patients. These are simple diseases, and this just highlights the difficulties we sometimes have using traditional tools.

Pneumonia, More Advanced Features for Distinction with Other Causes of Lung Consolidation

There are more than 10 signs in LUCI. With the lung pulse and the dynamic air bronchogram, it makes 12. These signs are used in the Extended BLUE-protocol.

Pneumonia means lung consolidation for some, but consolidations can be generated by hemodynamic pulmonary edema, pneumonia/ARDS, pulmonary embolism (sometimes even pneumothorax), and rare causes (atelectasis). Using the BLUE-protocol, it is possible to know what is the content of the alveoli: transudate (B-profile), exudate or pus (B', C, A/B, A-no-V-PLAPS profile), blood (A-profile plus DVT), or again nothing (atelectasis, not fully in the BLUE-protocol, see below).

In the strict sequence of the BLUE-protocol, consolidations "are" pneumonia, just because they are found either anteriorly (C-profile) or

Pneumonia, More Advanced Features for Distinction with Other Causes of Lung Consolidation 317

posteriorly after having ruled out pulmonary edema, pneumothorax, and pulmonary embolism.

Now that the BLUE-protocol has given a (likely) name to the disease, an Extended BLUE-protocol can be done at will, if required by the common sense, if able to help for the choice of the antibiotherapy.

The consolidation will be scanned (volume, windows, and body habitus permitting). A consolidation is (schematically) "gray." We have to search for darker and brighter areas. Dark areas mean necrosis (when they are not tubules, i.e., vessels). This is rather easy. Bright areas (gas) require some expertise since this gas can be air bronchograms (within bronchi), or pathological (abscess).

The Air Bronchogram

A consolidation can be homogeneous (see Fig. 17.5) or include hyperechoic punctiform or linear opacities: the air bronchograms (Fig. 35.5). The air bronchogram is certainly a specific sign of consolidation [10], but it is embedded within another specific sign (tissue-like sign and/or shred sign), therefore redundant. In the Extended BLUE-protocol, we deal also with exceptions, and this data can be of interest.

The Dynamic Air Bronchogram

Visualization of dynamics within an air bronchogram (Fig. 35.6 and Video 35.2) has clinical relevance: gas in the bronchi receive a centrifugal inspiratory pressure making them move toward the periphery. An air bronchogram that shows this dynamics is in continuity with the gas inspired by the patient (either spontaneously or through mechanical ventilation). The "dynamic air bronchogram" therefore indicates that the consolidation is *not* retractile. An obstructive atelectasis is quite ruled out, since the specificity of this sign for pneumonia versus obstructive atelectasis is 94 % [11, 12]. The dynamic air bronchogram is 60 % sensitive for the diagnosis of infectious consolidation [11].

Please do not confuse a real dynamic air bronchogram with an off-plane effect, where the air bronchogram suddenly appears and disappears. These patterns seem to light up, whereas air bronchograms are seen moving from one point to another, provided the bronchial axis is in the probe axis.

Fig. 35.5 The air bronchogram. Massive lung consolidation of the right lower lobe, PLAPS-point. Hyperechoic opacities are visible, punctiform (*arrowheads*) and linear (*arrow*), not generating acoustic shadows deeper. These are the features of air bronchograms. BLUE-consolidation index at least 11 cm, BLUE-consolidation volume of at least 1.3 l

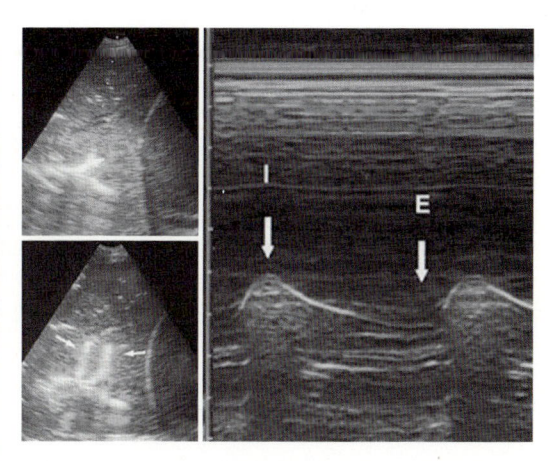

Fig. 35.6 Demonstration of the dynamic air bronchogram. Within this lung consolidation, the air bronchograms show an inspiratory centrifuge motion, highlighted on M-mode (*I* inspiration, *E* expiration). This demonstrates a nonretractile consolidation, pneumonia likely. No healthy mind will confuse this sinusoid with the one of a pleural effusion. Always see real time first, the M-mode is done only for having a paper track of what is seen on real time

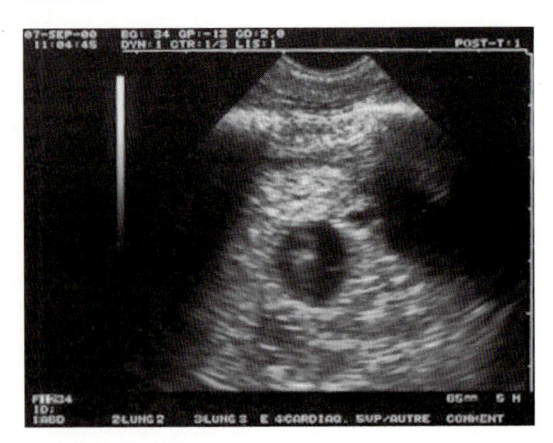

Fig. 35.7 Abscess within consolidation. A hypoechoic rounded image is visible, 12 mm below the pleural line (and just 30 mm below the skin), this abscess is ready for ultrasound-guided aspiration. No need for Doppler nor contrast-enhanced ultrasound for distinguishing it from an empyema. Lung sliding was abolished, which is usual in these diseases. This simplifies the puncture, highly decreasing any risk of laceration. The BLUE-consolidation index is at least 4.5 cm (since the depth is not visible) making a rough 90 ml (or more) volume. Note, in the Extended BLUE-protocol, such a pattern found at the PLAPS-point would definitely not come from a hemodynamic pulmonary edema

Abscess, Necrotizing Pneumonia

The abscess is an old application [13]. It can appear as either hypoechoic fluids, or hyperechoic gas.

Fluids

Detecting rounded hypoechoic areas amounts to diagnosing necrotizing pneumonia (Fig. 35.7) (see also Fig. 29.3 and Video 35.1). Ultrasound works on occasion better than CT [14].

Gas

Gas inside an abscess yields hyperechoic areas. These areas, if large, are easily distinguished from the punctiform or linear air bronchograms. If small, they need much more expert signs. In the case of poor window or small volume, distinguishing normal gas deeper to the consolidation or gas within an abscess may raise challenges. One more difficulty: detecting hyperechoic gas areas in a lung consolidation of a patient with marked pneumonia or ARDS raises an interesting problem. It may mean necrotizing changes. It may also mean re-aeration of a massive consolidation that begins to recover. Here, the clinical setting (Step 1 of the E-BLUE-protocol) helps: worsening, improvement?

Gas-Fluid Interface

The swirl sign. Several conditions must be present. We need a large consolidation with a frank posterior parietal contact. We need a gas-fluid level of the abscess within the consolidation. We need to catch this mass posteriorly (slightly turning the patient). The ultrasound flow, from a PLAPS-point toward the zenith (against gravity), traverses first a fluid area (pus) then a gas area (gas inside the abscess). At atmospheric pressure, the boundary has a characteristic, shimmering dynamic: the swirl sign, as we coined it (see Fig. 14.7). This sign is again seen in hydropneumothorax, in bowel occlusion.

Other Tools Used in the E-BLUE-Protocol

The next sections deal with the analysis of the pleural effusion (diagnostic puncture), and the puncture of the lung consolidation. Splitting a PLAPS into two distinct entities, PLApS (only consolidation) or PLaPS (predominant fluid) may bring some help (under study). Another tool considered in the E-BLUE-protocol is CT, if wisely used. Since the described signs can be expert-level, ordering for CT if an abscess is suspected is sometimes useful. This is perfectly in the scope of the LUCIFLR project, i.e., limiting, not eradicating CT (see Chap. 29). More details are available in our 2010 edition. Briefly, here, common sense and basic tools (inflammatory markers, etc.) up to sophisticated tools should be liberally used. In the countries where abscesses are frequent (Africa, India, etc.), CT and others are rarely available, and only the first tools of the Extended BLUE-protocol will be used.

Obstructive Atelectasis, a Diagnosis Fully Considered in the Extended-BLUE-Protocol

Atelectasis as a cause of acute severe dyspnea is part of the rare diagnoses of the BLUE-protocol, removed for the sake of simplicity.

Atelectasis means absence of peripheral expansion (*a-tele-ectasis*). Dealing with it makes didactic challenges. First there is a frequent confusion between the usual understanding and the physiopathology of this disorder. Many doctors label "atelectasis" any areas of basal alveolar consolidation seen on radiograph or CT. Fibroscopies are not done for these small, plane "atelectases" on radiography. Since the proof is missing, our research is progressing slowly. Second there are different causes. Third, atelectasis yields immediate, functional signs and late, anatomical signs. Temporarily, for decreasing the didactic challenge, we will not try to diagnose the small segmental atelectases. Not only is the volume small initially, but above all this volume shrinks. It would be chancy to apply the probe precisely at that small area (spending too much time violates the rules of fast ultrasound). Maybe these small atelectases are not a good application of lung ultrasound.

Which atelectasis are we speaking of?
1. Passive atelectasis?

    We are not sure of the existence of this nosologic entity. A pleural effusion compresses the lung, of course, but where does this effusion come, if not from a lung disorder? Apart from cases of chylothorax, picturesque cases of glucothorax from inadvertent puncture outside the subclavian vein, and the rare cases of pleural malignancies, we don't see where pleural effusions would come from. Concerned physicians may, if finding a huge amount of fluid with lung consolidation, first withdraw all the fluid, and see after.
2. Obstructive atelectasis

    This kind is secondary to bronchial obstructions and is the clinically relevant one. How to understand this disease? We can take again our healthy model of Chap. 10 and propose a less aggressive test that he will likely agree to do: just halt breathing. This creates however an experimental model of sudden, complete, bilateral atelectasis. A highly unstable situation is created: after 20 s, the oxygen saturation begins to decrease. After a few hours, a chest X-ray would show two white lungs with massive loss of volume, cupolas reaching claviculas. Far before this rather *theoretical* stage, ultrasound will observe immediate signs.

An Immediate, Functional Sign: The Lung Pulse

For keeping the textbook thin, we invite to read again the section on the lung pulse of Chap. 10. Very briefly, the cardiac beats, normally hidden by lung sliding, are immediately visible if lung sliding stops. They create vibrations at the pleural line, visible in real time (see Video 10.4), recordable in M-mode (see Fig. 10.7).

A lung pulse means that the heart transmits its vibrations through a motionless lung parenchyma.

Lung sliding is always and immediately abolished, within the first second of an obstructive atelectasis, with in 90 % of cases, a visible lung pulse [15]. The hemidiaphragm is standstill, a redundant sign (Video 35.1). A radiograph taken at this moment would show a normal lung of normal volume (cause apart).

The lung pulse is a disease (atelectasis), which allows to rule out another disease (pneumothorax). When ruling out pneumothorax, the lung pulse has been defined as an equivalent of lung sliding, which skips the need for long articles or changes in our decision tree. The lung pulse is on the top of the decision tree of it, not on the bottom; we just write "lung sliding, or equivalents."

Late Signs

(a) *The lung consolidation*

    With time, the alveolar gas is resorbed, and a lung consolidation appears on radiograph, CT, ultrasound.

(b) *Loss of lung volume*

    The narrowed intercostal spaces, the cupolas and abdominal organs (liver, spleen) found above the nipple line (usually at the PLAPS point), the heart shifted either at the right parasternal window (Fig. 35.8), or again all over the left anterior chest wall (a sign simply coined the *heart sign*) are signs that indicate loss of lung volume.

    The mediastinum, usually difficult to access, becomes analyzable, as during transesophageal examinations. This serendipitous phenomenon allows unusual analyses: superior caval vein (see Fig. 30.7), pulmonary artery, and its left and right branches, pulmonary veins. Before the treatment of an atelectasis, fast scanning of the mediastinum (even simply recording data), allows a posteriori quiet searching for thromboses or any other anomalies.

(c) *The static air bronchogram*

Within the consolidation, the absence of any air bronchogram is a rather indirect (or late) sign of atelectasis. The remaining, not yet resorbed gas, yields information of interest. The term of "static air bronchogram" is used when no dynamic is observed on air bronchograms. This can mean air bubbles trapped and isolated from the general air circuit (before being dissolved), fully consistent with obstructive atelectasis, a sensitive sign – unspecific, 40 % of cases of pneumonia with air bronchogram don't display any dynamic [11].

(d) *Other signs*

Fluid bronchograms (small anechoic tubular structures) would be observed in obstructive pneumonia only [16]. Some argue for Doppler for distinguishing them from vessels, but we fail to find a practical interest, up to now in the BLUE-protocol (in sophisticated lung studies, it may be possibly of interest). Doppler is again used by some for distinguishing atelectasis from inflammation. We think the signs we use may be redundant, meaning possibly that both approaches make the same conclusions, simplicity in addition for our approach. We are open to comparative randomized studies for fully clarifying this point.

Noninvasive Recognition of the Nature of a Fluid Pleural Effusion

We could make this section extremely short: little is brought at this step. Echoic effusions will likely be punctured by any team, with or without BLUE-protocol. Yet anechoic effusions can be transudates or exudates, this is long known [17]. In other words, in a complex patient, any pleural effusion should be tapped.

In acutely dyspneic patients, a pleural effusion can be a transudate (hemodynamic pulmonary edema), an exudate (embolism, infection), pus (purulent pleurisy), blood (trauma), gastric content (esophageal rupture), or anything else (glucothorax etc.).

In pneumonia, the pleural effusion can be anechoic, or septated (see Fig. 16.4), up to the hon-

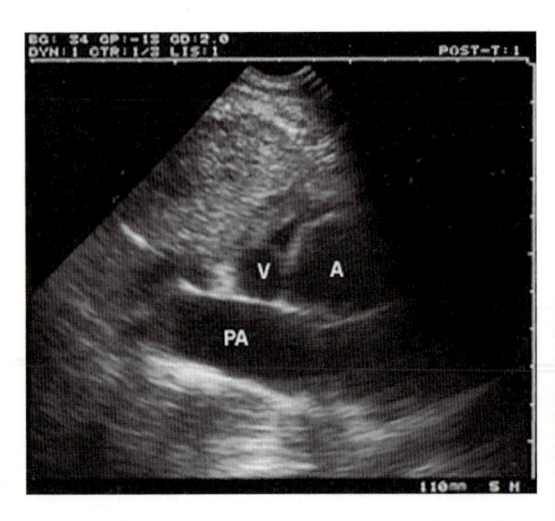

Fig. 35.8 Lung atelectasis at late stage. Complete atelectasis of the right lung in a ventilated 56-year-old man. Transversal scan of the right anterior lung for once. Through the complete consolidation, we can observe the ascending aorta (*A*), the superior caval vein (*V*), and a "beautiful" right pulmonary artery (*PA*), in brief, the mediastinum, here frankly shifted to the right, making diagnosis of lung consolidation with loss of volume, i.e., obstructive atelectasis in practice. Absence of air bronchograms, phrenic elevation, abolished lung sliding, and lung pulse were noted among others. BLUE-consolidation index 3.5 cm, i.e., rough BLUE-consolidation volume of 45 ml

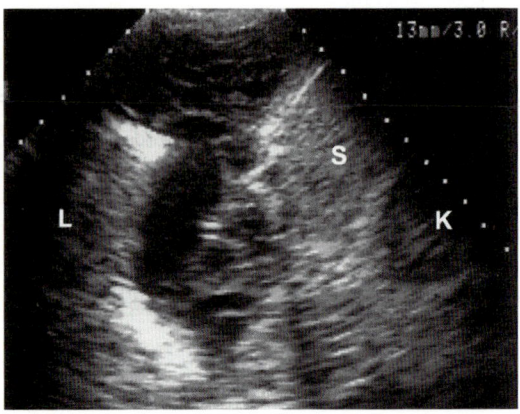

Fig. 35.9 Echoic pleural effusion. This effusion has a honeycomb pattern. It was found in a 37-year-old man with pneumonia due to *Clostridium perfringens*. White lung on X-rays. These septations are quite never seen on CT. *L* lung, *S* spleen, *K* kidney

eycomb pattern (Fig. 35.9), or again diffusely heterogeneous, echoic, with the plankton sign. The plankton sign (coined "signe des poissons" by Mezière) is defined by multiple randomly swimming echoic particles, shaken by respiratory and cardiac dynamics. This hectic dance is easily distinguished from the organized air bronchogram dynamics in rhythm with respiration, a distinction sometimes of value when anaerobic infections generate hyperechoic patterns (gas) within pleural fluid. Unlike ultrasound, CT misses the fibrinous septations [18]. Unlike many pulmonologic teams, we do not require Doppler for differentiating empyema from lung abscess – just using the quad sign and shred sign. Lung sliding is often abolished because of massive adhesions. Therefore, the sinusoid sign is not expected in severe infected effusions. Septated effusions do not always locate at the PLAPS-point, they can be encysted everywhere. Here is one clue: if lung sliding is detected anteriorly, an encysted effusion somewhere else in the thorax is unlikely, since it would suppose massive adhesions, i.e., mainly, abolished (anterior) lung sliding.

Hemothorax yields patterns from anechoic to echoic: the plankton sign (Fig. 35.10). Read Anecdotal Note 3.

We withdraw from this heavy chapter signs of pachypleuritis (see Figure 15.9 of our 2010 edition).

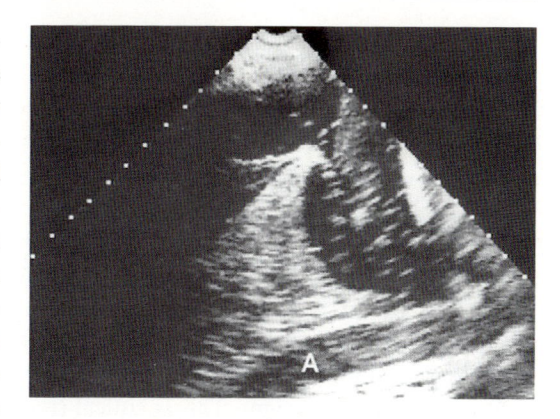

Fig. 35.10 The plankton sign. This nice picture (1982 technology) shows a few anatomical details: a fully consolidated lower left lobe, a huge pleural effusion, a nicely exposed descending aorta with many ghost echoes (*A*), and a bit of the cupola. The aorta is deep (for those who would insert a needle, it is far from any risk of inadvertent puncture). Countless elements within the pleural effusion have a whirling motion in real time, hence the label "plankton sign." BLUE-pleural index of 23 mm, with an uncorrected BLUE-pleural volume that should be 400–800 cc of fluid if the lung was dry, and corrected with a factor of 1.4, corresponding to the BLUE-consolidation index estimated at 5 cm, making a corrected BLUE-pleural volume of 560–1,120 ml. See if needed Chap. 28

One Tool Used in the Extended BLUE-Protocol: Bedside Early Diagnostic Thoracentesis at the Climax of Admission

Finding a germ in an effusion has a definite value [19]. In very critical patients with a challenge between ARDS and hemodynamic pulmonary edema, e.g., this procedure allows to see here an exudate, there a transudate. We found (unpublished data) a high rate of positive microbiology in our samples, up to 18 %, a rate that more than doubles when the procedure is ordered before any blind antibiotherapy. Each time the prognosis can be improved, we find it safer to consider anechoic effusions as possible exudates, and make liberal policy of thoracentesis. It allows to simplify endless debates and loss of time: the patient may be discharged earlier. Ultrasound-helped thoracentesis, one of so many potentials of critical ultrasound, is routine in our practice since 1989. Read Chap. 28 on ARDS.

For decades, the habits were to ignore pleural effusions, either because they were radioccult, or mainly for the fear of making more harm than good. So what happened? Usually, a probabilist antibiotherapy was given. With simple ultrasound, we can do much better.

Safety of Such Thoracentesis

The fear of inserting a needle within the thorax of a fragile patient is legitimate. What the Extended-BLUE-protocol fears is to prevent the patient to profit of this procedure. The benefit/risk ratio is major: Mayo reports 1.3 % of complications in a series of ventilated patients [20]. Our experience, done in ventilated patients usually receiving PEEP with radioccult effusions, has quite similar results: 0 % of complications [21]. This proves (repeat) that ultrasound allows safe puncture of small effusions, even if the patient is ventilated, even if the effusion is radioccult. In addition, the hypothetic risk of pneumothorax would be recognized immediately, just after the procedure.

Criteria for a Safe Thoracentesis [21]

They follow good sense.
1. The effusion must be definite, with quad and if possible sinusoid signs. This is critical (for not puncturing any nonsense image: heart, e.g., ectopic stomach, silicone breast, etc.).
2. A 15 mm inspiratory (i.e., minimal) interpleural distance was defined as a reasonable safety distance. It had to be visible at three adjacent intercostal spaces.
3. Care is done avoiding undesirable interpositions: lung, aorta, heart, liver, spleen (we assume that the modern reader, nowadays, does not need figures). Each of these organs must be clearly far from the puncture. If the lung is seen, appearing at the end of inspiration, the puncture must be done on another site, more posteriorly usually.
4. The puncture must immediately follow the ultrasound location, patient in strictly the same position. Sending patients to the radiologic department and seeing them coming back to the ICU with a landmark written on the skin belongs to the dark ages. In 48 % of cases, the fluid amount allows to keep the patient supine [21]. Obvious details are not reminded. The patient is (if needed) slightly turned, then the landmark is done (using ultrasound), and then the needle is inserted (unless loose skin may deviate the landmark). The site of puncture is usually not far from the PLAPS-point, but can be unusual, such as from time to time, in full hepatic area in the case the effusion is encysted there.

Which needle? The sinusoid sign indicates a low viscosity of the effusion, allowing to use fine, 21-G needles (gray 16-Gauge catheters would be for evacuation).

Once these points are checked, the procedure is fast, a few seconds are needed to obtain fluid sample in 97 % of the cases [21].

Technique

In order to keep this book thin, and for following the principle N°1 of lung ultrasound (simplicity), we limit the role of ultrasound to diagnose pleural effusions, define a site for the puncture, and check that the safety criteria are present. *CEURF does not use ultrasound during the needle insertion.* We assume that normal doctors insert the needle with a syringe under vacuum and stop its progression once fluid is filling the syringe (Anecdotal Note 4). Even small, pleural effusions make rather large targets, impossible to miss, making the use of ultrasound during the procedure a superadded complication. In order to foresee the unlikely case the needle gets obstructed during the wall crossing, it will be inserted up to a certain limit. We assume doctors are able to figure out the length of the needle. The green ones we use are 40-mm long. The chest wall is perfectly measurable, say, e.g., 2 cm. Fluid must be obtained just a little after this 2 cm insertion, i.e., a 2-cm visible outside needle. Once this 2-cm thickness of chest wall is crossed, after a minimal additional insertion (say 5 mm), fluid should be aspirated by the syringe under vacuum. These are common sense concepts. There are costly, sophisticated devices for those not at ease with these simple precautions. If there is a large safety distance (huge effusion), the needle can be inserted deeper (but this would not bring a lot, once the needle is in the pleural space). The needle is withdrawn and a simple familial dressing of 2×1 cm is applied. All in all, let us not, for an exceptional event, complicate a daily procedure.

The therapeutic thoracentesis was dealt with in Chap. 28.

Lung Puncture

Regarding community-acquired or ventilator-acquired pneumonia, it seems logical that the prognosis will be improved by an early bacteriological documentation. Yet the accurate diagnosis is a traditional challenge [22, 23].

We guess colleagues would be afraid to insert a needle within the lung itself. Clearly, we deal with extremely ill patients, and many of them die. They should be managed energetically (Anecdotal Note 5). Our approach is reasoned. It is based on logic and observation. Note that this concept does not scare the pulmonologists, who are accustomed to insert needles for lung biopsy. Lung abscesses are long managed this way [12]. Note that pneumothorax was a therapy of some diseases before antibiotics came. Some intensivists even tried lung puncture, without ultrasound, and with of course a high risk of pneumothorax [24]. With ultrasound, one can make much better. Consider two points. (1) The microbe is swarming within the lung tissue, i.e., just a few millimeters under the skin, ironically. (2) Traditional tools may furnish contaminated material (false positives) or no material (false negatives).

We propose a direct route, highly cost-effective, and to our experience safe. The physician must just be convinced of the interest of having the bacteriological diagnosis in terms of benefit/risk balance. The main hypothetical risk, i.e., pneumothorax, must be located at the right place. First, the criteria that follow reduce the risk deeply. Second, the risk exists with traditional procedures, either visual (fiberscope) or above all blind (plugged telescopic catheter). Third, would a pneumothorax occur, it would be recognized immediately at the postprocedure ultrasound – in other words, a near-zero risk, a high potential benefit.

Criteria for Performing a Safe Lung Puncture

1. A large consolidation. Take here Fig. 35.5. Through such a huge consolidation, a needle should provide far more information than risk. The consolidation should extend through the whole intercostal space between two ribs (i.e., 2 cm roughly). The depth should be sufficient in order that no doctor would have the idea of piercing it up to its aerated limit (i.e., traversing the fractal line). The dimensions of Fig. 35.5 are quite an invitation for this procedure. For fixing limits, for the beginners, we should write, if using a green, 40-mm long needle: if the chest wall is 1-cm thick, restrict the indication to the 4-cm deep consolidations; if the chest wall is 2-cm thick, restrict to 3 cm; etc.
2. Lung sliding must be abolished on mechanical ventilation: this demonstrates likely acute symphysis, an additional factor lowering the risk of pneumothorax.
3. Air bronchograms should be absent, or far from the puncture site – dynamic air bronchogram seems a logical contraindication.

Technique

The anterior lung surface is scanned before and after procedure. Like for thoracentesis, ultrasound does not need to be used *during* the puncture. We use a fine, 21-gauge green, 40-mm needle. For a BLUE-consolidation index superior to 3 cm, the risk of pneumothorax appears quite nil. A substantial vacuum is done in order to obtain a minute drop of brown material. Just do not squash the soft tissue with the syringe. Take care not to lacerate the tissue during the vacuum.

Results

With these described criteria being present, pneumothorax never occurred as a consequence of the puncture. The tap is positive in 50 % of our procedures. When positive, a pure culture of the responsible microbe is usually obtained. This may also change the habits in critical care.

Doppler in the Extended BLUE-Protocol?

Once the clinical setting, the BLUE-protocol, the extended signs of LUCI, simple cardiac sonography, +/− interventional ultrasound, etc., have been used, the non-redundant indications of Doppler are really poor. In these cases, use the DIAFORA approach in the suitable institutions (wealthy world). We think that using Doppler first-line, without having used even the simple BLUE-protocol, would be equivalent to shooting a spider using a bazooka, but we are permanently ready to revisit our position.

The Extended BLUE-Protocol, an Attempt of Conclusion

At the term of this chapter, one can make this temptative conclusion. The BLUE-protocol alone had a 90.5 % accuracy [7]. We calculated, according to the consideration that the gold standard was possibly not perfect, a corrected, officious value of 95 % (Chap. 20). With all or some of the elements of the Extended BLUE-protocol, mainly simple history and clinical signs, one may expect a substantial increase of this rate [25]. Common sense is a synonym of Extended BLUE-protocol, schematically. It helps us to remain doctors. The BLUE-protocol is only a protocol. At the pilot seat, there is first a doctor!

Anecdotal Notes

1. *Development of the C-profile*

    In the Extended BLUE-protocol, a distinction is made between a C-profile associated with lung sliding, which should be called the "sliding C-profile", and a C-profile associated with abolished lung sliding (which should be called logically C'-profile, but maybe for some decades, for avoiding any confusion, it should be wise to call it the "non-sliding C-profile") (since the term "C-profile" has been defined in the native article regardless of lung sliding). If we had to rewrite the BLUE-protocol, there would be the A, A', B, B', C, and C'-profile.

    In an expert version of the Extended BLUE-protocol, the C-on-A-profile indicates that the underlying artifacts are an A-predominance, and the C-on-B-profile when they are lung rockets. One can imagine also the C'-on-A-profile, etc. All these details, fully irrelevant in the native, preliminary version of the BLUE-protocol of 2008, are suitable for an expert extended version.

2. *Hemodynamic pulmonary edema* versus *septic cardiomyopathy*

    In this section, one can go more in detail. We make the assumption that most cases of hemodynamic pulmonary edema will have decreased LV contractility, and that *less* than most of cases of pneumonia (and maybe, *far less*) will have a decreased LV contractility (due to patent septic cardiomyopathy). In this hypothesis, adding the item of correct LV contractility would recognize those patients with those pneumonia with the B-profile, without the patent septic cardiomyopathy: this should alert the user. Of course, one can refine, i.e., focusing on causes of hemodynamic edema with normal LV contractility: search for a noise of mitral regurgitation, for a visible mitral valve anomaly, etc. Normally, a few points of specificity should be gained, i.e., the combination "B-profile plus impaired LV contractility" as a sign of hemodynamic pulmonary edema, should improve the accuracy of the BLUE-protocol.

    Read the small story of the BLUE-diagnosis of hemodynamic pulmonary edema of Chap. 24. – We remind the main point using the terms "strong" and "weak" heart for going fast. In 2.64 % of cases, strong heart plus B-profile indicated pneumonia. In 2.98 % of cases, weak heart plus absence of B-profile indicated the absence of hemodynamic pulmonary edema. If we had, just for a very charicatural demonstration, built a "red-protocol," just centered on the heart, we would have had more misleading than contributive results. This is why, remember, withdrawing the heart resulted in improving the results of the BLUE-protocol. Yet the gap between 2.64 and 2.98 is weak, and maybe large numbers will tell more. One more large study to design.

3. *Abdominal probes and trauma protocols*

    Some protocols have been developed for fast detection of traumatic hemothorax. We are concerned by the idea that the use of abdominal probes makes a limitation at the PLAPS-point, therefore a delay in the diagnosis of thoracic bleeding, unlike our short microconvex probe.

4. *Thoracentesis under ultrasound guidance*

    The use of ultrasound *during* the tap of pleural effusions may be apparented to, maybe not a mental disease, but a bad habit, where this elegant tool is used unnecessarily, and may complicate or infect a simple procedure.

5. *Agressive or conservative management of the critically ill*

    This is only an option, ours, greatly favored by the use of ultrasound. One frequent opinion argues that the more the patient is fragile, the less we should be invasive. This makes us puzzled. This is frequently heard too when an intensivist argues with a surgeon regarding a very critically ill patient. The classical "If we operate him, we kill him" should possibly be replaced by "If you don't rapidly operate him, he will die." We would like to see data supporting one of these two extreme managements.

References

1. Hoppin F (2002) How I review an original scientific article. Am J Respir Crit Care Med 166:1019–1023
2. Guyton CA, Hall JE (1996) Textbook of medical physiology, 9th edn. W.B. Saunders Company, Philadelphia, pp 496–497
3. West BJ (2012) Respiratory physiology. The essentials, 9th edn. Lippincott Williams & Wilkins, Wolters Kluwer, Philadelphia, Baltimore
4. Laënnec RTH (1819) Traité de l'auscultation médiate, ou traité du diagnostic des maladies des poumons et du cœur. J.A. Brosson & J.S. Chaudé, New York. Hafner, New York (1962)
5. Felson B (1973) Chest rœntgenology, 1st edn. WB Saunders, Philadelphia, pp 244–245
6. Gattinoni L, Caironi P, Valenza F, Carlesso E (2006) The role of CT-scan studies for the diagnosis and therapy of acute respiratory distress syndrome. Clin Chest Med 27:559–570
7. Lichtenstein D, Mezière G (2008) Relevance of lung ultrasound in the diagnosis of acute respiratory failure. The BLUE-protocol. Chest 134:117–125
8. Lichtenstein D, Axler O (1993) Intensive use of general ultrasound in the intensive care unit, a prospective study of 150 consecutive patients. Intensive Care Med 19:353–355
9. Jardin F, Farcot JC, Boisante L, Curien N, Margairaz A, Bourdarias JP (1981) Influence of positive end-expiratory pressure on left ventricle performance. N Engl J Med 304(7):387–392
10. Tuddenham WJ (1984) Glossary of terms for thoracic radiology: recommendations of the Nomenclature Committee of the Fleischner Society. Am J Roentgenol 143:509–517
11. Lichtenstein D, Seitz J, Mezière G (2009) The dynamic air bronchogram, an ultrasound sign of alveolar consolidation ruling out atelectasis. Chest 135:1421–1425
12. Lichtenstein D, Mezière G, Seitz J (2002) Le bronchogramme aérien dynamique: un signe échographique de consolidation alvéolaire non rétractile. Réanimation 11(Suppl 3):98
13. Yang PC, Luh KT, Lee YC, Chang DB, Yu CJ, Wu HD, Lee LN, Kuo SH (1991) Lung abscesses: ultrasound examination and ultrasound-guided transthoracic aspiration. Radiology 180:171–175
14. Lichtenstein D, Peyrouset O (2006) Lung ultrasound superior to CT? The example of a CT-occult necrotizing pneumonia. Intensive Care Med 32:334–335
15. Lichtenstein D, Lascols N, Prin S, Mezière G (2003) The lung pulse, an early ultrasound sign of complete atelectasis. Intensive Care Med 29:2187–2192
16. Yang PC, Luh KT, Chang DB, Yu CJ, Kuo SH, Wu HD (1992) Ultrasonographic evaluation of pulmonary consolidation. Am Rev Respir Dis 146:757–762
17. Yang PC, Luh KT, Chang DB, Wu HD, Yu CJ, Kuo SH (1992) Value of sonography in determining the nature of pleural effusion: analysis of 320 cases. AJR Am J Roentgenol 159:29–33
18. McLoud TC, Flower CDR (1991) Imaging the pleura: sonography, CT and MR imaging. Am J Roentgenol 156:1145–1153
19. Kahn RJ, Arich C, Baron D, Gutmann L, Hemmer M, Nitenberg G, Petitprez P (1990) Diagnostic des pneu-

mopathies nosocomiales en réanimation. Réan Soins Intens Med Urg 2:91–99
20. Mayo PH, Goltz HR, Tafreshi M, Doelken P (2004) Safety of ultrasound-guided thoracentesis in patients receiving mechanical ventilation. Chest 125(3):1059–1062
21. Lichtenstein D, Hulot JS, Rabiller A, Tostivint T, Mezière G (1999) Feasibility and safety of ultrasound-aided thoracentesis in mechanically ventilated patients. Intensive Care Med 25:955–958
22. Klompas M (2007) Does this patient have ventilator-associated pneumonia? JAMA 297(14):1583–1593
23. Torres A, Fabregas N, Ewig S, de la Bellacasa JP, Bauer TT, Ramirez J (2000) Sampling methods for ventilator-associated pneumonia: validation using different histologic and microbiological references. Crit Care Med 28:2799–2804
24. Torres A, Jimenez P, Puig de la Bellacasa JP, Celis R, Gonzales J, Gea J (1990) Diagnostic value of nonfluoroscopic percutaneous lung needle aspiration in patients with pneumonia. Chest 98:840–844
25. van der Werf TS, Zijlstra JG (2004) Ultrasound of the lung: just imagine. Intensive Care Med 30:183–184

Noncritical Ultrasound, Within the ICU and Other Hot Settings

36

This textbook deals mostly with critical ultrasound. The real ultrasonic revolution will regard the whole population in countless settings, in several decades or hopingly sooner, used by all up to the family doctor. Noninvasive ultrasound should be liberally performed each time there is a question regarding a macroscopic item.

Here is a (non-limitative) list of situations. We apologize for those who would find this chapter quite heterogeneous, but things came as they came. Not the aim of this textbook, this chapter is just a kind of appetizer on how far this method can go.

Noncritical Ultrasound Inside the ICU

Weaning Issues: Only the Diaphragm on Focus?

Weaning is a hot topic currently. Physicians devote a high energy for assessing the diaphragmatic work, the left heart, especially the diastolic function [1, 2]. We try to simplify what can be simplified. A failure of weaning can be explained by other factors.

- Diffuse interstitial changes. This is probably not a good condition for weaning, either from edema (fluid overload or inflammatory) or fibrosis.
- Substantial pleural effusion. It should be withdrawn. The technique is the same as the one described in Chaps. 25 and 28.
- Lung consolidations.
- Pneumothorax.
- Venous thrombosis, either from legs or recent catheters, may give small but iterative pulmonary embolism.
- Peritoneal disorders (substantial effusion) may create a hyperpressure, hampering diaphragmatic course.
- Maxillary sinusitis can generate pneumonia and keep it going.
- Vocal cord edema, laryngeal edema are sources of post-extubation dramas (stridor). Stridor can complicate from 2 to 15 % of extubations [3]. The cuff-leak test has good negative predictive value but poor positive predictive value. The ultrasound air-column width measurement should identify high-risk patients.

All these disorders can be radiocculent.

As to the diaphragmatic dysfunction, please read Anecdotal Note 1 of Chap. 21 on the excluded patients of the BLUE-protocol. We put here some notions in order not to frustrate those who find interest to this field. Just one technical word: getting interest to vascular (linear) probes only for this application would mean expenses for little benefit (especially since our microconvex probe makes the work). Here is the minimal we consider useful for assessing the diaphragm.

Electronic supplementary material The online version of this chapter (doi:10.1007/978-3-319-15371-1_36) contains supplementary material, which is available to authorized users.

The Diaphragm: Why and How to Analyze It

Why

In critical ultrasound, we never paid a lot of attention to this muscle, although a vital one. Our feeling is that, once an operator is aware of the potentials of lung ultrasound, the diaphragm appears slightly less interesting (Anecdotal Note 1). Said differently, we would advise this teaching only after priority targets are under perfect control. We remind the principle of critical ultrasound: Since we are unable to repair a paralyzed diaphragm in the night, we just give oxygen with noninvasive ventilation, or more (intubation, etc.), to these patients. Following this concept, for keeping the book thin, we devote a modest place to its analysis. The diaphragm is a real image. This is reassuring for those who are scared by lung artifacts. Therefore, the diaphragm is familiar to many intensivists today. They want to know, mainly, if a given patient can be weaned.

We do not search for looking at the diaphragm itself. Which interesting features should emerge from its vision? Tumors? Of course not. Inspiratory thickening (in spontaneous ventilation)? If it moves, it should thicken (see if necessary the subtle Fig. 16.11 of our 2010 edition). Assessing its function does not require direct visualization, and little energy is devoted in this. Indirect signs work as well as direct ones, see below.

How

How to locate it is schematically given by the BLUE-points, allowing minimal energy. The lower finger of the lower hand locates it. Observing lung items at the left of the image and abdominal items at the right ensures correct phrenic location. A location of this boundary image above the defined landmarks (phrenic line) is pathological. This being said, for those who really want to see the very diaphragm, ultrasound is probably the best tool at the bedside (and maybe the only, fluoroscopy remaining an exceptional referral). It just requires some skill, i.e., more energy. The diaphragm is a part of circle of roughly 22 cm of diameter in standard adults, for helping novice users to figure it out (see Figs. 16.4, 16.5, 16.7, and 17.5). One can apply the probe laterally (phrenic point) or two intercostal spaces below the PLAPS-point, or even posteriorly when the patient is turned laterally. The amplitude is the same.

How to assess its dynamic?
1. The detection of a lung sliding allows immediate recognition of a correct diaphragmatic function. Note that lung sliding is an item of the BLUE-protocol. The lung slides because the diaphragm contracts (read again how lung sliding is explained in Chap. 10).
2. Lung rockets, if present, enhance this dynamic since our image is sectorial.
3. One can also look for hepatic or splenic podal inspiratory excursion, and giving the same dynamic information maybe easier to measure.

Therefore, we don't require the presence of pleural effusions or atelectasis which are, according to some, necessary for a correct vision of the diaphragm. Care must be taken to be longitudinal. In spontaneous ventilation in a normal subject, or in conventional mechanical ventilation in a patient without respiratory disorder, the phrenic amplitude is roughly between 15 and 20 mm. A pleural effusion, even substantial, does not affect this amplitude even in mechanical ventilation.

A pathological diaphragmatic amplitude (using direct or indirect signs) is under 10 mm, for instance 5 mm, or null, or negative (paradoxical dynamic). Pleural symphysis, atelectasis, low tidal volume, neurological diseases, or abdominal hyperpressure explain a diminished or abolished phrenic amplitude. Phrenic palsy is a complication of cardiac or thoracic surgery and nerve blockade. It yields abolished lung sliding, elevated cupola, motionless cupola or paradoxical movement, absence of inspiratory thickening, for those who can assess this. For more information, read some excellent works [4, 5].

Outside the ICU

The Issue of Pulmonary Embolism in Standard Medicine

In many areas of medicine (internal medicine, emergency room, geriatrics, etc.), the spectrum of pulmonary embolism is an issue, quite an obsession. We have the feeling that the image of pulmonary embolism, which appears as a "monobloc disease," can be split into several subtle boxes thanks to ultrasound. Four different situations can be indeed described:

1. Severe dyspnea or shock plus visible venous thrombosis: extreme risk for sudden death
2. Severe state without visible venous thrombosis: major risk for sudden death
3. Good tolerance with venous thrombosis: risk for sudden death
4. *Good tolerance without visible venous thrombosis*

This last situation is interesting. Let us consider, e.g., the case of a young woman with isolated basithoracic pain, seen in the ER. The fear of the doctor to see such patients suddenly die is familiar. Yet the (laudable) energy invested in this diagnosis would imply night aggressive helical CT (without premedication), blind night heparin therapy, or blind thrombolysis, plus the remote consequences of irradiation. For decades before the advent of CT, we had the risk of the highly invasive pulmonary angiography, done day or night. At these times, ultrasound was fully operational. There is a price to pay for this behavior [6–11].

The Grotowski law speculates that, a few seconds before sudden death occurs from a massive pulmonary embolism, there is *always* a voluminous, floating, iliocaval, highly unstable deep venous thrombosis – easy to detect using simple ultrasound, in a patient with no or little thoracic complaint. De la Palice was said to be still alive 5 min before his death (in the year 1525). Usually, 5 min before death, people are in extremely critical shock. For drama such as massive embolism, de la Palice was possibly right: following his philosophy, we consider that massive pulmonary embolism should be anticipated – i.e., what the CLOT-protocol (described in Chap. 28) makes.

In a patient without thoracic distress (no major dyspnea, no underlying chronic respiratory disease), and no echovisible venous thrombosis, there is a reasonable safety margin. The Grotowski law (don't search for this law on Internet) is based on the speculation that thanks to simple ultrasound, such patients can be located far below the morbidity line. The balance between benefits and risks is completely modified using ultrasound. What is reasonable in one situation is no longer in another. Those who would exploit the Grotowski law to its extreme limits would simply estimate that such patients can make a pulmonary embolism anyway – since a *small* venous thrombosis was possibly missed. Such patients are assumed to present *moderate* chest pain, with *moderate* discomfort, i.e., time for scheduling usual investigations – or more pragmatically, the old scintigraphy, which will be relevant precisely in a patient without lung disorders (nude BLUE-profile). It can here be done at opened hours, is far less irradiating than the helical-CT, and therefore more elegant. Just respect pregnancy as a contraindication (because of the bladder concentration). We deeply think that the BLUE-protocol will give a new life to scintigraphy. When we schedule the patient for scintigraphy for the morning after, what can happen during the night of admission? Either no sudden change, and the patient is quietly referred to scintigraphy, or sudden changes indicating that the patient suffers in actual fact from something else, usually pneumonia (with fulminant evolution). Note that the patient can benefit from serial BLUE-protocols during the observation, showing early changes (interstitial, alveolar, pleural, etc.). Note last that sending such unstable patients to helical CT for a supposed pulmonary embolism makes really little sense (and may jeopardize the patient).

The Emergency Room

In the ER, the main problem is to decrease the chronic crowd of pseudo-emergencies. Less urgent and less life-threatening problems are seen. They are countless (from foreign body in soft tissues to social problems). Ultrasound will have the immense merit to expedite the discharge of the patients.

Lung

The case of mildly dyspneic patients, simply managed in the ER then discharged, can be seen here. These patients are not in the scope of the BLUE-protocol.

COPD asthma, and pneumonia: they have, roughly, regular BLUE-profiles.

Pulmonary embolism: mild cases should yield more C-lines, since minor emboli are more able to generate pulmonary infarctions [12]. Extensive venous thrombosis should be more frequent, logically.

Pneumothorax: for minute cases, one can use Stage-4 examinations, i.e., this comprehensive scanning that includes the apex in sitting patients. The apical scanning is difficult, since landmarks are less available as for standard intercostal views. However, discrete lung sliding can be clearly visible (a paradoxical feature since the apex is rather a starting block) and B-lines can be frankly visible. In these two cases, even a very small pneumothorax can be confidently ruled out. Note that only a microconvex probe has suitable ergonomy and resolution.

Pulmonary edema: some authors have found the absence of B-profile in mild cases [13]. This hypothesis may be explained by the physiopathology of pulmonary edema since fluids flow against gravity, yet our concept assumes that interstitial syndrome is complete before the patient complains (read the pathophysiological talk in Chap. 24). Rarely called for mildly dyspneic patients, we cannot make an opinion. Possibly, such patients initiated a beginning of recovery. Possibly, giant bullous dystrophy with anterior bullae partly explain this. Possibly, such studies may have the same irreducible proportion of wrong final diagnoses. Read again our gold standard in Chap. 20. We guess that in an emergency room, the conditions for an accurate diagnosis will not be more favorable.

Extra-Lung

Maybe in the ER Doppler should be a little more interesting, but we still consider that it has up to now killed maybe more lives than saved, for the reasons exposed in Chap. 37. When studying situations one by one, we *quite* always have an alternative, and still consider that the utility of Doppler can be balanced. We open again to the DIAFORA concept (see Chap. 2), which indicates that we respect Doppler, for moderate emergencies. Yet when we ask our emergency colleagues why they need Doppler so much, the answers are multiple and, interestingly, different from one doctor to another. Some want to diagnose deep venous thrombosis? The venous section of the BLUE-protocol showed it was not mandatory. Some want to know the cardiac output? The FALLS-protocol showed how to do without. Some want to distinguish abscesses from pseudo-aneurisms before puncture. In this case, simple clinical data (history, thrill), not to speak with simple ultrasound data such as a discrete systolic activity *and other signs*, the moderate degree of emergency make the doctor able not to insert a needle in these kinds of structures (see our note about round masses in Chap. 34), and ask for the classical Doppler analysis done by specialists.

Some would like to distinguish testicular torsion from orchiepididymitis. We develop this point a little (Fig. 36.1). First in order to locate its relevance, we must consider that the frequency of testicular torsion is low. It should be interesting to study the accuracy of combining simple but insufficient clinical tools (age, temperature) with ultrasound signs, simple (testis size) or more subtle (epididymal structure). Knowing that Doppler is not perfect (yielding false-negatives), it should be interesting to quantify the real relevance of

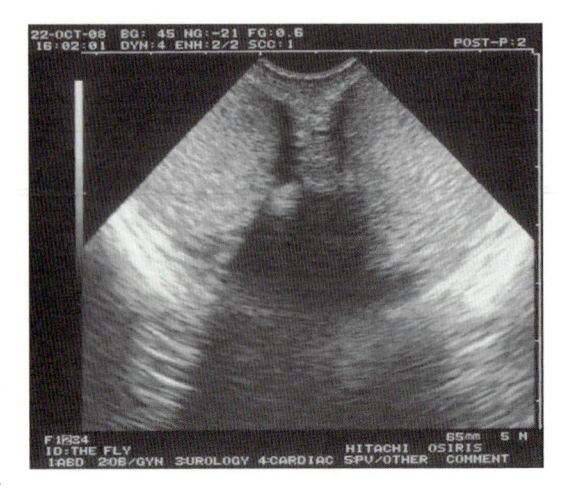

Fig. 36.1 The fly. This kind of fly with these voluminous bulging eyes is often seen wandering in the ER, but rarely reaches the door of the ICU – a domain not developed in this book. Healthy male fertility organs

Doppler. The DIAFORA approach can be used on open hours. The aim is to see a minimal rate of useless exploratory surgery. Meanwhile, lives are saved daily using simple ultrasound. This example illustrates a principle used with the BLUE-protocol: combining the clinical data with accurate ultrasound data makes a winning couple.

There are multiple examples where the DIAFORA approach will solve not very urgent or not very life-threatening problems, but we cannot deal with them in this volume.

The surgeon called at the ER may consider ultrasound a beneficial tool [14]. Thousands of articles show that this option is reasonable. Acute appendicitis [15], intestinal obstruction, and pneumoperitoneum are some openings among many.

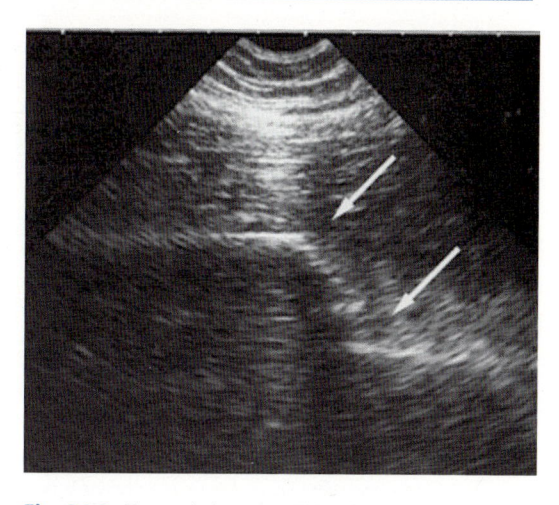

Fig. 36.2 Femoral fracture. This displaced fracture of the diaphysis cannot be missed. The proximal and distal segments are 20 mm distant, without overriding (*arrows*). Even a 1-mm rupture would be seen

A Bit from Other Fields

Bones

Just bone ultrasound may be the occasion for creating a whole discipline. Those willing to invest in it (there are 206 bones, more or less) will have a bright future. Basic knowledge allows to define two kinds of locations. At long bones, the diagnosis is really simple – femoral diaphysis, tibia, fibula, humerus, radius, cubitus, fingers, ribs, etc. (Fig. 36.2). At this area, minute ruptures (even 1 mm) are detected using soft scanning. This potential is at last used [16]. In bones with more complex anatomy (head of the femur, pelvis, carpe, etc.), advanced expertise is needed. Maybe a new type of specialist will arise, able to diagnose or rule out familiar situations. Let us consider, from the most vital (odontoid) to the most functional (scaphoid) the possibility of immediately documenting a cranial dish-pan fracture, a displacement of the cervical rachis (see Fig. 24.12, in our 2010 edition).

Orthopedic surgeons will one day use ultrasound for visualizing a bone after fixation. Just imagine the orthopedic world, where the surgeons depend so much on the radiologic technicians, and the students receive so much irradiation.

Pain

Pain would deserve a full chapter, and we apologize locating it inside a chapter labelled "noncritical ultrasound." Pain can indicate a diagnosis. A thoracic pain usually calls for an ECG. Coronary syndromes are not well seen using ultrasound but providentially, ECG usually corrects this. Most of the others yield ultrasound signs: pulmonary embolism, aortic dissection, aortic aneurism (no figure provided here for such a well-known pattern), tracheal rupture (E-lines, W-lines, bilateral abolished lung sliding), esophageal rupture (E-lines, W-lines, dirty pleural effusion), pneumonia, pneumothorax, pleurisy, rib fractures, etc. For pain management, apart from allowing early diagnoses (Anecdotal Note 2), apart from relieving pain by expediting procedures (venous cannulation, etc.), ultrasound can detect a nerve, helping in loco-regional anesthesia. This is now an exploding world market, and we are again sorry to see that this revolution was secondary to the laptop intrusion (whereas our machine was smaller 10 or 15 years before). Excellent books exist, too numerous for being cited [17, 18]. Note that, curiously, the radiologists denied this potential, which was, eventually, developed by physicians. Note also that our microconvex probe allows to see the nerves (Fig. 36.3). Last, note

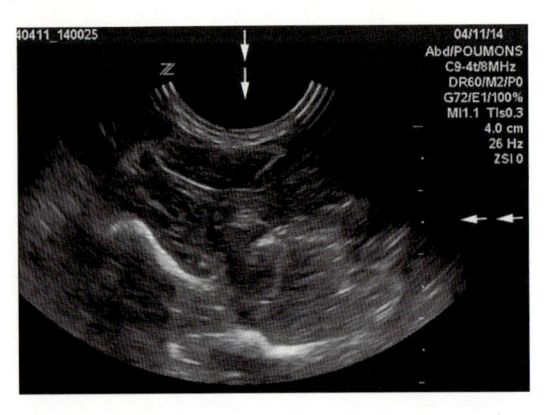

Fig. 36.3 The median nerve. Our median nerve (intersection of *arrows*) taken from a microconvex probe. This unit, available since a few years, has an even better superficial resolution than ours from the Hitachi-405. Note that the imaging quality is fully comparable to the one provided by traditional vascular probes

that we drive a study that should maybe conclude that the problems of anisotropy are possibly generated by these vascular probes.

Anecdotal Notes

1. The diaphragm

    We perfectly remember, while we tried during years and years to catch the interest of intensivists to lung ultrasound, we told to François Jardin, in a morning following a night shift, with a tired voice, that this patient was fine, just had an asymmetrical diaphragmatic function. He said to us that such an application would be of the highest interest for the intensivists. When we see the craze generated by this so simple field in the recent years, we must confess he was, once again, right. We however keep this important paragraph in the present chapter, as far as our work was to develop critical ultrasound in a priority.

2. Morphine

    For so many decades, so many patients suffered for the sake of the dogma (partially true) that morphine would decrease the clinical signs. This was Middle Age medicine when compared with the today's visual medicine.

References

1. Saleh M, Vieillard-Baron A (2012) On the role of left ventricular diastolic function in the critically ill patient (Editorial). Intensive Care Med 38:189–191
2. Papanikolaou J, Makris D, Saranteas T et al (2011) New insights into weaning from mechanical ventilation: LV diastolic dysfunction is a key player. Intensive Care Med 37:1976–1985
3. Ding LW, Wang HC, Wu HD, Chang CJ, Yang PC (2006) Laryngeal ultrasound: a useful method in predicting post-extubation stridor. Eur Respir J 27:384–389, De Taiwan, du Sumroc
4. Lerolle N, Guérot E, Dimassi S, Zegdi R, Faisy C, Fagon JY, Diehl JL (2009) Ultrasonographic diagnosis criterion for severe diaphragmatic dysfunction after cardiac surgery. Chest 135:401–407
5. Matamis D, Soilemezi E, Tsagourias M, Akoumianaki E, Dimassi S, Boroli F, Richard JC, Brochard L (2013) Sonographic evaluation of the diaphragm in critically ill patients. Technique and clinical applications. Intensive Care Med 39(5):801–810
6. Dalen JE, Alpert JS (1975) Natural history of pulmonary embolism. Prog Cardiovasc Dis 17:259–270
7. Stein PD, Athanasoulis C, Alavi A, Greenspan RH, Hales CA, Saltzman HA, Vreim CE, Terrin ML, Weg JG (1992) Complications and validity of pulmonary angiography in acute pulmonary embolism. Circulation 85:462–468
8. Diehl JL (2003) Should we redefine the threshold to initiate thrombolytic therapy in patients with pulmonary embolism? Reanimation 12:3–5
9. Brenner DJ, Hall EJ (2007) Computed tomography – an increasing source of radiation exposure. N Engl J Med 357(22):2277–2284
10. Berrington de Gonzales A, Darby S (2004) Risk of cancer from diagnostic X-rays: estimates for the UK and 14 other countries. Lancet 363(9406):345–351
11. Lauer MS (2009) Elements of danger – the case of medical imaging. N Engl J Med 361:841–843
12. Mathis G, Blank W, Reißig A, Lechleitner P, Reuß J, Schuler A, Beckh S (2001) Thoracic ultrasound for diagnosing pulmonary embolism. Chest 128:1531–1538
13. Volpicelli G, Cardinale L, Mussa A, Caramello V (2009) Diagnosis of cardiogenic pulmonary edema by sonography limited to the anterior lung. Chest 135:883
14. Lindelius A (2009) The role of surgeon-performed ultrasound in the management of the acute abdomen. Thesis for doctoral degree (PhD), Karolinska Institutet, Stockholm
15. Puylaert JBCM (1986) Acute appendicitis: ultrasound evaluation using graded compression. Radiology 158:355–360
16. Marshburn TH, Legome E, Sargsyan A, Li SM, Noble VA, Dulchavsky SA, Sims C, Robinson D (2004) Goal-directed ultrasound in the detection of long-bone fractures. J Trauma 57:329–332
17. Chan V (2008) Ultrasound imaging for regional anesthesia, a practical guide, 2nd edn. Ultrasound Booklet, Toronto
18. Eisenberg E, Gaertner E et al (2014) Echographie en anesthésie régionale. Arnette, Montrouge

Free Considerations

> If you hold a lighted candle, people in the darkness, attracted by your light, come near to you, stick their candle to yours, and they will have the light for them, and you will still have your light, noone has shadowed your area, everyone is rich from this light (heard from a lecture of Cédric Villani, 2010 Fields medal, from Thomas Jefferson).
>
> This is how we would like to see critical ultrasound widespread.

A man with a hammer in the hand finds a lot of objects which need to be hammered. (Mark Twain)

This sentence from our 2010 Edition referred to a US facility which is very used when present, whereas its absence would result in a non use of it. We just refered to… Doppler. Notwithstanding, a hammer can be useful on occasion.

If given time, the reader can glance this chapter in which we inserted free thoughts about a vision of critical ultrasound in the recent burst, how to explain some misconceptions that were (and still are) so widespread in this discipline, and how to locate ultrasound in the clinical approach. We take profit of this chapter to present the SLAM.

Critical Ultrasound, Not a Simple Copy-Paste from the Radiologic Culture

We are glad of having had the opportunity to enrich the discovery of Dénier and all founders of ultrasound [1, 2], for studying, since 1985, an unexplored field: critical ultrasound [3]. We remind that critical ultrasound was defined as diagnoses or procedures done in critical targets in the critically ill (echocardiography, then lung ultrasound, optic nerve, venous cannulation etc.), by the first-line physician on-site 24/7/365. This way to practice ultrasound was not a copy-paste of the radiologic culture, with some applications (aortic aneurism, biliary tract disorders, etc.) just transferred from the radiology department to the emergency room, nor from the cardiological cultures (heart function, a.m.o.). In this field, our main target was to define a simple unit and simple rules.

Lung Ultrasound in the Critically Ill: 25 Years from Take-Off, Now, the Sleepy Giant Is Well Awake (Better Late Than Never!)

Critical ultrasound was a silent volcano, which began to rumble since the early 1990s. Some pioneers tried to show during years to those who wanted to listen how to wake up this sleepy giant.

The prehistorical period ranged from the year 1946 (the birth) to 1982. The pioneers who created medical ultrasound were internists like Dénier [1] or surgeons like Wild [2]. Cardiologists and obstetricians immediately saw the interest and self-appropriated the method. The rest of the medical community did not move a lot. Why? How could intensivists not see the huge range of this weapon, this will remain a mystery (they are no longer here today for answering)? Since the tool provided images, it was given into the hands of the experts of medical imaging. They used their skills for creating a sophisticated discipline, immune to the non-initiated. Meanwhile, the frontline physicians (intensive care, emergency dept) did not see the interest of ultrasound but used their hands, X-rays, central venous pressures, etc. We have the absolute proof that with antique machines before the era of real-time (1974), it was possible to do lung ultrasound in the critically ill.

Ultrasound came on age, with the advent of the real time (1974, Henry & Griffith), but this was a discrete revolution which was not, once again, noticed by the critical care physicians – nor by some academicians whose work is to acknowledge the real innovations in medicine and biology.

In the 1980s, pioneering ICU teams developed the cardiac part [4].

Apart from cardiac uses, a *blackout* period extended from 1974 up to 1989. Suitable mobile machines were present, but used by nobody from the front line. We have no explanation regarding this period.

A really weird period ranged from 1989 to 2001. We had the opportunity to work since 1989 in a prestigious ICU, equipped with ultrasound, the first to our knowledge [4]. It is with the simple unit present there that we could define the whole field of critical ultrasound [3]. The intensivists around us were able to see its utility, but little happened. Human factors are unfathomable; intensive care (especially medical) is a prestigious discipline, and maybe these elites mastered their duty and did not feel the need to be better than excellent. When we used noncardiac ultrasound (an unusual image in 1989, fully inappropriate in this profession), and in addition pointing out that the most important to develop was the lung ultrasound, we can easily imagine what happened in the minds of doctors having been educated in the opposite way (ultrasound? "Not for us". Lung ultrasound?? "Impossible").

Therefore, the immediate change we were able to note was a complete standstillness (rather familiar in medicine), which resulted in an efficient stoppage of its widespread use.

Among incredible comments, one told us he would believe in lung ultrasound when the radiologists would give their endorsement. We guess the guy is still waiting.

During this time, other colleagues around us, less academic, learned immediately and use it today daily (Gilbert Mezière, Agnès Gepner, Philippe Biderman, Mohammad Siyam, Olivier Axler, and some others, efficient but discrete physicians). The university colleagues were less enterprising. We were "kings" of the night, but "outlaws" at daylight. Thus, we had to make a critical choice: devoting 100 % of time submitting in first priority the less known, i.e., lung ultrasound, instead of promoting "easy" fields (blood in the peritoneum). The period of these endless submissions took years and years (and is far from finished).

The *commercial period* (since 2002 to our days) was initiated by the laptop market, which quickly imposed these large machines in the emergency departments. In search for an acknowledgment of their hard work, the emergency physicians saw a unique opportunity for getting some light, an image favoring an explosive success. Possibly never in the history of medicine that so much money passed from one pocket to another has happened. Once ultrasound was in the hands of appropriate physicians, the content of our 1992 textbook (free blood in the abdomen, optic nerve, venous access, etc) exploded through countless publications, initiatives, etc. The candles of the start of this chapter were multiplied, exploded in a great light, nearly an uproar, a night bombing. We are rather happy to see that with this incredible story, we made many, many happy doctors, far more than saved patients in our night duties!

Seven Common Places and Misconceptions About Ultrasound

In no other field of medicine did we see so many dogmas. Let us select a few.
1. Laptop units: a key for the ultrasound revolution

The whole next section will show why this technological development was unnecessary.
2. "Lung ultrasound": a humbug?

One could also speak of oxymoron. Since this misconception originated the full textbook you now have in hands, we won't spoil space for arguing this. Now, this debate is completely obsolete.
3. Operator-dependency? Medicolegal issues?

In many minds, the performance of ultrasound depends on the operator's skill. On one side, those who don't use critical ultrasound, often academicians, repeat ad nauseam its highly operator-dependent feature, of limited interest when compared with CT, e.g. It is striking to hear these words still today by some. They just confused critical ultrasound with traditional ultrasound, which *is* difficult (echocardiography Doppler, obstetrics, abdomen). They confuse "difficult" with "new." Of course, turning the back to a method is the best way to never get the skill. If they had taken interest to this method since 1985, they would have, today, a huge proficiency. Just imagine, in the times when auscultation was not part of the clinical routine, physicians had to refer their patients to specialists in auscultation for detecting rales. Ultrasound is nothing more than a stethoscope, slightly heavier than Laënnec's invention. Lung ultrasound is not so easy, but far easier than the usual fields, and when the outcome is considered (immediate diagnoses, costs, a.m.o.), these academicians will not be able to hold such a behavior forever, no offense.

Especially when the medicolegal rules will be inverted, in 50 years or maybe tomorrow, physicians checking for the absence of a pneumothorax using the irradiating (and costly) CT may have to explain their choice to medicolegal experts. We humbly suggest them to anticipate this and take basic courses of LUCI.

4. "ECHO". What does this word mean? Have we time to decrypt it and its place in the ICU? Deciphering

The word "ECHO," a bit confusing but let us admit, is an abbreviation of expert echocardiography-Doppler US, popular in the US. The usual cardiologists were not especially trained to answering questions regarding shock, critically ill patients. As a striking example, they need standardized views, like policemen require strict front and profile ID views. Yet anyone is able to recognize a familiar face by any incidence, even not strictly frontal. First deep misconception. During decades, "ECHO" in the critically ill was a copy-paste of this culture: they were called at the bedside and used their science for providing advices in a field they ignored.

Little by little, intensivists have acquired their independency [4]. What we could see is that in some (but prestigious) ICUs, ultrasound is still today restricted to the heart and just the heart. "ECHO" is of high interest, and we fully understand that those who invested huge energy in this tool want to use it intensively. As a sign of respect to the heart, we published in 1992 a simple approach [3].

There are now four ways to use echocardiography. The regular one is done by cardiologists ever since. The ECHO is performed by intensivists of today (with Doppler TTE and TEE). The numerous simple protocols are recently developed such as FATE, RACE, and FOCUS and the CEURF approach, i.e., another simple to use but different approach, since it is fully coupled with lung ultrasound and venous ultrasound (BLUE-protocol, FALLS-protocol, etc.).

The readers may feel surprised to have in hands a textbook on critical ultrasound that does not deal with TEE. We appreciate TEE, a powerful technique providing high-quality imaging. Driving the reader to excellent and respectable textbooks, we recall some drawbacks. The cost makes TEE difficult to afford in most parts of the world. This cost includes that of the probe, scheduled for a limited number of examinations. The technique needs significant learning curve, full installation, long disinfection, etc. The introduction of this probe in the esophagus makes

TEE semi-invasive [5, 6]. The user has no choice but to study the heart and only the heart. One last drawback (only our opinion) is the absence of certitude that TEE is the gold standard for hemodynamic assessment – since it can be compared to no gold standard, currently. Aware of the rising place of TEE, not willing to make any fault, we will pay full attention to its value, if ever a gold standard can specify the exact place of each tool. Obviously, trained centers make a good job using TEE.

Now, the image quality of TTE is inferior to that of TEE, but as far as it remains acceptable, it fully pertains to our concept of the optimal compromise; read again Chap. 3. Other authors, and probably all users, are also willing to optimize the noninvasiveness in the first intention [7]. The examination is more democratic (cost, risk, etc.). The problem is now reduced to the interest of cardiac Doppler in the critically ill. See below the detailed (and long) paragraph.

Some believe in the heart (with no lung); we believe in the lung (with *simple* heart). Emergency cardiac sonography is a simple discipline. The organ is the same, but the user (cardiologist *or* intensivist) is different. A grand piano can be used for classical music (the cardiologic way) or popular music, as we do. Popular music is less "academic" than classical music, but obeys to extremely rigorous rules regarding harmony, rhythm, and layout. The rules are just different. Those who consider popular music as a precise discipline will be interested by critical ultrasound, which follows the same logic: a same instrument that makes a different music, not requiring the rigid training and scores of the traditional classical music, and a same tool (schematically), a fully different approach but, in both cases, a good music if we dare.

5. Doppler: let us closely see again its real usefulness in critical ultrasound

Doppler is interesting. The analysis of the flows provides a physiologic approach of high interest. In critical care, however, its incorporation without adaptation is a passive copy-paste maneuver, keeping the discipline complicated and costly. So what do we win?

Through this textbook (as well as the 1992, 2002, 2005, 2010, and 2011 editions), we took time for explaining the spirit of holistic discipline. In public (not private!) hospitals, the critically ill patients are found. Here, simple alternatives can be used.

The cost was long the main drawback. Out of reach for hospital budgets, the ultrasound units were not bought, keeping critical care doctors blind. A few avant-garde physicians had the conviction that ultrasound was possibly of interest in critical care. Yet they were intoxicated by the radiologic and cardiological culture. This restricted view did not make them immediately aware of the huge potential of simple ultrasound. Therefore, they wanted, candidly, Doppler machines or nothing. This belief that Doppler was mandatory has *costed lives*. Countless patients died of the absence of a simple visual diagnosis, accessible to real-time ultrasound. In this perspective, Doppler proved to be a *silent killer*, not Doppler really, but the belief in Doppler. Our 1982 ADR-4000 and our 1992 Hitachi-405, with the unique probe, were easy to purchase, a simple formality – a cheap revolution. With these simple machines in hands, intensivists of the world may have saved countless "dramatic" cases which came in at night and died in the same deep night. All these patients, the "forgotten souls of ultrasound," are all indirect victims of Doppler. For simplifying the debate, we don't even evoke the biological side effects of Doppler. Just take into consideration that it is now restricted during pregnancy [8–10].

Doppler does not mean *good* Doppler. Those who really need Doppler should know that its quality can be very different from one machine to another. In traditional machines swarming in the ERs, users are advised to check if the adequate quality is present (from non-academician but highly respectable sources).

And let us not forget, the best Doppler machine cannot cross gas (emphysematous lungs hiding the heart, bowel gas).

Inserting color Doppler images would have increased the cost of this textbook. The few color images are here in order not to make a too gray-tone textbook.

So which interesting data may Doppler provide?
- To show the direction of the flow is of little interest for us (as doctors, we guess that the arterial flow comes from the LV and the venous flow comes from the tissues).
- To determine whether a vessel is a vein or an artery is the least of Doppler interest (Chap. 18).
- To show a venous thrombosis is visual.
- To show an arterial obstruction may be interesting, but first, this is a rare occurrence in the intensivist's work, and second, we have developed a way of intervening without using a Doppler; see Chap. 18, section on calf veins.
- To see an impairment of cerebral perfusion may be redundant with the detection of an enlarged optic nerve (Chap. 34).
- For diagnosing the origin of an acute dyspnea, demonstrating a mitral regurgitation is maybe of interest, but lung ultrasound made the direct detection of pulmonary edema.
- A mitral valve destruction requiring immediate surgery at night is extremely rare – and often other tools can help (simple auscultation, simple visualization of the mitral valve).
- To assess the renal perfusion may be of interest, but likely redundant in terms of practical action with the FALLS-protocol.
- Even ultrasound-guided nerve blockade does maybe not so much require a Doppler; we are currently working on this (Chap. 36).
- The cardiac output? Let us read again the long Chap. 30, here a bit summarized: instead of values of cardiac output, lung ultrasound gave us the direct parameter enabling to initiate fluid therapy and to discontinue it. Therefore, a simple ultrasound approach, using the FALLS-protocol, may make the same work (if not *more*) than values of cardiac output, for deciding a policy of fluid. The lung plus veins plus simple heart may compensate (or *more*) the absence of Doppler – simplicity and rapidity in addition. A clinical study is at last ongoing.

This rarity of situations really requiring urgent Doppler without an alternative is central to our vision. Again, our DIAFORA approach was used since 1989 for these few cases. We would even accept to *transport* such rare patients to a specialized department if needed. The DIAFORA concept allows to purchase a cost-effective machine for a majority of daily tasks. Once its full potential is exploited, we promise that we will open to Doppler. Christian Doppler, from Salzburg, made his findings around 1852 and has his street in Serries, a small city at the east of Paris. We guess that coming back among us, he would be surprised to hear that his family name is probably the most often pronounced in the daily talks of all critical care disciplines. Keeping high respect to Doppler's works, we consider that the concerns mentioned above are substantial enough to invite the user to think twice.

A last point: as a researcher (more occupied in research than in politics), we don't prohibit the use of Doppler (and have no authority for doing so). We just open the minds, pointing out that each physician is free to use Doppler at will. We repeat that we can reconsider our position: we are not opposed to have Doppler on our next machine, provided it makes us happy with our seven requirements (size, image quality, start-up time, flat keyboard, simple conception, the universal probe, cost), and if Doppler inclusion does not create the slightest drawback, see again Chap. 2. The CU (CEURF units) conferred to the existing or upcoming machines are ready to be updated and even give positive points to such a progress (we envisage five points if such a Doppler is included, ten points if this Doppler has high quality).

6. The gel, a mandatory part of ultrasound

Ultrasound is gel. This gel is ultrasound, since ever. The gloomy spectacle of a *gooey* discipline. A kind of sauce, surrounded by amounts of crumpled wipes, it infiltrates everywhere, on the probe, the doctor's tie.... Sometimes, we see the whacky vision of a patient who was scanned in a haste and was not wiped. Other times, this distressing vision, not really glamour, of some hair stuck on the dried gel over the probe from the previous night. The correct word is "mess." Patients and colleagues accept this landscape, in view of the utility of ultrasound, but would possibly like to get rid of this nightmare (Fig. 37.1). In addition, this is not only a nightmare: in settings where time is of essence, using gel spoils precious seconds (see Chap. 2, and see its scientific relevance in

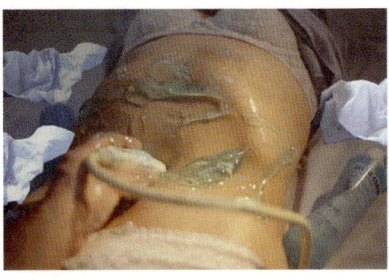

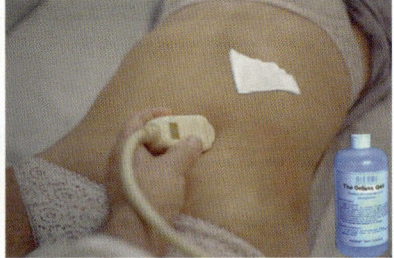

Fig. 37.1 The gelless gel. To the *left*, this sticky, whacky, gooey image, done thanks to the stoicism of Joëlle, is not our vision of ultrasound. Not only does it make a psychological barrier to a large widespread, but it extends the timing of fast protocols such as the BLUE-protocol and especially the SESAME-protocol, makes the chest wall slippery (an issue during resuscitation), and is a blessing for the microbes. To the *right*, ultrasound done with Ecolight®, soon available

Chap. 31). Gel? We don't use it. We long found the substitute for gel (Ecolight®, soon available). In our world, there is no gel, no wipes, no sticky skin, and no endless hours for (imperfectly) cleaning the skin. This is part of holistic ultrasound.

7. One probe for each territory

Only one probe is sufficient in the intensivist's use, as outlined throughout this book: our microconvex probe, the 0.6–17 cm range one. All others are good for each corresponding specialist, none of them being suitable for the main organ (the lung) and the main discipline (critical care).

See our detailed comments above.

Possibly one day (personal fear), sly manufacturers will propose a *liver* probe and a *splenic* probe. We are afraid by such a perspective, quite sure that they will succeed in convincing many that the performances of ultrasound will be enhanced. We advise interested colleagues to refer to doctors with extensive experience, not commercials, when buying a probe.

The Laptop Concept: An Unnecessary Tool for a Scientific Revolution, Why?[1]

One can do with any kind of machine, including laptops. Just, it was useless to wait for the laptop revolution, since we had much better, decades before… for introducing our philosophy of simplicity in the ICUs, ERs, ORs, and making a *scientifical* revolution, since 1992 (even since 1982).

We saw this first laptop machine and this strange, unadapted geometry and could do nothing, unable to prevent to see this philosophy invading our hospitals. Let us comment quietly, for readers who want to understand our point.

Some doctors are still persuaded that the modern laptop machines are small. The advocated "small size" was the only argument the manufacturers gave for having built these machines (Fig. 37.2). Some doctors strongly believe that it was the factor which initiated the revolution in medicine. Some do not hesitate to write such comments in stirring editorials at the occasion of world conferences (good friends, no offense). This would simply mean that this revolution was the fact of manufacturers and some engineers, not physicians. Would you accept this if you were part of the early ambassadors of critical ultrasound, using older and better tools, just used differently?

These manufacturers were, for sure, proud of their products. To answer the question "Did laptop units bring any interesting progress," we took simple but objective tools: an unsophisticated ruler, a chronometer, a bacteriologic swab, simple comparisons in costs, and simple thoughts. We describe again and shortly one by one our seven requirements (dealt with in Chaps. 2 and 3), which are in our 1992 Hitachi-405 (and most in our respected 1982 ADR-4000). So what may be the advantages of these new machines? At the

---

[1] Philippe Martin, a smart mind, inspired us a balanced editing of the sensitive paragraph devoted on laptop units. Our initial draft was more direct.

The Laptop Concept: An Unnecessary Tool for a Scientific Revolution, Why?

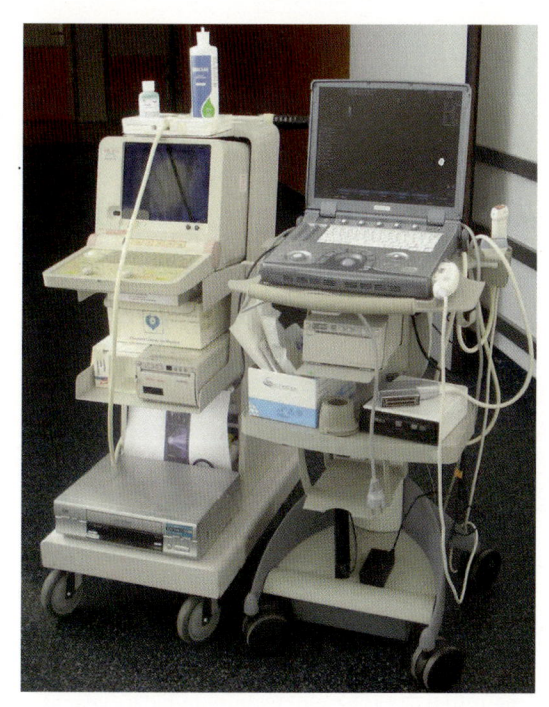

Fig. 37.2 Just measure and compare. Our Hitachi-405, smaller than a very widespread standard in laptop equipment, was perfect for a revolution which could have happened two decades before. This simple figure allows first an objective comparison of sizes. Note several features. One unit is much more compact than the other. One unit has an available top, useful for storing equipment (including our single probe) and avoiding these lateral stands. Note also the antique VHS recorder, which we still use (the videos of this textbook all come from here)

times where these lines are written, one popular brand of laptops has three or four of our seven criteria, resulting in a score of minus 260 CEURF units (CU), while another popular one has simply *none* of them (and minus 860 CU, an absolute record). How can it be possible? How could this happen? Beware; this is a sensitive section of the book.

1. Size of the machine: take a simple ruler and just see

We are always amazed when we see how long the necessary text for such a simple point is.

Laptop machines are small? The use of a simple ruler proves, scientifically, without emotion, that this argument is fully wrong. In a hospital setting, space lacks around the critically ill. Moving from bed to bed, from ICU to ER, etc., is a challenge. Each saved centimeter is a victory. The small height of the laptop machines was a good idea. Current laptop machines, naked, have a lateral width of 40–44 cm. This is smaller than more cumbersome machines, but we strongly believe that our 29-cm-width unit designed in 1992 (last update 2008) can even more rapidly reach the patient. Our material is higher (27 cm) than laptops (6 cm)? Not a problem, our ceilings are high enough! The critical dimension is the width, not the height. In this spirit, the respected 1982 ADR-4000® was near to perfect with its 42 cm width. For those who work in tiny places where ceilings are actually low (airplanes, e.g.), handheld machines are of major interest. Between 2000 and 2012, we used a 1.9-kg machine. We currently use a 0.4-kg unit.

Regarding the weight, they dared to propose a 6-kg machine for handheld use. We were charged to take one from one point to another for a Croatian course (probably May 2008, we took the train with it), and we still have the scar on our shoulder (at least psychologically).

Now let us add the cart and observe what happens. Now, the current laptops suddenly reach, laterally, up to 44, 52, and even 68 cm (current record). These machines were devoted to work in ICUs, ERs, and ORs. This is good because committed users can succeed with a 68-cm-width machine to cross all obstacles, to insert it between a patient and the ventilator, for sure. Our machine with the cart is now 32 cm width. Ask the question to a child: Is 32 cm more cumbersome than 44, 52, or 68 cm? Who would answer "yes"? Since 1992, we have the door opened to bedside visual medicine. With a gravity center at the bottom, this makes a 32-32-32 cm, i.e., dream mensurations for a mobile ultrasound unit. Note, even today, traditional echocardiographic machines have a 60 cm width (Fig. 37.3). Even nondoctors can see immediately this weird paradox (to use a balanced word).

How can a simple cart be so noxious? Because "imagination" was not at all "at work": the computer is large, but the cart is larger. In addition, you have these lateral stands which are used because the top cannot be used for storing objects because there is no top in a laptop. If we design a

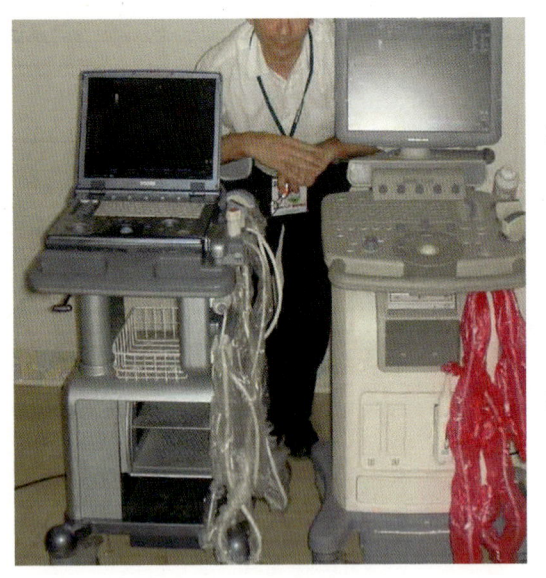

Fig. 37.3 Imagination: the fourth dimension. Mumbai, November 2008. Two machines from the same brand. The machine to our right (*dark screen*) is a laptop model (6 cm high). The left one is a traditional one (1 m high). Both have quite the same width. The laptop is even some cm larger, which means that in an emergency, the traditional machine would come faster at the bedside (thanks to the wheels). Laptop machines are a blessing for the warehousemen in ultrasound workshops, maybe their main interest

machine with a top (not a big technological challenge in 2015), we have space on this top for putting objects and can get rid of these cumbersome lateral devices. Figure 4.3 shows how precious lateral centimeters are saved, thanks to a simple top. Therefore, we still use our 1992 (last update 2008) system. Time saved.

For those who think that a laptop unit can be used without a cart in a hospital:

1. The cart is a highly practical tool. A physician using a laptop machine without cart, and called in an emergency, would be obliged to take (in a high haste) the unit in one hand, the contact product in another, the three usual probes at the neck, the procedural material between the teeth, and the disinfectant product between the knees and be obliged to jump through the corridors. Very trained doctors may arrive quickly on-site, sweaty and panting, but the image would not be fully elegant for the spectators, even a bit scary for the patient. With a smart cart, the whole material is transported using two fingers: really practical!
2. If not irreversibly fixed on the cart, the handheld unit is an easy prey, at the mercy of any predator. This means additional costs for paying the watchman who will have a 24/24 h work, unless machines may promptly vanish (a kind of honor, in one way). In the real life, look well: these machines remain always fixed on the cart – they never leave it.
3. Machines without a cart, simply laid down on the bed? This would imply very demanding disinfection maneuvers (if done). In addition, such machines can fall. Maybe they have been designed for falling; we don't let our machine fall (thanks to the cart).
2. Image quality: just see the enclosed images

One main result of the laptop revolution was to suppress the *cathode ray tube*. The quality of the initial 2000 machines initiated a 20-year step backward in the history of ultrasound (take time to see well Fig. 2.3). We learned that the manufacturers said to the new users (in the 2000s) that they "would get accustomed [to this new imaging quality]…." A full confession! Like vinyl music or fixed phones, which give a better acoustic quality than digital music or cell phones, the cathode ray tube of our unit gives the best quality. Now, the recent screens improve little by little the image quality, thanks to the work of our good engineers – although we are regularly dismayed when we visit ICUs and try to use these modern laptop machines, fighting with the filters and facilities for trying to optimize the image quality. How many times did we hear ICU colleagues through the world, afflicted by the image quality of their machines, once they know that one can scan not only the heart. We think that these units will be in some years as good as our 1992 reference. Up to now, the community has lost one quarter of century of technology, for no advantage.

We use again the term "harmony," since the concept of cathode ray tube results in a small size (in width), with an additional available top avoiding lateral devices which take useless place and no effort, thanks to the wheels of the cart.

3. Start-up time: take a chronometer

The start-up time of machines devoted to critical ultrasound is expressed in minutes, Half one for some, one or two, sometimes three for many others (reminder, 1 s costs one CEURF unit). This is short. Yet shorter is better in time-dependent patients, where each second counts. Our system starts-on in 7 s since 1992. The start-up time of the traditional machines shortens little by little (stabilizing around 1 min). We hope that in some years, technical progresses will make them able to reach our speed.

4. Disinfection issues: apply a bacteriologic swab on your laptop

Numerous buttons, cursors, hand levels, etc., of laptop machines are interesting for experts to make multiple manipulations. Yet these countless, prominent crannies and nooks are a godsend for microbes who can freely proliferate, sheltered from predators, waiting to jump on the next patients – unless the user carefully cleans each button. We go on using our *flat keyboard*, cleaned in a few seconds, since 1992. The concept of a unique probe favors efficient cleaning, since dense forests of cables and probes are again a blessing for the microbes. The buttons will disappear in the future (note, our 1982 and 1992 units had flat keyboards!); this is sure, which implies that all the previous machines which were built and bought before should be all sent to the garbage: an unprecedented waste.

5. Access to the ideal probe for critical ultrasound

We detailed the choice of the probe in Chap. 3. The new market uses traditional probes familiar to cardiologists, radiologists, angiologists, and gynecologists, and this is good because they are accustomed. Yet it is ironic that this new market, devoted for the critical care without mistake, did not care at developing the *intensivist's* probe (not the less important discipline!), the most suitable for the *lung* (the most vital organ!).

The probe of the intensivist is neither the phased array nor the abdominal nor the linear, etc., probe. The *microconvex* probe is a providence. We keep using this universal 5-MHz probe of our 1992 technology, perfect for access to any part of the whole body. No time is lost for changing the probe, cleaning it, and buying several ones. One can find microconvex probes in some laptop machines (probably built in a haste, probably subsequent to our reiterated comments); unfortunately, they have either really unsuitable resolution or unsuitable penetration, up to only 8 or 10 cm, which is once again a failure.

Since the lung was not considered, many variations can be seen, orchestrated by pure hazard. We don't congest this section; read again Chap. 3.

Our deep thought is that these tools were accepted by the same experts who proclaimed that the lung was immune to ultrasound.

6. Simple conception: take your common sense

Laptop machines have complete equipment, and this is a good point because experienced users can play with Doppler, harmonics, or other modes for suppressing the artifacts. However, these machines were developed using traditional concepts. The integration of the lung upsets the priorities of critical ultrasound: these sophisticated modes become of lesser relevance. Read all these chapters such as our hemodynamic approach (Chap. 30), all more or less futile technical details analyzed in Chap. 2. Countless misconceptions bothered nobody until users got aware of them – we hope the community will appreciate the work of those who try to bring the light (in Latin, lux, the light; fero, I bring) (from Jean-Luc Fournier). Sophisticated machines with too many buttons are not adapted to use by non-experts in time-dependent patients. In the crowd of buttons, the inadvertent use of some can create unexpected actions, such as sudden disappearance of the image! It happened to us (fortunately at a workshop, none was harmed). In the real life, the only solution for the user is to promptly find the correct page in the thick user's guide, while the team carries on the resuscitation.

7. Cost-effectiveness. Take now your purse

Simple conceptions yield low costs. Traditional laptop machines are less expensive (5 numbers) than traditional echocardiographic machines (6 numbers). Yet the first number can be a 1 or 9, a substantial difference. We think that the cost is a critical point: each saved Euro (dollar, rupee, etc.) makes a machine more easily bought, i.e., more saved lives. Our gray-scale 1992 (updated 2008) machine has the cost of one *simple automobile*.

Scoop 1: How 1 cm could have changed medicine

In our previous editions, we wrote: "The unit must be as small as possible. The idea of making any effort for moving it should in no case be a physical or psychological obstacle." This sounds a little obsolete now. The volume of our ADR-4000® unit was 40.000 cc. Such a volume could be dispatched in a 200×200×1 cm volume (with minor arrangements). Building ambulances with an additional length of *1 cm* could have made space for point-of-care ultrasound a reality since *the year 1982*. Countless patients did not arrive alive on the operating theater because the minds were not ready. This centimeter, not a lot, is the symbol that the revolution of ultrasound had nothing to do with technology.

Scoop 2: We found a fine advantage to the laptop technology

By trying by any means to write a balanced section, we found the main advantage of laptop machines: they are a godsend for the storekeepers of the congress workshops because they can move them easily from their trucks.

What do we want to express, eventually? Why is this tone slightly but desperately ironic? Our ultimate aim is to share with other doctors the pleasure we have every day to take our light unit, compact, always clean, ready after a few seconds, with no hard choice for having the perfect probe... and all details written and repeated through this textbook (we apologize of so many reiterations). The point is that very few key opinion leaders have used our equipment, whereas we perfectly know theirs, present everywhere (hospitals, workshops). This allows us to permanently compare, year by year.

What should modern physicians buy today? As a scientist, not a commercial, we will certainly not give any name, just some common sense advice. We hope to have convinced them that a laptop is of no interest (unless it is really small, without these huge empty spaces, with in addition the six other requirements for a visual medicine). Now that they have realized that they are not obliged to buy a "laptop," they have a really wide choice. Some machines are really suitable, although initially not at all "devoted to critical care" just because the manufacturers are not aware of this. Our Hitachi-405 was a great example of such a providence. One other paradox of critical ultrasound, one more. Some recent machines have quite the same features with our Hitachi-405. When they will have a slight real advantage on it with *positive* CU (with some Doppler, some modern connections, etc., all these details which make young doctors happy), we swear again that we will immediately throw our beloved machine to the trash compactor (or keep it just for sentimental reasons).

Critical Ultrasound, a Tool Enhancing the Clinical Examination

Some colleagues fear that ultrasound would replace the physical examination. They must catch the very dimension of this new tool. The extended BLUE-protocol was organized around physical examination. Taking the best of it, this is an example of synergic integration of these two weapons. For sure, once critical ultrasound and LUCI are widely used, the physical examination will not be the same. For sure, it will need to be deeply revisited. A giant round table should study all the physical signs and define, sign by sign, which ones are interesting (easy to find and clinically relevant) from those we may do without (difficult, plus doubtful usefulness – we suddenly think of the thumb-chin reflex – réflexe pollicomentonnier). This giant task of the new classification, made sign by sign, disease per disease, should deserve a whole book. It would be a real medical revolution. There would be surprises from both directions. There are excellent, useful clinical signs; there are less contributive, more difficult ones, not working so well [11]. There are easy patients; there are challenging ones (there are good and bad ultrasound signs, too). Simple images will illustrate this view and reassure pessimistic minds.

Good, contributive signs: the simple inspection of the patient, of the mottled skin, one among hundred examples, immediately diagnoses an acute circulatory failure. Some auscultation signs are excellent: the superiority of the physical examination when compared to radiography for diagnosing lung consolidations was already proven [12].

Difficult signs: the clinical detection of pulmonary edema without crackles, search for subtle pleural murmur for detecting small pleural effusions, urinary obstacle in obese patients… Featuring at the top of difficulty probably, the increase in precordial dullness in pericardial tamponade. Cardiologic signs seem to have been abandoned by the cardiologists. It is true that we rarely heard a splitting of protodiastolic heart sound in the crowded, noisy emergency room, for assessing a left heart failure. The difficulty of the physical examination was rarely assessed scientifically [13]. We, intensivists (emergency physicians, etc.), do not work like cardiologists, quietly, and must always have a plan B. Cardiac auscultation is part from it, and see below regarding a shock with the B-profile.

Absent clinical signs? The best example is the interstitial syndrome – where ultrasound plays a major role (see the BLUE-protocol and the FALLS-protocol).

The blood pressure? Read below.

Some clinical signs are good but painful. The percussion of the liver was for long one way of diagnosing hepatic abscess. This maneuver has no longer a raison d'être today, and the patient (if able to compare) will be grateful to you! During ultrasound, it is good to detect a parietal contraction in the maneuver shown in Fig. 28.7; this is why we do ultrasound with both hands (and fear pocket machines).

Among the hundred tools of physical examinations, the eyes for inspection and the hands for palpation (sometimes the nose) make a great part. The taste is fortunately no longer required: a nice advance, no? As regards the ears, by listening to the history, they make more than half the clinical work.

Now how about the ears for making diagnoses based on the body noises?

We speak here of the stethoscope, this respected symbol of medicine. Hung at the neck in a hospital corridor, it makes you a doctor, since centuries. We would like to succeed to write a balanced vision of its use, at the heat of an era where some begin to speak in contemptuous terms of this "old tool." Among many scientific answers, one may just say to them to visit the cockpit of any modern airplane: one can still find one antique magnetic compass, life saving when the high-tech tools fail. As evoked previously, rales make better than radiograph [12]. Now can we see ultrasound as a clinical tool, a modern stethoscope (i.e., not an "enemy" of physical examination, but a part of it)? Half of the answer is given if one considers that a test performed at the bedside is clinical (*clinos*, the bed). The other half is achieved if one looks into the etymology of the word *stethoscope* which, also a Greek root, was created by the French physician René T.H. Laënnec in the early 1800s [14]: a means of looking (*scopein*, to observe) through the lung (*stethos*, the chest wall). To "see" the lung, this is the duty of ultrasound, which should therefore be coined "stethoscope" rigorously. But let us keep this symbolic word as it is; let us not change history uselessly, too abruptly. "Free" provocation is not our cup of tea.

In his preface for the English translation of Laënnec's book of auscultation in 1821, Sir John Forbes wrote that the role of the stethoscope would be minor in medicine. We have used it thousand times. It has always been a fine companion, reassuring. In a fast, shallow approach, one may wonder when was the last time it allowed us to take an urgent therapeutic decision; one may dare the provocative contra-question: was Forbes completely wrong? LUCI allows us to give a more balanced answer. Especially in the light of the extended BLUE-protocol, we remind that the wheezes are heard using Laënnec tool and not seen using ultrasound, just one example. It helps to select the patients with the nude profile in the BLUE-protocol (with however a suspicion of pulmonary embolism) for scintigraphy or helical CT. Wheezes help in decreasing the global irradiation. The absence of a mitral murmur associated with a well contractile LV in a shocked patient with a B-profile probably indicates a noncardiogenic shock. The extended BLUE-protocol will hopingly rejuvenate our old good stethoscope, in spite of some issues now threatening its use. We don't evoke the laziness of some, but mainly the fact that in modern ICUs, each bed has its own stethoscope, of course a low-cost, low-quality piece, unless it would rapidly disappear. Taking back our excellent stethoscopes from the attics, using them wisely (read again the E-BLUE-protocol) and having the reflex of cleaning them after each use (what we did, student, in the year 1980, we remember our colleagues, Hospital Tenon, Paris, looking at us strangely – it was not on fashion), this would skip this minor issue. Briefly, don't panic [15]. Let us keep our stethoscope alive!

One tool has already threatened the use of clinical examination: CT. Like the GPS, e.g., the CT exempts physicians of thinking [16], with the risk of brain shrinking. Ultrasound is a didactic tool allowing to enhance one's physical examination – a unique opportunity to have self-improvement, since it shows diagnoses in real time. The physician who did not clinically detect this effusion can pay more attention to discrete signs such as pleuritic murmur, not recognized initially. These new doctors should be skilled in clinical examination, of precious help when the machine is suddenly not available (used by others, in breakdown, etc.) – the Internet did not kill TV, and TV did not kill radio, far from that.

We could show hundreds of examples, but this should deserve a specific book (we repeat, this will likely be a medical revolution).

Now how about the tensiometer? A continuous monitoring in a sedated patient is mandatory. Before this step, we must acknowledge that it never brought a lot to us. We take the blood pressure to look like a normal physician, yet in countless instances, we visit and fix a circulatory failure at night, then go for a little rest in our room, just write the report before the nap, and suddenly wonder: "But what was the blood pressure of this guy??" Regarding high pressures, for preventing brain hemorrhage, this is valuable, but for low pressures, other data (mottling, urine output, others) should be far more indicative; if we have very restricted space (airborne mission), we would favor without hesitation a pocket ultrasound machine instead.

Apart from its intrinsic utility, the physical examination is a strong moment for the awake patient. This direct contact with the hands of your doctor has major psychological impact. Ultrasound was a unique opportunity for the radiologists to get closer to the patients.

The SLAM

To slam: to close a door abruptly, with some disdain.

Acronym: sets of initials of a sequence of words organized (more or less artificially) for creating a new word.

The SLAM (Section for the Limitation of Acronyms in Medicine) was born on April 1, 2008 – not a hazard if creating an acronym assessing acronyms [17]). They are classified according to two simple criteria. First, are they really innovations or simple copy-paste of previously available methods done by certain doctors (e.g., radiologist/sonographer) for the use of other doctors (e.g., emergency physician)? Second, are they a source of possible confusion? Do they sound like words that we daily use in a discipline where communication must be fast? A third possible criterion, aestheticism, will maybe be added; we are working on it.

The SLAM would like to see a reasonable number – and quality – of acronyms, before the confusion rules. Some readers have sought in vain in this book (section Abdomen) a familiar acronym which is, still for some, a synonym of critical ultrasound (Fig. 37.4). The most famous acronym in emergency ultrasound would not have obtained an average note. First, it deals with an antique application done at the debuts of ultrasound: not an invention. Second, in our disciplines, some words are holy, because everything must be fast. Important words which are inopportunely spoiled would generate – have generated – deleterious confusions. In our 2010 edition, we warned that one day or another, doctors will, somewhere, search for an ascitic peritoneal fluid and pronounce the words of the protocol devoted

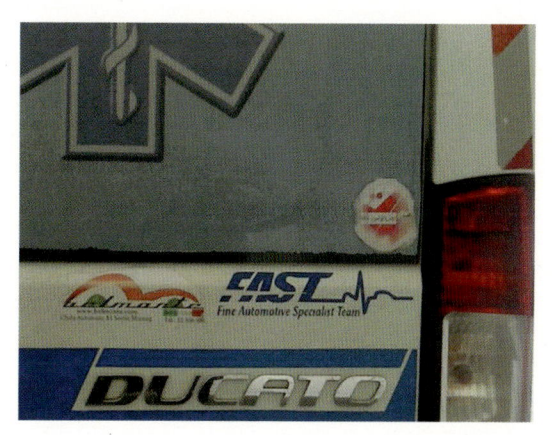

Fig. 37.4 A fast train (or ambulance) can hide another. Image taken at the back of an ambulance somewhere in the world during a medical mission. This fine automotive specialist team shows that in healthcare, everything must be fast. To reduce these precious words to a single application would make a restricted exercise

to finding blood in traumatized patients. And it happened. We fully respect the enthusiasm of these young doctors, but want also to show our respect to other teams which did not lose time for finding shiny acronyms for popularizing life-saving procedures. In our 1992 textbook on critical ultrasound, each line was important for saving lives. The aim was to define *what* was possible using this probe. In 1992, e.g., no book dealt with venous access in the critically ill. In our 1992 textbook, we did not search for an acronym, we just wrote that ultrasound can see a needle, so, just imagine. "Just imagine". The idea of adapting the signs of peritoneal effusion for the search of free blood did not take more than *12 lines* (and one line in our 1993 article sent in 1991). Now the SLAM apologizes in advance for close colleagues who could feel their hard contribution not fully considered. They should understand that the SLAM just tries to help CEURF recognition. No offense, but some familiar protocols have the peculiarity to be both focused and extended. The SLAM did not succeed to understand how a protocol can be extended and focused at the same time. The SLAM considers that it is not a big damage to add simple usual words, such as "pneumothorax" (anyone would understand). No offense, because these are precious friends, with respected commitment: the SLAM in some words

just tries to give respect to the work of the CEURF. The SLAM would be worried by knowing a posteriori that some doctors needed acronyms for realizing that ultrasound was a revolutionary tool. The SLAM regrets the number of deaths occurring between the first findings of pioneering teams (as to us, we began in 1985) and now simply because we did not find it mandatory to develop acronyms. No acronym, no marketing or flashy effects, just this idea: "Use ultrasound and be a visual doctor."

It is not difficult to create flashy acronyms.

We could have called our search for free blood the "assessment of blood using sonography in an emergency." But this is not all.

The Quality Ultrasound to Improve Current Knowledge protocol (under submission) aims at refining the traditional signs of the search for free peritoneal blood, using more than a copy-paste that was initially devoted to sonographers (i.e., technicians with a 3-year postgraduate). Such protocols require standardized views. We disdain these traditional five sites, making instead liberal scan of the belly. The QUICK-protocol is an original approach: it includes new signs (induced sinusoid sign, bat wing sign; see Figs. 5.7 and 5.8 of our 2010 edition), which are not to our knowledge in the traditional protocol.

Simple ultrasound devoid of complicated utensils is a game of strategy. At one side, there is a complex critically ill patient. At the other, there is a simple machine (with only one probe, fast switch-on, no Doppler, etc.). One must find the winning combination, for an immediate life-saving use.

Conversely, lung ultrasound in the critically ill (in the sky or not, with or without diamonds), simple emergency cardiac sonography, our limited investigation considering hemodynamic therapy, the ultrasound search for free blood, whole-body ultrasound in a few words, and all these applications using our simple critical ultrasound design (a long-distance weapon indeed), all these uses did not benefit from an acronym, for a symbolic reason: if the interest of an acronym is to save a few seconds, the use of ultrasound allows to save *hours* (when compared to the traditional management, CT, etc.). The wish for saving time using an acronym comes from a questionable intention.

We are currently working on a protocol designed for ultrasound distinction between a foot corn and a coryza that will be labeled the Algorithm of Bedside Screening Ultrasound to the Right Decision. It may be relevant. Maybe the SLAM will give an average note for it.

The SLAM is keen in some acronyms. The KISS, from Kathleen Garcia (Keep It Simple Sonography), summarizes our approach. The WINFOCUS is a rather elegant one, describing an original activity, not sounding confusing. The best acronym will probably be for long the VOMIT: those Victims Of Modern Imaging Technologies, would by the way be interested by critical ultrasound, precisely. We deeply hope that all these acronyms (one per day is maybe created, through countless articles) were not designed for creating territories and for gaining any power.

How about acronyms *at any price* (AAAP) (say "triple A-P" for being faster)? We suspect the ABCDE management of being an example of AAAP. "A" for airway is basic. "B" for breathing initiates a progression. "C" for circulation is an excellent sequel. A-B-C is nice, but suddenly, there is this "D" for disability. What has "disability" to do in a trauma patient? Was this "D" mandatory? We see rather another "B," for brain, without major damage to the concept. ABCBE (with E for "etc." rather than exposure, an artificial end for closing a flashy acronym) should have done a similar work. Do we really have to explain to young doctors that in a cardiac arrest, the search for abolition of osteotendinous reflexes is not a priority if the airways are obstructed?? These doctors are maybe young but not "disabled," after so many years of high-degree studies, among the hardest. As regards the "A," read in Chaps. 31 and 34 why we don't use ultrasound for intubating our patients.

Sometimes, acronyms can fight. Are the FATE, FEER, and FOCUS racing? Maybe the rather elegant RACE will arrive first? Some protocols used by close friends began by the abdomen, and little by little invade the lungs (those which are both extended and focused). We worry about a possible whole-body *vampirization*. Before the acronyms become too long, we would love to propose words such as "whole-body ultrasound" or simply "ultrasound."

We would like to see this BOA (Battle Of Acronyms) eventually dying by eating its tail.

So, why a BLUE-protocol? We saw at our very debuts, simultaneously, that fluids and air were critical targets in the critically ill. We took critical decisions: submitting a really interesting matter (air) or exploiting not innovative applications (fluids)? We could take the world leadership of nothing (at the beginning of any innovation, by definition you are alone!), but wanted instead to show the real potential of ultrasound. The BLUE-protocol was the conclusion of 20 publications which, brick by brick, rejection after rejection (the Editorial Boards were prudent), took 18 years. We did not know it would be so hard. A simple copy-paste of the simplest application (fluid in the abdomen) could have brought a complete revolution since 1985. What would *you* have done first? The BLUE-protocol, acute respiratory failure, was our nice answer to the revolution brought by the detection of peritoneal fluid. This label fulfilled the two conditions required from the SLAM: innovative work and not confusing terms (can be used without ambiguity in a doctor's talk in fast emergency settings). And mostly… it is not an acronym: it indicates that we deal with a cyanotic patient and that the venous network (usually blue) is associated with the lung analysis. The Pink-protocol and the Fever-protocol are not acronyms. The LUCIFLR project is here for limiting, not eradicating, radiations. Please no hasty acronym here.

CEURF develops a minimal number of acronyms, each answering to a specific setting: dyspnea (BLUE-protocol), shock (FALLS-protocol), cardiac arrest (SESAME-protocol), etc. As regards lung ultrasound in the neonates, we firmly hope to make use of no acronym [18]. Should acronyms be necessary for saving these lives? We find it disputable in adults, but for saving children? Here, doctors can do without any acronym. As a pacific wink, a symbol of serenity, the neonate's lung ultrasound will benefit from the "No Acronym Protocol."

And How About US?

Here, we leave the acronyms, which intend to create words, for the small world of abbreviations (ab.). The ab. that worries us mostly is certainly "US."

Ultrasound is the most critical word we have to use. As opposed to computerized tomography, or again the United States, which are groups of words, *ultrasound* is one word. The use of an ab. is therefore not allowed and does not make any sense. "Ultrasound" or "US" makes the same word count. Ultrasound has ten letters, a biblical symbol. Ultrasound is time (and life) saving. Please note we devote 2 s to type it in full letters versus 0.6 s for "US," i.e., a final investment of only 1.4 s. The ab. US is confusing with the success of US, now that political issues are raised – in the US mainly. When US use US, does it mean that the use of US will improve the global health level of the US? This makes the bed for confusions – what the SLAM wants to avoid. We wrote above that the SLAM will maybe give a note to the elegance of acronyms and even abs. If it does so, we guess the worst, inelegant, so ugly "LUS" would be the first to be flung into the fire.

Briefly, just as a homage, we go on writing ultrasound, with all letters. Ultrasound offers so much to us; we can make this small effort. "US" is not 100 % respectuous.

We also have a kind thought for Xavier Leverve, who took his precious time (in a congress in Bali) in advising us that without the manufacturers, nothing is possible. Although adopting a more flexible talk, we did not fully follow his pieces of advice and hope that he will see, from where he is now, that our vision was just announcing the future trend, based on our yesterday's tool, in answering the theme of the CEURF: "The tools of ever for tomorrow's medicine." An eternal rule will likely apply to critical ultrasound: if all manufacturers run in the same direction, there will be always *one* smarter and more visionary than the others, who will create the new standard, copying our 1992 unit. See the story of Apple. We hope it will be our historical Japanese one, which by providence made long ago a tool not at all devoted for critical ultrasound, but anyway the perfect tool for this use!

> **Anecdotal Notes**
>
> No anecdotal note here. This full chapter is an anecdotal one, since we know anecdotal thoughts would range among scientific ones: even the greatest experts (especially them) mingle high academic knowledge with a bit (or sometimes much more) of emotion.

References

1. Dénier A (1946) Les ultrasons, leur application au diagnostic. Presse Med 22:307–308
2. Wild JJ (1950) The use of ultrasonic pulses for the measurement of biologic tissues and the detection of tissue density changes. Surgery 27(2):183–188
3. Lichtenstein D (1992) L'échographie générale en réanimation. Springer, Paris, pp 1–200
4. Jardin F, Farcot JC, Boisante L, Curien N, Margairaz A, Bourdarias JP (1981) Influence of positive end-expiratory pressure on left ventricle performance. N Engl J Med 304(7):387–392
5. Jougon JB, Gallon P, MacBride T et al (1999) Esophageal perforation after transesophageal echocardiography. Eur J Cardiothorac Surg 16:686–687
6. Decharny JB, Philip I, Depoix JP (2002) Esophagotracheal perforation after intraoperative transoesophageal echocardiography in cardiac surgery. Br J Anaesth 88:592–594
7. Vignon P, Goarin JP (2002) Echocardiographie Doppler en réanimation, anesthésie et médecine d'urgence. Elsevier-Masson, Paris/New York
8. Taylor KJW (1987) A prudent approach to Doppler ultrasonography (editorial). Radiology 165:283–284
9. Miller DL (1991) Update on safety of diagnostic ultrasonography. J Clin Ultrasound 19:531–540
10. Barnett SB, Ter Haar GR, Ziskin MC, Rott HD, Duck FA, Maeda K (2000) International recommendations and guidelines for the safe use of diagnostic ultrasound in medicine. Ultrasound Med Biol 26:355–366
11. Lichtenstein D (2007) L'échographie "corps entier", une approche visuelle du patient en état critique. Bulletin officiel de l'Académie Nationale de Médecine (séance du 6 mars 2007), Paris, Tome 191, mars N°3, pp 495–517
12. Lichtenstein D, Goldstein I, Mourgeon E, Cluzel P, Grenier P, Rouby JJ (2004) Comparative diagnostic performances of auscultation, chest radiography and lung ultrasonography in acute respiratory distress syndrome. Anesthesiology 100:9–15
13. McGee S, Abernethy WB 3rd, Simel DL (1999) The rational clinical examination. Is this patient hypovolemic? JAMA 281:1022–1029

14. Laënnec RTH (1819) Traité de l'auscultation médiate, ou traité du diagnostic des maladies des poumons et du cœur. J.A. Brosson & J.S. Chaudé, Paris. Hafner, New York, 1962
15. Hubmayr RD (2004) The times are A-changin' (should we hang up the stethoscope?). Anesthesiology 100:1–2
16. Snyder GE (2008) Whole-body imaging in blunt multisystem trauma patients who were never examined. Ann Emerg Med 52(2):101–103
17. SLAM – Section pour la Limitation des Acronymes en Médecine (2009) – Déclaration 1609. 1er avril 2008. Journal Officiel de la République Française, 26 avril 2008 (N° 17), p 2009
18. Lichtenstein D (2009) Ultrasound examination of the lungs in the intensive care unit. Pediatr Crit Care Med 10:693–698

A Way to Learn the BLUE-Protocol 38

Adding *LUCI* in the armamentarium of critical ultrasound should result in a change of priorities, by training the intensivist (emergency physician, anesthesiologist, etc.) to the essential of the BLUE-protocol first. This physician should then be free to take as long time as needed for learning the complex expert echocardiography, during as many years as necessary, but will be ready to face night emergencies, using the best of the BLUE- or FALLS-protocol.

It seems wise to limit this initial training to the most basic alphabet: lung sliding and lung rockets. With just these two "letters," they will be able to compose countless "words," but we can limit this to one application: ruling out pneumothorax. The user must know that, each time this question is raised (i.e., *several times a day*), the simple unit can be used, with an immediate answer each time. Once these two "letters" are mastered, one can add another one (exponentially multiplying the number of possible applications) and so on for an indeterminate period.

Using this way, the intensivists will little by little change their way of working, with always the possibility to go backward in case of difficulty. Sudden changes are never good. Ultrasound mastery has a beginning but no end, and this author learns everyday.

How to train? Let us make a travel to the past. Since 1989, we had to choose between defining critical ultrasound (a full-time work) and training colleagues. We devoted 90 % of our time in defining the field, i.e., submitting manuscripts, hoping that this work would be easy. This was a mistake, but it is true that we found nobody during all our studies and after who told us how long it is, once a discovery made, to make it accepted. A training center was created, in order to modestly widespread our vision of simplicity (10 % of our time). The CEURF (Cercle des Echographistes d'Urgence et de Réanimation Francophones) was born from the absence of adapted structure at these remote periods, in 1989 [1]. Some courageous colleagues in the mid 1990s had to register to traditional diplomas, know about thyroid, obstetrics, liver segmentation, etc., but quite nothing about acutely ill patients and of course not a word on the lung. The CEURF (pronounce *surf*) describes new rules and does not sound confusing by itself; it was therefore accepted by the SLAM [2].

Making subsequently international courses, CEURF kept its initial label (just, the final F was first for France, then French-speaking countries, and now accounts for Foreign). It is a nonprofit association, which wants to be "99 % scientific and 1 % administrative."

CEURF is independent from the power of manufacturers or academicians' goodwill. CEURF focuses on personalized training, a slow but solid way to do. Our experiences have shown promising results. A 30 min session every week during 18 months covering the whole-body control has given an 18.5/20 accuracy [3]. Obviously, obtaining the value of 17.5/20 is shorter. A training for the limited BLUE-protocol, focusing only on an anterior analysis of lung sliding (yes/no) and lung rockets (yes/no), gives, after short sessions making a total of 90 min (90 min), an average accuracy of 19/20 (nineteen on twenty). A training focused on the lung part of the BLUE-protocol has given, after roughly seven sessions of 1 h, the accuracy of 19.5/20 (nineteen point five on twenty).

A Suggestion for the Training

There are now countless training centers, some world known, and we are glad to see this dynamism, so many years after our princeps publication [4]. CEURF remains different through seven peculiarities.

1. *A focused training*. Registrants benefit from a training focusing exclusively on points yielding *therapeutic management* of critical situations (that is, the definition of critical ultrasound). No energy is lost on noncritical points (physics of ultrasound, diaphragmatic visualization, no space for describing a steatosic liver, and many others), and it is carefully explained why. No time is lost for spectacular propaganda: we assume nowadays that physicians know "why" to use ultrasound and just want to know "how" to practice it.
2. *On-site training*. A unique *access at the bedside* of critically ill patients, in the ICU, i.e., not in healthy, vigorous but little informative models (but see below).
3. *Personalized training*. This bedside training is limited to two attendees – warranting a *personalized training*. One interest of the bedside step is to show optimal ways to hold the probe, have the best image, etc.
4. *Adapted training*. CEURF does not just copy traditional models of radiologic or cardiologic cultures (gallstones, use of Doppler, multiple probes, etc.). It provides a different approach, using an adapted unit, one universal probe, and adapted fields: the *lung* is the core of this approach, with respiratory *and hemodynamic* use. A traditional, expert approach to echocardiography with Doppler is *not* provided by CEURF. Adding simple emergency cardiac sonography, it shows an alternative approach for answering clinical questions, offering a direct parameter of *volemia* (FALLS-protocol) and a direct approach to respiratory failure (BLUE-protocol). Also is featuring the lung of the neonate, mesenteric infarction, pneumoperitoneum, optic nerve, the one-probe philosophy, the use of simplicity, mainly.
5. *Simplicity*. This is the keyword of CEURF, used at its extreme without compromise to the patient's safety. The consideration of the lung, with suitable machine and suitable approach, allows to simplify other fields (the heart). FALLS-protocol is a basic example.
6. *Homogeneous training*. It is warranted by the didactic potential coming from one lecturer. A one-author presentation is a drawback, since it expresses only one opinion. This drawback is balanced since this opinion (which is the one of simplicity anyway) is the one of a medical intensivist, with *26* years of ultrasound research at the bedside of critically ill patients seen between the ER and the ICU. Visiting professor, author of six textbooks, some dozens of publications, regularly invited in international congresses, he uses his didactic abilities for making critical ultrasound a *holistic* tool, centered by the lung.
7. *Long-term training*. The after-CEURF. Each CEURFer can use the line (infos@ceurf.net) without limitation of time for questions, comments, or advice. A *remote didactic refresher day* (included in the registration) allowed near CEURFers to see again, after several months of use, the didactic program. The personalized training favors contacts and makes way for future collaborations.

This textbook is usually fully dealt with in standard CEURF sessions.

CEURF has a fully autonomous system and is free from any commercial dependency (warranting its objectivity). CEURF makes all necessary efforts for making the participation lower each year, just because some attendees do not come with a hospital/academy help. The absence of advertisement makes one source among others of saving.

The registrants receive previously to the session a brochure detailing LUCI and the main protocols (BLUE, FALLS, SESAME).

Like the bat of our logo, who is as big as the last phalange of our thumb but gives birth to *one* baby each *year* (this is unique), we try to privilegiate quality (Fig. 38.1). The trained colleagues are then able to spread the method.

We give a simple clue to our attendees for making self-improvement.

First step: Once the attendee knows how to search for lung sliding, he or she must wait for a patient with confirmed pneumothorax. For the best didactic contribution, the pneumothorax should be complete in a quiet patient. The attendee must mandatorily find a stratosphere sign. If there is no stratosphere sign, there is a problem: Was the radiograph reversed by mistake? Is it the correct patient? Was the M-mode abusively used? After as many as possible examinations in known patients, the next step is aimed.

Second step: This step is searching for a stratosphere sign in a patient with an acute problem, making immediately the traditional management (X-rays, CT, etc., time permitting) and taking self-confidence little by little (but not yet taking any therapeutic decision based on sonography).

Third step: Facing a critically ill patient (with no time for confirmation) with clinical suspicion of pneumothorax, demonstrating a lung sliding should lead to *not* inserting a chest tube but driving the thought process in another direction. This softly initiates a life where the "traditional" losses (for difficult diagnosis) will gradually decrease, yielding to the ultrasound-enhanced critical care, a new discipline.

Training among colleagues in the same ICU is probably the best. Even if not many are trained per year, they transmit a solid knowledge in their next institution. If it had begun in 1982, using the quite perfect ADR-4000, critical ultrasound may be many decades old, completely included in the medical studies; the best way to teach is at school (see Anecdotal Note 1).

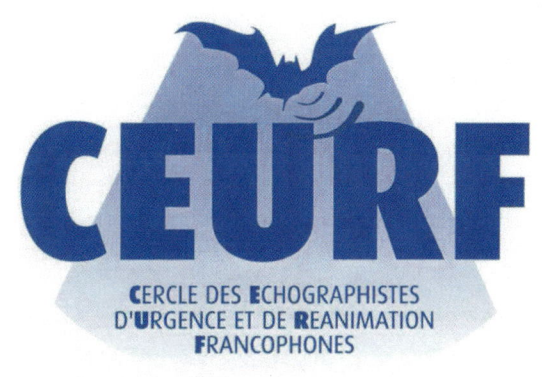

Fig. 38.1 The logo of our training center, the Cercle des Echographistes d'Urgence et de Réanimation Francophones (could be roughly translated as "Circle of Emergency Ultrasound for Resuscitation in French-speaking countries"). Pronounced *surf*. The benefits of this nonprofit association are used for spreading simple critical ultrasound development throughout the world. The bat is the only mammal who uses ultrasound, since 55 millions years ago. Apart from the popular dolphin (known for being rather smart), one bird also uses ultrasounds: the gray-rumped swift (the French word for swift is *martinet*), a really rare bird, who can fly while sleeping among others and was awarded Bird of the Year in 2003. For comparison, the bull has no ultrasound equipment for distinguishing the toreador from the cape – a providence for the toreador and the joyful crowd. Some people fear the bat, a nice and useful animal in the vast majority of cases. The snake in revenge killed many human beings but has been chosen as the symbol of medicine. For more details on this animal who looks like no other, see www. ceurf.net. The CEURF trains English-speaking colleagues but has kept its native label (just consider that the "F" became "foreign"). Small groups profit from a bedside training. The critically ill patient meanwhile profits from comprehensive ultrasound examinations, providing an ethical dimension to the CEURF

The Approach in Our Workshops: How to Make Our Healthy Models a Mine of Acute Diseases and How to Avoid Bothering Our Poor Lab Animals

We see with some concern that laboratory animals, pigs mainly, are used for simulation of lung diseases. We see with concern that simulators are sold by millions, in spite of the financial crisis. In our workshops, we have usually a young, normal slender model. How to take maximal advantage of his normality? We first build a whole scenario, imagining he just comes from a 14-h airplane travel (in economy class) from a wild area full of infectious diseases. He has major tobacco habits and allergy to airplane insecticides. Highly stressed during the flight by the prohibition of smoking, he took sleeping pills. The cabin crew found him comatose and woke him up. He vomited, then coughed a lot, then complained from sudden dyspnea and chest pain. You see him at the ER, severely dyspneic, near to encephalopathy. In the rooms behind, alcoholic folks generate major noise which prevents from serene auscultation. Our patient can have *all possible diseases*: pulmonary embolism, pneumonia (from the wild country or from aspiration), but also pulmonary edema complicating acute coronary syndrome, not to forget pneumothorax or again severe asthma.

1. We make an anterior examination, showing how to locate the upper and lower BLUE-points. We demonstrate the bat sign and the interest of longitudinal scans.
2. We demonstrate the half A-profile (expected in this model) at the right lung.
3. We check for the left lung sliding but insert our probe obliquely, *on the rib*, making profit of the M-lines, and demonstrate a motionless pattern with horizontal repetition artifacts, generating a stratosphere sign. This can look like a pneumothorax but without bat sign. This is simply a transversal technique that took a rib on purpose. We profit from this for explaining why we never use transversal or oblique scans, those details which would make ultrasound a confusing science.
4. Coming back to a correct technique, we demonstrate an A-profile (bilateral normal pattern). The A-profile invites to search for venous thrombosis. Using some black magic and a maneuver called the *Hypargonos* maneuver, so to speak, we insert a probe that has discretely been inverted at the internal jugular area, with a pressure sufficient for making the vein vanish. The screen displays the artery and, apparently outside, a tubular tissue-like structure: the body of the thyroid gland, used as a model of occlusive jugular internal venous thrombosis. The diagnosis of pulmonary embolism is done with a 99 % specificity [5].
5. Coming back to a correct technique, we search for B-lines at the physiologic locations. If no B-line at all is visible, we search for GB-lines in the abdomen, sometimes visible at the jejunal areas (and ask the attendees to imagine that these artifacts arise from the pleural line). We then search for Z-lines, usually always found, and point out the five basic differences. We ask the attendees to imagine three B-lines (i.e., lung rockets) per scan and diffuse lung rockets at the four anterior BLUE-points, making the diagnosis of hemodynamic pulmonary edema (specificity 95 %) [5].
6. We then illustrate a nude profile, making a rapid venous ultrasound scan at the V-point (this portion near the knee, reputed to be impossible to compress, a symbol in our vision of simple ultrasound), showing in 3 s a normal collapsibility – extrapolate to the rest of the venous system for saving time. The BLUE-protocol asks us to come back to the lung, searching for PLAPS.
7. With some more black magic (using the *Hypargonos* maneuver), we show at the left lateral wall a frank pneumonia at the lingula, tissue-like image touching the wall, with often air bronchograms, and the shred line. Podally is a normally aerated lung. The diagnosis of lingular pneumonia is done. Facing this A-no-V-PLAPS-profile, we conclude to a pneumonia. This is of course the simple spleen with an inversed probe.
8. Coming back to a correct technique, we analyze the PLAPS-point and demonstrate a nude profile (normal lung surface, normal venous system). This young man shows the profile of acute asthma, with a 97 % specificity [5].
9. Attendees want to see a pneumothorax? Just use your mouth (a cavity full of air) and don't bother the pigs! The probe inserted at the cheek will show an A'-profile, using the mucosa as the equivalent of the pleural line. They want to see a lung point? Just gently apply your *tongue* toward the cheek, with respiratory intervals; they will see quite

exactly what a pneumothorax looks like. Tongue in French is langue. This is, so to speak, the langue point.

It is at the time given difficult to simulate on-site pleural effusion, but we can show what pattern could be given by a pyothorax or again a hydropneumothorax (shaking our contact bottle). For those who are not tired and want to go beyond the BLUE-protocol, we can again simulate a peanut aspiration, by demonstrating a right abolished lung sliding with standstill cupola and the lung pulse, whereas the left lung sliding and cupola work correctly (we just talked previously with the model for agreeing on a signal to make him discretely halt breathing).

All in all, we are able to demonstrate, in our usual, healthy models and step-by-step pneumothorax, pulmonary embolism, pulmonary edema, pneumonia, acute asthma, empyema, and foreign body with complete atelectasis. This is acquired just using some imagination, i.e., for free, avoiding costly simulators, or murdering these (costly!) lab animals.

A more important detail, we prove that there is no magic in all that, just (intentional) bad technique, easy to avoid. Our main message is *do it yourself*, to avoid any kind of manipulation or clumsiness from unskilled young radiology operators.

We complete the training with hands on by ultrasound-guided catheterization in the lab, using tofu bricks, for cheap.

Anecdotal Note
1. Wild ultrasound

What is *wild ultrasound*? Many physicians had no choice but perform it in the solitude of a night shift in the hospital (what the author experienced too). Perfectly aware of his limited knowledge but facing an uncontrolled situation, a physician would be tempted to use the ultrasound machine (now that countless laptop machines have invaded our corridors). Aware of the deontology, which obliges any physician to use any means in case of extreme emergencies if there is no choice, barely remembering one or two lectures, he would try to do his best for taking again the situation under control. This is wild ultrasound. We hope that the number of situations clarified with ultrasound has exceeded the number of cases where the ultrasound unit should not have been switched on. We believe the intensivists and emergency physicians, who make a respectable work, will not tarnish the method [6, 7] and will use the way of humility and conscience above all.

References

1. CEURF (Cercle des Echographistes d'Urgence et de Réanimation Francophone) (2003) Journal Officiel de la République Française du 12 avril 2003, 135ème année, n°15:1808, p 2057. Association 1901 N° 0783011403 – www.CEURF.net
2. SLAM (Section for the Limitation of Acronyms in Medicine) (2009) Déclaration du 1er avril 2008. Journal Officiel de la République Française, 26 avril 2008 n° 17, p 2009
3. Lichtenstein D, Mezière G (1998) Apprentissage de l'échographie générale d'urgence par le réanimateur. Réan Urg 7(Suppl 1):108
4. Lichtenstein D, Axler O (1993) Intensive use of general ultrasound in the intensive care unit, a prospective study of 150 consecutive patients. Intensive Care Med 19:353–355
5. Lichtenstein D, Mezière G (2008) Relevance of lung ultrasound in the diagnosis of acute respiratory failure. The BLUE-protocol. Chest 134:117–125
6. Filly RA (1988) Ultrasound: the stethoscope of the future, alas. Radiology 167:400
7. Weiss PH, Zuber M, Jenzer HR, Ritz R (1990) Echocardiography in emergency medicine: tool or toy? Schweiz Rundschau Med Praxis 47:1469–1472

Lung Ultrasound: A Tool Which Contributes in Making Critical Ultrasound a Holistic Discipline and Maybe a Philosophy

39

Critical ultrasound is a bit more than a new tool – it is also a philosophy. Created from 1912 events (the sonar, born from the Titanic wreckage), adapted to the patient in the year 1950, adapted to the critically ill in the early 1990s, and becoming widely appreciated these recent years, lung ultrasound in the critically ill – LUCI – should first be considered through scientific appraisals: life savings, cost savings, and evidence-based medicine, which would definitely prove its value. It may also be considered a bit of a philosophy. The saved time, the spared irradiation, the increased comfort to the patient, and the comfort of the clinician facing critical situations, so to speak this kind of *elegance* used around the concept of point-of-care medicine, cannot be scientifically measured and are maybe as important.

To make ultrasound a kind of philosophy is a lesser problem. Some would love to make it a religion, and we should feel flattered to see our life's work turned into such a mystic glow. Yet if it is considered as a "religion" more than a tool, human factors may appear and uncontrolled events can happen. Blindness to some limitations and fights for power, all these obscure points would spoil its spirit. Critical ultrasound, lung ultrasound, BLUE-protocol, etc., are just tools. Powerful, elegant, allowing to see acute dramas through a visual approach it is true, but just tools, with limitations.

As regards LUCI, which is a major part of critical ultrasound (at least, our opinion!), most of these limitations could be taught from reading existing experience. Some will appear in the battlefield, since they are not yet known (probably because of their rarity), but this perspective should bring humility – and caution – in the concept. Conversely, we fully admit that we feel the triumph of simplicity in each case where LUCI is used *instead* of the giants of modern imaging (the newest multislice CT generations, RMI, sophisticated echocardiography) and answers the clinical question: one small drop of a philosophy. Again attached to this idea, this textbook could have been written in 1982; the ADR-4000 was at this remote period a perfect tool. Those who remain persuaded that CT is "fast" should see that (our) ultrasound is the fastest of all tools in medical imaging.

What is holistic ultrasound, by the way? This is maybe the time here to define this term we used countless times throughout the textbook! Far from mystical definitions, a discipline is holistic when the understanding of each of its components is necessary for understanding the whole. Each component interacts with the others, hence, this (rather) thick book. The word "harmony" should rule holistic ultrasound: one simple unit; one single probe, but not any probe (a microconvex) (our Japanese microconvex probe more precisely); the lung at the center of our use; a logic adapted to a visual medicine with the humble aim of simplifying critical care.

Critical ultrasound is holistic because it puts together several elements which, taken one by one, would be difficult to understand. We do not use Doppler; a reader not aware of all these potentials, including our hemodynamic assessment, would hardly accept this idea. No Doppler? All these elements make sense when they are considered altogether. Why are a simple unit and a single probe for the whole body suitable? Why does CEURF not use laptop machines? Why is ultrasound not used during a thoracentesis? There are dozens of examples.

The lines which follow were written as an exercise, where one line is linked to the next one. The reader will find a mingling between simplistic elements (wheels, lateral stands, etc.) and scientific ones (the science of lung artifacts). This mingling is one more typical example of holistic ultrasound. Let us begin:

Defining lung ultrasound allows to completely rebuild the traditional landscape of ultrasound.

Since the manufacturers do not know that the most important element is not fully developed in the up-to-date machines, the simplicity of older units is a vindication.

Incorporating lung ultrasound and refining venous ultrasound allow to simplify echocardiography.

This simplification contributes to the one-probe philosophy.

The one-probe philosophy allows, instead of several probes with lateral stands which increase the lateral size, to put the (single) probe on the top of the machine.

This top is found in a machine like ours (in laptops, no top for any object to be put above).

Without those lateral stands, this consequence: the unit arrives sooner at the bedside.

Such machines are possibly heavier than laptops; this is not a problem since they have wheels, a revolutionary technology (probably *disruptive* when it was invented in the Mesopotamian times, a really flashy word, on fashion, but which should not be reserved only to modern times!) which allows to transport heavy material without effort.

These wheels are intended for machines on a trolley, an excellent point which makes it so easy to transport for any hospital use.

This is a winning point regarding these following settings where space is an issue: ICUs, operating theaters, ERs, etc.

But paradoxically and probably far more, it regards all these settings where space is not at all an issue: the infinite (but austere) spaces where people live with minimal resources; those very ones who will appreciate the low cost of this single-probe unit and perform a cost-effective medicine.

These "undesirable" artifacts, always disdained, can build life saving diagnoses: pneumothorax, pulmonary edema, etc.

Poor and rich settings will profit of the simplicity (of the unit, of the technique) for training physicians more efficiently, mastering more rapidly a multifaceted tool. They will see critically ill patients as well as patients from pulmonology, pediatrics, cardiology ... a.m.o., and most of all: without any technical adaptation. Same unit, same approach.

Our tool since 1992, hopingly your tool tomorrow.

This also is holistic ultrasound.

Holistic ultrasound lastly considers a critical detail never to forget. Decades ago, before this magic era, before this mystical world, we, the doctors, did not kill them all! Some survived in spite of our (blind) care. Said differently, we have all made a good job without ultrasound (read Endnote 1). Now, this new tool will help us, just to make it better.

Endnote 1

In this book, we often spoke of these countless victims of pre-ultrasound medicine, these stars in the sky, etc., and now we use a more balanced vision. This is the simplest illustration that one can see everything and its opposite, even (especially) in medicine. This explains the duration of the morning visits, where the same management of the previous night can be laudated or shot down at will; all these pro-con debates and why a chair must be a leader for imposing a certain idea may be the opposed of the one of the hospital next door. It just reminds us that medicine is a philosophical occupation, and all these issues become clear. Knowing all details which define the B-line is one thing. But from time to time, succeeding in unsticking your sight from the screen, in looking your patients in the eyes and those who surround you in this room, including your colleagues, you will maybe, like Luke Skywalker, close the gunsight and just trust your instinct. Just from time to time, for keeping controlling clinical medicine. Making the correct diagnosis is the absolute basis, but remaining a doctor, i.e., a human being, should come immediately after. We feel, more and more, that the best use of ultrasound, the most gratifying, is when we can do a medical diagnosis without! This is for us the summit of elegance in medicine. We confirm usually with ultrasound, just for respecting its spirit: a fully noninvasive tool confirming we were right, another nice use of bedside ultrasound.

Maybe our next book will deal with philosophy, just trying to insert our life's findings within a philosophical "truth." In all fields, the best is possibly to see something with two visions. Ultrasound is our tool, used with passion but not religion. We have just to spend our time to understand, without any judgment, why this so simple tool took so much time to be accepted and controlled by the academy and become a standard of care. Maybe there is not a lot to explain; just taking back a word of Max Planck, the only secret is possibly to begin young. Beginning young was our best idea. Now, this book is quite over, resuming with technical notes (glossary, index...). We tried to delete any possible syntax mistake. If cautious readers find some errors anyway, they will for sure keep in mind that this book, fully devoted to a discipline which was not supposed to exist, erases a much bigger (and maybe historical) mistake!

Suggestion for Classifying Air Artifacts

40

Some artifacts are useless, others life-saving. The idea of suppressing all of them without discrimination is questionable. Technologies which will keep lung rockets alive will obviously keep alive the others, therefore, this short chapter. It intends to clarify the minds, describing all what can be encountered in the human being. Nothing is completely simple in medicine, and we aimed, in alphabetical order but some logic too, at decreasing the effort of memory. Remember that only two have a major clinical relevance, A-lines and B-lines (Fig. 40.1):

A-lines (A for the first letter)
  Lung
    Horizontal hyperechoic artifacts arising from the pleural line at regular intervals which are equal to the skin-pleural line distance – indicating physiologic gas as well as free gas– as shown in Chap. 9.
    A1, A2, etc., lines: Number of A-lines arising from the pleural line (not a very useful data).

B-lines (B for the second letter, also because this label is culturally linked to interstitial syndrome for the past 80 years. We specify in fact "ultrasound B-lines") shown in Chap. 11
  Lung
    Artifacts defined according to seven criteria:
      A. Constant criteria:
        1. Comet-tail artifacts
        2. Arising from the pleural line
        3. Moving with lung sliding
      B. Almost constant criteria:
        4. Well defined, laser beam-like
        5. Long, not fading
        6. Erasing A-lines
        7. Hyperechoic (like the pleural line)
b-line: one B-line visible between two ribs. The term b-line is always singular.
bb-lines: two B-lines.
B+ lines: three or more B-lines, again, visible between two ribs.
Septal rockets (ex-B7-lines): B+ lines separated in adults by 6–7 mm, i.e., the distance between two interlobular septa (interlobular septal thickening). Between two ribs, usually 3 or 4 B-lines.
Ground-glass rockets (ex-B3-lines): B+ lines separated in adults by 3 mm, i.e., twice as many B-lines, possibly explained by extreme cases of interstitial syndrome. They are correlated with CT ground-glass lesions.
Birolleau variant: so many B-lines that the Merlin's space appears homogeneously hyperechoic.
Sub-B-lines: see below.

C-lines (like centimetric cupuliform consolidation) shown in Chap. 17
  Lung, real image (the exception in this chapter)
    Curvilinear centimetric piece of alveolar consolidation abutting the pleural line. "Pleural-based" small lung consolidation, in other words.

D.A. Lichtenstein, *Lung Ultrasound in the Critically Ill: The BLUE Protocol*,
DOI 10.1007/978-3-319-15371-1_40, © Springer International Publishing Switzerland 2016

Suggested classification of thoracic artifacts

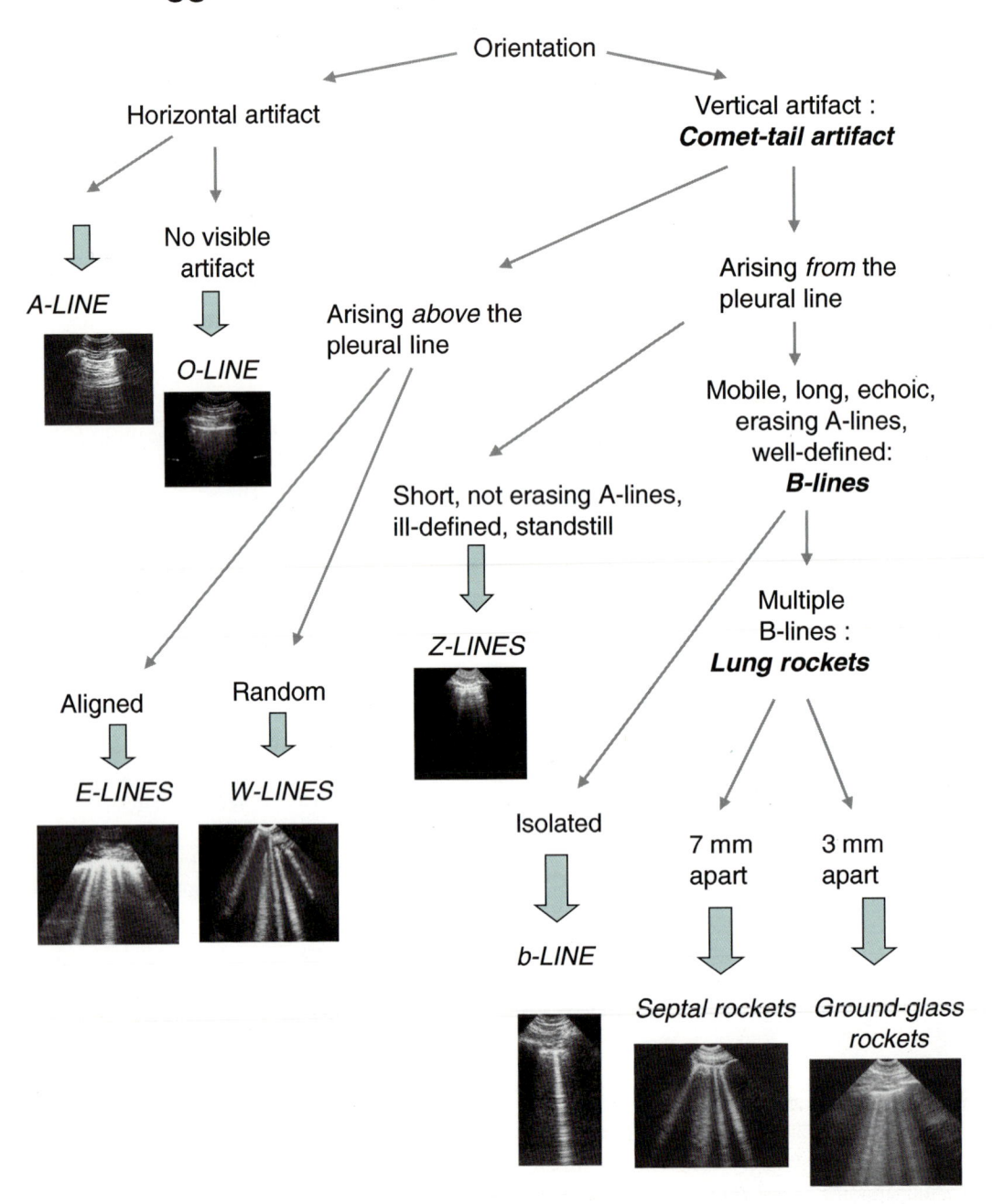

Fig. 40.1 Filiation between comet-tail, B-lines, and lung rockets. The main thoracic artifacts. This figure shows the scientific filiation between names sometimes confused in the brains. Lung rockets are a certain kind of B-lines. The B-line is a certain kind of comet-tail artifact. This figure aims at showing that lung ultrasound is a simple discipline, where confusions should not exist once the field has been standardized

40 Suggestion for Classifying Air Artifacts

D-lines
  Available space

E-lines (for emphysema) shown in Chap. 14
  Subcutaneous tissues
    Comet-tail artifacts laser-like, hyperechoic, and spreading to the edge of the screen, but arising *not* from the pleural line, but from a hyperechoic line horizontally located above the pleural line (erased by these E-lines). Stripe of subcutaneous emphysema. No bat sign is visible: we are not in lung ultrasonography.

F-lines (from Fabien Rolland, a CEURFer)
  F like Fantôme (ghost) also. Designates all these punctiform or oblique lines sometimes found in the Merlin's space at normal lung surface and mimicking, for novice eyes, air bronchograms (Fig. 40.2).

G-lines (like guts)
  Extra lung
    G-A-, G-B-, and G-Z-lines (Fig. 40.2)
      Describes any kind of artifact (horizontal, comet-tail, ring down) visible at the abdomen. They look exactly like A-lines, B-lines, and Z-lines, but arise from abdominal structures. Main relevance: the G-B lines can act as (lung) B-lines, which are useful in workshops with too "healthy" models who have no B-line at all.

H-lines (for the geometric, symmetrical shape of the H)
  Roughly horizontal lines (in fact, bended lines using microconvex probes but appearing roughly horizontal at the center) arising from any air area (a probe on its stand, the air of the ICU room), demonstrating that air generates horizontal lines (such as A-lines at the lung area) (Fig. 40.2).

I-lines (like the letter i)
  Lung. Comet-tail artifacts. Rare pattern. Have the features of the B-lines but are short (2–3 cm). Unknown meaning (seen in healthy subjects).

J-lines (for Julie) shown in Chap. 11
  Lung artifacts
  Small horizontal hyperechoic lines (1–3 mm width) superposed from the pleural line to the bottom of the screen, each 1–2 mm, and generating the B-line

K-lines (K for Klingons).
  Any location
  Designates parasite artifacts due to environmental electric interferences (Fig. 40.3).

Lung rockets
  See B-lines.

L-lines
  Available space

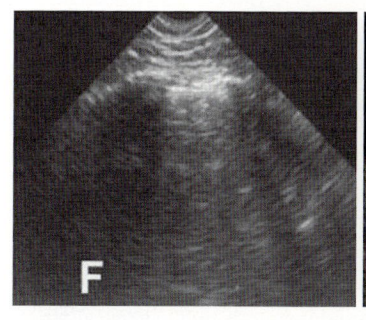

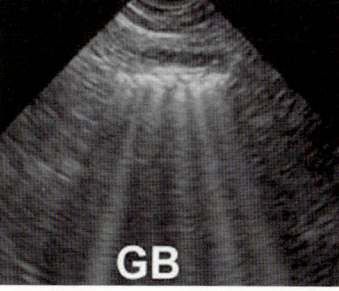

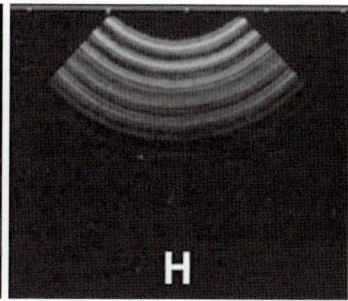

Fig. 40.2 F-lines, GB-lines, and H-lines. *F* F-lines. These hyperechoic punctiform artifacts, if standstill whereas a lung sliding is identified, have no other meaning than parasites – and should never be confused with air bronchograms. Such "air bronchograms" should be very static. Very because not only they do not show the pattern of the dynamic air bronchogram, but above all because they do not move, whereas lung sliding is identified. Real air bronchograms should follow lung sliding. In addition, the Merlin's space never displays a shred sign in these cases (nor a frank tissue-like sign or the mediastinal line): all signs of lung consolidation. *GB* No bat sign? This is not lung ultrasound. It helps however in workshops, on occasion. GB-lines are abdominal artifacts, possibly indicating jejunal loops. *H* H-lines. When the probe lies on its stand, horizontal hyperechoic lines are generated, remember from far to the A-lines

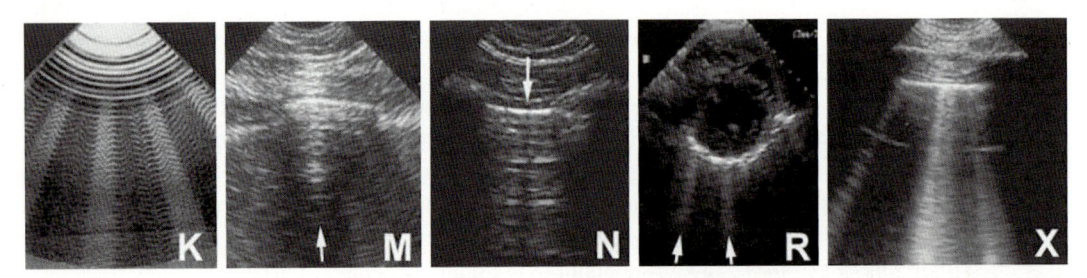

Fig. 40.3 Some comet-tail artifacts are not to be confused with B-lines. *Left*, K-lines, coming from rough parasites from the sector (need filter between the ultrasound machine and the electric socket). *More right*: M-lines, small horizontal artifacts often seen arising from the rib, within its acoustic shadow (*arrow*). *Middle*, N-line (*arrow*). *More right*: the R-lines, those comet-tail artifacts arising from the pericardium at the lung interface. *Full right*, X-lines, a (rare) variant where some typical B-lines are however erased by A-lines

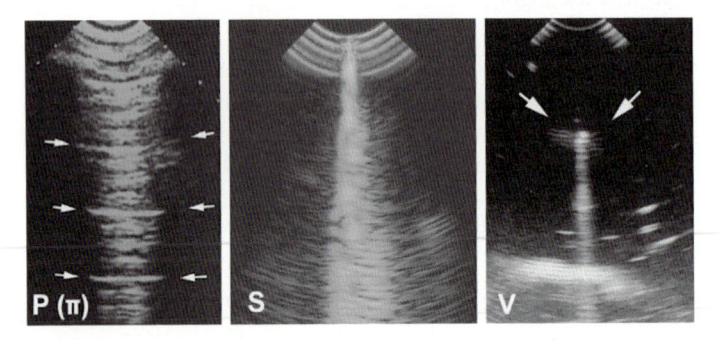

Fig. 40.4 Pi-lines, S-lines, and V-lines. *P* From a distance, some observers may describe a vertical artifact. Yet it is done here by three A-lines clearly identified (*arrows*). Between two A-lines, two smaller horizontal artifacts are visible: the sub-A-lines. When a normal anterior lung surface (also visible in some cases of pneumothorax) displays this pattern, we speak of Pi-lines. This patient had, by the way, a pneumothorax. *S* Look at this sinuous artifact. Metallic bar of an ICU bed here. *V* The tip of this needle (*arrows*) generates also a comet-tail artifact, near the B-line, but not tributary of any pleural line

M-lines (for Fernand Macone)
  Small horizontal hyperechoic artifacts sometimes generated below the rib surface. Cannot be confused with A-lines (search for the bat sign) (Fig. 40.3). We sometimes use the M-lines for didactic applications (simulating a pneumothorax).

N-lines (for Noir, black; also for Neri)
  Lung
    Artifacts with roughly 6 of the 7 patterns of B-lines, just they are hypoechoic. Nothing to do with B-lines. Probably devoid of pathologic meaning. Wink to Luca Neri, who witnessed them once (Fig. 40.3).

O-lines (for non-A-non-B) shown in Chap. 9
  Lung
    Absence of any visible artifact either horizontal or vertical nor anatomical image of pleural or alveolar change arising from the pleural line. Assimilated clinically with A-lines.

P-lines or Pi-lines or π-lines (look like the Greek letter π)
  Lung
    In some (usually skinny) patients, the A-lines can be numerous, associated with sub-A-lines and even sub-sub-A-lines. Candid eyes would see a roughly vertical structure – reminder of the letter π. Yet they

40 Suggestion for Classifying Air Artifacts

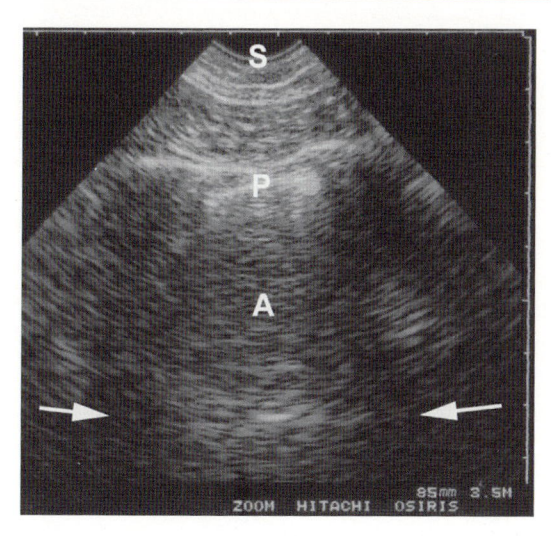

Fig. 40.5 Powell-lines. Sometimes, an oblique artifact (arrows) is visible in Merlin's space. It is not parallel to the pleural line, not at the expected location of the A-lines (*A*), i.e., in a distance equal to the skin (*S*) – pleural line (*P*) distance. No known meaning

are at the foreseen distance (skin/pleural line), their length is roughly the one of the pleural line (B-lines are roughly one-tenth of the pleural line distance), and the A-lines are clearly identified, between all these sub-A-lines and sub-sub-A-lines (Fig. 40.4).

Powell-lines (from Elisabeth Powell, CEURFer from Toronto)
  Lung
    Oblique hyperechoic line sometimes visible in the depth of the Merlin's space (Fig. 40.5)

Q-lines
  Available space

R-lines (from Roberta Capp)
  Comet-tail artifacts having quite all the features of the B-lines but arising from the deep pericardium at the interface with the lung in short-axis left ventricle views (Fig. 40.3).

S-lines (look like S-shaped lines)
  Extra-lung
    Characteristic sinuous propagation generated by large metallic structures (pacemakers). Round metallic bars generate beautiful S-lines (Fig. 40.4).

Sub-A-lines
  These are horizontal lines sometimes visible between A-lines or between the pleural line and an A-line. There can be one, two, or more. Limited relevance. See Pi-lines in Fig. 40.4.

Sub-B-lines – shown in Fig. 16.3
  They really look like B-lines, and all novice users make the confusion (the "butterfly" syndrome). Yet, if all other criteria are present, they arise not from the pleural line but from the lung line. This distinction is important since the BLUE information are hierarchized. If we see sub-B-lines, it means that there is a pleural effusion, an information superior to the one of interstitial syndrome.

T-lines (they look like the letter T) shown in Fig. 10.8
  Lung
    M-mode concept. Fine vertical lines that strictly arise from the pleural line (or, seen from downstairs, strictly stop at the very pleural line). They are a very narrow equivalent of the lung pulse and mean absence of pneumothorax.

U-lines
  Abdomen
    Arciform artifact generated by bowel loops, shaping a reversed U. Found at the colon areas (see Fig. 6.1 of our 2010 edition).

V-lines
  Labelled in August 2014. Chosen because of the shape of the letter V (sharp like the tip of a needle). The V-line is an artifact

generated by a metallic structure, usually a needle inserted in a biological, hydric space. Like the B-line, it is a comet-tail, well-defined, long without fading, and hyperechoic. Unlike the B-line, it does not of course erase from the pleural line, does not move with lung sliding, and does not erase A-lines (Fig. 40.4).

W-lines (shape of the letter W)
    Comet-tail artifact
    Subcutaneous tissues
        Variety of artifacts looking like E-lines, but not aligned. They are the consequence of multiple air bubbles randomly located within the soft tissues (parietal, subcutaneous, surgical emphysema) (Fig. 40.1).

X-lines (like the shape of an X)
    Lung
        Infrequent case where B-lines and A-lines are simultaneously visible, resulting in a crossing image (Fig. 40.3).

Y-lines
    Available space

Z-lines (for the last letter of the alphabet)
    Lung artifacts
        Parasites having two common points with the B-lines (comet-tail artifacts, arising from the pleural line) and five opposed points: not hyperechoic (rather gray at the onset), not well defined, not long (3–4 cm), not erasing A-lines, and not moving with lung sliding. No known meaning, genuine parasites to our knowledge, and in no case to be confused with B-lines. Shown in Fig. 11.4 and Video 11.1.

Glossary

41

Here most of the technical words coined or used for the BLUE-protocol and LUCI are featured. The artifacts, benefiting from Chap. 40, are just listed.

A-lines Please refer to Chap. 40.

A/B-profile (BLUE-protocol) Predominance of A-lines at one lung and of B-lines at the other, in Stage 1.

Anechoic Free of echo. The tone is black by convention.

A-predominance (FALLS-protocol) Detection of either an A-profile, A'-profile, or A/B-profile.

A-profile (BLUE-protocol) Association of predominant A-lines and lung sliding in Stage 1.

A'-profile (BLUE-protocol) Association of predominant A-lines and abolished lung sliding in Stage 1.

A-DVT profile (BLUE-protocol) Association of an A-profile with a deep venous thrombosis. Association quite specific to pulmonary embolism.

A-no-V-PLAPS-profile (BLUE-protocol) The longest label. Association of an A-profile with an absence of deep venous thrombosis and the presence of a PLAPS.

Artifact Artificial image created by the physical principles of propagation of the ultrasound beams. The shape is always geometrical with precise symmetrical axes. Artifacts do not correspond to real anatomical structures.

Avicenne's sign In the case of a pneumothorax (generating absence of movement) in a dyspneic patient (generating muscular movements), the use of M-mode allows to detect the standstillness of the pleural line through the dynamic of the muscular recruitment. When the column of sand which appears above the pleural line crosses the pleural line and remains fully unchanged, this demonstrates that lung sliding is definitely abolished. This is the Avicenne's sign.

Bat sign In the initial and basic step of any lung ultrasound, the bat sign identifies in a longitudinal view the upper and lower ribs (the wings) and, deeper, the pleural line (the belly of the bat). This step makes it possible to correctly locate the pulmonary structures in any conditions.

Bat wing sign Special pattern displayed by a peritoneal effusion, surrounded by convex limits. This sign is of interest for detecting non-anechoic effusions (i.e., the most severe cases).

Bed level (at) When the probe explores the lateral chest wall in a supine patient and cannot explore more posterior (without moving the patient) because of the bed, the probe is said to be applied at bed level (or FDL). If pleural effusion is visible at bed level, this means that this effusion has substantial volume.

B-lines Please refer to Chap. 40.

BLUE-hands Two hands applied on the thorax, one above another, thumbs excepted, beginning just below the clavicle immediately show the lung location (the lowest finger being usually at the chest/abdomen junction. The term "BLUE"-hands means that the hands are those, theoretically, of the patient (from any size, any age).

BLUE-consolidation index, BLUE-pleural index Approximate way to rapidly and simply estimate the volume of a lung consolidation or a pleural effusion (Chap. 28). A standardized area of measurement in a standardized position of the patient (supine, slightly turned to the opposed way), a standardized location (the PLAPS-point), and a standardized probe (a microconvex probe that can be inserted far to the posterior wall). The expiratory distance between pleural line and lung line roughly correlate with the abundance of the effusion.

BLUE-protocol This is a fast protocol for diagnosis of the cause in acutely blue patients. It associates bedside lung ultrasound in an emergency and a venous scanning adapted to the critically ill. The BLUE-protocol proposes simple profiles helping in assessing the cause of an acute respiratory failure.

BLUE-points Standardized locations immediately accessible and allowing immediate diagnosis of the main life-threatening disorders. In the BLUE-protocol, two anterior points and one subposterior point are used.

B-predominance (FALLS-protocol) Detection of either a B-profile or a B'-profile.

Carmen maneuver This basic probe movement makes critical ultrasound easier. The probe is applied on the skin, without excessive pressure. It is gently shifted like a large paintbrush, i.e., to the left then right when the probe is in a longitudinal position or to the top then to the bottom in a transversal position, taking advantage of the gliding of the skin over the underskin, i.e., staying at the same position. It allows to control the three dimensions: in a longitudinal scan, it shows lateral images, i.e., scans transversally, without losing the target.

B-profile (BLUE-protocol) Association of predominant lung rockets and lung sliding in Stage 1.

B'-profile (BLUE-protocol) Association of predominant lung rockets and abolished lung sliding in Stage 1.

C-lines Please refer to Chap. 40.

C-profile (BLUE-protocol) Detection of alveolar syndrome in Stage 1 (anterior chest wall, supine patient, Earth level).

CLOT-protocol (Catheter-Linked Occult Thromboses protocol) Daily analysis of the venous areas which have received cannulation in long-staying patients, performed routinely and after any acute worsening. By making early detection and follow-up of the deep venous thromboses, it allows to help in the diagnosis of pulmonary embolism in these challenging patients.

Comet-tail artifact This term designates a repetition artifact which is hyperechoic and roughly vertical. It can arise *or not* from the pleural line. It can move in concert with the pleural line *or not*. It can be long *or not*. It can be well defined *or not*. It can erase other underlying structures *or not*. It can be hyperechoic like the pleural line *or not*. Many comet-tail artifacts can be described, the B-line (for interstitial syndrome) being one of them.

Consolidation index Simple measurement of an alveolar consolidation using an area at a given point and assuming that the consolidation has roughly three similar dimensions.

Culminating (sign, point) This term refers to the sky-Earth axis and indicates something near the sky.

Dark lung (ultrasound dark lung) A situation where a diffusely hypoechoic pattern is recorded at the chest wall, with no static or dynamic element that can affirm a solid or fluid predominance. The radiograph usually shows a white lung.

Dependent (sign, point) This term refers to the sky-Earth axis and indicates something near the Earth.

DIAFORA approach This term describes the use of Doppler when necessary, using an outside machine and an outside operator and, if necessary, transporting the patient (as done for the CT examinations). DIAFORA means Doppler Intermittently Asked From Outside in Rare Applications. It allows the physician to, meanwhile, rapidly benefit from a cost-effective machine which will be of daily help. The concept is based on the rarity of these situations and based also on the degree of emergency, which usually allows to wait open hours.

Doppler hand This designates the free hand of the operator, which will replace the Doppler function for compressing the veins, even at reputedly noncompressible areas (see V-point).

Dynamic air bronchogram Alveolar consolidation within which hyperechoic punctiform particles (indicating the air bronchograms) have a centrifuge inspiratory movement. This is characteristic of nonretractile consolidation (pneumonia in clinical practice).

Echoic In principle, a tone with the same echostructure as a reference structure (classically, the liver). Usually, "echoic" designates a structure rather "hyperechoic," i.e., near a white tone.

E-lines Please refer to Chap. 40.

Escape sign When suspecting occlusive venous thrombosis, a slight pressure of the probe makes the whole of the soft tissues move, but the proximal and distal walls of the vein do not change. The vein seems to escape from the probe. This indicates the noncompressibility of the vein, when compared to the surrounding soft tissues which receive appropriate pressure.

F-lines Please refer to Chap. 40.

G-lines Please refer to Chap. 40.

Gain Setting the device to provide a well-balanced reference image. The upper parts of the screen can be lightened or darkened (near gain), as can the lower parts (far gain). The gain can be standardized (see Fig. 1.3).

Grotowski law This is an adaptation of the probability law when sequentially organized in the critical care setting, here using the help of the visual medicine (ultrasound). In this field, death is a frequent event. Using a multiplication of probabilities, enhanced by the use of ultrasound, the risk of deleterious management appears more and more infinitesimal. For instance, the error risk of the ultrasound approach of the BLUE-protocol, combined with the clinical data and basic tests, can be advantageously compared with approaches using usual tools which can have side effects (helical CT in each dyspneic patient for instance).

If a diagnosis is rare, and if precisely the patient has an atypical presentation of this (presumed) rare disease, another disease, more frequent, should be sought for.

As last example, if a common procedure based on a potential mistake can anyway be of help to the patient, its use should be considered. Aeroportia is a rare diagnosis. Mistakes can be done (confusion with aerobilia, usually of lesser severity) but hesitations at this moment should be deleterious. In a patient with septic shock plus abdominal pain plus possible aeroportia, a laparotomy may (in this rare event, reminder) make more good than harm. Even if the ultrasound sign of aeroportia was misleading, it should be considered that laparotomy is often useful in the management of septic shock of unknown origin – for a precise evaluation of the real risk.

Gut sliding Dynamic generated by the visceral peritoneal layer against the parietal layer in rhythm with respiration. Rules out pneumoperitoneum.

H-lines Please refer to Chap. 40.

Hyperechoic Tone located between the reference pattern (classically the liver) and what is called the white tone.

Hypoechoic Tone located between the reference pattern and a black (anechoic) tone.

I-lines Please refer to Chap. 40.

Induced sinusoid sign A peritoneal effusion can be echoic (mimicking tissue), but the probe pressure decreases the thickness of this image, demonstrating its fluid and free nature.

Interpleural variation See "sinusoid."

Iso-echoic Tone equal to a reference structure (classically, the liver).

J-lines Please refer to Chap. 40.

Jellyfish sign Visualization of particular dynamics of the inferior pulmonary strip within a substantial pleural effusion. In rhythm with respiration and heartbeats like a jellyfish.

K-line Please refer to Chap. 40.

Keyes' space In an M-mode image, rectangle limited downward by the pleural line (from Linda Keyes, CEURFer).

Keyes' sign Accidents visible at the Keyes' space, normally stratified. It indicates substantial dyspnea.

Lateralization maneuver Maneuver of placing the arm of the supine patient at the contralateral shoulder. Several centimeters of the posterior aspect of the lung are thus accessible and can be explored using ultrasound, probe pointing toward the sky. This is in actual fact an extended PLAPS-point, a maneuver allowing to see a small effusion with more sensitivity.

Lower BLUE-point When the BLUE-hands are applied on the thoracic wall, point defined by the middle of the lower palm – for immediate diagnosis of pneumothorax and interstitial syndrome.

LUCIFLR project Also LUCIFLR program, since many physicians using LUCI enter into it, aware or not. Lung Ultrasound in the Critically Ill Favoring Limitation of Radiation. This acronym has been thoroughly worked in order to show that the idea of eradicating the radiographies would not be a scientific thought process.

Lung line Deep border of a pleural effusion, regular by definition (see the quad sign), indicating the visceral pleura.

Lung point Sudden and fleeting appearance, generally on inspiration, of a lung sign with lung sliding and/or lung rockets and/or alteration of A-lines, at a precise area of the chest wall where abolished lung sliding and exclusive A-lines were previously observed. Specific sign of pneumothorax.

Lung pulse Visualization at the pleural line of vibrations in rhythm with the heart rate. Means abolished lung sliding, rules out pneumothorax, possibly indicates massive atelectasis.

Lung rockets They designate several B-lines (more than two) between two ribs. Have the meaning of interstitial syndrome.

Lung sliding Dynamics – a kind of to-and-fro twinkling – visible at the whole of the Merlin's space, beginning at the very level of the pleural line.

M-lines Please refer to Chap. 40.

Merlin's space An image framed by the pleural line, the shadow of the ribs, and the lower border of the screen. The Merlin's space can be artifactual (normal subject, interstitial edema, pneumothorax) or anatomic (alveolar or pleural syndrome). From Elisabeth Merlin, CEURFer

M-mode Analysis of dynamics passing along a precise line. A posteriori, the reading of the image alone detects the observed dynamics. M-mode is opposed to two-dimensional observations.

N-lines Please refer to Chap. 40.

Nude profile (BLUE-protocol) Normal lung examination, with A-profile, absence of PLAPS and free venous axes.

O-lines Please refer to Chap. 40.

Out-of-plane (effect) An image that leaves the plane of the ultrasound beam can give a false impression of dynamics. To be distinguished from true dynamics.

Phrenic point One of the four standardized points of lung ultrasound, used to analyze phrenic function. Intersection between the middle axillary line and the horizontal line prolongating the lowest BLUE-finger (see BLUE-hands).

Plankton sign Numerous punctiform echoic images within an anechoic or echo-poor collection. These images have slow, whirling dynamics, as in weightlessness.

P-lines Please refer to Chap. 40.

PLAPS Posterior and/or Lateral Alveolar and/or Pleural Syndrome. In other words, detection of either consolidation or effusion or both at the posterior wall.

PLAPS-point One of the three BLUE-points. Area of investigation delimited by horizontally the lower BLUE-point and vertically the posterior axillary line (or more posteriorly if possible, without moving a supine patient), accessible using a short probe. The PLAPS-point indicates all free pleural effusions and most alveolar consolidations in the critically ill.

Pleural line Normally echoic line located between two ribs, slightly deeper (0.5 cm in

41 Glossary

adults), in a longitudinal view of an intercostal space. It shows the interface between parietal tissues and thoracic gas. See bat sign.

Posterior shadow Anechoic image with an artifactual shape, located behind a bony structure.

Quad sign Quad shaped by the four borders of a pleural effusion, when seen in intercostal approach: pleural line, shadows of ribs, and the deep lower border, called the lung line (visceral pleura).

R-lines Please refer to Chap. 40.

Seashore sign M-mode pattern of a normal lung sliding. The parietal layers are motionless and generate horizontal lines (reminiscent of quiet waves) at the upper part of the screen, called the Keyes' space. The image above and from the pleural line generates a homogeneous granular pattern (reminiscent of sand) since it reflects lung sliding, which spreads homogeneously through the Merlin's space.

SESAME-protocol A simple new word indicating a pragmatic way to immediately manage a cardiac arrest or a shock with imminent cardiac arrest, by mingling at the same level the signs of the mechanism of circulatory failure (e.g., A-profile) and the signs of the cause of the circulatory failure (e.g., hemoperitoneum). From the beginning of "sequential emergency sonographic assessment of mechanism or origin of shock of indistinct cause."

Shred line The deep border of a non-translobar lung consolidation, which makes a shredded line with the aerated deep lung tissue. This sign is specific to lung consolidation.

Shred sign A shredded boundary with aerated lung seen in the depth of nontranslobar consolidations (the shred line).

Sinusogram Ultrasound visualization of the walls of the maxillary sinus.

Sinusoid sign In a free pleural effusion, the lung line has a centrifuge inspiratory dynamic toward the motionless pleural line. In M-mode, this displays a characteristic sinusoid.

Sky-Earth axis The axis where gravity rules. This is useful for understanding the logic of the BLUE-points (see this term) and critical for understanding lung pathophysiology.

Splanchnogram Direct visualization of an abdominal organ when the probe is applied in a supine patient, which means that no free gas (pneumoperitoneum) collects at the abdominal wall.

Stage 1 examination (lung ultrasound) Anterior lung analysis in a supine patient at the Earth level.

Stage 2 examination (lung ultrasound) Adjunction of the lateral wall to Stage 1.

Stage 3 examination (lung ultrasound) Insertion of a small microconvex probe at the posterior wall in a supine patient, as posterior as possible.

Stage 4 examination (lung ultrasound) Comprehensive lung examination, with lateral positioning for complete posterior analysis, plus analysis of the apical areas.

Static air bronchogram Lung consolidation within which hyperechoic punctiform particles (indicating the air bronchograms) are present and have no visible movement.

Stratosphere sign M-mode pattern composed of horizontal lines in an intercostal view. This pattern is reminiscent of a flying fortress squadron in the stratosphere, a pattern characteristic of pneumothorax (some colleagues use the term of barcode sign, which is confusing since modern barcodes look like the seashore sign).

Tissue-like sign Label indicating that lung consolidation (a fluid disorder) yields a tissue-like pattern, reminiscent of a liver in mesenteric ischemia (with possible gas collections).

T-lines Please refer to Chap. 40.

Two-dimensional A two-dimensional image provides a view in two dimensions, as opposed to a M-mode acquisition (see this term). Also see "Real time."

U-line Please refer to Chap. 40.

Ultrasound-aided procedure A procedure is ultrasound aided when done after ultrasound location, as opposed to a procedure carried out with permanent ultrasound guidance.

Upper BLUE-point When the BLUE-hands are applied on the thoracic wall, the point between the origin of the middle and ring finger of the upper hand indicates a location for immediate diagnosis of pneumothorax and pulmonary edema.

V-line Please refer to Chap. 40.

V-point A precise location at the thigh (posterior aspect just above the knee) where the "Doppler hand" should be located for efficient compression of the lower part of the "superficial" femoral vein.

W-lines Please refer to Chap. 40.

X-lines Please refer to Chap. 40.

Z-lines Please refer to Chap. 40.

Index

A
A-line, 48, 65, 84, 232, 359
  A-line sign, 101
A-profile, 67, 187, 190
A-profile plus, DVT, 158
A-no-V-PLAPS profile, 158, 179
A'-profile, 75, 97, 160
A/B-profile, 160, 204
ABCDE, 303
Abdominal probe, 31
Abolition of lung sliding, 98
Abscess (parenchyma), 296, 303, 318
Acoustic shadow, 302
Acronym, 344
Acute circulatory failure, 91, 227
  and cardiogenic shock, 236
  and distributive shock, 238
  and hypovolemic shock, 148, 153, 231, 236, 243
  and obstructive shock, 236
  and septic shock, 237, 252, 254
  in neonate, 305
Acute hemodynamic pulmonary edema.
  See Hemodynamic pulmonary edema
Air, 66
Air bronchogram, 120, 317
Air-fluid ratio, 46
Airplane, 19
Airway management, 91, 303
Alveolar-interstitial syndrome, 87, 117
Alveolar edema, 232
Alveolar recruitment, 206
Anaphylactic shock, 238
Anesthesiology, 291
Angio-CT, 189
Animals, 294
Anisotropy, 32, 332
Anterior tibial vein, 140
Anuria, 296
Aortic aneurism, 297
Aortic rupture, 304
ARDS, 79, 91, 93, 203, 238, 312
  quantitative assessment, 204
  story, 215
Arterial blood gas, 165

Artifacts, 7, 79, 365
  classification, 360
Asepsis, 23, 38, 220
Asthma, 90, 161, 187
Asymmetrical heart, 248
Asystole, 269
Atelectasis, 74, 117
  obstructive, 318
Avicenne sign, 100, 365
Australian variant (pneumothorax), 197

B
B-line, 48, 80, 232, 359
  unstable, 85
B-profile, 95, 160
B'-profile, 95, 160, 204
Bariatric patient, 61, 292
Bat sign, 62, 365
Bladder, 296
Bleeding, 253
Blood letting (and FALLS-protocol), 246
BLUE-consolidation index, 207
BLUE hands, 365
BLUE-pleural index, 205
BLUE-points, 51, 121, 366
  and neonate, 278
BLUE-profile, 158
BLUE-protocol, 157, 366
  and absence of diagnosis, 168
  and acronym, 346
  and decision tree, 159
  and excluded patients, 167
  and frequently asked questions, 171
  and gold standard, 158
  and neonate, 279
  and non blue patients, 174
  and multicentric studies, 174
  and multiple diagnoses, 167
  and pathophysiology, 162
  and rare causes, 167
  and user's guide, 163
Bone, 331
Bradypnea, 72

Brain, 9
Brain edema, 251, 303
Bronchiolitis, 283
Bronchopulmonary dysplasia, 283
Burn, 293

C
C-line, 119, 359
C-profile, 117, 160, 178, 204
Cable (of probe), 16, 55, 264
Calf venous thrombosis, 138
Capillary pressure, 232, 243
Cardiac anatomy, 146
Cardiac arrest and SESAME-protocol, 35, 98, 148, 261
Cardiac asthma, 90, 181, 315
Cardiac gallbladder, 296
Cardiac output, 250
Cardiac probe, 31
Cardiac window, 151
    absent, 151
Cardiogenic pulmonary edema.
    See Hemodynamic pulmonary edema
Cardiogenic shock, 235
Cardiology, 291
Carmen maneuver, 5, 366
Cart, 16, 339
Cathod ray tube, 13, 340
Caval vein, 237
    inferior, 135, 211, 239
    superior, 211, 240
Cellulitis, 303
Central venous access, 269, 297
CEURF, 349
CEURF unit, 28
Challenging patient, 56
Child and critical ultrasound, 305
Cholecystitis, 296
Chronic interstitial syndrome, 79, 167, 173, 182, 291, 312, 315
Clinical volemia, 254
CLOT-protocol, 208, 366
Coffee sign, 121
Comet-tail artifact, 81, 366
Common femoral vein, 133, 210
Compound filter, 73
Confusion, 45
Convention, 4, 150
COPD, 90, 161, 187
Corridor (talks), 166
Coronary circulation and perfusion pressure, 247, 272
Cost, 17, 33, 195, 218, 263, 341
Critical ultrasound, 333
CT, 177, 217, 287, 335
Cystic fibrosis, 291

D
D-dimer, 190
Deep venous thrombosis, 123, 190, 266
    catheter-linked, 301
Depth, 263
Desert, 288
DIAFORA concept, 15, 26, 144, 150, 337, 366
Diaphragm, 53, 91, 168, 169, 288, 305, 328, 332
Diastolic ventricular dysfunction, 149, 185
Dilated cardiomyopathy, 149
Disinfection (of unit). *See* Asepsis
Distension, 188
Doppler, 5, 14, 15, 21, 31, 121, 124–127, 134, 136–138, 140, 141, 143, 144, 147, 150, 152, 153, 165, 175, 182, 193, 211, 236, 237, 243, 268, 289, 294, 297, 300, 304, 310, 320, 323, 330, 331, 333, 335–337, 341, 342, 356
    and silent killer, 336
Doppler hand, 131, 367
Dynamic air bronchogram, 317, 367
Dyspnea, 70

E
E-line, 84, 104, 361
Early Goal-Directed Therapy, 242
ECG, 57
Echolite, Ecolight, 5, 17, 37, 69, 172, 263, 268, 338
Ectopic stomach, 115, 298
Electro-mechanical dissociation, 273
Elite, 173
ELSISSCEC-protocol, 297
Emergency physician, 290
Emotion, 271
Emphysema (bulla), 197
Empyema, 48
Endocarditis, 150
Endovenous ultrasound, 193
Epigastric vessels, 303
Escape sign, 132, 367
Esophageal intubation, 304
Esophageal abscess, rupture, 151, 297
Ethics, 174
Extended BLUE-protocol, 309
Extravascular lung water, 208
Exudate, 320

F
Facility, 15
FALLS-endpoint, 237
FALLS-protocol, 85, 227
    and anesthesiology, 291
    decision tree, 235
    synthesis, 251
FALLS-PLR-protocol, 254
FALLS-responsiveness, 236
Family doctor, 293
Fantasy, 97
Fast, 344
Fast protocols, 29
    and BLUE-protocol, 264
    and cardiac arrest, 262
    and FALLS-protocol, 227

Index

and neonates, 283
and trauma, 304
Fat, 121, 293
Fat embolism, 316
Fat-protocol, 292
Fever, 213
and extended BLUE-protocol, 310
Fever-protocol, 213
Filters, 15, 69, 73, 98, 263
Filter, inferior caval vein, 193
Fissure (lung), 82
Flat (keyboard), 14
Floating thrombosis, 210, 214, 242
Fluid overload, 79, 230, 251
Fluid responsiveness, 230
Fluid therapy, 91, 231, 264
Flying doctor, 19, 288
Foreign body, 290
Fractal sign, 48, 118
Frank-Starling curve, 245
Freeze function, 9
Fulminans sepsis, 244

G

G-line, 361
GA-line, 295
GB-line, 295
GZ-line, 295
Gain, 6, 77
Gallbladder, 296
Gap, 71
Gas, 66
Gas embolism, 151, 300
Gas tamponade, 151
Gastric dilatation (acute), 296, 316
Gastro-intestinal hemorrhage, 297
Gel, 17, 172, 268, 337
Gel (traditional), 41
Ghost, 115, 129, 321
Gooey sign, 93
Gravidic hypertension, 290
Grotowski law, 86, 136, 141, 178, 255, 273, 329, 367
Ground-glass rockets, 89, 359
Gut point and pneumoperitoneum, 295
Gut sliding, 295, 367
Gyneco-obstetrics, 290

H

Hand (second), 6
Harmonic filter, 15, 73, 263
Harmony, 340
Heart and BLUE-protocol, 171
Helicopter, 20
Hemodialysis, 292
Hemodynamic assessment, 227
Hemodynamic pulmonary edema, 79, 89, 95, 161, 171, 181, 184, 232, 236, 238, 244, 312

and mild cases, 330
and pathophysiology, 182
Hemopericardium, 304
Hemoperitoneum, 304
Hemothorax, 48, 304, 321
HICTTUS, 223
HIRTUS, 223
Holistic ultrasound, 33, 35, 143, 144, 148, 152, 213, 241, 293, 355
Hyaline membrane disease, 283
Hydro-aeric artifact, 80
Hydropneumothorax, 103, 353
Hyperthermia, 303
Hypertrophic cardiomyopathy, 149
Hypervolemia. *See* Fluid overload
Hyponatremia, 91
Hypovolemic shock, 148, 153, 231, 235, 243

I

I-line, 85
Iliac vein, 210, 215
and iliocaval thrombosis, 135
Image quality, 13
Imagination (at work), 16, 273
Industrial era (of ultrasound), 31
Infections (crossed). *See* Asepsis
Inferior caval vein. *See* Caval vein
Instant response, 73
Interlobular septa, subpleural, 82
Internal mammary vessels, 303
Internal medicine, 292
International consensus conference, 53, 300
vascular access, 302
Interstitial edema, 232, 237
Interstitial pulmonary fibrosis, 291
Interstitial syndrome, 87, 227, 245
physiological, 92
Intracardiac thrombosis, 150
Intracranial pressure, 302
IPF, 291
Irradiation, 193, 195, 208, 217, 288, 329, 331
and cancer, 219
and neonate, 287

J

J-line, 83, 361
Jugular internal vein, 135, 210
canulation, 301
thrombosis, 209, 214

K

K-line, 85
Kerley line, 80, 89
Keye's sign, 70, 100
Keye's space, 63
Knobology, 3

L

Laënnec, 343
Lag, 71
Laptop machines, 19, 262, 338
Left renal vein, 240
Left ventricle contractility, 148
Linear probe. *See* Vascular probe
Liver (acute), 296
Liver point, 107
Lower BLUE-point, 54
Lower femoral vein (and V-point), 134
LUCI, 1–370
LUCIFLR-project, 68, 164, 198, 208, 217, 312, 368
   and neonate, 283
   and Extended BLUE-protocol, 318
Lung abscess, 321, 323
Lung cancer, 291
Lung comets, 253
Lung compliance (expansion), 76, 91, 204
Lung consolidation, 48, 109
   and pulmonary embolism, 191
   nontranslobar, 118
   translobar, 119
   volume, 206
Lung exclusion, 291
Lung line, 48
Lung point, 102, 197, 266, 368
Lung pulse, 74, 264, 319
Lung puncture, 322
Lung rockets, 79, 87, 182, 233, 237
Lung sepsis, 236
Lung sliding, 48, 67, 220
   and euphonia, 78
   in pulmonary edema, 183
   maximal type, 70
   minimal type, 72
   quantification, 76, 204
Lung water, 208, 242–243
   interstitial lung water, 242–243
LUS, 86
Lymph node, 126

M

M-line, 85
M-mode, 16
Mangrove variant, 73
Maxillary sinusitis, 213
Medical studies, 173
Medicolegal issues, 335
Merlin's space, 63, 368
Mesenteric ischemia, infarction, 296
Mess, 263, 301, 337
Metabolic dyspnea, 316
Mickey Mouse, 133
Microconvex probe, 13, 23, 267, 341
Midfemoral vein, 135
Missed patients of the BLUE-protocol, 162
Model (workshops), 351

Morrison's pouch, 267
Multibeam mode, 15
Multiple organ failure, 243
Muscular sliding, 70
Myocardial infarction, 149, 262
Myocarditis, 168
Myonecrosis, 303

N

N-line, 85
NASA, 294
Neonatalogist, 287
Neonate, 277, 305
Neonate ICU, 284
Nephrology, 292
Nerve, 32, 133, 331
Noncritical ultrasound, 327
Norepinephrine, 251
Nude profile, 159, 187

O

O-line, 65, 362
Obstructive shock, 235
Operator-dependency, 335
Optic nerve, 302
Optimal compromise (concept), 26

P

Pachypleuritis, 321
Pain, 331
Pancreatitis, 296, 304
Pantographic ultrasound and lung ultrasound, 215
Paradox, 79
Parasite, 84
Pediatrics (and critical care), 287
Pericardial tamponade, 33, 147, 152, 236, 268
   and pericardiocentesis, 33, 274
Peritoneal blood, 297
Peritoneal sliding, 295
Permeability-induced pulmonary edema, 79
Phantom. *See* Ghost
Philosophy, 355
Physical examination, 157, 342
Physician-Attended ambulance, 289
Physiologist, 292
Physiotherapist, 293
PICCO, 228, 253
Pink-protocol, 203
Plankton sign, 321
PLAPS, 109, 117, 175, 368
PLAPS-point, 54, 368
Pleural effusion, 48, 109
   anechoic, 111
   massive, 167
   nature, 320
   septated, 113
   volume, 204
Pleural line, 61

Index

Pleural symphysis, 105
Pneumonia, 95, 161, 177, 182, 313
    amiodarone, 316
    aspiration, 316
    necrotizing, 221, 318
    pathophysiology, 181
Pneumoperitoneum, 295, 304
    and aerogram, 296
    and splanchnogram, 295
Pneumothorax, 74, 76, 90, 97, 151, 162, 195, 264, 294, 319
    after venous line insertion, 301
    and LUCIFLR project, 283
    delayed, 198
    in pre-hospital medicine, 288
    minor cases, 330
    pathophysiology, 196
    radioccult, 103, 195, 208
    septated, 105
    tension pneumothorax, 236
    volume, 207
Popliteal vein, 135, 139
Portal gas, 296
Pregnancy, 224, 290
Pre-hospital medicine, 288
Principles of lung ultrasound, 45
Probe, 341
Procedure, 297
Prone positioning, 56, 207
Pseudo A'-profile, 74
Pseudomembranous colitis, 296
Psychology, 271, 344
Pulmonary artery (right), 135, 190, 267
Pulmonary artery occlusion pressure, 91, 228, 255
Pulmonary edema. *See* Hemodynamic pulmonary edema
Pulmonary embolism, 90, 161, 178, 187, 189, 208, 214, 235, 247, 264
    and deep venous thrombosis, 123
    and Extended BLUE-protocol, 314
    and letter to the Editor, 167, 254
    and LUCIFLR project, 283
    and noncritical settings, 328
    and venous thrombosis in cardiac arrest, 266
Pulmonary hypertension, 247
Pulmonectomy, 291
Pulmonology, 291
Pulseless electric activity, 273
PUMA, 21, 289
Pyothorax, 353

Q
Quad sign, 48, 112

R
R-line, 85
Radial artery, 269
Radiation, CT irradiation, 195, 218, 223
Radiography
    in neonate, 277

Radiologists, 334
Real time, 215
Red-protocol, 324
Remote areas, 293
Repetition artifact, 7
Resolution of ultrasound, 220
Retina, 302
Rhabdomyolysis, 303
Rib, 61
Right ventricle dilatation, 147
Right ventricle failure, 247
    chronic, 149
Right ventricle infarction (with shock), 244

S
S-line, 85
Safely, 220, 283, 336
Scintigraphy, 224, 329
Seashore sign, 68, 369
Septal interference, 247
Septal rockets, 89, 359
Septic cardiomyopathy, 248, 324
Septic shock, 237, 251, 254
Septic venous thrombosis, 212
SESAME-protocol, 31, 98, 148, 261, 369
    decision tree, 264
Setting, 3, 263
Setting "lung", 16
Shock. *See* Acute circulatory failure
Shred sign, 48, 118
Shrinking sign, 131
Silicone (breast), 115
Simple emergency cardiac sonography, 143, 165, 172, 253
Sinusitis, 213
Sinusogram, 213
Sinusoid sign, 114
Size (of the machine), 12, 339
Sky-Earth axis, 46
SLAM, 344
Sleepy giant, 129
Snake (and medicine), 351
Soft tissues, 302
Spinal tap, 290, 302
Spinal shock, 238
Stalingrad, 252
Standard ultrasound report, 39
Start-up time, 13, 341
Static air bronchogram, 320
Stethoscope, 188, 335, 343
Story (small) of
    ARDS, 215
    BLUE-protocol, 165
    critical ultrasound, 42
    FALLS-protocol, 251
    lung rockets, 92
    medicine, 334
    pulmonary edema, 185
Stratosphere sign, 48, 98, 369
Sub-A-line, 65, 102

Sub-B-line, 85, 363
Subclavian vein, 135, 210
  and cannulation, 298, 306
Subcutaneous emphysema, 62, 84, 104, 361
Subpleural lung consolidation, 193
Sudden death sign, 130
Systolic heart function, 185
Swan-Ganz catheter, 151, 228
Swirl sign, 104, 115, 318

T
T-line, 75
Tell, 100
Thoracentesis, 114, 177, 205, 321
  and safety, 322
Thoracic surgery, 291
Thrombophlebitis, 212
Thymus, 282
Time lag, 73
Timing, 38, 140, 164, 172
Tissue-like sign, 119
Tofu, 28, 32, 272, 299
Torsade de pointe, 269
Trachea, 26
Tracheal rupture, 304
Tracheal stenosis, 168, 316
Training, 349
Transesophageal echocardiography, 234, 268, 335
Transient tachypnea of newborn, 282
Transudate, 320
Trauma, 304
Traumatologist, 287
Triage, 290
Trojan horse, 195

U
ULTIMAT-protocol, 289
  standard report, 290

Ultrasound, 1–370
UK, 110
Unit, 11
Universal probe, 23
Upper BLUE-point, 54
US, 347

V
Valvular disease, 150
Vascular probe, 31, 32, 124, 209, 301
Venography, 193
Venous access. *See* Central venous access
Ventricular fibrillation, 269
Veterinarian, 294
Volemia, 243
  in the neonate, 305

W
W-line, 104
Weaning, 91, 327
Wheels (of unit), 16, 263
Wheezing, 187, 312, 315
Whole body ultrasound, 295
Wild ultrasound, 353
Workshop, 351
World, 174, 293

X
X-line, 81

Z
Z-line, 84, 364
Zebra, 66, 90
Zero pressure, 5